BLACKWELL'S NEUROLOGY AND PSYCHIATRY ACCESS SERIES

Adult
Psychiatry

SECOND EDITION

Other books in Blackwell's Neurology and Psychiatry Access Series

BLACKWELL'S NEUROLOGY AND PSYCHIATRY ACCESS SERIES

Adult Psychiatry

SECOND EDITION

EDITED BY

Eugene H. Rubin, MD, PhD

Professor of Psychiatry
Washington University School of Medicine
Department of Psychiatry
St Louis
Missouri

and

Charles F. Zorumski, MD

Professor of Psychiatry and Neurobiology
Washington University School of Medicine
Department of Psychiatry
St Louis
Missouri

SERIES EDITOR

Ronald B. David, MD, FAAP, FAAN

Richmond
Virginia

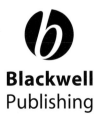

Blackwell
Publishing

Blackwell Publishing, Inc., 350 Main Street, Malden, Massachusetts 02148-5020, USA
Blackwell Publishing Ltd, 9600 Garsington Road, Oxford OX4 2DQ, UK
Blackwell Publishing Asia Pty Ltd, 550 Swanston Street, Carlton, Victoria 3053, Australia

First published 1997
Second Edition 2005

Library of Congress Cataloging-in-Publication Data

Adult psychiatry / edited by Eugene H. Rubin & Charles F. Zorumski. 2nd ed.
    p. ; cm. – (Blackwell's neurology and psychiatry access series)
  Rev. ed. of: Washington University adult psychiatry / Samuel B. Guze, editor.
  Includes bibliographical references and index.
  ISBN-13: 978-1-4051-1769-2
  ISBN-10: 1-4051-1769-9
  1. Psychiatry.
  [DNLM: 1. Mental Disorders–diagnosis. 2. Mental Disorders–therapy.
3. Primary Health Care–methods. WM 140 A2434 2005] I. Rubin, Eugene H.
II. Zorumski, Charles F. III. Washington University adult psychiatry. IV. Series.
  RC454.W35 2005
  616.89–dc22

                                                                    2005012232

ISBN-13: 978-1-405-117692
ISBN-10: 1-4051-1769-9

A catalogue record for this title is available from the British Library

Set in 9.25/12pt Palatino by SNP Best-set Typesetter Ltd., Hong Kong
Printed and bound in India by Replika Press PVT Ltd, Harayana

Commissioning Editor: Stuart Taylor
Development Editor: Nick Morgan
Project Manager: Kate Bailey
Production Controller: Kate Charman

For further information on Blackwell Publishing, visit our website:
http://www.blackwellpublishing.com

Contents

Contributors

Dr Deanna M. Barch
Washington University
Department of Psychology
Campus Box 1125
One Brooking Drive
St. Louis, MO 63130

Dr Laura J. Bierut
Washington University School of Medicine
Department of Psychiatry
Campus Box 8134
660 S. Euclid
St. Louis, MO 63110-1093

Dr Kevin J. Black
Washington University School of Medicine
Department of Psychiatry
Campus Box 8134
660 S. Euclid
St. Louis, MO 63110-1093

Dr Kelly Botteron
Washington University School of Medicine
Department of Psychiatry
Campus Box 8134
660 S. Euclid
St. Louis, MO 63110-1093

Dr Robert M. Carney
Behavioral Medicine Center
4625 Lindell Blvd
Suite 420
St. Louis, MO 63108

Dr C. Robert Cloninger
Washington University School of Medicine
Department of Psychiatry
Campus Box 8134
660 S. Euclid
St. Louis, MO 63110-1093

Dr Wilson M. Compton
Director, Division of Epidemiology, Services and
    Prevention Research
National Institute on Drug Abuse
6001 Executive Boulevard, MSC 9589
Bethesda, MD 20892-9589

Dr John N. Constantino
Washington University School of Medicine
Department of Psychiatry
Campus Box 8134
660 S. Euclid
St. Louis, MO 63110-1093

Dr John G. Csernansky
Washington University School of Medicine
Department of Psychiatry
Campus Box 8134
660 S. Euclid
St. Louis, MO 63110-1093

Dr Stephen H. Dinwiddie
University of Chicago
Department of Psychiatry
MC 3077
5841 S. Maryland Ave.
Chicago, IL 60637-1470

Dr Wayne C. Drevets
Senior Investigator
Chief, section on Neuroimaging in Mood and Anxiety Disorders
Mood and Anxiety Disorders Program
National Institutes of Health, NIMH/MIB
15K North Drive, MSC 2670
Bethesda, MD 20892-2670

Dr Peter Fahnestock
Washington University
School of Medicine
Department of Psychiatry

Campus Box 8134
660 S. Euclid
St Louis, MO 63110-1093

Dr Nuri B. Farber
Washington University School of Medicine
Department of Psychiatry
Campus Box 8134
660 S. Euclid
St. Louis, MO 63110-1093

Dr Kenneth E. Freedland
Behavioral Medicine Center
4625 Lindell Blvd
Suite 420
St. Louis, MO 63108

Dr Keith S. Garcia
Washington University School of Medicine
Department of Psychiatry
Campus Box 8134
660 S. Euclid
St. Louis, MO 63110-1093

Dr Dan Haupt
Washington University School of Medicine
Department of Psychiatry
Campus Box 8134
660 S. Euclid
St. Louis, MO 63110-1093

Dr Gitry Heydebrand
Washington University School of Medicine
Department of Psychiatry
Campus Box 8134
660 S. Euclid
St. Louis, MO 63110-1093

Dr Anja Hilbert
Department of Psychology/Clinical Psychology and
Psychological Therapies
Philipps University of Marburg
Gutenbergstrasse 18
D-35032 Marburg, Germany

Dr Barry A. Hong
Washington University School of Medicine
Department of Psychiatry
Campus Box 8134
660 S. Euclid
St. Louis, MO 63110-1093

Dr Richard W. Hudgens
Washington University School of Medicine
Department of Psychiatry
Campus Box 8134

660 S. Euclid
St. Louis, MO 63110-1093

Dr Keith E. Isenberg
Washington University School of Medicine
Department of Psychiatry
Campus Box 8134
660 S. Euclid
St. Louis, MO 63110-1093

Jennifer Ivanovich, MS
Washington University School of Medicine
Department of Surgery
Campus Box 8100
660 S. Euclid
St. Louis, MO 63110-1093

Dr Mark C. Johnson
BJC Behavioral Health
1430 Olive Street, Suite 500
St. Louis, MO 63103

Dr Patrick J. Lustman
Washington University School of Medicine
Department of Psychiatry
Campus Box 8134
660 S. Euclid
St. Louis, MO 63110-1093

Dr Richard E. Mattison
Stony Brook University School of Medicine
Department of Psychiatry and Behavioral Science
161 Potnam Hall
Stony Brook, NY 11794-8790

Dr George E. Murphy
Professor Emeritus of Psychiatry
Washington University School of Medicine
Department of Psychiatry
Campus Box 8134
660 S. Euclid
St. Louis, MO 63110-1093

Dr Elliot C. Nelson
Washington University School of Medicine
Department of Psychiatry
Campus Box 8134
660 S. Euclid
St. Louis, MO 63110-1093

Dr John W. Newcomer
Washington University School of Medicine
Department of Psychiatry
Campus Box 8134
660 S. Euclid
St. Louis, MO 63110-1093

Dr Carol S. North
Washington University School of Medicine
Department of Psychiatry
Campus Box 8134
660 S. Euclid
St. Louis, MO 63110-1093

Dr Devna Rastogi-Cruz
Washington University School of Medicine
Department of Psychiatry
Campus Box 8134
660 S. Euclid
St. Louis, MO 63110-1093

Dr Eugene H. Rubin
Washington University School of Medicine
Department of Psychiatry
Campus Box 8134
660 S. Euclid
St. Louis, MO 63110-1093

Andrea B. Schnur
Washinton University School of Medicine
Department of Psychiatry
Campus Box 8134
660 S. Euclid
St. Louis, MO 63110-1093

Dr Dragan M. Svrakic
Washington University School of Medicine
Department of Psychiatry
Campus Box 8134
660 S. Euclid
St. Louis, MO 63110-1093

Dr Melissa Swallow
Washington University School of Medicine
Department of Psychiatry
Campus Box 8134
660 S. Euclid
St. Louis, MO 63110-1093

Dr Katrin Tobben, MSW, LCSW
Barnes-Jewish Hospital
Psychiatric Services

Mailstop 9071356
One Barnes-Jewish Hospital Plaza
St. Louis, MO 63110

Dr Richard D. Todd
Washington University School of Medicine
Department of Psychiatry
Campus Box 8134
660 S. Euclid
St. Louis, MO 63110-1093

Dr Richard D. Wetzel
Washington University School of Medicine
Department of Psychiatry
Campus Box 8134
660 S. Euclid
St. Louis, MO 63110-1093

Dr Alison J. Whelan
Washington University School of Medicine
Departments of Internal Medicine and Pediatrics
Campus Box 8073
660 S. Euclid
St. Louis, MO 63110-1093

Dr Denise E. Wilfley
Washington University School of Medicine
Department of Psychiatry
Campus Box 8134
660 S. Euclid
St. Louis, MO 63110-1093

Dr Sean H. Yutzy
University of New Mexico
Department of Psychiatry
2400 Tucker Blvd, NE
Albuquerque, NM 87131

Dr Charles F. Zorumski
Washington University School of Medicine
Department of Psychiatry
Campus Box 8134
660 S. Euclid
St. Louis, MO 63110-1093

Foreword

Traditional textbooks convey knowledge. It is the goal of this text in the Blackwell Neurology and Psychiatry Access Series to convey not only essential knowledge but also the collected wisdom of its many highly regarded contributors. To achieve the goal of conveying not only knowledge but wisdom, each book in this series is built on a structural framework that was well received by critics and readers alike in David: *Pediatric Neurology for the Clinician* and the first editions of *Child and Adolescent Neurology*, *Adult Neurology*, *Child and Adolescent Psychiatry* and *Adult Psychiatry* (Mosby). Each volume is divided into three sections:

- tools for diagnosis
- diseases and disorders
- common problems.

Also included to facilitate a physician's use of this book are:

- Nosologic diagnosis tables
- "Pearls and perils" boxes
- "Consider consultation when . . ." boxes
- selected annotated bibliographies
- a complete bibliography
  and (new in this edition)
- "Key clinical questions and what they unlock."

The Nosologic Diagnosis tables are based on a discriminator model to promote clearer understanding.

> Whoever having undertaken to speak or write hath first laid for themselves some [basis] to their argument such as hot or cold or moist or dry or whatever else they choose, thus reducing their subject within a narrow compass.
>
> Hippocrates

As Hippocrates has suggested, structure is the key to learning. Unless there is a structure onto which knowledge can be built, confusion and disorganization are the inevitable consequences.

Classification systems induce orderliness in thinking and enhance our ability to communicate effectively. A review of the most enduring hierarchical classification systems, particularly that of Linnaeus (that is, phyla, genera, species), makes clear the value of grouping according to discriminating features, as well as the value of simplicity, expandability, and dynamism.

The goal, whatever the classification system, is to seek the most powerful discriminating features that will produce the greatest diagnostic clarity. Discriminating features should avoid crossing domains. Much of the confusion that arises in diagnosis may be the result of the clinician who unwittingly crosses the anatomic, pathologic, pathophysiologic, phenomenologic, and etiologic classification domains used in medicine (for example, the inclusion of anatomically oriented "temporal lobe seizures" in a phenomenologically based classification system that includes complex partial seizures). Some conditions, such as brain tumors, are classified according to their histopathology and lend themselves well to this classification system. Others, such as headaches and movement disorders, are classified phenomenologically and are therefore much less easily classified. In other cases, discriminators must encompass inclusionary, as well as, exclusionary features. At times, we can only use a criterion-based system or construct tables to compare features.

Arbitrarily, we label as consistent features those which occur more than 75% of the time; features are considered variable when they occur less than 75% of the time. The diagnostic tables should be viewed, therefore, only as a beginning in the extremely difficult effort to make diagnosis more precise and biologically based. How well this book accomplishes the goals of identifying the most powerful discrimination features for maximum diagnostic clarity is limited by the current state of the art in psychiatry and neurology. In some areas, several features, when clustered together, serve to discriminate.

This text is designed to be pithy, not exhaustive, as there are already many available of this ilk. Each text in this series reflects appropriate stylistic differences among content editors. However, each is built upon the same structural framework, hence the value of this text to the users.

As a part of this foreword, I would like to acknowledge some of the people who have made key contributions to this effort. They include: Craig Percy, who initially saw the potential of this effort; the National Institute of Neurological Disorders and Stroke (NINDS)[1] for its support in nosologic research; and the investigators who were involved with this NINDS project; Dr Grover Robinson, a long-time friend (who suggested the "Consider consultation when..." boxes); Ms Laura DeYoung, Mr Stuart Taylor and all the Blackwell team who made this vision a reality.

Last, but certainly not least, I would like thank Eugene Rubin and Charles Zorumski who saw and shared this vision.

Ronald B. David, MD

[1] NINDS 1PO1NS20189–01A1 (Nosology, Higher Cortical Function Disorders in Children)

Preface to Second Edition

Psychiatry lost a great leader when Sam Guze, MD, the editor of the first edition of this text, passed away. We were honored and pleased to have the opportunity to update and revise the first edition of this text. This book, as was the case with its predecessor, is aimed squarely at the primary care practitioner. Our objective is to provide a readable, reasonably concise, medical model approach to patients with psychiatric disorders. Since the publication of the first edition, it has become apparent that primary care physicians are becoming increasingly responsible for the treatment of the majority of psychiatrically ill patients. There are several reasons for this trend: first, psychiatric disorders are often comorbid with other medical disorders and strongly influence the morbidities associated with concurrent medical disorders; second, psychiatric disorders are among the most disabling illnesses, and primary care doctors are beginning to recognize the need to aggressively diagnose and treat these illnesses; third, there is an inadequate number of psychiatrists, which is resulting in a shift of responsibility for the management of psychiatrically ill patients to primary care physicians; and fourth, managed care and insurance issues continue to make it difficult for many patients to receive long-term care from psychiatrists.

Many health care professionals are involved in treating psychiatrically ill patients. Although this book is aimed at primary care physicians, the information is presented in a conceptual format that medical students and junior residents may find useful. In addition, this book may help psychologists, social workers, and counselors, including members of the clergy, better understand the nature and treatments of psychiatric illnesses.

The field of psychiatry is advancing at a rapid pace. We have tried to integrate knowledge from these advances with pragmatic presentations of clinical information. The didactic tools used in the Access Series are designed to allow clinicians to upgrade their psychiatric and neurological clinical skills efficiently and effectively.

Finally, we would like to acknowledge the outstanding organizational and editorial contributions of Dorothy A. Kinscherf.

Eugene H. Rubin, MD, PhD
Charles F. Zorumski, MD
Richard W. Hudgens, MD
Keith E. Isenberg, MD
Barry A. Hong, PhD

Preface to First Edition

This book has certain distinctive attributes. First, it is directed to generalists or primary care practitioners, physicians who nearly always need to know a good deal concerning psychiatric conditions and how to think about and manage them. For the same reason, it is also directed to medical students and residents. We of course hope that it will, at the same time, be of use to psychiatrists and other mental health professionals. For all such potential readers, we have tried to make clear that psychiatric disorders are very common, widespread, and often disabling; have great impact on the victim's life and family; and often carry risk of premature death. *No illnesses cause more widespread suffering and devastation to the victims and their relatives.*

We have tried to make clear that the most appropriate approach for dealing with psychiatric conditions is to use the concepts and strategies from general medicine: emphasizing diagnosis and differential diagnosis, course, outcome, complications, treatment, etiology, pathogenesis, and epidemiology. This approach is what is meant by the term *Medical Model*, which encapsulates the above concepts and strategies.

Because this Department of Psychiatry has played a central role in the application of the Medical Model to psychiatry and in its gradual acceptance by the field, we concluded that drawing our authors from the Department's faculty would maximize the likelihood of a consistent and useful book.

Our readers will not be surprised by our conviction that the future of psychiatry will increasingly depend on research in the neurosciences (including of course neuropharmacology), genetics, and neuroimaging, as well as continued improvements in clinical skills, epidemiology, and the organization of medical care (including psychiatry) generally.

Finally, but of great importance, we have tried to make clear that psychiatric conditions are the most characteristically human of medical problems, dealing as they do with temperament, personality, thinking, emotion, learning, perception, motivation, sexuality, interpersonal relationships, and character. No medical conditions require more sensitivity and compassion from the physician. These attributes in turn depend on significant knowledge and training because physicians must understand, recognize, and accept the validity of psychiatric disorders to reflect to the patient and family the understanding and sympathy that are essential for good medical care. If our book helps achieve these goals, we shall be truly gratified.

Samuel B. Guze, MD
Richard W. Hudgens, MD
Eugene H. Rubin, MD, PhD
Charles F. Zorumski, MD

SECTION 1

Assessment and Evaluation

Richard W. Hudgens, MD

CHAPTER 1

Psychiatry and the Medical Model

Kevin J. Black, MD

Why psychiatry matters

The most disabling illnesses in America are not cancer, heart disease, or infections. Rather, the most disabling illnesses are psychiatric illnesses, including substance abuse (Table 1.1(a)).

These are also among the most costly illnesses in America, whether measured by medical costs or lost productivity. A full 2.5% of the country's gross national product is consumed by the annual costs of mental illness. When measured by mortality, more young people die from suicide than from homicide (Table 1.1(b)).

People are less likely to consider psychiatric illness as a major public health problem in developing countries, yet even in Africa, psychiatric illness contributes one-sixth of all disability. Mental disorders account for over half of all primary health care visits in Santiago, Chile, a third in Rio de Janeiro, and a fifth in Bangalore, India. Suicide is the leading cause of death among 15–34-year-olds in China. These observations would suffice to highlight the public health importance of the major psychiatric illnesses, but additionally, these illnesses contribute immensely to human suffering. The inability to hope for the future, to trust loved ones, or even to trust one's own senses may comprise the most human form of suffering. For all these reasons it is crucial to deliver effective treatment of mental illness and to improve our knowledge about mental illness.

Why the medical model matters

Psychiatry is the medical specialty concerned with disturbances of thought, emotions, perception, and behavior. This definition may seem simple and obvious, but it is a product of a long and contentious history. Over the years, mental illnesses have been assessed, explained, and treated in very different ways. This textbook uses an approach to mental illness that has been called the medical model of psychiatry.

This is simply the consistent application, in psychiatry, of modern medical thinking and methods.

Some readers may feel that how one views psychiatric symptoms is irrelevant or that now 'everyone agrees' with the medical model. However, assumptions about psychological symptoms can dramatically influence how physicians learn, practice, and teach medicine. Consider the following patient scenarios.

A 72-year-old man with no psychiatric history is sad, listless, insomniac, and disinterested in food since a stroke the previous month. He prays for God to end his life because he feels he is not only a terrible sinner but also useless to his family. The nurse caring for him at the rehabilitation center sympathizes: "Who wouldn't be depressed after a stroke?" His son notes that his father has always been fiercely independent and attributes his symptoms to frustration with his new role as recipient of help. His granddaughter says she used to feel the same way and feels better since taking an antidepressant drug. His physician wonders whether the patient's beta-adrenergic blocker might be causing the fatigue, sadness, and insomnia. Each suggests a different intervention.

A 28-year-old woman consults the third physician in as many weeks because her left leg 'feels funny'. There is no objective neurological deficit. She is told that stress can cause physical symptoms, like headache or upset stomach or unusual sensations, and she is referred for counseling. The patient and family reject this explanation because she was under much more stress a year ago during a divorce and job change, while over the past six months her life otherwise has been going well. Her therapist notes that her upbringing may have led her to preferentially report physical symptoms rather than psychological symptoms. A psychiatrist tells the patient that there is no clear evidence of any specific psychiatric illness, and the patient understands this to mean that she must have a neurological problem. The patient's boyfriend becomes frustrated with her for not returning to work, but she eventually receives disability income.

TABLE 1.1

The burden of psychiatric illness

(a) Disability due to illness, US, 2000, ages 15–44

Disease	YLDs*, % of total
1 **Unipolar depressive disorders**	**16.4**
2 **Alcohol-use disorders**	**5.5**
3 **Schizophrenia**	**4.9**
4 Iron-deficiency anemia	4.9
5 **Bipolar affective disorder**	**4.7**
6 Hearing loss, adult onset	3.8
7 HIV/AIDS	2.8
8 Chronic obstructive pulmonary disease	2.4
9 Osteoarthritis	2.3
10 Road traffic accidents	2.3
11 **Panic disorder**	**2.2**
12 Obstructed labor	2.1
13 Chlamydia	2.0
14 Falls	1.9
15 Asthma	1.9
16 **Drug use disorders**	**1.8**
17 Abortion	1.6
18 Migraine	1.6
19 **Obsessive-compulsive disorder**	**1.4**
20 Maternal sepsis	1.2

* Years lived with disability.
Psychiatric disorders listed in bold face.

(b) Deaths from all causes, US, 2000, ages 15–44

1 Accidents	26%
2 Cancer	14%
3 Heart disease	11%
4 **Suicide**	**10%**
5 Homicide	8%

Sources:

(a) World Health Organization: The World Health Report 2001: Mental Health: New Understanding, New Hope. http://www.who.int/whr2001/. Accessed 3/12/04. Reproduced with permission.

(b) National Vital Statistics Report, vol. 50, no. 16, September 16, 2002.

A 25-year-old man with lifelong tics visits his family doctor for anxiety and is treated with diazepam. After modest benefit and annoying side effects, he goes to a psychiatrist and is diagnosed with obsessive-compulsive disorder. With high-dose fluoxetine he has partial improvement but his tics are more noticeable. He calls his psychiatrist to ask about the tics but is referred to a neurologist. She adds risperidone and both the tics and obsessions improve substantially. He asks the neurologist about switching his care to her for all his symptoms but is told that she doesn't treat psychiatric problems. He goes back to the family doctor and tells him what to prescribe.

In each of these cases, the patient's care is substantially affected by different views about what causes symptoms and how they should be treated. Clearly, how one conceptualizes psychological symptoms still matters to patient care. This chapter briefly describes some alternative views to the medical model of psychiatry. Then, after considering several practical benefits of the medical model, some common myths about psychiatry are discussed.

Models of mental illness

As Western civilization has changed and science has progressed, theories of illness have changed. Mental illness is no exception. The history of these changes explains a great deal about current popular opinion regarding mental illness. A brief and selective synopsis of this history follows.

Pre-1800s

Hippocrates wrote:

> From the brain, and from the brain only, arise our pleasures, joys, laughter, and jests, as well as our sorrows, pains, griefs, and tears . . . . It is the same thing which makes us mad or delirious, inspires us with dread or fear . . . and [produces] acts that are contrary to habit. These things that we suffer all come from the brain when it is not healthy, but becomes abnormally hot, cold, moist, or dry.

In other words, psychological symptoms, like physical symptoms, were ascribed to alterations in bodily elements or humors. The term 'melancholia' (literally, 'black bile') reflects this conception. Other ancient cultures also attributed emotions and thought, like sensation or movement, to bodily dysfunction. The brain was sometimes implicated, but so were the heart, bowels, and uterus. However, bodily disease was not always presumed. Mental illness in several cultures was ascribed to mystical or supernatural influence. These same influences, however, were often felt to cause somatic illnesses as well. In other words, mental and physical illnesses have often been thought to have similar causes.

However, a competing idea over time has been that mental illnesses are by their nature different from other, "physical," illnesses. In this view, the causes, treatments, and study of mental illnesses are assumed to be very different from those of physical illnesses. This concept derives in part from a philosophical view, represented by René Descartes, that mind and body are of two different genera, neither knowable by the methods used to study the other. This concept of mind-body duality has been prominent for the last several centuries and underlies much of the debate mentioned in succeeding paragraphs.

Origins of the medical model

The late 19th century was a time of great strides in medicine. Koch and Pasteur, among others, elucidated the role of bacterial pathogens in infectious disease. Virchow developed modern pathology, and, with clinical-pathological correlation, laid the foundations of a new specialty, internal medicine, which relied on the application of biology to everyday clinical medicine. The English surgeon, Hunter, tested the safety of new treatments before they were applied to patients. These and other advances in basic medical science led to the dramatic medical discoveries of the 20th century.

Perhaps more important than the scientific discoveries themselves, however, was a new approach to illness. After all, many specific discoveries or treatments have come and gone over the last century. However, the empiric approach to medical research has remained more constant. This approach to illness had roots in the late 1600s, when Sydenham championed the idea that symptoms with a given cause fell into natural groupings, or syndromes, and that study of such syndromes was the best approach to uncovering the causes of the presenting symptoms. Koch, Pasteur, Virchow, Hunter, and others contributed specific important discoveries to medical science, but they changed medicine in a broader way by beginning to use controlled studies that tested hypotheses. In the early 20th century, Fisher and others laid the statistical groundwork that allowed quantitative testing of a hypothesis. The scientific method soon spread to clinical medicine. Case studies, personal experience, and authority were no longer the unquestioned basis of medical epistemology. This attitude has gradually solidified until now one might say that thinking scientifically is the very core of modern medicine.

Even before modern research methods had matured, psychiatry shared in these advances. Philippe Pinel, considered by his contemporaries to be the leading French authority in general medicine, is often credited with founding psychiatry as a medical discipline. His 1801 textbook on insanity discussed psychosis as properly falling within the purview of medicine. He felt that mental illness should be classified by a "deep study of the symptoms" rather than by an expert's assumptions about etiology. Antoine Bayle linked general paralysis of the insane to the pathological lesions of neurosyphilis. Later he suggested that other forms of insanity should also be studied with clinical-pathological correlation. Karl Friedrich Kahlbaum contributed careful, longitudinal study of psychiatric symptoms, seeking to find commonalities among groups of patients with similar course and outcome. Emil Kraepelin, motivated by Sydenham's assumption that etiology could best be discovered by studying syndromes, used this longitudinal approach to divide dementia praecox (schizophrenia) from manic-depressive illness. As chair of an influential department of psychiatry, Kraepelin also brought together several renowned psychiatric scientists, including Alois Alzheimer, to study mental illness with scientific methods. Julius Wagner-Jauregg developed the fever therapy for neurosyphilis that won him the Nobel Prize and made fundamental contributions to the treatment of endemic cretinism (a psychiatric complication of hypothyroidism). Hans Berger invented the electroencephalograph, which had tremendous implications for the diagnosis and treatment of epilepsy and sleep disorders.

Not surprisingly, these discoveries led to great hope for further advances in the treatment of other forms of psychosis through continued biological investigations. Leading physicians such as Griesinger, Maudsley, Schneider, and Wernicke felt that insanity was a disease of the brain, best studied by the methods of neuropathology.

The specific discoveries of 19th-century psychiatry are not the focus of this chapter. Rather, they are important as examples of applying the philosophy and techniques of general medicine to psychiatry. This approach, i.e., the medical model approach to psychiatry, is based on a few key assumptions. First, the same approach should be used for mental illnesses as for other illnesses. One corollary of this assumption is that there exist different psychiatric illnesses with different causes, courses, and optimal treatments. Second, empiric proof is the best way to test a medical theory. In other words, the scientific method should be medicine's approach to knowledge. A third assumption of medical model psychiatry is that an increased understanding of the physiology of the brain will eventually improve the care of patients with mental illness. Different 19th-century psychiatrists accepted these assumptions to greater and lesser degrees. However, it is hard to resist the impression that this medical model of psychiatry was responsible for the intellectual climate in which the important psychiatric discoveries of the late 19th century were made.

The psychoanalytic school

Increasing knowledge of neuroanatomy confirmed that some patients had signs of neurological dysfunction that did not correspond to anatomical pathways—in current terms, conversion symptoms. The neurologist Sigmund Freud (a contemporary of Wagner-Jauregg's) had a special interest in these cases. He eventually developed an extensive theory of human behavior that did not depend on altered brain function to explain abnormal behavior. In the early and mid-20th century, American psychiatry turned almost wholly to the psychoanalytic theory of Freud and his followers. Psychiatry's interest in 'organic' illnesses such as pellagra, epilepsy, and neurosyphilis all but disappeared.

Psychiatry's loss of interest in the brain was firmly entrenched when the encephalitis lethargica epidemic struck in

1917. Some physicians felt that the unusual psychological and motor signs of encephalitis reflected abnormal brain functioning. As a result, they learned a great deal about basal ganglia physiology. However, similar signs had long been described in patients with schizophrenia, and psychodynamic explanations of these unusual postures and movements were already available. Consequently, many other physicians of the day largely ignored these valuable clues to abnormal brain function.

Psychodynamic theory has a voluminous literature and has changed over time, including division into several schismatic viewpoints. It cannot be thoroughly covered in the space available. Briefly, however, psychodynamic theory presupposes that some record of past experiences is maintained by the individual but is inaccessible to ordinary recall. These unconscious parts of the mind are thought to greatly affect one's day-to-day actions and can be noted through properly interpreting slips of the tongue, the content of recurring dreams, free association, and symptoms. These effects are also thought to be reflected in several aspects of culture. According to this theory, the unconscious not only influences daily life but also produces pathological behavior, especially if difficult early life conflicts involving powerful emotions have not been correctly resolved. Unconscious motives are perhaps most evident in certain situations that either obviously or symbolically recapitulate important situations from early life. One such situation is the special relationship between doctor and patient, especially during the course of psychoanalysis. Often the patient's actions toward the therapist appear to be re-enactments of relationships with powerful figures of the patient's past rather than truly appropriate responses to the present situation. Interpretation of this transference—that is, explaining the symbolism of these actions to the patient—is thought to have powerful therapeutic potential.

It is more relevant to the present discussion that "above all, psychodynamic psychiatry is a *way of thinking*" (Gabbard, 1990). This way of thinking characterized American psychiatry for much of the 20th century. Many psychoanalytically trained psychiatrists now accept at least some role for the scientific method in clinical psychiatry, but this acceptance was not common until recent years. For our purposes, the following features of traditional psychodynamic thought are worth noting: (1) emotions and behavior are thought to have similar causes in both health and illness, (2) most psychiatric symptoms can be explained within the constructs of psychodynamic theory without reference to neuroanatomy or physiology, (3) the form of a symptom, e.g. a hallucination versus a dream, is not considered as important as the specific content or the meaning attributed to the symptom by the patient or therapist, (4) there is a relative emphasis on individual precipitants to an illness rather than common features among groups of patients, (5) the optimal mode of treatment is thought to be similar for many different psychiatric symptoms, and (6) knowledge is acquired by special training and is heavily influenced by personal experience, single case studies, expert opinion, and tradition; the empiric methods of scientific inquiry are generally considered unnecessary or inappropriate.

The reader may note that these beliefs differ radically from the assumptions of the medical model and drastically lessen the urgency of diagnosis, biological investigation, and controlled studies of causation and interventions. The consequences for day-to-day clinical management of patients are significant, compared with the medical model view that accurate diagnosis, recognition of clinical uncertainty, and reliance on treatments with proven efficacy are essential to good patient care.

Psychology

While psychoanalysis dominated American psychiatry for much of the 20th century and was essentially limited to physicians, others continued to study behavior from other perspectives. Experimental psychology began to make substantive contributions to scientific knowledge about cognition, especially about normal learning of narrowly defined tasks. Theories derived from investigations of animal learning were extrapolated to human learning, and methods were devised for reproducibly testing certain aspects of mental function. Abnormality was often viewed as quantitative variation from the norm rather than categorical difference.

Naturally, the observations of experimental psychology were extrapolated to abnormal human behavior and emotional states. Neuropsychology developed as the application of experimental testing methods to humans, especially neurological patients. Several clinical tests originated as elaborations of the bedside neurological and mental status examinations. These methods proved clinically useful in helping to localize abnormalities of brain structure or function. A field with related interests is behavioral neurology, which examines alterations in cognition and behavior in patients with known brain pathology. Behavioral theory discusses mental illnesses in terms of experimental psychology, drawing attention to observable undesired behaviors and the observable antecedents and consequences of such behavior. Cognitive-behavior therapy extends these techniques from strictly externally observable phenomena to include patients' self-reported thought content. Thus, correcting habitual errors of logic is a technique used to treat causes of depression, anxiety, and personality disorders. Cognitive psychology is a newer science that attempts to study both actions and inferred mental activities. With this approach, specific steps in mental processing can be examined in healthy subjects or in patients.

These approaches, when applied to mental illness, share important features with the medical model, including an emphasis on consistent application of the scientific method. However, there are some differences, such as a relative focus on symptoms rather than syndromes and on pathophysiology rather than etiology or treatment.

Psychosocial and cultural models

Some have held that "mental illness" is only the expected, or normal, response to living in an increasingly abnormal world. For example, advocates of this view have attributed depression to intolerable role demands in society. The fact that schizophrenia is more common in inner cities was interpreted as evidence that poverty, crowding, and other conditions of urban life produced schizophrenia. These explanations are intuitively appealing, but empirical support is less clear. "That psychiatric disturbances arise from the social and psychological environment appears to be so plausible that hypotheses often are not critically examined" (Guze, 1992).

Even when such questions are studied scientifically, methodological issues can make meaningful studies difficult. However, careful epidemiological research can be done and has addressed some of these issues. For instance, the balance of evidence concludes that schizophrenia is more common in the inner city not because it is born there but because it migrates there. That is, people who develop schizophrenia come from approximately equivalent social environments as those who do not, but as the illness progresses, they often move into less privileged settings. Perhaps the main difficulty with the psychosocial model of mental illness is that it fails to explain why some individuals become ill in certain environments, while most do not.

More extreme versions of the psychosocial model of mental illness include claims that there is no such thing as mental illness. Eccentricity, in this view, is interpreted as pathological solely because society tends toward ethnocentric bigotry. According to this argument, people intentionally choose to report hallucinations, delusions of persecution, or depression and hence should not be forced to conform. Some advocates of this position claim that there is no justification for reifying schizophrenia as an illness when there are no clearly consistent chemical or anatomical abnormalities.

One argument against this position is that many people affected by mental illness suffer greatly. To view these illnesses as voluntarily chosen lifestyles seems incomprehensible to those who work daily with such suffering. Furthermore, the major mental illnesses are quite similar in their clinical features and prevalence across a wide range of cultures. Most compelling, it is hard to reconcile this view of mental illness with the facts. Bipolar disorder, for instance, is largely a genetic illness.

What about the complaint that these are not illnesses because their causes remain unknown? A little historical reflection may persuade the reader that, a century ago, the causes of general paresis or pellagra were equally unknown. To imagine that they suddenly became illnesses when their causes were discovered is hard to accept. Equally untenable is the supposition that the pathology, or cause, for all "real" brain diseases has already been discovered. Migraine, torticollis, and other neurological illnesses remain equally baffling.

The psychosocial view of mental illness more often surfaces in a less strident form. When discussing major depression in a patient with a stroke, for instance, it is common to hear medical personnel state, "I'd be depressed, too." This sympathetic view unfortunately falls short of the facts, since most stroke victims never experience major depression. The specific factors that lead to major depression in some but not all stroke patients might never be elucidated if the cause is assumed to be obvious. This example also highlights the common confusion of "understandable" and "normal." Post-stroke depression may seem understandable, but that has nothing to do with whether it is normal. By comparison, it is entirely understandable when an elderly smoker with diabetes and a strong family history of coronary disease suffers angina after shoveling his walk in cold weather. That does not make angina "normal."

Resurgence of the medical model of psychiatry

Since the 1970s, there has been a dramatic change in American psychiatry. The psychodynamic way of thinking about mental illness is gradually being replaced by a more empiric approach to validation of diagnosis and treatment. To a large extent, this can be attributed to four practical benefits derived from applying the medical model to psychiatry. Perhaps the first impetus for change was the discovery of dramatically effective somatic treatments for mental illness. One of the criticisms of psychoanalysis from Abraham Myerson, a leading mid-20th-century neurologist, was that it was not very effective for treating serious mental illness. By contrast, many psychiatric hospitals were virtually emptied during the two decades following the discoveries of electroconvulsive therapy in 1938, lithium salts for mania in 1949, and chlorpromazine in 1952. These somatic treatments had clear, significant efficacy.

These therapeutic discoveries coincided with several discoveries that reminded psychiatrists that the brain was involved in mental illness. For instance, reserpine, which depletes the brain of monoamines, was found to precipitate melancholia, while drugs that inhibited degradation of monoamines were found to treat melancholia. As another example, when computed tomography became available, the cerebral ventricles were found to be enlarged in people with schizophrenia compared with controls. These findings offered an alternative etiologic view to psychodynamic theories, and the strict methods used to test biological hypotheses suggested that psychological theories should be subjected to equal rigor.

Another advance that helped to reform psychiatry was the development of reliable diagnostic criteria that followed the outline of diagnostic rules in general medicine. The Washington University criteria for research diagnosis, published in 1972, rapidly became the most frequently cited of all psychiatric publications. These criteria had demonstrably high reliability, paving the way (as intended) for meaningful etiologic research. On the clinical front, physicians were hungry for a reliable way of communicating about their patients. When the American Psychiatric Association introduced the third revision of its *Diagnostic and Statistical Manual* (DSM-III) (1980), derived from the Washington University criteria, it rapidly became a bestseller. (See the following chapter for more on diagnosis.)

Finally, psychiatry was the beneficiary of (and often the originating force behind) powerful new research tools. These included modern epidemiological methods, mathematical tools for the genetic study of common diseases and quantitative traits, and imaging techniques to examine the structure and function of the living brain. These research tools further boosted hopes that the causes of mental illness might eventually be uncovered.

What the medical model of psychiatry is and is not

These four major advances are well known, but the medical model of psychiatry has spread more slowly. Perhaps because of this, some have erroneously concluded that the medical model means insisting on biological causes for all mental illness or even has "an exclusive focus on body chemistry and the prescribing of psychoactive drugs. Nothing could be more incorrect" (Guze, 1992). Instead, the medical model is a way of thinking about patients.

We believe this way of thinking to be critical. Physicians swear an oath to "first, do no harm," but unscientific thinking can harm patients. When clinicians uncritically accept hypotheses about a patient's illness, they tend to feel the cause of his symptoms is "obvious," and this comforting fallacy can lead to major—even fatal—errors in treatment. This error can be made whether the clinician favors a biological, dynamic, cognitive, or biopsychosocial etiology and can be avoided only by recognizing that clinical hypotheses must be treated as critically as research hypotheses. Skepticism about etiology and treatment is as crucial for the clinician as it is for the researcher.

The medical model of psychiatry does not assume that all mental illnesses will turn out to have biological causes. Rather, medical model psychiatrists critically examine the evidence for any proposed etiology. Theoretical speculation can be useful "if it produces testable hypotheses" (Goodwin and Guze, 1989). However, experience has taught us that many theories have been plausible but wrong, and many

more theories remain altogether untested. In the words of one critical physician, "one good experiment is worth a dozen subtle theories piled dubiously and uncertainly" (Myerson, [1944] 1994). In other words, for a theory to be attractive or plausible "is not enough; systematic and controlled data are necessary" (Guze, 1992). Thus, medical model psychiatry makes no specific assumptions about etiology. It does share the assumptions of general medicine: namely, that there are different causes for different illnesses, and that careful study of patients and of normal physiology will continue to elucidate those causes, just as it has in the past.

Similarly, the medical model does not condone uncritical acceptance of pharmacological treatments, or uncritical rejection of psychotherapy. On the contrary, specific psychotherapeutic techniques have demonstrated efficacy for many patients, and available somatic treatments have shown little or no efficacy for some conditions. The emphasis is not on choosing a treatment congruent with the illness's presumed etiology, but rather on a demand for empiric demonstration of safety and efficacy. Evidence-based medicine has long been at home in medical model psychiatry.

Beyond specific treatments, an ongoing compassionate, supportive, educational dialog with the patient is also part of the physician's role for all patients. We could hardly recommend any clinical practice in which patients were "simply medicated" and not "listened to" (Gabbard, 1990).

The medical model of psychiatry

- The medical model is the consistent application of modern medical thinking and methods to psychiatry.
- Medical model psychiatry is a way of thinking about mental illness that relies on empiricism rather than theory.
- The medical model does not assume that all psychiatric illnesses have only genetic or biochemical causes.
- Optimal knowledge of psychiatric disorders requires continued study of brain physiology.
- Psychotherapy is an important part of psychiatric practice.
- The medical model is largely responsible for many research and clinical advances in psychiatry.
- The medical model of psychiatry has several important, practical benefits for the physician and the patient.

PEARLS & PERILS

Some have characterized the empiric approach to psychiatry as superficial. This charge of superficiality seems to come in three flavors. First, some have interpreted the research focus on objective signs of illness as synonymous with a lack of curiosity about the inner workings of the mind. This hardly fits our experience with medical model psychiatrists. A fascination with the varieties of mental experience is nearly ubiquitous among such clinicians. Medical model psychiatrists tend not to be satisfied with explanations of symptoms at the superficial psychological level. Rather, they wish to understand the underlying pathophysiology responsible for the psychological manifestations. Furthermore, medical model psychiatrists tend to be frustrated with superficially plausible explanations of causality, preferring instead provable hypotheses that may lead to firm etiologic knowledge.

Others have claimed that medical model psychiatry is not interested in the subjective psychological experience of the patient, and hence is superficial in that sense. This misconception may result from the medical model's reliance on objective findings as a basis for diagnosis. For instance, somatization disorder (Briquet's syndrome) was defined by a pattern of lifelong unfounded physical complaints largely because this produced reliability of diagnosis. Yet the overall clinical presentation of such patients, including their psychological and interpersonal difficulties, was a central motivation for studying this disorder. It is after all the subjective experience of symptoms of illness that commonly motivates patients to seek treatment. The subjective perceptions of the patient are the common working material of the psychiatrist. They are also, largely, the basis for his or her empathy. The difficulty is that such perceptions have rarely been precise enough to have any solidly demonstrated value in guiding treatment. Basing treatment decisions for patients on any unproven theory, no matter how plausible, is risky, and rarely likely to be in patients' best interests.

Medical model psychiatry also has been called superficial for focusing on illness. This scientific approach to patient care, some feel, does not fully appreciate the human condition. Clearly, a medical approach to psychiatry does not explain all of human behavior. But this was never its intent. Its hope, though less grand, is no less worthwhile: namely, that an empiric approach to psychiatric diagnosis and treatment will prove to be in patients' best interests. Besides, there are risks to any model of mental illness that attempts to also explain all of normal mental and social life. Although psychiatrists naturally benefit from broad interests in these directions, claims for special knowledge and expertise that are too broad run the risk of diluting credibility. It is sheer hubris to expect that psychiatrists have discovered not only the best approach to mental illness but also the best view of normal mental life as well as the answers to many serious philosophical and religious questions.

Finally, medical model psychiatry has been accused of fostering a superficial understanding of our patients. But this is a misunderstanding. Black (1994) wrote:

Diagnosis, after all, is "the careful examination and description of the patient's condition" (Guze). Both our ability to provide good care and our enjoyment of

psychiatric practice depend on how well we know our patients. So much of compliance, motivation, and therapeutic success hinges on the doctor-patient relationship, rather than on knowledge of a particular piece of data. In fact, thinking scientifically about one's patients obliges one to know more, not less, about them because so many questions of diagnosis and management remain unanswered by controlled studies.

Knowing one's patients well is crucial in psychiatry but may be equally important in general medicine. "A mental disease is a disorder of the person following the laws of general pathology like any other disease" (Meyer, [1897] 1994).

The most serious charge against the medical model is that an empirical approach to patient care somehow precludes empathy. Our belief is that nothing could be farther from the truth. "Scientific skepticism is in no way incompatible with compassion for the sick or disabled. In fact, it is the desire to help patients that causes one to be frustrated by the lack of definite knowledge about what really helps and what does not. There are few things more humanitarian than the effective use of knowledge to relieve suffering" (Guze, 1970).

Practical benefits of the medical model

This chapter has taken a good bit of space to discuss philosophical issues relating to psychiatry. The primary justification for this is the belief that a consistent application of the scientific method to clinical psychiatry is in our patients' best interests. Thus, this medical model underlies all subsequent chapters in this volume. This approach to psychiatry also has a number of practical benefits for psychiatrists, neurologists, and other physicians at all levels of training. A description of some of these benefits follows.

A common, accessible language for education and collaboration

Implicit in the medical model is an insistence on reliable diagnostic methods. One practical benefit is that the experience of more senior clinicians can be more easily shared with students and residents. Obviously, students must still gain clinical experience to identify signs of illness, such as tangential speech or an Argyll Robertson pupil. With defined diagnostic criteria, however, they can already have some idea what is meant by paranoid schizophrenia or secondary mania.

If this benefit were limited to medical novices, reliable diagnostic methods could serve as a temporary nursemaid and then be abandoned. However, modern diagnostic criteria also make a physician's continuing medical education much easier. Before widespread acceptance of research diagnostic criteria, it was very difficult to know whether treatment studies reported in the literature had any relevance for one's own patients, since different investigators meant very different things by even such common terms as schizophrenia. Now, on the other hand, one can read a study of a new treatment for schizophrenia and know whether one's own patients share important features with the patients studied. Finally, using specific diagnostic criteria, psychiatrists can discuss patients with collaborators and have some hope of communicating clearly.

A hope for discovery of etiology and treatment

The hope for successful research into the causes and treatment of mental illness is a significant *raison d'être* for the medical model of psychiatry. Some historical support for the success of this approach has already been discussed, but it bears repetition that the major discoveries of psychiatry can be attributed largely to the assumptions of the medical model.

A unified general approach to all patients

Internists, neurologists, and other physicians spend years in training, learning among other things a tried and true approach to their patients. This approach includes gathering careful historical information from the patient, conducting a general or focused exam, matching the patient's symptoms and signs with those of a known syndrome if possible, and then turning to controlled studies to support one's diagnostic and therapeutic actions. Special techniques have developed in each specialty appropriate to its needs, but this underlying approach is nearly universal in medicine. Patients with psychiatric illnesses constitute a large share of the practice of physicians in other specialties. If a completely different approach were required for psychological as opposed to bodily complaints, then physicians of other specialties would understandably feel at a loss when faced with these patients. If, on the other hand, physicians adopt a medical model approach to mental illness, then their general medical skills — careful history and examination, identification of a syndrome, and reference to the diagnosis and treatment of similar illnesses in the literature — will serve equally well for "psych patients" as for all other patients.

A medical approach to all patients helps not only physicians but patients. For instance, several studies show that non-psychiatrist physicians often overlook important psychiatric syndromes such as dementia or major depression. When evaluation is not limited to "physical" complaints, patients receive better care. Similarly, many idiopathic psychiatric illnesses include physical signs (such as the motor retardation of major depression), which are more prone to be overlooked if their cause is assumed to be psychological.

No need for unreasonable illness boundaries

Many common clinical situations defy the dualistic supposition that mental and physical illnesses should be separated. For instance, obsessive-compulsive symptoms are likely an integral part of Tourette's syndrome. Similarly, depressive symptoms can be the earliest manifestations of Parkinson's disease, and psychosis is a common side effect of antiparkinsonian medication. Depression and dementia are as much a part of Huntington's disease as is chorea. It seems arbitrary and wasteful for a clinician to need to "change gears" mentally when assessing affective or cognitive signs compared with motor signs of the same illness. Also, many clinicians have shared the frustration of dealing with disparate insurance coverage for the same patient, depending on whether psychiatric or neurological symptoms are more prominent at the time.

Differential diagnosis

Almost all major mental illnesses have a broad medical differential diagnosis. Although not the most common causes of psychological symptoms, secondary psychiatric illnesses are far from rare. For instance, delusions can result from Lewy body dementia, adult metachromatic leukodystrophy, phencyclidine or amphetamine. Fatigue and depression are very sensitive indicators of hypothyroidism and other endocrine disorders. In fact, for most psychiatric presentations one can generalize the words of Gelenberg (1976) regarding catatonia: "Like hypertension . . . catatonia discovered on physical examination should spur a medical investigation to uncover the probable cause."

Aside from the fact that differential diagnostic considerations provide much of the enjoyment of medical practice, psychological symptoms can be significant clues to general medical illnesses. However, these symptoms are common enough that a good working knowledge of psychiatry is required to sort out their likely cause. If psychological complaints are simply assumed to result from life stressors or intrapsychic conflict, rather than as symptoms whose differential diagnosis should be pursued as warranted by the rest of the history and exam, many patients will not receive optimal treatment.

The enjoyment of medical practice

The excitement of evaluating a new patient is one of many factors that can make medical practice an enjoyable vocation for a lifetime. Considering that a large fraction of patients seen in primary care practices have psychiatric illness, one's approach to these patients becomes important. If the non-psychiatric physician approaches symptoms of depression, somatization disorder, or anxiety with the medical model, he or she may be more likely to view these complaints as part of the challenge of medical science and part of the healing art of helping those who are suffering. If patients with psychological complaints are instead seen as an extraneous distraction from "real illness," one suspects that much of medicine, especially primary care medicine, may become very frustrating.

Saving lives

Schizophrenia, major depression, panic disorder, and mania are diseases with high morbidity and mortality. They are also among the most treatable of medical conditions. Their treatment success rates are comparable to those of hypertension, angina, and other common general medical disorders. If these conditions are viewed as separate from other medical conditions, the physician may miss an opportunity for sharing in very rewarding clinical results. If the primary care physician does not see these diseases as part of his or her duty, the physician may even unintentionally contribute to a death.

Societal considerations

There are many practical repercussions of how physicians, as a group, view mental illness, including effects on psychiatric research and insurance for mental illness. Research funding for mental illness often has not received the public financial support it would merit on a basis of societal cost, extent of disability, or even prevalence. To some extent this may be attributed to public perception that cancer and stroke are "real" and dreadful diseases that strike indiscriminately, while mental illnesses are not illnesses but weaknesses which one can avoid by personal effort. When physicians support this dichotomous view of illness, we slow research for its prevention and cure.

On another front, the nearly ubiquitous discriminatory policies that underinsure mental illnesses as compared to other illnesses, if not the result of greed and exploitation of ignorance, must be due largely to a view that mental illnesses are not real. Physicians should be patients' best advocates. When physicians support such discriminatory policies, they share in the responsibility for the pain and suffering these policies cause. Instead physicians can spread the knowledge that treating serious psychiatric illnesses actually saves money.

> We may have to control the growing costs of health care, but we should not do it by discriminating against a particular category of illness that can be as painful, disabling, and life-threatening as most other serious medical conditions, and that is often long-lasting and broadly pervasive in its manifestations (Guze, 1992)

Myths about psychiatry

Considering the difficulties psychiatry has faced in defining itself over the last century, it is perhaps no surprise that there are a number of common misconceptions about the field. Below we briefly address a few of the more prevalent myths.

Myth: Psychiatric illnesses aren't real

This issue is hard to address in a few sentences, and the serious reader is referred to the discussions by Kendell (1975) or Guze (1992). However, a few points answer many arguments commonly given to support this assertion. (1) If "real" illnesses always have identifiable pathology, then several general medical problems today (such as hypertension or migraine) are not diseases, and "most of the great scourges of mankind have only become diseases during the last hundred and fifty years" (Kendell, 1975). Furthermore, to require known pathology implies the bold assumptions that our current methods for finding pathology are already perfect, and that we already know exactly where to apply which tools. In fact, whether one associates a given illness with pathology depends largely on the power of one's research methods.

(2) If only serious illnesses are "real," then the major mental illnesses certainly qualify. They are associated with a great deal of suffering, and they cause death and disability to a greater extent than many "physical" illnesses. Another way of judging the seriousness of an illness is to consider its effect on the biological fitness of the individuals affected. Judged in this way, schizophrenia (for instance) is clearly a serious illness.

The fact that this question is raised in psychiatry more often than in general medicine largely reflects the tacit assumption of mind-body duality. Kendell (1975) wrote:

> Most doctors, after all, never give a moment's thought to the precise meaning of terms like illness and disease, nor do they need to. They simply treat the patients who consult them as best they can, diagnose individual diseases whenever they can, and try to relieve their patients' suffering even if they can't. At times they are well aware that they are dealing with matters other than illness [e.g. childbirth], but rarely do they pause to consider what is the essential difference between the two. The practical nature of medicine is not conducive to theorizing.

Myth: Psychiatry is an inexact science

Of course psychiatry is an inexact science, just like all of clinical medicine. The only myth here is the implicit idea that other medical specialties somehow escape this charge. In fact, medicine itself is an inexact science.

Myth: Even psychiatrists can't agree on diagnosis

This is a special case of the previous myth. The best brief answer is perhaps that diagnostic dilemmas are not limited to psychiatry but are part of the reality of all of clinical medicine. In diagnostic studies of many general medical conditions, it is apparent that perfect diagnostic concordance is nearly impossible (see Table 2.2). Research on the major psychiatric illnesses, for which specific laboratory tests are generally unavailable, has had to face this difficulty head-on. As a result, recent studies of psychiatric diagnosis show high diagnostic reliability. The methods developed by psychiatric researchers to improve clinical judgments and quantify diagnostic concordance have since been recognized and adopted by other specialties for illnesses in which laboratory tests play a minor role (e.g., headache). Chapter 2 further addresses the reliability of psychiatric diagnosis.

Myth: Psychiatric illnesses are diagnoses of exclusion only

This unfortunate idea seems to come from three prevalent fallacies: (1) psychiatric means unexplained, (2) psychiatric disorders are not treatable, and (3) psychiatric disorders are not medically serious. Two facts replace these fallacies. First, undiagnosed illness does not imply psychiatric illness. For instance, follow-up of single conversion symptoms occasionally reveals a neurological or systemic disease. Conversely, diagnosing a valid syndrome, even if its cause is not completely known, provides a degree of certainty about prognosis including response to treatment. Sometimes the psychiatric diagnosis provides much more information than the less well-validated physical disorder being assessed (for example, major depression vs. irritable bowel disease). Often the psychiatric disorder under consideration is at least as treatable as the physical disorder (e.g., panic disorder vs. coronary artery disease). And often, treatment of the psychiatric disorder is more important than treatment of the "rule-outs" for preventing disability or even death. In short, psychiatric illnesses should be considered early in the medical evaluation, not as a last resort.

Consider the common clinical situation of a middle-aged woman with atypical chest pain. An abnormal stress test has about the same positive predictive value as a coin flip, whereas a clinically definite diagnosis of somatization disorder has roughly a 94% chance of still explaining her chest pain on follow-up years later. If this disorder is identified, the clinician now has diagnosed a condition, known to cause complaints of chest pain, which can explain the presentation. If instead of a careful record review, history, and psychiatric exam, one had a laboratory test with this success rate, no doubt the test would be used early in the evaluation.

Myth: Psychiatry is concerned only with psychologically-caused symptoms

The introduction to this chapter defined psychiatry as a medical specialty concerned with disturbances of thought, emotions, perception, and behavior. Notice what this definition does not say. There is no reference to what causes the disturbed thinking, mood, perception, or behavior. Psychiatry is not concerned only with illnesses whose causes are "psychological."

One reason for this is that many different illnesses can cause the same symptoms, and treatment and prognosis are often quite different. For instance, depressed mood can be caused by a primary mood disorder, personality disorder, alcoholism, hypothyroidism, stroke, bereavement, or everyday disappointments. The differential diagnosis of these mental symptoms is a medical question for which psychiatrists are best suited by nature of their education and training.

Conversely, treatment for some psychiatric syndromes can be similar regardless of the etiology, and psychiatrists have expertise in these symptomatic treatments. For instance, the manic syndrome can be effectively treated with hospitalization, medication, or electroconvulsive therapy whether it is a consequence of bipolar disorder or steroids. Few, if any, illnesses have a purely psychosocial etiology. For most major mental illnesses, there is strong evidence that genetic and biochemical components contribute to causation.

In other words, psychiatry is best defined by the clinical manifestations of its patients, not by what causes these manifestations. Hallucinations are psychiatric symptoms whether they result from drug use, brain tumors, or schizophrenia, and major depression is a psychiatric syndrome whether it is a result of reserpine, stroke, or bipolar disorder.

Issues regarding general psychiatry

- Psychiatry is a medical specialty concerned with disturbances of thought, emotions, and behavior.
- "Organic" disorders of cognition and mood remain part of psychiatric practice.
- Psychiatric illnesses can be reliably diagnosed.
- Most psychiatric illnesses can be effectively treated, but often go untreated.
- Psychiatric illnesses are real, common, and serious, yet they remain stigmatized.
- People with mental illnesses deserve a physician's care as much as people with other equally severe illnesses.

PEARLS & PERILS

Myth: The difference between psychiatry and neurology is that neurology deals with real brain disease

Another medical specialty, neurology, is also concerned with disturbances of thought, emotions, perception, and behavior. Naturally, there is a considerable overlap of interests. For instance, there are conditions for which expertise is shared by the two specialties (e.g. Tourette's syndrome, Alzheimer's disease, or sleep disorders). There are illnesses in each specialty without clear pathology (e.g. torticollis or panic disorder) and illnesses in each specialty with clear pathology (e.g. stroke, or disinhibition in Wilson's disease). There are several conditions that were treated by psychiatrists a century ago but are now treated by neurologists (such as epilepsy and neurosyphilis). Others have taken the reverse route (e.g., neurasthenia). There are illnesses that take patients to both neurologists and psychiatrists (such as depression or somatization disorder). Obviously there are differences: neurologists do not commonly treat mania or personality disorder, and psychiatrists usually are not the primary doctor for epilepsy or multiple sclerosis. However, there is enough overlap between the two specialties to discredit the simplistic notion that pathology and etiology reliably distinguish them. In practice, neurology and psychiatry are demarcated primarily by medical and social convention.

Myth: People with mental illnesses don't need a physician

The usual answer to this invidious myth is this: Who else is properly trained in differential diagnosis, triage, and both psychological and somatic treatments? This is a crucial point, and for many observers it settles the question.

However, another part of the answer lies in society's expectations for its medical care. The current extensive training of physicians arose in the very early years of the 20th century. At that time, physicians had few if any effective treatments, and very little was known about the pathophysiology of disease. Doctors often had brief courses of practical study and informal apprenticeships. However, the influential Flexner report in the early 1900s revolutionized medical training by its radical suggestion that medical schools require basic science education before matriculation and again before graduation. Formal internships were required even after this extensive education. The underlying reason for these changes was the hope that training in the biological sciences would make for better doctors. Not only would they be better situated to find causes and treatments of disease, but they could better analyze new research findings of others and think scientifically about their patients' problems. These reasons are arguably more important now than ever, given the vast body of scientific facts available to support the modern practice of medicine and the overwhelming rate at which new biomedical knowledge is being acquired.

The exigencies of wartime in the 1940s, and later the rising costs of medical care, have led to a number of other professionals taking roles traditionally filled by physicians. Psychologists and social workers are not alone in seeking a more direct role in providing patient care; they are joined by nurses, physicians' assistants, physical therapists, optometrists, and others. Society now has an important question to answer. Without a doubt these professionals have important roles to play in the efficient delivery of medical care, but should they supplant the physician? Put another way, we feel that extensive scientific and medical training is still the best way to train for providing competent psychiatric care.

Finally, to say that people with mental illness don't need a physician is really simply a form of discrimination against a minority. People with mental illnesses already face enough stigma and discrimination. Denying them access to a physician when no such denial is made for other illnesses is only adding injury to insult.

Conclusion

Mental illnesses are real. They are common. They cause a very human form of suffering. They can cause disability and even death. Yet they remain undertreated, stigmatized, and widely misunderstood.

However, applying the methods of modern medicine to psychiatry has led to exciting advances. Several major mental illnesses of the 1800s, such as endemic cretinism, neurosyphilis, and pellagra, have been largely eliminated. Psychiatric illnesses can now be reliably diagnosed. The safety and efficacy of many psychiatric treatments have been clearly established, and treatment outcomes in psychiatry are among the most rewarding in all of medicine. There are almost daily advances in our understanding of how the brain functions in health and disease. The medical model approach to psychiatry, which is largely responsible for many of these advances, offers a proven approach for continuing to help those affected by mental illness.

Annotated bibliography

Guze, SB (1992) *Why Psychiatry is a Branch of Medicine*, New York, Oxford.
  This short book offers an introduction to the medical model of psychiatry, explaining its advantages and discussing its implications.
Kendell, RE (1975) The concept of disease and its implications for psychiatry, *Br J Psychiatry* 127:305–315.
  A clear, brief discussion of what defines a disease.
National Institute of Mental Health: The impact of mental illness on society, NIMH Publication No. 01–4586. Available at http://www.nimh.nih.gov.

This source summarizes important data showing that psychiatric illnesses cause substantial cost, disability, and death.

Pichot, P (1994) Nosological models in psychiatry, *Br J Psychiatry* 164:232–240.

A brief history of psychiatric classification.

Rogers, D (1992) *Motor Disorder in Psychiatry: towards a neurological psychiatry*, New York, John Wiley & Sons.

A challenge to the simplistic idea that neurology treats the brain and psychiatry treats the mind (see especially pp. 1–10 and 113–114).

Shorter, E (1997) *A History of Psychiatry: from the era of the asylum to the age of Prozac*, New York, John Wiley & Sons.

This very readable book discusses the roots of modern psychiatric medicine in the 1800s and 1900s.

CHAPTER 2

Diagnosis

Kevin J. Black, MD

Introduction

Consider the following typical case.

> Mr A is a 30-year-old man who visits his family doctor for "a checkup." Soon it becomes obvious that Mr A is very worried that he may have cancer. He has quit work to take care of his health. A careful physical examination and a long discussion do not seem to reassure him. He requests various lab tests, imaging studies, and referrals to specialists. He asks about taking various food supplements to counteract toxic substances in the environment. As the doctor tries to end the visit, Mr A asks, "Doc, why won't you just tell me what's wrong with me?" He refuses an invitation to return for further discussion, saying, "You already said you didn't find anything wrong."

Mr A probably doesn't have cancer, but he probably does have a very treatable illness that is disabling him and destroying his quality of life. The appropriate treatment will be very different depending on whether he has major depression, obsessive-compulsive disorder, or schizophrenia. Unfortunately, as discussed in Chapter 1, Mr A will likely get mixed messages unless psychiatric diagnosis is seen as an important part of his medical care.

In this chapter, we address the questions of why psychological symptoms are categorized into diagnoses, how diagnostic criteria for psychiatric illness are useful, and how psychiatric diagnoses are made.

Why make diagnoses for psychological symptoms?

Among the core goals of medicine are treating illnesses successfully, predicting their outcome, and finding their causes. The process of diagnosis has become fundamental to meeting all three of these goals. From early times, physicians have observed that afflictions tend to fall into *syndromes*—patterns of signs and symptoms that are fairly stable across patients. Identifying a syndrome may address each of these three goals. Usually those with similar signs and symptoms have a similar prognosis. Often, the cause of an illness can be found by comparing similarities among the backgrounds of different patients with the same syndrome. Treatments that help one patient with a given syndrome often help others with the same syndrome. The process of carefully listening to the patient, examining him, and classifying symptoms and signs into recognized syndromes is called *diagnosis*.

Diagnosis began with clinical observations alone. However, the advent of modern pathology in the 19th century had two significant effects on diagnosis. First, many diagnoses made by purely clinical criteria (such as pneumonia) were validated by laboratory findings and autopsy. Second, new diagnostic subcategories arose when different laboratory findings in the same clinical syndrome tended to help predict outcome (e.g., streptococcal pneumonia). These new diagnoses based on pathology enjoyed great popularity for a simple reason: they were generally superior to purely clinical diagnoses in the three functions of diagnosis mentioned above—explaining illness, suggesting treatment, and predicting outcome.

These were enormous advances. Unfortunately, however, they helped change the common concept of disease from clinical syndromes to specific pathology or abnormal laboratory tests. This had a profound effect on psychiatry because American psychiatrists in the early and mid-1900s largely abandoned illnesses with pathological or laboratory findings. They turned to alternative models of disease which assumed that mental processes were similar in health and illness. They also turned their attention from syndromal commonalities among patients and instead emphasized factors unique to an individual. As a result, two widespread misconceptions arose. One was that meaningful diagnoses are always associated with laboratory or postmortem abnormalities. A second was that diagnosis for "physical" illness is meaningful, while diagnosis for mental illness is nothing but an arbitrary label. These fallacies are still common among physicians. For instance, the problem list for patients seen in other specialties may include the entry "psych problem," when one can hardly imagine the entry "kidney problem." Such a vague label is nearly useless given the wide variety of causes, outcomes, and appropriate treatments for different psychiatric illnesses. The truth is that diagnosis in psychiatry has invaluable benefits for clinical care, medical education, and research.

All diagnoses are not created equal

In medical diagnosis, valid diagnoses ideally would reflect a natural classification in which each diagnostic syndrome indicates a single disease entity. For many illnesses the cause is still not completely known, yet an interim classification is needed. In some diseases (like rheumatoid arthritis), the validity of clinical diagnosis can at least be judged with reference to autopsy or laboratory findings. For other diseases (like migraine or schizophrenia), there is no visible pathology.

Fortunately, there are clinical observations that can suggest validity even for purely clinical diagnoses. Robins and Guze (1970) discussed five clinically relevant ways of testing diagnostic validity (see Box 2.1): clinical description, delimitation from other disorders, follow-up studies including response to treatment, family studies, and laboratory studies.

TABLE 2.1

Selected psychiatric diagnoses with more and less well-established validity

Validity well established	Validity debated
Alzheimer's disease	Hypochondriasis
Alcoholism	Primary insomnia
Schizophrenia	Generalized anxiety disorder
Bipolar disorder	Dissociative identity disorder
Major depression	Borderline personality disorder
Somatization disorder	Seasonal affective disorder
Antisocial personality disorder	Psychological factors affecting
Obsessive-compulsive disorder	medical condition
Anorexia nervosa	Intermittent explosive disorder
Panic disorder	

BOX 2.1

Steps to establishing diagnostic validity

1 Clinical description.
2 Delimitation from other disorders.
3 Follow-up study (including response to treatment).
4 Family study.
5 Laboratory studies.

Adapted from Robins and Guze, 1970.

The importance to the clinician is that often these features of a diagnosis also predict its clinical utility. For instance, if a diagnosis overlaps almost entirely with another diagnosis, it may add little information. By contrast, if follow-up studies of patients with a given diagnosis show a reasonably consistent outcome, we can predict a patient's prognosis; and if we can quantify heritability for a given disease, we can better predict risk to a patient's relatives. Diagnoses for idiopathic illnesses tend to be most useful when they are based on careful study of these illness features. If instead "diseases" are invented arbitrarily, they may or may not be valid and often are less clinically useful. Again, note that diagnostic validity and

utility do not depend on the existence of a pathognomonic laboratory or autopsy abnormality. Angina predicted heart attacks long before the EKG was invented.

Some psychiatric diagnoses have met these tests. Schizophrenia, major depression, and somatization disorder are examples of psychiatric diagnoses supported by numerous validity studies (see Table 2.1). Not coincidentally, there is also substantial information about prognosis and treatment for these disorders. On the other hand, validity has not been demonstrated for a number of other psychiatric diagnoses. Fortunately, increasing attention is being paid to diagnostic validity, and there are now numerous research studies that address the points in Box 2.1.

Reliability is a different concept that indicates how likely different observers are to give the same opinion. Diagnostic reliability is crucial to both the clinician and the researcher. In clinical medicine, a diagnosis is hardly worth making if it fails to consistently describe the patient, and a diagnosis that describes different patients to different colleagues can hardly aid communication between physicians. Etiologic research on less valid diagnoses may be pointless, but research without diagnostic reliability is nearly impossible.

DSM-IV: what, why, and how good?

One of the most important psychiatric advances in the last three decades of the 20th century was the development of rules for psychiatric diagnosis based on clearly defined disease features. These criteria had a dramatic effect on both research and clinical practice. With them, physicians could meaningfully communicate about a patient by saying (for example) that he or she met Washington University criteria for schizophrenia or ICD-10 criteria for bipolar affective disorder. Studies of treatment, natural history, or etiology from another institution suddenly became relevant to one's own patients. This approach has proven so valuable that it has been adopted by other specialties when dealing with clinically defined illnesses. For instance, the International Headache Society modeled its diagnostic criteria for various headache syndromes on those used by American psychiatrists. In the United States, the current standard is to use the American Psychiatric Association's *Diagnostic and Statistical Manual of Mental Disorders, 4th Edition* (usually referred to as DSM-IV; minimal changes were made to the diagnostic criteria in a 2000 revision, referred to as DSM-IV-TR).

Reliability and validity have been extensively studied for many DSM-IV diagnoses. Diagnostic reliability tends to be higher for broader diagnostic categories (anxiety disorders vs panic disorder with agoraphobia) and more severe illnesses (mania vs hypomania), but reliability is still acceptable for most diagnoses. In fact, modern psychiatric research studies demonstrate very good reliability for major DSM-IV diagnoses, in a range at least comparable to that for other medical diagnoses made by clinical criteria (Table 2.2). In other words, disagreement about diagnosis is not unique to psychiatry but is part of clinical medicine in general.

Validity is a separate question. There are disagreements between different researchers as to the validity of various DSM-IV disorders. However, discussions of validity increasingly benefit from data that address the points in Box 2.1, and there is widespread acceptance that certain diagnoses are valid (see Table 2.1).

DSM-IV will not be the ultimate iteration. Preparation for DSM-V has already begun, though its release is not envisioned prior to 2010. In any case, nosology should continue to improve over time as knowledge accrues. It has in the past. For instance, clinical definitions of general paresis of the insane were largely supplanted when laboratory tests for syphilitic infection became available. More recently, several genetic subtypes of degenerative dementias have been identified. One may reasonably expect that the causes of bipolar disorder will be better elucidated with time, so that specific laboratory tests or different clinical criteria will be adopted for diagnosis. Alternatively, future research may demonstrate that some of our clinical diagnoses correspond poorly to biological reality. In the meantime, using widely available, reliable standardized diagnostic criteria, even if imperfect, still affords the clinical and research advantages discussed above.

DSM-IV divides psychiatric diagnoses into several categories and suggests listing diagnoses according to five "axes" corresponding to different aspects of illness and health. Most major psychiatric illnesses, such as substance abuse, cognitive disorders, mood and anxiety disorders, and psychoses are listed on Axis I. Axis II is reserved for mental retardation and personality disorders and Axis III for nonpsychiatric medical illnesses. Life stressors can be described on Axis IV, and overall psychological and social functioning is rated on Axis V according to a numerical scale. For example:

Axis I. 1. major depression, recurrent, moderate severity;
    2. obsessive-compulsive disorder
Axis II. no diagnosis
Axis III. congestive heart failure
Axis IV. chronic cardiac disability, recent job loss
Axis V. current: 20 (recent suicide attempt); best past year: 70 (mild symptoms)

The process of modern psychiatric diagnosis

Most psychiatric diagnoses are made by clinical criteria alone. Clinical diagnosis in any specialty involves gathering information through history and examination, and then choosing an appropriate diagnosis. The following paragraphs briefly discuss key aspects of this process for psychiatric illness in modern medical practice.

Gathering information

Accurate diagnosis begins with accurate fact-finding. Reliability of diagnosis is poor if different information is available to different diagnosticians, and a diagnosis is only as valid as the information supplied. These observations apply to all of medicine, but assume special importance in the absence of a laboratory "gold standard." Spitzer coined the term "LEAD standard" (Longitudinal, Expert, All Data) to describe one way of addressing this problem as applied to psychiatric research. Several suggestions follow for applying this idea to clinical practice.

Psychiatric diagnosis is based on reliable facts and not merely on a patient's reported symptoms. Although an individual's view of his life is meaningful, and may even have diagnostic importance, often it does not accurately reflect objective history. The physician must define whether he or she is dealing with verifiable history or with subjective history, as exemplified by the following fairly typical case.

> Mr B reports lifelong depression to his physician. However, close friends and family members say that he sleeps and eats well, enjoys his usual activities, and usually appears happy. He does have brief periods every few days, lasting from a few minutes to two hours, when he feels hopeless in a difficult interpersonal situation and may cry.

This patient's distress may be an appropriate focus of clinical attention but does not reflect a major depressive episode. Discrepancies between symptom self-report and observation by others exist in all medical specialties. After all, different observers recall different facets of an experience, and time blurs memory of past events. However, these discrepancies assume special importance in psychiatry, where patients often have disorders of perception, mood, cognition, or insight, and where many important diagnoses require

TABLE 2.2

Reliability of selected diagnoses

Diagnosis	Diagnostic criteria	Means of assessment	By whom?	Kappa*
Restless leg syndrome	International RLS criteria	Johns Hopkins Telephone Diagnostic Interview (TDI)	Expert interviewers	0.95**
Alcohol abuse, alcohol dependence	DSM-IV	Structured Clinical Interview for the DSM (SCID), adapted for teenagers	Five clinical raters	0.94
Schizophrenia	DSM-III-R	SCID	Three trained raters	0.94
Obsessive-compulsive disorder	DSM-IV	Anxiety Disorders Interview Schedule: lifetime version (ADIS-IV-L)	Clinical psychologists and psychology doctoral students	0.85
Rotator cuff disorders (full thickness tears)		MR images of the shoulder	Radiologists	0.74–0.92
Major depressive episode	DSM-IV	Composite International Diagnostic Interview (CIDI)	Two psychiatrists	0.82
Chorioamnionitis and umbilical vessel vasculitis	Clinical judgment	Review of slides	Two senior pathologists	0.78–0.81
Panic disorder (with or without agoraphobia)	DSM-IV	Anxiety Disorders Interview Schedule: lifetime version (ADIS-IV-L)	Clinical psychologists and psychology doctoral students	0.79
Social phobia	DSM-IV	Anxiety Disorders Interview Schedule: lifetime version (ADIS-IV-L)	Clinical psychologists and psychology doctoral students	0.77
Endometrial thickness		Transvaginal ultrasonography (≤5.0mm vs >5.0mm)	Two gynecologists	0.74
Acute myocardial infarction	Clinical judgment	Serial serum enzyme concentrations	Two cardiology specialists, two internal medicine specialists, two trainees	0.74
Personality disorders	DSM-IV	SCID-II, version 2.0	Eight trained clinicians	0.48–0.98
Pneumonia		Chest radiograph	Radiologic panel and a radiology specialist	0.71–0.72
Transient ischemic attack		Standardized protocol	Neurologists and neurology residents	0.65–0.77
Personality disorders	DSM-IV	Diagnostic Interview for DSM-IV Personality Disorders (DIPD-IV)	Twelve trained MA- or PhD-level raters	0.4–1.0
Dysplasia in Barrett's esophagus		Review of slides	Gastrointestinal pathologists	0.70
Generalized anxiety disorder	DSM-IV	Anxiety Disorders Interview Schedule: lifetime version (ADIS-IV-L)	Clinical psychologists and psychology doctoral students	0.67

Continued

TABLE 2.2 (continued)

Reliability of selected diagnoses

Diagnosis	Diagnostic criteria	Means of assessment	By whom?	Kappa*
Personality disorders	DSM-IV	SCID-II	Ten cognitive-behavioral psychotherapists and trainees	0.63
Adolescent idiopathic scoliosis	King classification	Radiographs	Orthopedic surgeons	0.61
Cutaneous melanoma	Clinical judgment	Review of slides	Experienced histopathologists	0.61
Oral lichen planus and leukoplakia	WHO 1978 classification (OLP), Uppsala definition (leukoplakia)	Photographs	Clinicians	0.43–0.77
Sleep disorders (various diagnoses)	DSM-IV	Standard clinical interview	Two clinicians, one a sleep specialist	0.35–0.56
Renal cell carcinoma	Furhman nuclear grading scheme	Review of slides	Pathologists	0.45
Osteolysis	Clinical judgment	Radiographs	Joint arthroplasty surgeons	0.28–0.44
Endometrial hyperplasia	Snomed system	Review of slides	Histopathologists with interest in gynecology	0.25
Insomnia (various diagnoses)	DSM-IV	Semistructured sleep disorders interview	Sleep disorder specialists (3 MDs, 2 PhDs)	0.23–0.25
Schizoaffective disorder	DSM-IV	CIDI	Two psychiatrists	0.22
Suspicious for prostate cancer	Clinical judgment	Digital rectal exam	Urologists	0.22

* A κ (kappa) value of zero indicates that any diagnostic agreement is purely due to chance, while κ = 1 means that diagnostic agreement is perfect. Generally, κ > 0.75 is interpreted as excellent reliability and 0.60–0.74 as good reliability. The κ statistic is not an ideal measure of diagnostic concordance, but it is probably the most commonly reported. References for entries in this table are available from the author.

** This entry is an intraclass correlation coefficient.

accurate delineation of past episodes of illness and health. For clinical purposes it is often crucial to gather information from other sources.

Medical records can be particularly valuable, since they contain written observations from trained examiners "on the spot." However, medical records can include omissions or errors; for instance, alcohol history is rarely recorded in most medical records. Family members, close friends, co-workers, or even casual acquaintances can be better sources of information about a patient's functioning outside the hospital or office. Even when there is no inaccuracy in the patient's history, others often notice things about an individual that he does not notice about himself. Of course, a patient's permission must be obtained before the physician divulges confidential information *to* third parties. However, often patients will help the physician obtain information *from* third parties once they understand how important this information can be to their diagnosis and treatment.

Whether or not third party observations are available, the physician is a trained observer. Good medical practice dictates examining for signs of illness in addition to eliciting symptoms. The mental status examination nearly always includes assessment of certain signs: the patient's appearance, behavior, speech, spontaneous movements, flow of speech, and emotional behavior. Memory and language are also examined. Certain presentations dictate further examination for other signs of illness, such as tachycardia, dilated pupils, goiter, apraxia, rigidity, catalepsy, or ataxia. When there is marked disparity between reported symptoms and visible signs, the physician should use caution in assigning a diagnosis.

Identifying signs of illness requires expertise from the examiner. Gathering historical data also requires expertise. Patients may give some types of information more accurately on a questionnaire or in an interview with a stranger, especially information about illegal or other stigmatized behavior. However, patients can hardly be blamed if they withhold information about their thoughts, hopes, mood, and intimate relationships from a cold or uncaring interviewer. Developing trust is part of the physician's art and duty, along with developing other skills needed for effective interviewing. With these caveats, diagnosing schizophrenia is no more a rote checklist exercise than diagnosing rheumatic fever, since the examiner must know how to elicit and identify the symptoms and signs that form the criteria.

Sometimes the patient, his medical records, or third parties can supply adequate historical information for a confident longitudinal diagnosis even at a first interview. However, often patience and follow-up examinations are required.

Depending on the setting, one may benefit by supplementing the usual clinical examination with tools originally developed for clinical research. Signs of illness may be more reliably determined by standardizing severity ratings or examination techniques. Well-studied clinical rating scales (such as the Hamilton Depression Rating Scale or Brief Psychiatric Rating Scale) help anchor clinical descriptions to a standard rating of severity. Standardized examination techniques have been developed for the neurological examination and for ratings of psychomotor retardation, to give two examples.

Symptoms can also be elicited in a highly reproducible way using standardized interviews. Important examples include the Structured Clinical Interview for Axis I DSM-IV (SCID), the Schedules for Clinical Assessment in Neuropsychiatry (SCAN), the Diagnostic Interview Schedule (DIS), and the Composite International Diagnostic Interview (CIDI). These standardized interviews have been extensively tested and applied widely in psychiatric research. Self-report questionnaires (such as the Beck Depression Inventory, Michigan Alcoholism Screening Test, or Minnesota Multiphasic Personality Inventory) are highly reliable and can be added to the usual clinical evaluation at low cost. These approaches also make sure that important diagnoses are not forgotten, which can happen often in the usual busy clinical setting. On the other hand, some illnesses are poorly diagnosed by standardized interviews or self-report questionnaires. This happens because some diagnoses may require historical information from medical records or third parties for diagnosis (e.g., somatization disorder), others may require expert interpretation of self-report (e.g., obsessive-compulsive disorder or pseudoseizures), others are better defined by physical signs than by symptoms (e.g., catatonia, or melancholic subtype of major depression), and others are poorly remembered or described by patients (e.g., hypomania or dementia).

Finally, psychological testing and clinical laboratory tests can add valuable diagnostic information for certain presentations. Further discussion of how to elicit history, perform the mental status examination, and request psychological or laboratory testing is available in the next chapter.

Choosing an appropriate diagnosis

Chest pain has numerous causes and outcomes, depending largely on whether the pain syndrome is angina, heartburn, pleuritic pain, or so on. Similarly, most psychiatric symptoms, taken singly, are very nonspecific. The symptom of sadness, for instance, is nonspecific. It has many causes, and vastly different prognosis and treatment depending on the cause. On the other hand, well-defined syndromes (like major depression with melancholic features) have more uniform prognosis and treatment response. When a complete syndrome is present, one has greater certainty in treatment decisions.

As discussed above, each clinical syndrome of an ideal nosology would have a single cause. However, in medicine many syndromes seem to represent "final common pathways" of clinical expression, so that even though recognition of a syndrome narrows the etiologic considerations considerably, there often remain several known causes for a given syndrome. In psychiatry, this is most obvious with the syndromes traditionally called "organic," such as dementia or delirium, and many physicians appreciate that these cognitive disorders have a broad differential diagnosis.

However, the same can be said of most other psychiatric syndromes. Autism, mania, major depression, and catatonia are examples of psychiatric syndromes with many medical causes. DSM-IV lumps these as "[syndrome] due to [disease or toxin]," e.g., "mood disorder due to Huntington's disease" or "psychosis due to ketamine." The DSM-IV manual tries to help the physician remember differential diagnosis by grouping most of the "due to" diagnoses with the appropriate syndromal category; e.g., "mood disorder due to . . ." is listed in the same section of the DSM-IV as bipolar disorder. These differential diagnostic considerations do not mean that every patient needs dozens of diagnostic procedures. Rather, if the physician has a good knowledge of which nonpsychiatric conditions can cause which secondary psychiatric illness, then diagnosis can often be made by a prudent consideration of the clinical setting, the medical history, and findings on the psychiatric and neurologic examinations. When laboratory testing is indicated, a few well-chosen studies are often adequate. Diagnostic criteria can help by identifying presentations that differ substantially from the idiopathic syndrome (see the case of Ms C. at the end of this chapter).

Most physicians agree that criteria-based psychiatric diagnoses have clear advantages. However, many are uncomfortable with bringing research criteria into day-to-day practice. Two common concerns are addressed here.

1 *Do I have to look up (or memorize) the criteria?* Using accepted diagnostic criteria can improve patient care. But this presumes the criteria are used correctly. Unfortunately, this is far from universal. One common misconception is that a DSM-IV diagnosis is simply a new name for an old concept: a label to be applied to a patient not based on clear rules but rather on a gestalt impression of the patient's presentation. When this is done, the benefits of communicating accurately with other physicians, or of applying research from the literature to the patient, are lost. An example from another specialty may clarify this. Compare the two statements, "I think this patient's joint inflammation is probably due to rheumatoid arthritis" and "this patient meets revised ARA criteria for rheumatoid arthritis." Both statements have their place, but they are not at all identical. If clinicians commonly confused the two and diagnosed "ARA-criteria rheumatoid arthritis" based solely on pattern recognition or a vague clinical impression, the research diagnosis would lose much of its meaning.

Some clinicians feel that the use of written diagnostic criteria is too time-consuming. This is sometimes true. Occa-sionally the treatment plan does not hinge on the complete accuracy of a diagnosis. Just as with rheumatoid arthritis, given a typical clinical picture with good treatment response, one may not need to turn to research criteria for diagnosis. But often substantiating a diagnosis is critical, and the extra time it may take to gather additional history and consult the written criteria is well spent. Another reason for referring to the diagnostic criteria is that even when physicians believe they are following certain rules for diagnosis, often their clinical diagnosis is actually based on information outside those rules. Obviously one need not page through the entire DSM-IV manual for each patient. Common clinical sense can usually eliminate all but a few important "rule-outs." The decision trees in Appendix A of the DSM-IV-TR can also be very helpful.

2 *What about cases that don't seem to fit the criteria for anything?* Although research often limits a study to classic or typical cases of an illness, physicians in practice take care of a number of patients whose presentations are atypical. These atypical presentations are part of the excitement of clinical medicine, but can also present the physician with difficult diagnostic dilemmas. Commonly, an incomplete clinical database can give the impression that the patient's presentation is atypical, when in fact further inquiry reveals characteristic "missing" features. However, many cases remain atypical after thorough evaluation. Sometimes unusual presentations are a result of comorbid conditions. General medical illnesses, psychoactive substances, and mental retardation commonly alter the usual signs and symptoms of psychiatric illness. Furthermore, some conditions appear to change in presentation at different times during the course of illness, or at different ages. Specific strategies for dealing with comorbid illness and age effects are discussed in the relevant chapters later in this volume. Here are two general considerations.

The first is that definite diagnosis should be deferred for many patients. Although it is human nature for physicians to feel uncomfortable with uncertainty, it is usually in the patient's best interest to avoid premature insistence on a diagnosis when features are atypical or information is lacking. This avoids the automatic repetition of an unjustified diagnosis by those who review the medical record in the future. Since *some* diagnosis often must be recorded for various purposes, DSM-IV provides NOS ("not otherwise specified") categories, which may be used liberally in these situations. When one is more confident, the label "(provisional)" can be appended to a diagnosis, or the phrase "rule out" can be prefixed to it.

The second general consideration arises from the frequent need to do *something* in medical practice in the face of diagnostic uncertainty. For instance, acutely psychotic patients usually need some form of intervention before there is enough information to make a definite diagnosis. In this situation it is useful to recognize when one is expressing a hunch, and when one is giving a diagnosis based on standard criteria and supported by clear evidence. Recording both diagnoses in the medical record may support one's treatment decisions in the face of insufficient data. For instance, one may suspect that a patient has major depression, even though it may not be clear yet whether the symptoms persist for most of the day, are a consequence of alcohol use, or result from a general medical condition such as hypothyroidism. Still, it may be prudent to start psychotherapy, or prescribe an antidepressant, or hospitalize the patient before such information can be obtained. In this case one might think as follows: "From currently available history, I believe this patient probably has mild recurrent major depression. However, tests of thyroid function and further history from family members regarding his mood symptoms and alcohol use will be important in firming up the diagnosis. The DSM-IV diagnosis at present is depressive disorder, not otherwise specified."

An example of psychiatric diagnosis: the case of Ms C

Before closing, we describe a fictitious but fairly typical case that illustrates many of the points discussed in this chapter.

Ms C is a 30-year-old, previously healthy woman who presents to the emergency room complaining of shortness of breath and inability to walk properly. She is agitated and appears frightened. Physical exam is otherwise normal except for tachycardia and abnormal gait. She falls consistently into the examiner, but can walk normally after much reassurance. The symptoms resolve while diagnostic studies are under way. Chest X-ray and electrocardiogram are normal, and arterial blood gases reveal only acute respiratory alkalosis.

A similar episode occurs the following week. She is admitted to the hospital and undergoes pulmonary function testing and studies to rule out recurrent pulmonary embolism. An intern elicits a history of several stressful events on the day of the first emergency room visit and wonders whether the patient might have a psychiatric illness, but is told that psychiatric illness is a diagnosis of exclusion only. However, after further testing and consultation with specialists, no "organic disease" is found and Ms C is referred to a psychiatrist for hysteria.

At this juncture, although Ms C has had thousands of dollars worth of medical investigation, she still has occasional episodes of dyspnea and anxiety and has taken a leave of absence from work. The psychiatrist, Dr D, tries to substantiate the referring diagnosis. He knows that although the word "hysteria" tends to be a vague concept, criteria-based somatization disorder is a valuable diagnosis that can help avoid further costly or invasive laboratory testing. However, a systems review uncovers only a few medically unexplained symptoms. Other than the anxiety and difficulty walking, the patient's symptoms are largely limited to pulmonary and cardiovascular complaints. Her illness does not even approach DSM-IV criteria for somatization disorder. Dr D could make a case for a diagnosis of conversion disorder, given the temporary inability to walk, but knows that some patients diagnosed with conversion disorder turn out to have an underlying medical illness on follow-up. Thus, hysteria does not explain Ms C's presenting symptoms, and there is a concern that some serious or treatable illness may have been overlooked.

As several of the complaints were common symptoms of anxiety, Dr D probes deeper into possible anxiety diagnoses. Further questions reveal typical panic attacks in varied settings. The remainder of the mental status examination uncovers no surprises. Dr D makes a presumptive clinical diagnosis of panic disorder, initiates treatment and schedules a return visit in a few weeks.

After Ms C leaves the office, the psychiatrist looks up the DSM-IV criteria for panic disorder, since the exact defining symptoms are hard to remember, and finds that Ms C. does in fact meet criteria for panic disorder with agoraphobia.

However, Dr D still feels uncomfortable with a definite diagnosis because of the patient's trouble walking, an unusual symptom in panic disorder. Also, Dr D knows she still may have somatization disorder, since this diagnosis is often not detected on a single interview or by self-report alone. In his notes, he describes this concern and qualifies the DSM-IV diagnosis: "panic disorder with agoraphobia (provisional)."

With the patient's prior permission, he reviews her medical records and gathers diagnostic information from her family. These sources agree that she was quite healthy until recently and so does not meet criteria for somatization disorder. He briefly considers insulinoma, pheochromocytoma, and other less common causes for recurrent anxiety attacks, but there is sufficient clinical information from the patient and the hospital chart that no further laboratory testing is indicated.

After several weeks of pharmacologic treatment and appropriate psychotherapy, Ms C has only rare, limited panic attacks, her fear of public places is greatly improved, and she is able to resume work. Over the ensuing years, she returns about twice a year and remains essentially symptom-free on modest doses of an antidepressant.

Conclusion

This case demonstrates many important messages about

psychiatric diagnosis (see *Pearls & Perils*). Most importantly, the integration of psychiatric diagnosis into routine medical practice could have saved Ms C time, expense, invasive studies, and suffering. Accurate psychiatric diagnosis can provide gratifying results in daily clinical work. Considering that good psychiatric diagnosis is really nothing more than a careful application of well-informed medical thinking to psychological symptoms, we owe our patients nothing less.

PEARLS & PERILS

- Psychiatric diagnosis is based on clinical syndromes.
- Most psychiatric syndromes have a medical differential diagnosis.
- Psychiatric diagnosis is imperfect—just like diagnosis in any other medical specialty.
- Some psychiatric diagnoses are more useful than others.
- The physician should do the following:
  — consider psychiatric illnesses early in the differential diagnosis of medical patients;
  — gather longitudinal history from more than one source;
  — conduct a careful mental status examination, including appropriate items from the physical examination;
  — refer to the exact diagnostic criteria when accurate diagnosis is crucial;
  — exercise diagnostic humility in the form of NOS or provisional diagnoses.
- The physician should not do the following:
  — think of psychiatric illnesses only as diagnoses of exclusion;
  — lump all psychiatric patients together, denying them the benefits of careful diagnosis;
  — make a firm diagnosis based on symptoms alone;
  — make a firm diagnosis based on a cross-sectional presentation.

Annotated bibliography

Goodwin, DW and Guze, SB (1996) *Psychiatric Diagnosis*, 5th Edition, New York, Oxford.
A comprehensive review of the diagnostic validity of major psychiatric illnesses. The brief prefaces discuss the importance of psychiatric diagnosis.

Robins, E and Guze, SB (1970) Establishment of diagnostic validity in psychiatric illness: its application to schizophrenia, *Am J Psychiatry* 126:983–987.
Discusses the rationale for the validation method summarized in Box 2.1.

Robins, LN and Barrett, JE (eds) (1989) *The Validity of Psychiatric Diagnosis*, New York, Raven Press.
A multiauthored review of the evidence.

Sox, HC Jr, et al. (1988) *Medical Decision Making*, Boston, Butterworths.
This excellent text brings clarity and relevance to mathematical decision-making methods.

Widiger TA et al. (1994–1998) *DSM-IV Sourcebook, vols 1–4*, Washington, D.C., American Psychiatric Association.
This multivolume work documents the rationale for the nosologic changes in DSM-IV. It serves as a convenient compilation of the literature on DSM-III, -III-R, and -IV diagnoses. These volumes include reviews of the literature on all major diagnostic categories, reanalyses of pre-existing data sets to answer specific questions, and results of the DSM-IV field trials of new diagnostic criteria.

CHAPTER 3

Examination of Patients and Evaluation of Common Chief Complaints

Keith S. Garcia, MD, PhD and Richard W. Hudgens, MD

Introduction

Psychiatric illnesses are brain diseases that affect mood, thinking, and behavior. While often a degree of specialization is required to accurately diagnose and treat these illnesses, patients with psychiatric illnesses usually present first to primary care settings, and they make up a sizable minority of the patients treated in these settings. In addition, by finding comorbid psychiatric conditions in medically ill populations, physicians can have a profound impact on treatment outcome, as psychiatric illness can impair judgment, motivation, and the ability of patients to adhere to medical treatment. It is therefore important for primary care physicians to know how to identify and initiate treatment of psychiatric conditions and when to refer to a specialist. This chapter outlines a specific approach to diagnosing patients who are suffering from psychiatric illness.

Making a diagnosis

A physician's approach to the evaluation of patients with psychiatric illness should be no different from their approach to any other patient. The goal is to obtain information necessary to make an accurate diagnosis. This information may come from historical narrative provided by the patient or collateral sources, from physical exam, or from laboratory tests. The evaluation process begins with careful exploration of the patient's chief complaint. From this complaint a broad differential diagnosis is developed. In gathering information about this complaint and the symptoms associated with it, the physician narrows the differential diagnosis to arrive at a diagnosis that most parsimoniously explains the constellation of presenting symptoms.

The diagnostic process is not always straightforward. The focus of the chief complaint may not obviously suggest the underlying pathophysiological process nor dictate the entire focus of treatment. For example, a presenting complaint of foot pain in a patient with undiagnosed type II diabetes mellitus, and a resulting neuropathy, would warrant treatment for the diabetes as well as the pain. Unexplained somatic complaints may be part of a psychiatric syndrome. Likewise, symptoms of mood, thinking, and behavior may be caused by non-psychiatric illnesses. Thus the chief complaint serves as a point of departure in the development of a differential diagnosis, not as an endpoint. A complete differential for any presenting complaint should consider multiple pathological processes, including primary psychiatric illnesses.

When to suspect a psychiatric illness

Several circumstances may lead a physician to entertain the possibility that a patient is suffering from a psychiatric disorder. Patients may present to their physicians complaining of symptoms such as depression or anxiety. Patients may also present with concerns about somatic symptoms that are secondary to a psychiatric illness, such as insomnia associated with major depressive disorder, or shortness of breath associated with a panic attack. Still other patients may present with psychiatric illnesses that mimic medical illnesses such as somatization disorder or factitious disorder. Finally, physicians may elicit evidence that suggests a psychiatric illness during a review of systems in the course of a routine medical interview.

A physician should be alerted to the possibility of a psychiatric illness in the following circumstances:

1 Complaints about persistent emotional distress, such as depressed mood, fearfulness or excessive worrying, anger or irritability, suicidal or homicidal thinking, or behavior

that suggests such distress, are indications that a psychiatric disorder may be present. Do not be dismissive of these symptoms in the context of an obvious medical disorder. Such symptoms do not automatically accompany even the most serious medical illnesses and demand further investigation. Major depression in people who are very sick with a medical illness requires the same active treatment as major depression occurring by itself. On the other hand, it is important to explore possible non-psychiatric etiologies of psychiatric complaints. For example, anxiety may be the presenting chief complaint in patients with diseases of the cardiac, pulmonary, or endocrine systems. Remember to start with a broad view of possibilities, even if the chief complaint has a psychiatric "flavor."

2 Disturbances in perception, memory, cognition, concentration, or communication may occur in a number of psychiatric disorders including major depressive disorder, bipolar affective disorder, schizophrenia, and dementia. These may also be a feature of delirium, a psychiatric emergency in which underlying medical illness affects the brain and behavior (see Chapter 11).

3 Several psychiatric illnesses may be accompanied by physical symptoms that may be the patient's principal complaint. Fatigue, sleep disturbances, and changes in appetite with associated changes in weight may be symptoms associated with mood or anxiety disorders. Panic attacks can present with chest discomfort, feelings of breathlessness, dizziness, gastrointestinal distress, or tremor. Muscle tension and headaches are often features of generalized anxiety or depression. Complaints about libido or sexual performance may be a symptom of a mood disorder, or a manifestation of a urologic or endocrine disorder.

4 Some psychiatric syndromes, particularly the somatoform disorders and factitious disorder, mimic medical illnesses. Consider psychiatric illness in the differential diagnosis of any patient who has an extensive or vague medical history of illnesses or pain complaints for which there are no objective findings, especially when the presentation is overly dramatic or biologically implausible. Patients who have engaged in extensive "doctor shopping" and will not consent to a release of information should arouse suspicion. Avoid elaborate diagnostic procedures in these patients until you have collected enough data to rule out a psychiatric diagnosis.

5 Changes in behavior, even in the absence of complaints by the patient, often indicate that a psychiatric disorder is present. Irritability and temper outbursts occur in depression, delusional disorder, schizophrenia, and drug and alcohol dependence. This behavior may appear before any other symptoms. Lethargy, slovenliness, irresponsibility, or neglect of self-care may also be early symptoms of one of these disorders. In contrast, increased energy, excessive talkativeness, multiple projects hastily launched, lack of

self-restraint, and intense spiritual zeal in a person who was previously casual about religion may herald the onset of mania.

6 Special attention should be paid to seeking psychiatric disorders in patients suffering from medical illnesses. Comorbid psychiatric disorders frequently occur in endocrine illnesses such as diabetes or thyroid disease; coronary artery disease; any illness of the central nervous system including cerebrovascular disease, head trauma, Parkinson's disease, Huntington's disease, neoplasm, or seizure disorder; autoimmune illnesses such as systemic lupus, rheumatoid arthritis, or inflammatory bowel disease; and some cancers such as pancreatic carcinoma. Psychiatric illness in such patients should be treated, not written off as an inconsequential result of the medical disorder.

7 Finally, whenever a prominent aspect of the history is peculiar or does not make sense, the physician should be alert to the possibility that a psychiatric disorder is present, even if other symptoms of such a disorder are denied. In such cases further observation or information from reliable informants often reveal the patient is suffering from delusions, is abusing drugs or alcohol, or is consciously making up stories for some gain of his own. The physician should always follow up histories that seem conspicuously odd. Something may be going on that the patient does not want to disclose to the physician.

The initial interview

The interview is the most important tool that physicians have to diagnose psychiatric illness—there are few diagnostically revealing laboratory tests or physical examination findings. Psychiatric diagnoses are made by gathering information from the interview of the patient and informants and from direct observation of the patient's behavior during the interview. The physician should allow adequate time to explore symptoms relevant to the chief complaint, and, ideally, to screen for disorders that are not encompassed by the chief complaint and history of the presenting illness. Even in situations where one clearly identified problem dominates the clinical picture and requires urgent attention, a comprehensive history should be obtained as soon as possible. Important problems are often overlooked simply because physicians did not ask about them. The following information should be obtained during the interview:

Identifying information

The patient's age, gender, and race are important to note because, just as with non-psychiatric illnesses, major psychiatric disorders have different epidemiological risk factors. Most psychiatric illnesses have an age of onset prior to 30 years of age, for example. Females are more predisposed to certain mood and anxiety disorders. Males are more likely to complete suicide. The identifying information helps a physician to begin the diagnostic process even before he or she has met the patient.

Referral source and source of information

Knowing how the patient arrived at the treatment setting provides information regarding his or her motivation for treatment. Often patients initiate treatment at the request of others, in which case they may have poor insight into their illness, and are less likely to provide an accurate history. Additional information should be solicited from other sources such as family members, previous physicians, or hospital records in order to better understand the context of the presenting illness. The patient's permission should be obtained before contacting collateral informants unless the absence of information poses a threat to the safety of the patient or another person.

History of present illness

The history of present illness flows from the chief complaint. If the patient is articulate and capable, he or she should be allowed 5–10 minutes without interruption to give a spontaneous account of his/her illness. Unnecessary interruptions by the physician can derail the patient and result in the loss of important information. After the patient has completed his/her account of the present illness, the physician can ask questions to fill in missing information.

A complete history contains information regarding not only the pertinent symptoms, or absence of symptoms, that suggest a particular diagnosis but also previous diagnostic impressions by other physicians; information regarding treatments that have been offered in the past and their effectiveness; and the biological, psychological, or social factors that have complicated treatment or diagnosis such as treatment resistance, noncompliance to treatment, substance abuse or dependence, medical complications, homelessness, or poverty. The history specific to a psychiatric illness should also include presence or absence of mood symptoms (including manic symptoms), psychotic symptoms, previous suicide attempts, and hospitalizations. Finally, the physician should gather information regarding the type of treatment or disposition the patient or referral source expects.

Medical history

The physician should gather information about medical illnesses, surgeries, current medications, and drug allergies. As discussed above, he or she should pay special attention to conditions and medications that are known to be associated with psychiatric illness or symptoms.

Family history

The physician should inquire about a family history of diagnosed mental illness, "nervous breakdowns," psychiatric contact, substance use, criminal or other antisocial behavior, suicide or suicide attempts. Most psychiatric illnesses have a genetic risk associated with them—the offspring and siblings of people with mood disorders, psychotic disorders, anxiety disorders, and substance use disorders are more likely to develop these illnesses than the general population.

Knowing the patient's family psychiatric history allows the physician to better anticipate the patient's needs. (Consider an obstetrician who is attending the first pregnancy of a patient with a family history of postpartum psychosis.) Also, family treatment history can be used to guide the patient's treatment, as there may be a genetic component to treatment response.

Social history

The social history is the environmental and developmental context in which the illness presents. This context can modulate the presentation of the illness and have profound influence on the delivery of care. Social history should include information about where the patient was born, educational history including behavioral or learning difficulties, history of childhood psychiatric illness or delinquent behavior, the nature of early relationships with friends and family, history of physical or sexual abuse, stability of adult relationships including marriages and children, current intimate relationships, work history, current source of income, current residential status, whether or not the patient feels this environment is supportive, and history of substance use including alcohol, drugs, and tobacco.

Review of systems

The fact that some patients present with comorbid illnesses that have overlapping symptoms makes diagnosis difficult. It is critical that the diagnostic process includes a systematic exploration of each organ system including behavioral aspects of brain function. In addition to questions about constitutional, cardiovascular, pulmonary, gastrointestinal, urogenital, musculoskeletal, and neurological symptoms, every patient should be asked about mood, sleep, sexual function, cognition, and perception.

When interviewing patients with suspected or identified psychiatric complaints, there are additional areas for the physician to explore. He should ask about feelings of hopelessness, preoccupation with death, death wishes, and suicidal ideation. If such wishes are present he should ask about their rationale. Death wishes based on distortions of reality such as delusional guilt or driven by command auditory hallucinations are most ominous. Patients who are suicidal should be asked about their specific plans, the availability of a means to carry out these plans, and motivations that have prevented them from acting thus far. The physician should not avoid asking difficult questions for fear of putting ideas in the patient's head — suicide cannot be prevented unless the intent is disclosed, and the information gathered may govern the choice among types of treatment and treatment settings.

Obsessions and compulsions are often omitted from patients' spontaneous accounts of their histories for fear of sounding foolish or crazy. Obsessions are involuntary, intrusive, irrational thoughts that provoke anxiety, which are alleviated through the performance of repetitive behavioral or mental rituals (compulsions) such as counting, praying, washing, or checking. The presence of obsessions and compulsions warrants treatment that differs from that of other anxiety disorders.

Similarly, diagnoses of eating disorders are often missed because physicians fail to ask. Physicians should ask anxious or depressed young women in particular questions about body image or fear of gaining weight. They should enquire about unusual dietary habits such as binging on food or restricting intake. They should ask whether the patient engages in behaviors directed at losing weight such as vomiting, or the abuse of laxatives, enemas, or diuretics.

The physician should ask about delusions and hallucinations in any patient who is severely depressed, agitated, suspicious, hostile, or confused. A delusion is a fixed, false belief. Typical persecutory delusions that a patient may have include the perception that people are spying, following, or talking about him or her. Manic patients may feel that they have special powers or wealth, while depressed patients may have delusions that they are contaminated, unworthy, or guilty of unpardonable sin. Delusions that people are controlling a patient's thoughts or behavior are typically seen in schizophrenia. Primary care physicians may see patients who have hypochondriacal delusions that they have a serious illness despite no evidence of illness after medical evaluation and subsequent reassurance by the physician. Hallucinations, false perceptions in the absence of physical stimuli, may occur with any sensory modality but are usually auditory in primary psychiatric illnesses such as depression, mania, or schizophrenia. Auditory hallucinations can be of one or more voices commenting on the patient's behavior, arguing about the patient, calling the patient derogatory names, or directing the patient to act in a certain way. Vivid visual, tactile, olfactory, or gustatory hallucinations suggest a toxic or organic etiology. The presence of hallucinations or delusions should prompt referral to a psychiatrist.

When hallucinations or delusions are suspected, the subject should be approached with tact but not avoided. The physician may begin by asking questions that are neutral and proceed to asking about more bizarre content. For example he could first ask the general questions, 'Is there anything upsetting, strange, or scary going on in your life?' or 'Is there something making you feel unsafe?' and if this is confirmed follow by asking open-ended questions about what that may be. Facilitating or normalizing questions can be used to obtain information about bizarre content that the patient may not want to disclose, for example, 'Sometimes when people get very depressed they can hear people talking when no one is around. Has that happened to you?' When asking about psychosis it pays to be empathetic, nonjudgmental, and persistent. Often the physician can improve the yield of information by asking the question in more than one way.

The mental status exam

Mental status is not assessed by tacking on a set of questions about the date, current events, calculations, and proverbs at the end of a diagnostic interview. The mental status exam begins the moment a physician meets the patient. It is an assessment of the way the patient interacts with the physician and the environment. The first observation that is made is of the patient's general appearance and behavior. The physician notes the patient's grooming or level of self-care. People with depression or schizophrenia may be disheveled or dirty. People with mania may be wearing excessive jewelry or makeup haphazardly applied. The patient's motor activity is assessed, as well as body language such as posture and eye contact. Changes in psychomotor activity (either speeded up or slowed down) are associated with many psychiatric illnesses. Evidence of movement disorders can suggest to the physician that the patient has been treated with antipsychotic medication.

The patient's speech is noted. Abnormalities in rate, amount, or volume may be evidence of a mood disorder. Odd word choices or word-finding difficulties may be suggestive of dementia or schizophrenia. Flow of thought is a reflection of the patient's ability to abstract and manipulate information. Patients with schizophrenia or mania may have difficulty providing a sequential and logical history and may stray off topic. Patients with dementia may be excessively concrete. Deviant or pathological thought content is noted including hallucinations, delusions, obsessions, compulsions, suicidal or homicidal ideation. The physician notes the mood that is reported by the patient and his manifest emotional state, or affect. Parameters of affect may include the average affect, the range, and how well it matches the patient's stated mood. Insight and judgment are often assessed from their perception of the severity and impact of their illness. The status of the patient's sensorium and intellect can be inferred from the patient's behavior during the interview. If the patient's sensorium or intellect appears impaired, formal questioning to assess orientation, memory, concentration, calculation, and language should be undertaken.

Rapport

Behavior by physicians that promotes good rapport, mutual trust, and respect is not only the kindest way of dealing with patients, it is also the most medically effective way. In such circumstances patients are more comfortable, more likely to tell physicians what they need to know, and more likely to be compliant with treatment. Rapport is best established not by small talk about irrelevant pleasantries but rather by listening to the patient talk about things that are troubling them and taking their complaints seriously. The patient has come to see the doctor because of a problem; nothing is more reassuring at the outset than the knowledge that it is this problem and nothing else in which the doctor is most interested. If the physician approaches patients with a genuine desire to understand their problem and to help them with it, rapport will be established as a natural result.

Follow-up appointments

If a primary care physician is treating a patient for a psychiatric disorder, it is important to schedule sufficient time for each follow-up appointment. Follow-up evaluations should include an assessment of the interval history that includes current symptoms, important life events, current mental status, and the therapeutic and toxic effects of the medications. Even if the patient is receiving psychotherapy from another provider, this can rarely be accomplished in less than 15–30 minutes. If a physician's busy schedule does not allow time for such an assessment, he or she should refer the patient to a psychiatrist.

On asking questions

The psychiatric interview should not be conducted like a checklist interrogation. Patients are often unwilling or unable to disclose information regarding their symptoms for various reasons. They may be embarrassed, afraid, too disorganized, suspicious, or distracted by hallucinations. They may simply understand the symptoms in a context that differs from how the question was phrased. For example, a patient with schizophrenia may answer "no" to the question "Do you ever feel as though people are trying to harm you?" because he is quite sure they are trying to harm him—it's not just a feeling. Thus the psychiatric interviewer must be attuned to the patient and flexible in the way that he phrases questions so as to improve the information yield.

Different types of questions can be used to obtain information. Open-ended questions such as "What brings you here?" promote narrative answers and provide the most valid information. Open-ended questions should be phrased carefully so that they are nonjudgmental and pose no challenge to the patient's belief system. Open-ended questions allow the patient to talk about the part of the problem they think is important. Patients, however, may omit pertinent facts that are clinically relevant.

Directed questions such as "Has your sleep changed?" can be used to fill in the history or to verify the physician's interpretation of open-ended answers. They should be followed with open-ended questions such as "How has it changed?" to get more detailed clinical information. Because directed questions may draw the patient's focus away from the problem that is really bothering them, they should be reserved for the latter part of the interview.

Finally, a questioning style that compares the patient's experience to the common experiences of others can be used to elicit endorsements of symptoms that the patient may be reluctant to mention. For example, the physician may say, "Sometimes when people get depressed they feel like they would be better off dead. Have you ever felt like that?" The caveat to this approach is that it may lead to over-endorsement of symptoms, and thus it is important to follow up with open-ended questions to verify the information.

> **PEARLS & PERILS**
> - Psychiatric illnesses are brain diseases.
> - By finding comorbid psychiatric conditions in medically ill populations, physicians can have a profound impact on treatment outcome.
> - Diagnosing psychiatric illnesses requires a high degree of suspicion.
> - During an initial patient evaluation, questions about psychiatric symptoms should be included as a part of the general review of systems.
> - Psychiatric illness in patients with medical illnesses should be treated, not written off as an inconsequential result of the medical disorder.

Conclusion

Psychiatric symptoms and illnesses are common in patients treated by primary care physicians and are associated with substantial functional disabilities. Such illnesses also may worsen impairments from other medical disorders. By incorporating the evaluative techniques reviewed in this chapter, the primary care physician can have a major impact on a psychiatrically ill patient's quality of life.

Annotated bibliography

American Psychiatric Association (1994) *The American Psychiatric Glossary*, 7th Edition, Washington D.C.
This is an alphabetical listing, with definitions of almost all the technical terms in current use in psychiatry.

CHAPTER 4

Psychological Testing

Gitry Heydebrand, PhD and Richard D. Wetzel, PhD

Introduction

The role of the psychologist in a medical setting is not merely to administer and interpret tests but to use them as part of a comprehensive assessment, which may also include systematic interviews of patients and informants. Communication between psychologist and referring physician following the assessment is the key to the psychologist's helpfulness to the patient.

Psychological testing in any branch of medicine is best understood when a psychological test is considered to be an expanded, detailed version of part of the patient's general examination. Depending on the type of test, the results can amplify the clinical history, the mental status examination, or the neurological examination. Table 4.1 provides examples of this process.

Memory assessment is a convenient example of the difference between the process a physician ordinarily uses during a clinical exam and the process a psychologist uses when doing formal testing. A physician typically tests memory by telling the patient the names of three or four objects and asking the patient to repeat them. After an interval of 3–5 minutes, the physician asks the patient to repeat the names of the items again. A failure to perform the task is very informative clinically. The psychologist may utilize a test like the Logical Memory Scale from the Wechsler Memory Scale-III. The stories in the Logical Memory Scale each contain 25 pieces of information. This allows the psychologist to obtain a wide distribution of scores on the scale. The advantage is that the psychologist can describe a range of verbal memory capacity from superb to markedly impaired. Which type of evaluation is most useful cannot be decided until the clinical issue has been defined.

Data from formal psychological tests are gathered in greater detail, with more attention to procedure and comparison to explicit norms (standards). Having developed a spread or range of scores, the psychological tester uses normative data, that is, statements about the distribution of scores (mean, standard deviation, skew, and kurtosis—see Table 4.2) in specific groups. Physicians tend to rely on implicit norms (for example, normal people should be able to do this, and slow patients should be able to do that). The increased precision in measurement obtained from psychological tests is sometimes valuable, depending on the clinical decision to be made.

Once the physician has decided to obtain the more precise measurement available with formal psychological testing, he or she must decide whether or not to be satisfied with the additional information provided by the test alone or to obtain consultation with a psychologist.

If the physician knows what information is desired from testing and has enough experience with a test to know its clinical strengths and weaknesses, there may be no need to involve a psychologist (see *Consider consultation when . . .*). Test makers and vendors recognize this and classify tests in terms of the training and experience required to purchase and use them (see Box 4.1). Many tests are immediately available to physicians; more may be obtained if training requirements (e.g., workshops) are met.

Test authors and publishers increasingly offer computerized assessment tools with printed reports based on scoring sheets. Comments about the patient are offered on the basis of the relative frequency of characteristics in a previously studied population or group. While reports of this type generally are very helpful, they can be misleading in some cases. These reports become problematic when there is not an integrated evaluation that has accounted for all pertinent factors in a patient's case, which can be of particular importance in forensic cases.

TABLE 4.1

Examples of the role of tests in medicine

Purpose	Test	Measure
Clinical history	Beck Depression Inventory	Symptoms of depression
	Minnesota Multiphasic Personality Inventory—2	Symptoms of anxiety, depression, psychosis, suicidal ideation, etc.
Mental status examination	WAIS-III Information subscale	Fund of information
Physical examination	Finger tapping test	Motor speed
	Hand dynamometer	Strength of grip

CONSIDER CONSULTATION WHEN...

- The physician is unable to make decisions about diagnosis and treatment from the clinical interview and the physical examination.
- Advice is needed about which tests to administer.
- The test results alone do not provide an adequate answer.

BOX 4.1

How to find out about a test

1 Consult the manual for the test. The makers of psychological tests are required by ethical standards for test construction to publish the relevant information about the reliability and validating studies done on the test.

2 Consult the Buros Institute's *Mental Measurements Yearbook*. This reference book is published every few years. It contains critical reviews (usually by more than one expert) of 300–400 tests. These are short, technical, and point out the flaws in a test in detail. This is a fast way to obtain information. *The Fifteenth Mental Measurements Yearbook* was published in 2003. The Buros Institute also has an online source for individual test reviews.

3 Call the author of the test, especially if it is an obscure test. Authors are usually glad when someone has heard of their tests and will discuss them willingly. They usually provide selected reprints. The addresses and phone numbers of the authors can be obtained from the *Directory of the American Psychological Association*. The directory is available in many university libraries. Many psychologists also have one.

4 Almost all research on psychological tests can be found by consulting *PsychINFO* (computerized) or *Psychological Abstracts* (book), either online with a computer or in university libraries. This is the hard but thorough way.

Psychological consultation

While it is not difficult to understand the results from a single test if one is sufficiently motivated and spends enough time examining the findings, integrating and synthesizing a number of test scores with interview data and behavioral observations is much more complex. A consultation with a clinical psychologist or neuropsychologist can provide detailed information on the patient's clinical history, mental status, cognitive functioning, and aspects of behavior as they relate to diagnosis and treatment planning.

A psychological consultant can answer many questions in the psychological report, including:

1 Psychosocial factors that may be interfering with functioning. Examples include stressors at home or at work that the patient may not report during a medical intake but that may be elicited during a clinical interview with a psychologist.

2 Psychological factors that may be contributing to physical illness. Depression, anxiety, and certain types of personality traits may compound the physical problems that a patient encounters. In some cases, somatization may be a primary feature of the clinical picture. One of the major contributions offered by a psychological assessment may be an increased understanding of the patient's attitudes and beliefs regarding his illness.

3 Differential diagnosis of psychiatric disorders. Patients may report many different mood and behavioral symptoms that may require detailed, comprehensive assessment. Patients and/or their families often regard psychological testing as more objective and more convincing than the opinions of either psychologists or psychiatrists without such support. This is also true of judges and juries.

4 Confirmation of clinical impressions. The physician may often have a sense or hunch regarding particular problems, dysfunctions, or issues that are pertinent to diagnosis and treatment. The psychological assessment can confirm this hypothesis in some cases while in others it may support the conclusion that the patient's symptoms do in fact present a diagnostic problem. Sometimes, the

TABLE 4.2

Key terms in tests and measurements

Reliability	A measure (from 0.00 to 1.00) of how often the same answer is achieved under the same conditions of measurement. (When one uses a yardstick to measure a table, one expects to get the same answer time and again.) Giving the same test twice is the usual way to measure reliability. Some variables, such as depression, are expected to change over time. Statistical methods exist to estimate reliability in a variety of ways. Reliability is never a function of a test by itself; it is a function of a test being given under certain conditions to a certain population. A high reliability in the general population does not necessarily imply a high reliability in a special population; this is always an empirical question. The reliability of a test sets the upper limit of the validity of a test.
Validity	The degree to which a test measures what the tester wants it to measure with reasonable accuracy. A depression scale should measure depression and not anxiety or neuroticism. The validity of a test can be developed by using differing criterion groups and future outcomes or by the predictability from scientific theory of scores obtained on the test.
Distribution	If a useful test is given to a number of people, they will not all have the same score. The tester can sort or order these scores and describe the way they spread out. The distribution of scores can be described in terms of their mean, standard deviation, skew, and kurtosis.
Mean	The mathematical mean of the scores, which is found by adding all the scores and dividing the total by the number of scores.
Standard deviation	A measure of how far the scores fall from the average. The differences between each score and the average are squared (the unsquared differences always add up to zero) and then added. The sum is divided by the number of scores and then changed back to the original units of measure by taking the square root.
Skew	A measure of whether one tail of the distribution is longer than the other.
Kurtosis	A measure of whether the distribution is too narrow or too wide. In other words, did the tester squeeze the distribution in or sit on it and flatten it out?
Normal curve, bell curve	A statistical or mathematical abstraction describing a theoretical distribution of scores. This is the result one would expect if scores have an infinite number of causes, all of which have a small effect. Scores on psychological tests never fit a normal curve perfectly. With a large enough number of scores, a statistically significant deviation from normality can always be found.
Standard score, T-score	Standardized or transformed score. Remembering the mean and standard deviations of a number of different scales is difficult and bothersome. Test makers try to help by converting raw scale scores to a more easily remembered set of numbers. This is done by subtracting the mean score on the scale from the obtained score. The difference is then divided by the standard deviation. The original score has now been converted to a *Z-score*, with a mean of zero and a standard deviation of one. The Z-score is then multiplied by a constant. Then another constant is added. The Wechsler Intelligence Quotient [IQ] score is a standard score, or a T-score, with a mean of 100 and a standard deviation of 15.
Norms	The distribution (mean, standard deviation, skew, and kurtosis) of scores on a test in a specified population (for example, white males, college graduates, or patients with low back pain and no demonstrable pathology).
Standard error of measurement	Just as there is a distribution or range of scores within a large group of people taking a test, there is also a distribution or range of scores when a person (or a group) takes a test over and over again. The standard deviation in this situation is called the standard error of measurement. This is ordinarily much smaller than the standard deviation. The size of this statistic is a function of the number of times the test is taken or the number of people taking the test.
Difference scores	People like to compare a score on one test to that on another, for example, a person might like to say that he is better at math than spelling. This poses some problems, since the tester would like to be sure a difference between two scores is meaningful. In classic testing theory, a score on the first test is thought of as having two parts — a true measure of one trait and an error component. The score on the other test is a true measure of the second trait and its error component. When the two scores are compared, the result is the true difference between the first trait and the second trait plus two error terms. Difference scores are inherently less reliable (more influenced by error) than the scores from which they are derived.
State	A short-term condition, such as depression; a quickly changing trait.
Trait	A long-term condition or a slowly changing state. The distinction between state and trait is essentially arbitrary.

assessment also provides the documentation to justify the treatment approach.

5 Neuropsychological dysfunction. In addition to assessment of cognitive function following neurological disease or injury (e.g., stroke or head injury), issues such as attention deficit disorder, learning disorder, and dementia may be addressed by a neuropsychological assessment.

6 Possible symptom exaggeration or malingering. A psychologist with training and experience in assessment of primary or secondary gain can assist with identifying this type of problem.

The psychological report

The psychological report provides information about the patient that has been gathered according to specific methods, presented in an integrated format that draws conclusions about the patient's functioning based on data/evidence from many different sources. These include:

- The clinical interview. The psychologist may rely on a structured interview, schedule or format, or use personal guidelines to obtain information on the patient's childhood (including psychosocial factors), education, employment history, relationships, and other background information, all of which can have an impact on current functioning.

- Review of records. When feasible, the psychologist relies on patient records to investigate factors that may contribute to symptomatology and performance, such as medical history and current medications. Review of records is particularly important when malingering or somatization disorder are possible explanations for the patient's complaints.

- Measures. Psychological measures (described further below) are standardized and normed assessment instruments that determine a variety of aspects of functioning. The psychologist's expertise in determining which instruments are appropriate to answer the referral question is one of the strongest advantages to requesting a psychological consult.

- Behavioral observations. The psychologist may offer comments on appearance, physical responses, interaction style, and mental status that support the conclusions presented in the report.

Types of assessments

There are literally thousands of different psychological and neuropsychological tests and measures. The particular skills psychologists bring to testing are experience and knowledge about the administration of the tests according to standardized procedures, the appropriate context in which to use a test, and the interpretation of the scores in the context of other information. Psychologists also have

expertise in conveying the findings in a relevant and useful manner.

Psychological tests or measures are designed to address specific questions. Measures are standardized, which means they are administered in a specific format following a specific, delineated protocol. The purpose is to reduce testing bias and error. Even minor deviation from established procedure significantly diminishes the utility of test findings.

One of the greatest advantages of psychological testing is that the data provide an objective comparison between the patient's performance and that of other individuals of similar background (usually, age, educational history, etc.). The issue of what is "abnormal" has been controversial to some extent. Psychologists have become more aware of the need to be sensitive to socioeconomic, psychosocial, and other host factors that can have an effect on response. However, norms are very useful in determining an expected range of performance for the individual; e.g., the 62-year-old woman who worries that her memory is deteriorating can be reassured that her performance on memory tests is the same as those of other people in their sixties with no known psychiatric or neurologic problems.

The form and structure of a psychological report is likely to vary according to individual clinical style, the referral question, and the psychologist's experience with the referring physician. Generally, a report might be expected to include the following information:

- A statement of the purpose of the evaluation and what focus the conclusions and recommendations will have.

- A fairly comprehensive and detailed presentation of the patient's history, in order to identify or rule out factors that might contribute to current functioning and to track apparent discrepancies (e.g., noting that a patient's current job is not commensurate with his level of education). Failure to understand the history undermines the opinions of psychologists just as much as it affects those of physicians.

- Behavioral observations that describe speech, movement, affect, and other clinical states that support or contradict the issue at hand (the referral question).

The presentation of test results differs according to the clinician's training and orientation but is likely to report on performance and patterns of functioning according to the psychometric tests used in the assessment. Many psychologists include a statement about whether test results can be considered reliable and valid, based on several factors noted during the assessment administration. Ordinarily, a psychologist will integrate the findings and relate them to the question posed by the physician. The report may give a diagnosis and/or provide interpretations or suppositions about the patient's functional capacity. Many psychologists tend to use language such as "appears to be," "seems," "points towards," and "suggests" in their psychological reports. This merely reflects a difference in the training of psychologists and physicians.

If asked, the psychologist will provide recommendations in the report. Depending on the referral question, a diagnosis may be given and suggestions provided for placement (e.g., independent vs. supported living), referrals for additional evaluation (e.g., EEG, psychiatric intervention), possible topics to be addressed in psychotherapy, adaptive techniques, possible compensatory approaches for deficits or problems, and prognosis.

- The opinions offered by a psychological consultant need to be evaluated in terms of the clinical history of the patient.
- The diagnosis of mental retardation cannot and should not be made solely from an IQ score. Social functioning is as important or more important than IQ scores.
- Screening for brain dysfunction with only one test—usually a drawing test like the Bender-Gestalt Test or Benton—is not competent psychological or medical practice.
- The most important decision a neuropsychologist makes when looking for cognitive deficits is the estimate of how well the patient should be able to do on a test. The validity of all other conclusions depends on this conclusion.

Common questions

How intelligent is my patient?

Patients have to cope with the world, their diseases, and the medical regimen prescribed by physicians. Intelligence helps. The concept of intelligence is somewhat controversial, particularly when the issue becomes politicized. Most people have a sense of what they mean when they speak of intelligence, but they may have more difficulty defining and (particularly) operationalizing it.

Wechsler, who developed a widely used IQ test, defined intelligence as "the aggregate or global capacity of the individual to act purposefully, think rationally, and deal effectively with the environment" (Matarazzo, 1972). Spearman proposed a "g" factor of intelligence as a way to explain why some people seemed to have the ability to do well across a range of functions. Clinical neuropsychologists find it helpful to think of intelligence as consisting of fluid intelligence (basic reasoning ability that is dependent on current neurological functioning) and crystallized intelligence (acquisition of skills and information relevant to the person's culture and background). Others have added additional components or factors, such as emotional or social intelligence. The exact position of common sense in these theories is unclear.

Measurement of IQ was first developed in part to predict which children would require special help in middle-class grade schools. IQ tests are considered most accurate at the cut-off point between mental retardation and borderline intelligence. IQ tests were not intended to discriminate well at the higher ranges in adults, which is why they are not used to select students for law school or medical school. Current IQ tests are culture bound and are designed to measure both fluid and crystallized intelligence; IQ tests that are not as culture-laden do not predict school success as well. Doing well academically is a function of both the biological potential for intelligence and the acquisition of culturally (and subculturally) valued skills and knowledge. For example, it has been well documented that, as a group, pupils from lower socioeconomic status (SES) groups tend to have lower IQ scores than those from higher SES levels, though there is considerable individual difference. Kline (1991) noted:

> The bright and well-adjusted child who attends a good school and receives encouragement at home will invest most of her fluid ability in the crystallized skills of the culture. On the other hand, the equally bright child in a home where education is not valued and who attends a school of indifferent quality will not thus invest his fluid ability.

To say that the apparent difference in IQ scores between groups differing in race, nationality, or SES is primarily the result of the biological determinants of intelligence is quite unsophisticated and naive. It can be hurtful and damaging. Less culturally laden IQ tests have been developed, but they do not work as well. This explains the continued use of scientifically problematic (factorially impure) tests.

What does an IQ score tell me?

An IQ score gives one a general sense of functional capacity, but the test taps a relatively limited range of abilities or skills. People with a "normal" IQ may have difficulty functioning due to personality factors. Alternatively, a patient may have a normal IQ with focal deficits in specific areas (e.g., memory); in such cases, an IQ score does not give a full picture of their capacity. In contrast, a person with a "below-average" IQ score might still have good decision-making abilities even though they don't "test" well.

If the physician is meeting a patient for the first time and determines that the patient has been having difficulties at school, at work or in day-to-day functioning over a long period of time (i.e., it is not a sudden change), then below-average intelligence may be a contributing factor. IQ scores can predict educational and occupational success with fair accuracy (about 10–25% of the variance is explained), as well as social functioning. At times, the estimate by both physicians and psychologists of a patient's IQ is poor. Clinicians are generally not aware of how much and how easily they adapt to the vocabulary and cognitive level of their patients. Clinicians also adapt their subjective norms to their patient population rather than the general population as an average or reference point. If determining the patient's IQ is clinically relevant and important for treatment, placement, or competency issues, then a referral for an IQ assessment is indicated.

Is my patient mentally retarded?

The criteria for the diagnosis of mental retardation have changed over the years. The diagnosis is based on how much the patient knows, how well he or she can function, and the age at which the problem started. Adaptive functioning has always been considered to be more important than IQ score alone, and in recent years there has been even more emphasis on functioning. At the present time, the diagnosis is based on verification of difficulty functioning in two or more of the following areas: communication, self-care, home living, social/interpersonal skills, use of community resources, self-direction, functional academic skills, work, leisure, health and safety. A person who can care for herself in an age-appropriate way is not mentally retarded, whatever the IQ score.

There are adaptive behavior scales widely used in the field. Some assess only the skills needed for activities of daily living, while others also assess maladaptive behaviors that interfere with living in the community.

IQ scores should not be used in a mechanical or arbitrary way; of course, this is true of any other score, value, or finding a physician uses. When the presence or absence of mental retardation is a question, both IQ and social adaptive behavior should be carefully evaluated. Keyes *et al.* (1998) stated, "A low IQ score without deficits in adaptive functioning is not defined as mental retardation. Conversely, poor adaptive skills in the presence of average intelligence is not mental retardation, either."

Since the Supreme Court decision that the mentally retarded may not be executed (Atkins v. Virginia 06/20/2002), there has been an apparent effort to expand the definition of mental retardation from about 2.3% (IQ < 70) of the population to 5.0% (IQ < 75). Criminals are much more likely to have a history of poor social or maladaptive behavior than others. They are also less likely to have been deeply invested in school, reducing their IQ scores. As a result, 15–20% of the criminal population could meet these relaxed criteria.

The causes of mental retardation are multiple and can include prenatal, perinatal, and postnatal events. For most causes, psychological testing will not be informative. There are some particular patterns of deficits that are more common with some types of mental retardation (Pulsifer, 1996). However, none of them constitutes a signature or is definitive in identifying a biological cause.

Does my patient have a learning disability?

The practice parameters of the American Academy of Child and Adolescent Psychiatry (1998) state, "When the clinician suspects or determines that the child has a language or learning disability, referral for psychoeducational and speech testing is essential, particularly if prior school assessments are incomplete or inconclusive. At a minimum, current or recent testing (within the last year) should include individual tests of IQ, academic achievement, and speech and language functioning." They note that the central clinical feature of a learning disorder is a lack of normal development of a particular cognitive skill. Learning disabilities range in severity from subtle to marked. Some are easily observable on clinical assessment, while others are diagnosable only through standardized testing.

A learning disability can be diagnosed by comparing achievement in particular areas such as reading, arithmetic, spelling, or writing to the IQ score (one standard deviation below the IQ score is the threshold in most states) or by a significantly lower level of achievement than expected for the student's age (two to three years behind). It has been correctly noted that a discrepancy large enough to cause clinical problems may not be large enough to meet the thresholds qualifying for special help.

The IQ score is derived from typical individual tests of intelligence. Achievement scores are derived from academic tests like the Woodcock-Johnson, the Wechsler Achievement Test, the Peabody Individual Achievement Test, and the Kaufman Test of Educational Achievement. Additional testing may be done with a wide range of neuropsychological tests to identify specific deficits.

The discrepancy approach to diagnosis has been criticized by some authors because it does not identify a group of students with a homogenous problem. These authors propose that the emphasis should be placed on phonological (single word) processing skills, the most common problem associated with learning disabilities. The discrepancy approach also has been criticized because the diagnosis is more difficult to establish in slower children and because it takes a significant amount of time to develop, requiring several years of poor performance (Mathias and Denton, 2002) before diagnosis.

Doing poorly in school can impair students' self-esteem. Many children will also have problems with attention deficit disorder, with or without hyperactivity. Psychological evaluations of this disorder should be considered by the clinician when a learning disability is suspected.

Does my patient have attention deficit/hyperactivity disorder?

Attention deficit/hyperactivity disorder (ADHD) consists of symptoms in three categories: inattention, hyperactivity, and impulsivity. Symptoms in one category may dominate the clinical presentation, or the patient may show a mixed picture. The key problem in all cases of attention deficit disorder is that the patient is less able to control attention and avoid distraction than other people at the same developmental stage and ability level. The disorder is usually diagnosed clinically through inquiry about key symptoms, using information provided by patients, family, and sometimes teachers. Formal psychological testing, while often helpful, is not essential for making the diagnosis.

Multiple tests are available to measure attention and to assess the symptoms of ADHD. This disorder has been approached psychometrically through tests assessing neglect in part of the visuospatial field, tests requiring continuous attention, and tests requiring selective attention. Other approaches involve parent questionnaires, teacher questionnaires, clinician checklists, self-report measures, and other similar evaluations. Research has shown relatively poor agreement among different approaches to problems with attention and concentration.

It is generally accepted that the key to appropriate diagnosis of problems with attention and concentration is a multimodal approach, with multiple sources of information. Any single measure of attention is easily affected by transitory causes. The physician's goal should be to establish that the patient's problems with attention exist relatively often in multiple settings under multiple conditions. If psychological assessment is used, it should be comprehensive and performed by an experienced practitioner with an interest in this area.

As awareness of attention deficits and other neurologically based problems has increased, more people have begun to question whether they have undiagnosed ADHD. Often, when a child is diagnosed, adult family members perceive similarities to their own childhood experiences and begin to wonder whether they have ADHD, too. An Internet website may seem to explain all the problems they have been having at home and at work. The site may indicate they should be taking medication. However, a more thorough clinical evaluation is warranted before initiating treatment. There are many different types of tests and assessment protocols useful for supporting a diagnosis of ADHD. In a clinical assessment, the psychologist may typically inquire about the history of childhood symptoms of ADHD and other childhood psychological and psychiatric disorders. It is common to administer psychometric measures in order to assess visuospatial functioning, continuous attention, and selective attention skills. Deficits in these areas can impact overall processing, memory, and reasoning, as there is insufficient intake of information to use other cognitive processes effectively.

There is also evidence suggesting that many individuals with ADHD, perhaps even half of those diagnosed, may have mild learning disabilities, which may be useful to identify. The physician can determine whether a referral for ADHD would be useful if the patient presents with chronic problems (rather than a sudden change) that manifest in multiple settings. Sometimes, a patient may have developed compensatory techniques without realizing it, but a change

in job or other circumstances may cause a "system overload." The ADHD assessment should provide not only diagnosis but also recommendations for adaptive approaches.

What kind of psychiatric disorder does my patient have?

There are many objective tests used to assess anxiety, depression, obsessive-compulsive disorder (OCD), phobias, panic disorder, and somatization disorder. Some widely used psychological tests still lump these disorders together under the old term "neurosis," while others split them into separate entities. Many of the standard personality tests used to find neurosis also serve to identify personality features, traits, or disorders that may be relevant to managing a patient's problem.

The most widely used clinical tests in psychology are objectively scored tests to describe the presence or absence of Axis I psychiatric disorders. These include the Minnesota Multiphasic Personality Inventory (MMPI), the MMPI-2, the Millon Clinical Multiaxial Inventory-III (MCMI-III), the Neuroticism, Extroversion, and Openness Personality Inventory (NEO), the Personality Assessment Inventory, and the like. Each of these tests has its adherents. These tests typically have validity scales, which assess the patient's approach to the test and take such factors as exaggeration, malingering, or defensiveness into account. There is also usually another measure of the care with which the patient is reading the items. If the test shows that

1 the patient has read the items carefully,

2 and has answered them with some consistency,

3 and is trying to tell the truth as the patient knows it,

then the rest of the findings on the tests are likely to be useful.

Most of these tests relate to the symptoms and complaints associated with different psychiatric disorders. The list of disorders assessed ordinarily is between 10 and 20. We are not aware of any tests that attempt to measure all 300+ diagnoses in DSM-IV.

These tests are usually used as part of a more general psychological or psychiatric assessment. They make a statement about a particular patient on the basis of the most frequent correlates of the scores that the test computes. Frequently, these are accurate and helpful. Usually most, but not all, of the correlates are correct. On occasion, however, the most common correlate in the group producing a specific profile is not the best for some of the individuals in the group. The second or third most common correlate may fit better.

Psychologists are well aware that the name of a scale does not necessarily indicate that the scale measures what its name implies. For example, the schizophrenia scale on the MMPI-2 is virtually uncorrelated with *current* concepts of schizophrenia (Ben Porath *et al.*, 1991). Psychologists use the same procedures as other scientists to test how well their instruments measure what they purport to measure.

Multiple tests have been developed to measure the severity of a single syndrome—anxiety, depression, etc. Their virtue is that they are quick and require little time from the clinician. These tests are extremely useful in tracking response to treatment after the diagnosis has been established. Their flaw is their lack of discriminative ability, i.e., high anxiety or deep depression will lead to high scores on both anxiety and depression scales. They also are transparent and easily faked. They are very useful in the right hands for the right purpose, but they are not diagnostic.

Psychological testing can be particularly helpful in identifying somatoform disorders. Patients with these disorders typically overreport symptoms in many different organ systems and do so with a dramatic and histrionic flair. These patients are willing to consume as much time as the physician will allow to present their elaborate and debilitating complaints. Personality tests give them the opportunity to do this without consuming too much physician or staff time. These test results are easily interpreted by experienced psychologists.

There are scales that predict vulnerability to alcohol or substance abuse with a fair degree of validity. Others assess the admission of substance abuse. There are many specialized tests that assess substance abuse in its different forms. All are easily administered, short, require little staff time, and identify people with these problems with some degree of accuracy. The substance abuser who wishes to escape detection can usually do so on these short tests, however.

Does my patient have psychotic symptoms?

The noun "psychosis," which once broadly included several psychiatric disorders, is dropping from use as a diagnostic term in modern nomenclature. The compound phrase "psychotic features" is now used to designate the presence of delusions, hallucinations, thought disorder, and bizarre behavior in whatever psychiatric illness they occur.

While the presence of psychotic symptoms is fairly obvious in the majority of cases, there are times when the presentation is less clear, particularly in cases of paranoia, new-onset psychotic disorders, or psychiatric illnesses with contributing organic etiologies (e.g., substance use or metabolic encephalopathy). Clinicians may use the MMPI-2 and/or Rorschach, which have been shown to be useful in distinguishing between depressed patients who are psychotic and those who are not. Patients who are very upset or who wish to appear to be very upset often have very high scores on psychological tests that would suggest psychosis, even though it is not present. False positives for psychosis often occur in patients with somatization disorder, borderline personality disorder, and dissociative identity disorder. Such scores also can occur in patients with factitious disorder or malingering.

Some psychologists use projective techniques as part of their battery to diagnose schizophrenia or other psychotic illnesses. Projective techniques are tests that do not elicit structured, objectively scored answers. The Exeter system for coding the Rorschach ink blot test responses has proven to be fairly reliable, more so than most would expect. The indices on that test to identify schizophrenia are fairly valid. Experienced psychologists are usually better at identifying patients with schizophrenia by relying on history, observations, and a clinical interview than on psychological tests alone.

Does my patient have a traumatic brain injury?

Neuropsychological evaluation can be particularly helpful in assessing whether or not a traumatic brain injury has occurred. This is one of the few areas in which a detailed formal psychometric evaluation can be more accurate than the clinical mental status examination performed by a physician.

The diagnosis of traumatic brain injury requires an event that could cause brain injury and some indication of brain dysfunction or injury at the time of injury. This almost always includes a loss of consciousness or a persisting alteration in cognitive functioning. It may include, on occasion, a focal, abnormal neurologic examination or positive findings on CT scan or MRI. The best predictor of residual cognitive impairment from a head injury is the length of peritraumatic amnesia. The next best predictor is the duration of unconsciousness.

If an event occurred that could cause brain damage, the extent of damage can be inferred from radiologic findings or persistent neurological or neuropsychological findings. If such an event did not occur, the explanation of deficits on neuropsychological examination is likely to be a psychiatric disorder or malingering. The great advantage of a neuropsychological examination is the precision of measurement of cognitive skills. Subtle to mild impairments not detectable on gross mental status examination can be appreciated. The most common findings in subtle to mild traumatic brain injury involve the abilities to concentrate and to recall information.

The exact level at which the patient performs is not crucial in the diagnosis of mild traumatic brain injury. The crucial element is the difference between how well he should perform and how well he did perform. Estimation of the prior level of ability is central to the diagnosis of residual cognitive impairments. The gold standard is testing prior to the injury. When that information is unavailable, reasonable estimates can be made from performance on IQ tests or from performance on specialized reading tests (the Wide Range Achievement Test [WRAT-3], North American Adult Reading Test [NAART], etc.). Estimates based on occupational success or educational levels are much less reliable.

The presence of symptoms associated with "post-concussive syndrome" can be assessed with a variety of checklists.

While reliable, these procedures are not very informative or diagnostic. Many patients endorse symptoms of post-concussive syndrome without experiencing any injurious event. The symptoms overlap with typical symptoms seen in anxiety, depression, or somatoform disorder. "Post-concussive" symptoms are as common in patients suffering orthopedic injuries as they are in those suffering head injuries. The frequency of these symptoms decreases with increasing severity of symptoms. Symptoms reported by patients who have suffered a mild traumatic brain injury overlap considerably with symptoms of depression. A thorough neuropsychological evaluation looks for underlying depression or anxiety.

The use of tests like the MMPI or other standard personality inventories is quite helpful in our opinion. Some neuropsychologists use different schemes to "correct" for the fact that some individuals with mild head injury report problems with concentration and memory. We prefer not to use these systems. These symptom complaints are not seen in patients with readily evident brain injury, but rather are seen in many people with pre-existing personality or psychiatric disorders. As in any other diagnosis, one needs to consider all the evidence and all the findings before reaching a conclusion.

Is my patient with a closed head injury ready to return to work or school?

Neuropsychological testing is particularly useful when the patient has a known or diagnosed neurologic disorder and the question is, "What effect does that disorder have on his or her current level of functioning?" Neuropsychological testing attempts to measure the patient's current level of fluid intelligence, i.e., current ability to learn, remember, think abstractly, solve problems, draw, and complete other similar tests. In addition, it is often useful to know whether or not performing these cognitive activities unduly fatigues the patient.

A complete neuropsychological examination takes a long time and taps many different areas of cognitive functioning. Performing sequential and complicated tasks using multiple brain areas is more like the demands of school or work than the neurologic examination, which focuses on each individual brain function one at a time. If the patient is able to perform at the level expected for his or her IQ or education without undue fatigue, the answer is clear: the patient can function and is able to return to school or work. If minor difficulties are detected, cognitive rehabilitation or a delay in return to work or a partial return to work may be indicated.

Does my patient have dementia?

As people age, their capacity for rapid information processing and response, as well as their ability to retain information, decreases. The degree of loss is related partly to continued use of the mind in intellectual pursuits; people forget unused knowledge more than regularly used information. This "loss" is offset to some extent by breadth of knowledge and ability to rely on experience and reasoning ("wisdom"). However, older adults may become concerned that because they don't always remember where they left their car keys, they may be developing Alzheimer's disease. At the same time, as awareness of the symptoms of early-stage dementia has increased, diagnostic capacity has improved.

Except for research and legal purposes, neuropsychological evaluation is usually unnecessary in moderate to severe cases of dementia. The situation is obvious. However, comprehensive neuropsychological batteries in conjunction with careful histories of psychological and social functioning at home and at work can detect subtle degrees of cognitive impairment in the early stages of senile dementia of the Alzheimer's type. Our colleagues in neurology have reported that careful interview by well-trained clinicians at the very earliest stages of the disease detects the disease more accurately than the neuropsychological test battery they used. The battery they used was much more abbreviated than that used by most neuropsychologists. Of course, good neuropsychologists also do interviews. There is no doubt that even brief neuropsychological batteries identify more severe degrees of dementia.

Confounding conditions
Depression
One of the more common causes of real or perceived decreased cognitive capacity in older adults is depression. Depression can cause impaired concentration and "pseudodementia." (We prefer the British term "the cognitive impairment of depression.") The degree of depression can be assessed with a depression inventory; some have been developed specifically for an older adult population, in which depression may be experienced in physiological terms.

Depression also exists comorbidly with dementia in a substantial minority of patients. Some clinicians note that depressed individuals with the awareness to worry that they have dementia usually do not have significant deficits. A lack of awareness of deficits of functioning apparent to the family may be a hallmark feature of moderate to severe dementia.

Medication effects
As individuals age, they may develop more physical problems requiring pharmacological treatment. These can sometimes interfere with cognitive functioning, e.g., anticholinergic properties associated with various medications can impair memory. These factors should be ruled out as much as possible.

Physical condition

Medical status can interfere with cognitive functioning for a variety of reasons, from stress due to pain, decreased energy and malaise, the effects of sleep apnea, impaired blood flow, and toxic factors. The advantage of a neuropsychological assessment is that testing challenges the patient to respond in a variety of cognitive spheres and allows for more precision in describing performance outside the normal range. If a patient performs poorly in only one area of cognitive ability, this is not considered sufficient for a diagnosis of dementia.

Is my patient competent?

A variety of specialized tests have been developed to assist clinicians in evaluating patients' competency to make decisions about their personal medical choices and their ability to assist counsel in the legal forum. Testing to support a medical opinion of competency/incompetency is usually done only when the physician anticipates going to court because of the competency decision. Testing is usually not considered until a supporting opinion has been obtained from a neurologist or a psychiatrist.

Is my patient exaggerating, embellishing or malingering?

People with a medical illness usually describe only the symptoms of one syndrome. They may report a few other complaints. People with somatization disorder and personality disorders usually report everything is wrong and has been for years. Their complaints are not limited to the illness at hand. Their complaints are also malleable. They develop in whatever direction the physician seems to find interesting. This is easily picked up by objective personality tests used by psychologists.

Malingering is an especially interesting problem for psychologists. People faking psychiatric disorder usually overdo it and endorse more symptoms than psychotic patients endorse. Naive people faking cognitive problems usually underdo it; they perform too well. Psychologists, like physicians, are not particularly good at identifying when someone lies. The best way for clinicians to detect malingering is a careful review of the medical history. However, in addition, psychologists have developed special tests to evaluate malingering. They generally use a forced choice methodology (between a right answer and a wrong one) on a relatively easy task. Detection of malingering on neuropsychological testing without standardized assessment for lack of effort or malingering is difficult to perform. The malingering must be unusually poorly done or blatant to be detected. In medical–legal contexts, it has been estimated that about 40% of those examined malinger.

Special problems to avoid

A lack of definition of the referral question

When asking for a consultation, it is very helpful to specify the question, not the test. The psychologist is best able to provide an effective consultation if the reason for the referral is clearly stated. If a physician orders a specific test like the MMPI-2 but does not note the purpose of its administration, the psychologist is likely to describe the patient in general terms but may not respond to pertinent issues that would be helpful. Also, if the physician has a hunch that the patient is dealing with considerable anxiety, then ordering only the MMPI-2 may prevent the psychologist from using the appropriate assessment instruments (e.g., the MMPI-2[1] is not the best choice as a measure of anxiety). Similarly, a screening for neuropsychological dysfunction may be a good first step if cognitive dysfunction is suspected, rather than ordering a full (and expensive) neuropsychological battery.

The psychologist who works in consultation with the physician, rather than as a psychometrician, is best able to help in providing optimal patient care. The more precise the question, the more efficient, inexpensive, and helpful that testing will be.

Incomplete assessments

Incomplete assessments can be confusing. At one time, most psychologists screened for neuropsychological dysfunction or brain damage by using one test (the Bender or Benton) assessing praxis. This is not an adequate basis for making an informed opinion. Reliance on such a report leads to erroneous medical decision-making. Knowledge about test validity and the effort expended on the test is very important. Reports should have a statement commenting on reliability and validity of administration. The interpretation of a psychological test result is only a hypothesis to be considered in the context of all available information. This is particularly true of computerized test interpretation. All test statements or hypotheses must be checked against the complete clinical picture.

Several professional associations, including the American Counseling Association, the American Psychological Association, the American-Speech-Language-Hearing Association, and the National Association of School Psychologists, have generated standards for the responsible use of tests by their members. The first principle of competence espoused by the psychologists, counselors, and speech pathologists is

---

[1] Faithful to the concepts of the time when it was developed, the MMPI-2 lumped obsessive-compulsive disorder, generalized anxiety and panic disorder into one category — psychasthenia. Posttraumatic stress disorder (PTSD) was unknown.

complete assessment. Testing should always be integrated with all pertinent patient history and findings. This should always be done by the physician and should usually be done by the psychologist is well.

Projective tests

These are generally relevant only if the physician has some interest and training in psychodynamic principles. Examples of projective tests include the Rorschach ink blot test, the Thematic Apperception Test, sentence completion tests, and drawing tests (the House-Tree-Person Test and the Draw-a-Person Test). Except for the Rorschach, the scoring, coding, and interpretation of these tests is generally unreliable. These tests have been abused by untrained or poorly trained people working in the mental health field.

Rachel Klein, a well-known researcher and scholar in child psychiatry, has questioned the usefulness of projective testing with children, either for the purpose of describing personality or for clinical diagnoses. Klein (1987) states:

In fact, there is very little evidence to document the belief that children's personality characteristics are well estimated by projective testing. . . . It is a grave error to make diagnostic or psychotherapeutic decisions on the basis of projective testing . . . It is important to repeat that the very negative picture presented here pertains only to projective testing. There are other psychological testing procedures, such as tests of cognitive ability, that have great merit.

The diagnosis of child physical or sexual abuse offered to a physician solely or primarily on the basis of projective tests, art therapy products, or sand play should lead the physician to suspect that the person proffering the opinion is ignorant of the clinical and scientific literature, biased, or practicing out of their field of competence. An inquiry as to the person's experience in interpreting such material should confirm the suspicion.

Cost of testing

Some tests are inexpensive, while other batteries can cost thousands of dollars. The key to controlling cost is clearly defining the request for testing and providing as much information as possible to the consulting psychologist. A discussion with the psychologist prior to initiation of testing is often beneficial. Increasingly, managed care requires justification and review of requests for testing.

Conclusion

The reasons for requests for psychological testing should be as explicit as possible in the minds of both the referring physician and the psychologist receiving the referral. Reports back to the physician should also be as explicit as possible, clearly stating any qualifications about the validity of the testing. The patient's behavior and cooperation should be described sufficiently to allow the referring physician to evaluate the validity of the test.

Physicians typically review MRIs and CT scans with radiologists. They very infrequently go over psychological reports with psychologists. However, that process allows physicians to understand what has been done and why, and it allows psychologists to refine their appreciation of what physicians need to know and how they plan to use the information.

The results of psychological testing should always be evaluated as part, and only as part, of a comprehensive clinical evaluation.

Annotated bibliography

Greene, RL: Assessment of Malingering and Defensiveness by Multiscale Personality Inventories, in Rogers, R (ed.) (1997) *Clinical Assessment of Malingering and Deception*, 2nd Edition, New York, Guilford Press.
This is an excellent discussion of validity scales on a number of different tests in a very good book about malingering.
Kline, P (1991) *Intelligence: the Psychometric View*, London, Routledge.
This book presents a careful argument about the nature of intelligence as revealed by factor analytic studies. It is not technical and it can be readily understood by the nonexpert.
Placke, BS, Impara, JC, and Spies, RA (2003) *The Fifteenth Mental Measurements Yearbook*, Lincoln, Nebraska, Buros Institute of Mental Measurements.
This is the latest in a series of books containing critical reviews of several hundred tests, usually by more than one expert. It is one place to start in looking up a test.
Spreen, O and Straus, E (1998) *A Compendium of Neuropsychological Tests: administration, norms and commentary*, 2nd Edition, New York, Oxford University Press.
This is an excellent source for reviewing neuropsychological tests with basic technical information.
Ziskin, J and Faust, D (2000) *Coping With Psychiatric and Psychological Testimony*, with 1997 and 2000 supplements (three volumes) 5th Edition, Los Angeles, Law and Psychology Press.
This is a biased, three-volume set of books that results from a careful search of the literature to cull negative evidence about psychological testing. If one wants to find out what is wrong with a test, this is a good and easy place to start. It offers little about the strengths of a test.

CHAPTER 5

Clinical Rating Scales

Devna Rastogi-Cruz, MD and John G. Csernansky, MD

Introduction

In this chapter, the phrase *psychiatric rating scales* refers to standardized instruments used to quantify the symptoms and signs of psychopathology. Such scales facilitate the description of patients and their symptoms in terms that are replicable and easy to communicate. (This definition does not include typical neuropsychological tests or instruments used to arrive at diagnoses; see Chapter 4 for further information in this area.) There are three main types of rating scales: patient-rated, informant-rated, and professional-rated, which may also be called observer-rated. Although all of these scales are subject to certain biases, professional-rated scales are often felt to be the most objective.

All rating scales have certain advantages and disadvantages. Patient-rated scales render direct assessment of subjective internal states; however, the process of self-monitoring may have an effect on the target symptoms. These scales may also be more sensitive in identifying less severe pathological conditions. They require less professional time and are therefore less expensive. Disadvantages of patient-rated scales include difficulties completing the scales because of a patient's illiteracy, illness, unwillingness, or false answers. Completion of patient-rated scales may also be problematic in cases where there are memory and attention problems.

Informant-rated scales, which can be completed by anyone who knows the patient well, have some of the same advantages and disadvantages as patient-rated scales. The main advantages include the ability to evaluate patients in their usual environments and distinguish between current symptoms and premorbid behavior. The shortcomings of informant-rated scales are similar to those of patient-rated scales and are related to biases of the rater.

Professional-rated scales can be done in different formats, including structured, semistructured, and unstructured interviews. Unstructured interviews may allow different interviewing styles, experience, and theoretical beliefs to interfere with the reliability of assessment. Completely structured interviews that are standardized and involve specific ordering and wording of questions reduce variability and increase reliability.

Psychiatric rating scales are used in clinical practice, in research, and for teaching. In everyday clinical practice they can be used to document changes in symptoms during treatment. The practice of using such scales may become more prevalent as third-party payers require "hard" evidence of treatment benefits. The primary use of psychiatric rating scales is in research. In such settings, they are used to characterize patient populations and to systematically evaluate the effects of experimental treatments. Rating scales are also helpful for teaching residents and students ways to evaluate particular groups of symptoms.

It is important for practicing physicians to be familiar with clinical rating scales in order to properly interpret clinical trial reports of new psychotropic drugs. Physicians should also be familiar with these scales because they are useful in everyday practice. The use of a clinical rating scale may clarify the patient's most prominent symptoms and the degree to which they change during treatment. Additionally, patients themselves may find it difficult to articulate their symptoms without the benefit of being asked specific questions. When asking specific questions, it is difficult to find more appropriate ones than those recorded on a widely used scale. Reviewing such a list before and after treatment may offer the patient insight into the degree of her improvement. Anyone who has reviewed medical records and searched for a record of a patient's prior response to treatment appreciates that in many records there are few specific or usable statements. A series of rating scales documenting the type and degree of the patient's response to a series of treatment interventions can become an invaluable record for review by the original physician or by others at a later date.

Psychiatric rating scales can evaluate symptoms selected *a priori* or the overall psychiatric picture. They can be used to assess internal states or observable behavior for a specific time period. It is important that the answer scale is explicit. Clinical benchmarks to elucidate numerical scores are helpful in this regard. Rating scale scores may be either dichotomous (for example, absent or present and true or false) or continuous, where the rater has to describe frequency (never, rarely, occasionally, often, very often, always) or severity (absent, slight, mild, moderate, severe, extreme).

There are numerous psychiatric rating scales, and there are often many different types that can be used to evaluate the same symptoms or disorders. There is not a single best scale for each psychiatric disorder, so the first step in assessment is choosing the most appropriate scale. The choice of a rating scale should be based on its ability to accurately and reliably evaluate the specific symptoms and signs of the patient groups or disorder under consideration and depends on whether the rater is the patient, an informant, or a professional. It is also important to consider why a rating scale is being used. Rating scales should be used to evaluate and monitor symptoms and signs; they should not be used for the purpose of establishing or supporting a diagnosis unless that is the intended purpose of the instrument.

It is beyond the scope of this chapter to discuss the merits and disadvantages of all psychiatric rating scales. Instead, the discussion will focus on the more widely used scales for use in particular patient groups and for assessing general psychopathologic states. In the interest of space, the scales themselves are not reproduced but references are provided for all those discussed.

Rating scales

The Mini-Mental State Examination

The Mini-Mental State Examination (MMSE) is the most popular mental status screening examination. It is a quantitative assessment of the cognitive functioning and capacity of a patient. The MMSE assesses orientation, memory (registration and recall), attention, calculation, language (naming, repetition, ability to follow complicated commands, reading, and writing), and constructional ability. The instrument consists of 11 questions and takes only 5–10 minutes to administer. Therefore, it can be used serially and routinely. It has been found to validly and reliably evaluate cognitive processes and distinguish patients with and without cognitive disturbances. It is reasonably sensitive to changes in cognitive state.

As with other scales discussed in this chapter, the MMSE should not be used diagnostically because it cannot determine the cause of cognitive difficulties. Additionally, it may be insensitive to cognitive problems where the severity of the symptoms is slight (as in schizophrenia). There are different disorders in which cognitive impairments are present, and

there are many other reasons for a low MMSE score besides delirium and dementia. These reasons include sensory deprivations such as blindness, deafness, mutism, aphasia or other language barriers, mental retardation or an education level less than the eighth grade, or uncooperativeness. These factors should always be taken into consideration when administering the MMSE, and patients should have their usual sensory aids such as glasses and hearing aids available during testing. The test is not timed, and the maximum total score is 30. Mungas has proposed that a score of 25–30 indicates intact function or questionable impairment; 20–25 signifies mild impairment; 10–20 points to moderate impairment; and 0–10 implies severe cognitive impairment.

The Brief Psychiatric Rating Scale

The Brief Psychiatric Rating Scale (BPRS), developed in the 1960s by John Overall, remains among the most widely used clinical rating scales. It was originally intended for use in controlled clinical trials of new psychotropic drugs. However, it has also been widely employed in studies of the clinical (that is, symptom) correlates of cognitive and neurobiological phenomena.

Eighteen individual items, each describing a fundamentally different element of psychopathology, are rated by the physician on the basis of a semistructured interview. Each item is scored on a seven-point scale (from 0 to 6 or from 1 to 7 depending on the particular version being used). Using factor analysis, the BPRS items can be divided into five factors (hostility-suspiciousness, withdrawal-retardation, thinking disturbance, depression-anxiety, and activation). These factor scores, as well as the total score, are often used to evaluate changes in specific symptom groupings during treatment.

The Hamilton Rating Scale for Depression

The Hamilton Rating Scale for Depression (HAMD) is the most popular professional-rated scale used to evaluate the severity of depression and to demonstrate changes in depressive symptoms during treatment. The HAMD is not intended to be used as a diagnostic tool. Completion of this scale is based on a patient interview together with observations of the patient.

The classic HAMD consists of a 21-item list of symptoms that are evaluated on a severity rating scale of 0 to 4 or 0 to 2. Alternate 17- or 18-item versions (the last three or four items have been omitted) are also used. Guidelines are stated for each category to aid the rater in assigning a number to a symptom. For example, for agitation 0 corresponds to none; 1 equals fidgetiness; 2 is playing with hands, hair, etc.; 3 is moving about, can't sit still; and 4 equals hand-wringing, nail-biting, hair-pulling, and biting of lips.

The HAMD has been commonly used for clinical and

research purposes to quantify change in depressive symptoms and to evaluate the benefits of various treatments, including antidepressant drugs, psychotherapy, and electroconvulsive therapy (ECT). Decreasing scores indicate improvement of symptoms.

The Beck Depression Inventory

The Beck Depression Inventory (BDI) is the most broadly used self-rating scale for depression, and, like the HAMD, it is a standard in its class. It was designed to measure the behavioral manifestations of depression based on the characteristic symptoms and attitudes of depressed patients in the literature. Patients select the statement in each question that best describes their condition. In doing so, they have a total of 84 statements to consider. The total score ranges from 0 to 63. A particular score reflects both the number and severity of symptoms. Six of the 21 questions involve vegetative symptoms, and the rest refer to mood and cognitive symptoms.

Categories of symptoms covered by the BDI include mood, pessimism, sense of failure, lack of satisfaction, feelings of guilt, sense of punishment, self-hate, self-accusations, self-punitive wishes, crying spells, irritability, social withdrawal, indecisiveness, body image, work inhibition, sleep disturbance, fatigability, loss of appetite, weight loss, somatic preoccupation, and loss of libido. When the BDI is used correctly to quantitate changes in the intensity of depression, it has been found to be internally consistent and stable and to have high degrees of reliability and validity.

The Hamilton Anxiety Rating Scale

The Hamilton Anxiety Rating Scale (HAMA) is intended to assess the severity of anxiety symptoms and signs, and to measure changes in anxiety in patients who have previously been diagnosed as having an anxiety disorder. It is a professional-rated scale that is recommended to be administered before treatment is started and periodically during treatment. The symptoms evaluated include anxious mood, tension, fear, insomnia, cognitive functioning, depressed mood, behavior at interview, somatic (sensory) symptoms, somatic (muscular) symptoms, cardiovascular symptoms, respiratory symptoms, gastrointestinal symptoms, genitourinary symptoms, and autonomic symptoms. The rating scale ranges from 0 to 4, with 0 equal to no symptoms and 4 corresponding to severe or grossly disabling symptoms.

Although there is no other specific scale for generalized anxiety disorder (GAD), there are specific scales for phobias, panic disorder, posttraumatic stress disorder (PTSD), and obsessive-compulsive disorder (OCD). The only scale for a specific anxiety disorder discussed in this chapter is the Yale-Brown Obsessive Compulsive Scale (Y-BOCS).

The Yale-Brown Obsessive Compulsive Scale

The Y-BOCS is a professional-rated scale that is designed to assess the severity of obsessive and compulsive symptoms, the cardinal manifestations of obsessive-compulsive disorder (OCD). Again, it is not intended to be a diagnostic tool. The Y-BOCS has become the standard outcome measure in drug trials involving patients already diagnosed with OCD.

Before administering the Y-BOCS for the first time, the rater should define the patient's specific obsessions and compulsions to generate a Target Symptom List. The Y-BOCS contains a Symptom Checklist that has more than 70 examples of obsessions and compulsions to aid in the process of enumerating symptoms. Avoidance behaviors, which are often indictors of OCD symptoms, are also part of the Target Symptom List. Following completion of the Target Symptom List with the identification of avoidance behaviors, the interviewer uses the questions provided in the listed order to do the evaluation.

The main section of the Y-BOCS is a ten-item scale. Each item is rated from 0 (equal to no symptoms) to 4 (signifying extreme symptoms). The total range is from 0 to 40; the subtotal of items 1 through 5 assesses the severity of obsessions and the subtotal of items 6 through 10 assesses compulsions. Symptoms are generally evaluated weekly, so the rating is based on the average occurrence of the symptom during the previous week. Both obsessions and compulsions are evaluated by how much they interfere with normal functioning, cause distress, take up the patient's time, are resisted by the patient, and can be controlled by the patient. The total Y-BOCS score is not directly affected by the type or number of obsessions or compulsions present. It is indicative of the total severity of the illness, which is based on the combination of the individual target symptoms and their effect on the patient. This characteristic enables the comparison of severity of illness in patients with different types of obsessions and compulsions. Another advantage of the scale is that it allows changes in obsessions and compulsions with treatment response to be evaluated separately. Decreases of 35% in the total Y-BOCS scores from the baseline are usually selected to signify clinically significant improvement.

Mania rating scales: the Beigel and Petterson scales

All of the more widely used mania rating scales are professional-rated scales, since using self-rating scales for a disorder characterized by uncooperativeness, poor judgment, distractibility, cognitive impairment, and denial of illness is not feasible.

The Manic State Scale, developed by Beigel, was designed to be used by trained nursing staff and consists of 26 items that are rated from 0 to 5 to indicate intensity and frequency. The scale has been criticized for being too extensive to be serviceable, requiring too much time to finish, having some ambiguous items, and excluding some core features of mania, such as sleep changes.

The Petterson Scale is a shorter mania rating scale that consists of seven items and uses a five-point severity range. Behaviors evaluated include motor activity, pressure of speech, flight of ideas, noisiness, aggressiveness, orientation, and elevated mood. Because the scale is brief, it can be readily used for even closely spaced serial ratings. The Petterson Scale rates fewer symptoms than the Manic State Scale, but the items are more explicitly defined. It does not assess mixed states and does not address important aspects of mania, such as sleep and work disturbance.

SAPS and SANS in schizophrenia

The Scale for Assessment of Positive Symptoms (SAPS) and the Scale for Assessment of Negative Symptoms (SANS) provide standardized definitions and measurements of the positive and negative symptoms of schizophrenia, respectively. The positive symptoms of schizophrenia include hallucinations and delusions. The negative symptoms include flat affect and lack of volition. Recently, experts have suggested that illogical thinking, which is also characteristic of the disease, probably represents a third and separate dimension of the illness. Presently, different forms of this symptom are represented in both of the scales.

Neither the SAPS nor the SANS is intended as a diagnostic device. They have been used primarily in studies of the neurobiological correlates of symptom groupings. They are increasingly being used in drug treatment studies. The SAPS contains 34 items divided into four *a priori* subscales: hallucinations, delusions, bizarre behavior, and formal thought disorder (that is, loose associations among thoughts). The SANS comprises 25 items divided into five *a priori* subscales: affective flattening or blunting, alogia (paucity of apparent thinking and thought content), apathy, asociality, and inattention.

The Clinical Global Impression Scale

The Clinical Global Impression Scale (CGI) is composed of three general items and is almost always used in the evaluation of new psychotropic drugs. The first item asks the rater to score the patient on a six-point scale according to the severity of illness in this patient compared with the physician's total prior experience with this type of client. The second item asks the rater to score the patient on a six-point scale describing the degree of change since the last rating. The third item cross-tabulates the degree of improvement with the global severity of side effects. In this way, the total utility of the drug treatment can be assessed.

During a clinical drug trial, patients may improve in ways difficult to detect using the scales of psychopathology chosen for the study. This may occur because the drug has unan-

ticipated benefits and the scales required to assess them were not selected ahead of time, or because the changes in the patients' conditions cannot be recorded on any existing scales. At such times, the CGI can be invaluable and its use may ultimately lead to the refinement and improvement of other clinical rating scales.

The Nursing Observation of Inpatient Behavior

The Nursing Observation of Inpatient Behavior (NOSIE) was developed so that nurses' observations about the behavior of inpatients in clinical trials or other neurobiological studies of psychiatric illness could be recorded. The NOSIE measures a variety of individual and social-interactive behaviors, as well as the severity of particular symptoms. It can be highly useful for recording the psychopathologic conditions of patients who cannot always articulate their own symptoms or whose behavior is changing rapidly.

Rating scales for drug side effects

Rating scales are available for a variety of specific drug side effects. In particular, there are scales for the neurological side effects of antipsychotic drugs, such as pseudoparkinsonism (the Neurological Rating Scale), akathisia (the Barnes Akathisia Scale), and tardive dyskinesia (the Abnormal Involuntary Movement Scale [AIMS]). These scales can divide the symptoms of a complex side-effects syndrome such as pseudoparkinsonism into components (for example, tremor and gait disturbance), as do the Extrapyramidal Symptom Rating Scale (ESRS) and the Simpson-Angus Scale. Alternatively, the scales can divide the assessment across the areas of the body, as does the AIMS. Global scores are usually also rated.

In addition to side-effect rating scales for known and defined syndromes, there are side-effect scales designed to rate common complaints (such as sedation and dizziness) regardless of the type of psychotropic drug being tested. The most common scales in this category are the Treatment Emergency Symptom Scale (TESS) and the Systematic Assessment for Treatment Emergent Events (SAFTEE). In both cases, the physician explicitly inquires about a long list of potential side effects. Another approach to eliciting side-effect complaints is for the physician to ask a nonspecific question, such as, "Have you noticed any unusual or troublesome sensations?" The latter approach is more likely to highlight serious (and unexpected) side effects, although many problems, such as complaints of sexual dysfunction, are notoriously underreported.

Limitations of using clinical rating scales in research

Changes in the scores of particular rating scales, even those developed to rate the symptoms of a particular psychiatric disorder, do not always truly reflect a change in the severity of the target syndrome. This can occur because different clinical syndromes can overlap empirically. For example, many symptoms in patients with mood disorders and anxiety disorders are similar and nonspecific. Sleep disturbance in particular, although a specific symptom of depression, is also found in a variety of anxiety disorders and can be improved by any sedative drug. Therefore, any sedative would appear to have antidepressant effects if a change in this item were improperly interpreted.

As another example, aspects of depression and the negative symptoms of schizophrenia also overlap. In patients who have schizophrenia and no major mood disorder, assessments of decreased work, activities, and energy level can appear increased on scales used to assess either depression or negative symptoms. To avoid the interpretation of non-specific drug effects as specific improvements for the intended disorder, overlaps among such clinical syndromes should be kept in mind when evaluating the results of clinical trials.

Rating scale guidelines

- Nonspecific side effects of drugs (such as sedation) can affect the scoring of specific items on rating scales.
- Symptoms of specific psychiatric disorders can overlap.
- Statistically significant changes in rating scale scores may not be clinically significant.
- Rating scales can be used in everyday practice to record patterns of symptoms for review in the future.

PEARLS & PERILS

Another caveat that must be kept in mind when evaluating clinical rating scale data is that a statistically significant change in the scale score does not always indicate a clinically significant change. In studies where the sample size is large, a statistically significant change may represent a difference of only 10–15% in the severity of the targeted group of symptoms. Whereas such changes may be important in the design of future drugs and future clinical trials, most physicians would be unimpressed. Additionally, physicians must keep in mind that in studies where the sample size is small, the measurement of change is unreliable, even when a reliable scale is used to assess it. This problem can often be encountered when reading small, uncontrolled, and unblended trials or series of case reports.

Conclusion

Clinical rating scales are widely used in epidemiological and neurobiological research to describe the characteristics of patients with psychiatric disorders and to record responses to treatment. Rating scales are available for specific psychiatric syndromes and treatments, and for global evaluations as well. Care should be exercised in the selection of rating scales so the goals of the study can be best achieved. Clinical rating scales can also be used in everyday practice to help the physician and patient articulate the most prominent symptoms of the patient and to make a record for the future.

Annotated bibliography

Brook, S, Lucey, JV, and Gunn, KP, for the ziprasidone I.M. Study Group (2000) Intramuscular ziprasidone compared with intramuscular haloperidol in the treatment of acute psychosis, *J Clin Psychiatry* 61:933–941.
This article demonstrates the use of psychiatric rating scales to compare the efficacy and tolerability of IM Ziprasidone versus haloperidol in the treatment of acute psychotic agitation.

Guy, W (1976) *NCDEU Assessment Manual for Psychopharmacology*; U.S. Department of Health, Education and Welfare Publication (ADM) 76–338, Rockville, MD, Alcohol, Drug Abuse and Mental Health Association.
This manual contains example versions of a large number of the most commonly used clinical rating scales. The manual also contains reviews of reliability data for those scales available at the time.

Potkin, SG, Saha, AR, Kujawa, MJ, Carson, WH, Ali, M, Stock, E, Stringfellow, J, Ingenito, G, and Marder, SR (2003) Aripiprazole, an antipsychotic with a novel mechanism of action, and risperidone vs. placebo in patients with schizophrenia and schizoaffective disorder, *Arch Gen Psychiatry* 60:681–690.
This article is a multicenter trial demonstrating use of psychiatric rating scales to help establish the efficacy, safety, and tolerability of aripiprazole in the treatment of schizophrenia.

Prien, RF and Robinson, DS (eds) (1994) *Clinical Evaluation of Psychotropic Drugs*, New York, Raven Press.
This book contains an exhaustive review of information related to the design and implementation of clinical drug trials, including the selection and use of clinical rating scales.

CHAPTER 6

Neuroimaging in Psychiatry

Wayne C. Drevets, MD, Kelly Botteron, MD, and Deanna M. Barch, PhD

Current applications of neuroimaging in psychiatry

The application of modern neuroimaging technology to investigations of psychopathology holds the potential to transport psychiatry into a new era in which pathophysiology, rather than signs and symptoms, guides the nosology of psychiatric disease. A variety of imaging techniques affords unprecedented opportunities to examine brain structure and function noninvasively, permitting elucidation of the neuroanatomical correlates of psychiatric disorders and the emotional and cognitive processes disturbed in such disorders. In addition, the trajectory of technology development in nuclear magnetic resonance spectroscopy and ligand development for neuroreceptor imaging indicates that these neuroimaging techniques will provide increasingly powerful means of assessing the brain's chemistry, as well as its anatomy and physiology.

Because the sensitivity and specificity of imaging measures for determining psychiatric diagnosis and guiding treatment decisions have not yet been established, the greatest utility of neuroimaging in psychiatry is currently found in its research applications. Therefore, this chapter emphasizes principles that are relevant to the interpretation of research findings that utilize imaging techniques. Some of the consistently replicated findings in the literature are reviewed, and methodological issues germane to the resolution of apparent discrepancies across studies are discussed.

Neuroimaging research

Neuroimaging encompasses techniques for mapping both the structure and the function of the brain. Structural imaging evaluates morphology and elements of tissue composition using magnetic resonance imaging (MRI) or computed tomography (CT). These techniques have revolutionized clinical diagnostic evaluation by affording the ability to noninvasively visualize gross neuropathology *in vivo*, thus facilitating differential diagnosis in cases where psychiatric signs and syndromes may constitute manifestations of lesions or degenerative processes. Moreover, whereas qualitative inspection of MRI or CT images reveals gross structural pathology in only a minority of cases involving primary psychiatric disorders, research using quantitative neuromorphometric methods (that is, methods that quantify the size and shape of cerebral structures) has provided compelling evidence that subtle differences in the volumes of cerebral structures exist between subjects with psychiatric disorders and healthy controls. Such studies have dispelled the notion that the major psychiatric disorders are purely "functional" in nature, and their results have begun to guide postmortem neuropathological assessments to identify histopathological correlates associated with some of these conditions.

Functional imaging techniques permit noninvasive assessments of neurophysiology and neuroreceptor/neurotransmitter function. Compared with techniques involving lesion effects, electrical stimulation and recording, postmortem neuroreceptor assessment, cerebrospinal fluid chemistry, or neuropsychological test performance, functional imaging affords superior spatial resolution and the ability to simultaneously measure the function of multiple brain structures *in vivo*. State-of-the-art functional imaging studies generally employ either functional MRI (fMRI), which detects nuclear magnetic resonance signals related to blood flow, oxygen extraction, and blood volume, or positron emission tomography (PET) imaging of blood flow or glucose metabolism using scanners that detect radiation emitted from the decay of radionuclides administered by inhalation or intravenous infusion. A more recently developed technique is magnetoencephalography (MEG), which measures magnetic fields generated outside the scalp by neuronal activity.

Finally, one of the most promising areas for PET and single photon emission computed tomography (SPECT) imaging involves the quantification of neuroreceptor binding. Ligands have been developed that permit imaging of dopamine, benzodiazepine, opiate, serotonin, and acetylcholine receptors, and for some neurotransmitter precursors. In some cases, the neuroreceptor radioligands available for such studies have proven sensitive to endogenous neurotransmitter concentrations, permitting investigation of dynamic neurotransmitter function.

Clinical applications of neuroimaging

The clinical utility of neuroimaging in psychiatry is currently confined to differential diagnosis, where it is used to rule out coarse brain diseases that present with psychiatric signs or symptoms (Chapter 27). The most useful technology in this regard is neuromorphological MRI, which can sensitively detect areas of infarction, atrophy, tumors, or white matter lesions. Cases where anatomical MRI is generally indicated as part of the clinical evaluation include new onset of psychosis, new onset of mania after age 40, or new onset of psychiatric signs/symptoms in patients who also have focal neurological deficits, seizures, cognitive impairment, or suspected metastatic disease.

In rare cases, functional imaging has also been used in differential diagnosis. Examples have included cases in which PET was used to distinguish schizophrenia or mania from psychotic behavior associated with seizures when the EEG was equivocal. However, functional brain imaging has generally not yet proven clinically useful in psychiatry. Although abnormalities in regional blood flow and metabolism have been consistently reported in carefully selected subgroups with psychiatric disorders, few studies have assessed the diagnostic sensitivity and specificity of such findings. This is partly because the magnitude of resting differences between psychiatric and control samples has been relatively low (between about 2% and 20%) and the variability of such measures has been high enough that the respective distributions of patient and control values overlap. Finally, repeated scanning of large numbers of subjects has not been performed to evaluate test-retest variability, duration of confounding medication effects, or the effects of nonspecific factors such as sleep deprivation and timing within the menstrual cycle.

In contrast to the relatively subtle resting blood flow and metabolic abnormalities identified in patients with psychiatric disorders, imaging techniques that quantify neuroreceptor binding or assess neurophysiological responses to pharmacological challenges may ultimately prove sufficiently robust to distinguish healthy and ill cases. For example, one study reported that in 9 of 10 subjects scanned in various phases of bipolar disorder, dopamine D1-receptor affinity fell outside the distribution of control values. Another study found dramatic reductions in serotonin type 1A (5-HT1A) receptor binding in subjects with panic disorder (irrespective of the presence of comorbid major depression or previous psychotropic drug treatment) when compared with healthy controls. While such findings await replication in larger samples and assessments of specificity, they suggest that differences of the magnitude needed to differentiate target and normative populations may be achievable with neuroreceptor imaging techniques.

Overview of structural imaging technology

Computed tomography (CT)

The development and application of x-ray CT afforded the first capabilities for *in vivo* examination of soft tissues such as the brain. In 1979 Cormack and Hounsfield described the analytical technique of projection reconstruction imaging that enabled the development of CT and the other tomographic imaging techniques, MRI, PET, and SPECT. Although these technologies differ in the origin of the signals they detect, they share in common the reconstruction of two-dimensional views of a tissue slice from a set of one-dimensional projections taken at multiple angles. CT is based upon delineation of the differential attenuation of x-rays by distinct tissue types.

CT is the preferred imaging modality when bony disease or lesions involving calcified tissue are suspected. However, CT is also susceptible to artifacts near bony surfaces that obscure visualization of the brain stem, the basotemporal cortex, and the posterior fossa. Other disadvantages of CT relative to MRI include its low contrast resolution between gray and white matter, the risks associated with exposure to ionizing radiation, and the inability to acquire image slices in coronal or sagittal orientations.

PEARLS & PERILS

- CT scans can identify gross neuropathological lesions such as structural malformations, ventricular enlargement, infarction, hemorrhage, and tumor.
- CT involves exposure to ionizing radiation.
- The intravenous contrast agents sometimes used in CT techniques may produce serious allergic reactions.
- CT is preferred over MRI for visualizing bony abnormalities.
- CT has poor gray-white matter contrast resolution, and some brain structures are poorly visualized with CT because of bony artifacts.

TABLE 6.1　Tissue appearance of magnetic resonance images

	T1-weighted	T2-weighted
Gray matter	dark gray	light gray
White matter	light gray	dark gray
CSF	black	white
Inflammation/ demyelination	darker	brighter
Infarction	darker	brighter
Edema	darker	brighter
Solid tumor	darker	brighter
Hemorrhage—chronic	brighter rim	brighter

- MRI produces images that can be visualized in any orientation.
- Anatomical MRI is not susceptible to the bony artifacts associated with CT imaging, permitting visualization of the entire cerebrum, posterior fossa and brain stem.
- MRI does not involve exposure to ionizing radiation.
- Compared with CT, MRI affords higher tissue contrast between gray and white matter, superior delineation of white matter lesions, and greater spatial resolution (that is, small structures are better visualized).
- Image acquisition can be accomplished in minutes.
- Subjects may develop claustrophobic anxiety in MRI scanners that have a narrow cylindrical aperture.
- MR images are sensitive to motion artifacts, so patients who are unable to remain motionless may require sedation.

Magnetic resonance imaging (MRI)

Of the *in vivo* brain imaging techniques, nuclear magnetic resonance imaging (MRI) provides the highest spatial and tissue contrast resolution for neuroanatomical structures. MR images are generated using the inherent magnetic properties of atoms, which are amplified and enhanced for detection and visualization. The most common nucleus targeted for clinical MRI is hydrogen because of its abundant distribution in living tissue. Tissues with different hydrogen concentrations and tissue relaxation parameters produce distinct resonance signals that underlie the characteristic appearances of cerebrospinal fluid (CSF), gray matter and white matter in MR images (Table 6.1). Moreover, alterations in the acquisition sequences can enhance the ability to examine particular types of tissue pathology. For example, T2-weighted images are more useful than T1-weighted images for examining white matter pathology.

MRI does not involve exposure to ionizing radiation and has no significant known biological risks to tissues at the magnetic field strengths currently employed for clinical use. Other advantages of MRI over CT include its higher spatial resolution (about 0.5 mm in all planes for 3 tesla scanners), superior gray-white matter contrast, ability to acquire images in any orientation, superior depiction of white matter pathology, greater flexibility of image acquisition parameters to vary tissue contrast, and improved accuracy for volumetric measurements. The disadvantages of anatomical MRI include its expense and sensitivity to motion artifacts. The known risks associated with MRI relate to the potential of the magnetic field to dislodge metallic objects (for example, metal intracranial or aneurysmal surgical clips or intraocular metallic objects) and interfere with the operation of electrically or magnetically activated devices (for example, cardiac pacemakers and cochlear implants).

Overview of functional imaging technology

Nontomographic methods for imaging regional blood flow

Nontomographic methods used to measure regional blood flow in humans rely upon the principles of inert gas exchange. After inhalation of air containing xenon-133, the gamma rays emitted during ^{133}Xe decay are counted by crystal multidetector systems placed over the scalp. Detector sensitivity declines rapidly as tissue depth increases, and the recorded activity originates almost entirely from brain surfaces lying within 2 cm of the detector face. For this and other technical reasons, nontomographic methods employing ^{133}Xe measure blood flow exclusively from the cortical gray matter lying near the scalp. This is a major limitation in psychiatric studies since measures cannot be obtained from the deep cortical (such as ventral and medial portions of the frontal and temporal lobes), limbic, and basal ganglia structures that appear to participate in emotional processing, psychosis, and psychomotor activity.

Positron emission tomography (PET)

The PET camera images the annihilation radiation generated as positrons are absorbed in matter. Thus, it records highly accurate spatial representations of the distribution of a radionuclide that has been inhaled or injected (Fig. 6.1). The PET image is effectively equivalent to a quantitative tissue radiogram in laboratory animals, but it affords the advantage of being non-invasive, permitting imaging in humans. The various positron-emitting radiopharmaceuticals

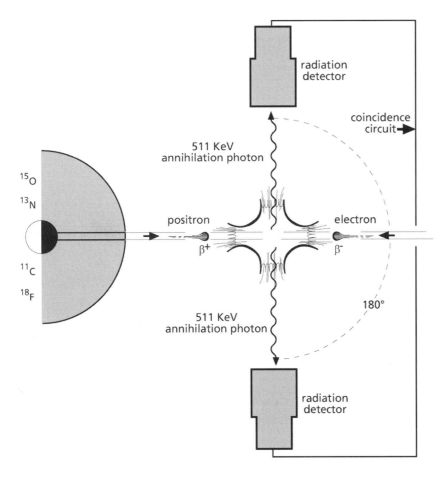

Fig. 6.1 Detection scheme for positron emission tomography (PET). Radionuclides employed in PET decay by emission of positrons from a nucleus unstable because of a deficiency of neutrons. Positrons lose their kinetic energy in matter after traveling a finite distance (~1 to 6 mm) and, when brought to rest, interact with electrons. The two particles are annihilated, and their mass is converted to two annihilation photons traveling at ~180 degrees from each other with an energy of 511 keV. Annihilation photons are detected by the imaging device, using opposing radiation detectors connected by electronic coincidence circuits that record an event only when two photons arrive simultaneously. A major factor determining the ultimate resolution of PET is distance traveled by the positron before its annihilation.
Reproduced with permission from Raichle (1983), *Annual Reviews of Neuroscience* 6: 251.

currently available provide capabilities for imaging blood flow, blood volume, glucose or oxygen metabolism, neuroreceptor binding, or water extraction across the blood-brain barrier. Radioisotopes that decay by positron emission (and their respective half-lives) include ^{15}O (122 seconds), ^{13}N (10 minutes), ^{11}C (20 minutes) and ^{18}F (110 minutes).

PET is superior to nontomographic measurements using ^{133}Xe inhalation in that it provides three-dimensional data and the ability to image deep structures. Compared with SPECT, PET affords higher spatial resolution, greater sensitivity for deep structures, fewer artifacts from the scatter and attenuation of radiation, the ability to make both absolute and relative measures, and the potential for a greater variety of measurements. Finally, unlike fMRI, PET has potential for measuring characteristics of biological compounds (such as neuroreceptors) that exist in minute concentrations. The limitations of PET include its high expense and dependence upon radiolabeled tracer administration.

Single photon emission computed tomography (SPECT)

SPECT systems measure the distribution of statically distributed radiopharmaceuticals (tracers trapped in the brain with a stable distribution over time) that reflect perfusion patterns. The radiopharmaceuticals used for SPECT emit single gamma rays, in contrast to the two simultaneous gamma rays emitted by PET radiopharmaceuticals. This distinction leads to instrumentation differences between SPECT and PET, as SPECT cameras are designed to determine the point of origin of single photons (gamma rays) based solely upon their trajectory. The spatial resolution of SPECT is nearly as high as that of PET, as recent innovations in SPECT instrumentation have led to systems capable of 8 mm resolution and imaging times as short as 2–3 minutes. Nevertheless, several technical problems reduce the sensitivity of SPECT for measuring changes (especially increases) in regional blood flow, particularly in deep structures.

The major advantage of SPECT is that the necessary equipment and radiopharmaceuticals are routinely available in most nuclear medicine departments. The radiopharmaceuticals can be obtained from commercial manufacturers, obviating the need for an on-site cyclotron. Consequently, SPECT imaging is lower in cost than PET.

Functional magnetic resonance imaging (fMRI)

A variety of methods have been developed to image

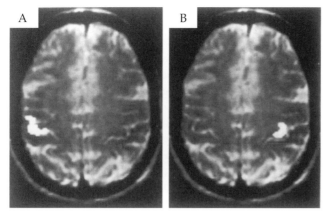

Fig. 6.2 Activation of the contralateral motor cortex by repeated squeezing of a sponge with each hand separately, detected by fMRI. Decreased deoxyhemoglobin concentration caused by increased local cerebral blood flow and blood volume was putatively responsible for the bright regions in the motor cortices contralateral to the exercising left (A) and right (B) hands. The two images shown were produced by acquiring 16 single-excitation gradient echo images during left hand squeezing, in alternation with 16 others made during right hand squeezing. Images were obtained every 15 seconds, resulting in a total acquisition time of 8 minutes. The two groups of 16 images associated with left or right hand squeezing were summed separately and compared with each other by t-test mapping. Voxels different at a level of *P*<0.01 comprise the bright regions, which are superimposed on a two-excitation spin echo anatomical image of the same brain made in the same session. (From Prichard, JW (1995) *The Neuroscientist*, 1: 84–94.)

hemodynamic activity using fMRI. The fMRI techniques for identifying anatomical correlates of sensory or cognitive processing show regional changes that are similar in location to those identified using PET measures of cerebral blood flow (CBF) (Fig. 6.2). The most commonly applied fMRI method for mapping brain function putatively detects shifts in local deoxyhemoglobin concentration. Unlike hemoglobin, deoxyhemoglobin is paramagnetic, a property that causes it to suppress the nuclear MR signals from other substances in its immediate vicinity. When local neural activity increases sufficiently, local oxygen uptake, blood flow and blood volume also increase. However, the increases in the latter two variables outpace the concomitant rise in oxygen utilization, causing the deoxyhemoglobin concentration to fall. The local water signal consequently becomes stronger than it was prior to the onset of the increased neuronal activity, providing a map of brain areas recruited by the experimental task.

fMRI offers several advantages over PET and SPECT for dynamic brain mapping studies. For example, fMRI permits measurements at a spatial resolution of less than 1 mm, although the technical difficulties in distinguishing signal from noise are magnified at such high spatial resolutions, and most fMRI applications in clinical populations use somewhat lower spatial resolution sequences (e.g., ~3 mm). The temporal resolution of fMRI is also superior to that of PET; an approximately 0.5 second time period is required for the physiological signal to develop. [MR scanners are capable of faster measurements, but the blood flow rise does not develop until about 0.5 sec after the increase in cortical electrical activity (Fig. 6.3)]. Although this temporal

Fig. 6.3 Activation of cerebrovascular changes by real and imagined visual stimulation, as detected using fMRI. The time course of signal intensity changes in visual and nonvisual cortex during two periods of actual photic stimulation by light flashing at 16 Hz and an intervening period during which the subject imagined the lights to be flashing. Images were obtained by pulse sequences sensitive to deoxyhemoglobin concentration in each voxel; the 5% intensity increases during actual photic stimulation and the 3% increase during imagined stimulation are all thought to reflect local increases in cerebral blood flow and blood volume related to neural activity in visual cortex. (From Le Bihan, D, *et al.* (1993) *Proc Natl Acad Sci USA*, 90:11802–11805.)

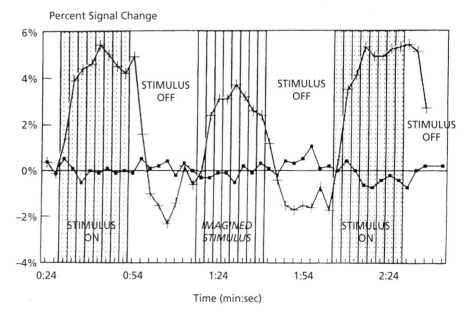

resolution is not as good as that achieved with techniques such as EEG and MEG, it does offer the ability to address questions about the time course of cognitive and emotional processing that cannot be answered using techniques such as PET. In addition, fMRI does not expose subjects to radiation and no deleterious effects have been associated with the magnetic and radiofrequency fields applied, so subjects can undergo repeated study without risk. This noninvasive aspect of fMRI is particularly beneficial for studies examining the development of neuropsychiatric disorders; it is also useful for tracking changes in functional brain activity over time or as a function of treatment. Finally, fMRI tends to be more cost effective than PET.

The limitations of fMRI include uncertainties regarding the nature of fMRI signals (i.e., vascular rather than direct neuronal activity, presynaptic versus postsynaptic activity, which may alter interpretations of the functional significance of the signal), an inability to interpret absolute differences in fMRI signals among groups (as compared to methods such as quantitative PET) because a number of extraneous factors can influence absolute fMRI values, and greater susceptibility to artifacts created by subject movement and signal susceptibility.

Magnetic resonance spectroscopy (MRS)

In addition to the capabilities of nuclear magnetic resonance imaging for examining anatomy and physiology, MR techniques exist that provide *in vivo* information about the neurochemistry of brain tissue. MRS assays atoms that possess a net charge (e.g., ^{31}P, ^{1}H, ^{19}F, ^{13}C, ^{7}Li, and ^{23}Na) and are present in sufficient concentration to produce an adequate signal. For example, ^{31}P-MRS can explore brain energy metabolism through assays of adenosine triphosphate (ATP) and related metabolites. MRS also permits investigations of the distribution of certain antidepressant and antipsychotic drugs via the use of ^{19}F-tagged medications.

MRS can be performed using standard MRI magnets with magnetic fields of 1.5 Tesla or greater. MRS is technically demanding and requires rigorous standardization and prolonged scanning time. The latter constraint limits its utility for investigating rapid changes in metabolism related to neuronal activation. Nevertheless, MRS may be applied in comparisons across longer time frames (such as before and following treatment).

Methodological issues in structural imaging research

A wide range of qualitative and quantitative image analysis techniques have been applied in structural imaging studies. Qualitative evaluations rely upon either standard clinical impressions or structured rating scales that are insensitive to subtle volumetric abnormalities. Quantitative techniques range from linear or area measures (for example, the ventricle-to-brain ratio, obtained by dividing the ventricular area in the axial slice where the ventricles appear largest by the area of the entire brain in that slice) to more sophisticated volumetric measures. Neuromorphometric techniques for measuring the volume of cerebral structures generally rely upon either manual outlining of structures on sequential MR image slices or stereological sampling (point counting) methods. Semi-automated and automated techniques have also been developed that either combine simple thresholding with manual editing or employ fully automated multispectral analytic methods to trace boundaries with uniform pixel intensity. However, the utility of these methods has been limited since the MR signal intensity is inhomogeneous across an MR image. Automated techniques are under development that involve image warping (global deformation) models that reduce dependence upon pixel intensity by utilizing shape information.

All of these methods struggle with problems of boundary definition for brain structures. The precise boundary of brain structures cannot be determined in MR images because, unlike tissue sections, a CT or MRI pixel has a signal intensity that reflects an average of the signals from all of the tissues it contains. Consequently, structural borders are blurred. Boundary definition becomes more difficult as image slice thickness and voxel size increases, since more tissue types are included within and located adjacent to larger pixels.

Volumetric measures obtained by different techniques for a particular structure vary substantially, and individual laboratories have developed guidelines for defining regions that have adequate inter-rater and intra-rater reliability within their own laboratory. Other experimental design issues critical to the interpretation of results from structural imaging studies involve subject selection and sample size. Biological heterogeneity within a psychiatric disorder may result in dissimilar findings across studies. For example, in investigations of mood disorders, the polarity (unipolar versus bipolar) and age-at-onset of the subject sample profoundly influence the results of both structural and functional imaging comparisons. Adequate matching of psychiatric and control subjects is also critical, since recent studies have shown that differences in age, sex, intelligence, socioeconomic status, or psychiatric comorbidity can lead to morphometric differences among groups. Finally, the high variability of human neuroanatomy reduces the sensitivity for detecting abnormalities in small subject samples or individual cases, contributing to apparent discrepancies across studies.

Principles of functional neuroimaging

In 1890 Roy and Sherrington published their pioneering observations that an "automatic mechanism" exists in the brain such that local variations in functional activity are accompanied by local variations in blood supply. This hypothesis has been corroborated by numerous experiments both before and since the development of modern tracer methodology, which have additionally demonstrated that increases in neuronal activity are associated with rises in regional metabolism as well. By mapping regional blood flow or metabolism, functional imaging thus provides detailed pictures of local neuronal work.

The ability to image regional blood flow and metabolism non-invasively has afforded unprecedented opportunities to map the brain areas involved in cognitive processing. Using strategies that compare dynamic images obtained during experimental and control tasks, imaging studies have identified the anatomical correlates of motor, somatosensory, visual, auditory, linguistic, attentional and memory tasks (for example, see Figs 6.2, 6.3, and 6.4). Such techniques are also helping to elucidate the functional anatomy of human emotion, hallucinations, psychomotor activity, individual differences in personality, and intelligence. Brain mapping studies involving induced emotional states have been particularly illuminating. Although animal research provides insights into the neural substrates of emotional behavior and autonomic expression, establishing the correlates of subjective emotional experience depends upon human research.

Brain mapping studies using PET are generally limited to measurements of blood flow using ^{15}O-labeled water or butanol. This is because the short half-life ($t_{1/2}$) of ^{15}O (2 min.) permits image acquisition over a sufficiently short time period (40 sec) to capture physiological changes related to neuronal activity before the blood flow signal decays. In addition, the short half-life of ^{15}O permits repetition of measurements at several minute intervals, so scans can be acquired in multiple cognitive-behavioral states during the same session (Fig. 6.4).

In contrast, PET measures of glucose or oxygen metabolism or utilization are less suitable for activation paradigms. This is because such measurements employ radionuclides with long half-lives (about two hours for ^{18}F), limiting the ability to repeat measurements during the same session, or because they require sequential administration of three ^{15}O-labeled tracers, O_2, CO, and either H_2O or CO_2. In contrast, the longer period for counting radioactive emissions during glucose metabolism imaging is an advantage in studies comparing resting neurophysiology between groups, since the larger number of radioactive counts per pixel in glucose metabolism as compared with blood flow images improves the statistical quality of metabolic images.

In current research, the most frequently employed method for elucidating the brain systems involved in human cognition and emotion is fMRI measures of blood oxygen level dependent (BOLD) signals. fMRI does not require the use of radioligands, so it can be applied repeatedly with the same subjects and can be used in children. This allows a larger amount of data to be acquired for each participant and allows multiple cognitive and emotional processes to be imaged in the same individuals. These advantages of fMRI have allowed its use in generating information about healthy human cognitive development. In addition, fMRI's relatively good temporal resolution (compared with PET) allows researchers to begin to disentangle brain activity associated with different aspects of cognitive and emotional processing that can occur in relatively close time with each other.

A disadvantage of fMRI is that the source of neural activity generating the BOLD signal remains uncertain. fMRI takes advantages of the well-known coupling of neuronal activity and changes in blood flow and oxygenation. However, the source of the fMRI signal is vascular rather than neuronal activity. As reviewed by Heeger and Ress, the fMRI signal may reflect a variety of physiological signals, including changes in the firing rates of local neurons, subthreshold neuronal activity, or even modulatory inputs from other regions of the brain. Because the factors influencing the relationship between neuronal activity and change in blood flow and oxygenation are not fully understood, the interpretation of results of brain imaging studies using fMRI techniques are not entirely clear.

Brain mapping during cognitive activation

The experimental strategies employed in brain mapping studies rely upon paired comparisons between dynamic scans acquired in two different cognitive-behavioral states. Typically blood flow images in each task state are superimposed and then subtracted from one another to highlight regional blood flow changes associated with the neural activity that distinguishes the two states (Figs 6.2, 6.3, and 6.4). Since subjects serve as their own controls, nonspecific variations related to differences in anatomy and head positioning are minimized.

The number of possible interpretations for each area of observed blood flow change rises with the number of mental operations that differ between the experimental and control tasks. Thus complex cognitive processes are dissected into a series of simple, component steps. These elemental steps are imaged in successive control-activation subtraction pairs so that the distributed neural networks involved in each aspect of the more complex task can be isolated from one another.

This strategy for brain mapping studies is exemplified by the investigation of the cortical anatomy of single-word processing reviewed in Fig. 6.4. In this experiment, knowledge from cognitive psychology, linguistics, and clinical neurology was used to parse single-word processing into three component steps, which were isolated from one another by scanning subjects in each of four behavioral conditions. The four behavioral tasks were used to form a three-level

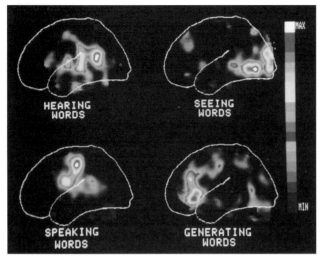

Fig. 6.4 PET images of changes in regional blood flow show the cortical areas activated during single word processing. The image sections shown here are from composite images of mean blood flow changes in which images acquired with PET during the experimental task and the control task are superimposed and subtracted, and the resulting blood flow difference images from several subjects are then summed to enhance the signal-to-noise ratio. All of the sections shown are from sagittal slices through the lateral left hemisphere (the subjects were right-handed). The *seeing words* image demonstrates areas in the occipital cortex where flow increases in scans acquired as subjects passively view nouns presented on a video screen, as compared with ones acquired as they view a cross-hair on the same screen. These blood flow responses indicate the functional anatomical correlates of passive sensory processing for visual input (striate cortex) and modality-specific word-form processing (extrastriate cortex; see text). The *hearing words* image reveals areas in the temporal cortex where flow increases as nouns are presented aurally, rather than visually, during the experimental task. Thus, at the level in which verbal input is passively received, distinct systems are activated for visual vs. auditory processing. In contrast, the *speaking words* comparison shows that as subjects repeat the nouns aloud, the same areas related to motor output and articulatory coding become activated whether the nouns have been presented visually or aurally. These areas include the mouth area of the primary sensorimotor cortex, the dorsal insular cortex (both shown) and the supplemental motor area (not shown); the task in which subjects passively view nouns served as the control task for comparison with this higher level "repeat words" task. Finally, as subjects view or hear nouns and generate aloud a verb related to each noun (*generating words*), flow increases in the dorsolateral and inferior PFC (shown) and the dorsal portion of the anterior cingulate gyrus (not shown); the repeat-words task serves as the control task for this comparison. The anterior side is toward the left, and the dorsal aspect is toward the page top. (From Raichle, ME in Pechura, CM and Martin, JB (eds) (1991) *Mapping the Brain and its Functions*, Washington D.C., National Academy Press.)

subtractive hierarchy such that each task state added a small number of mental operations to the previous task state.

The first level of comparison involved the subtraction of a blood flow image acquired as the subject passively viewed nouns presented on a video screen from an image acquired while the subject viewed a cross-hair on the same screen. The blood flow changes were interpreted as indicating two levels of computation: passive sensory processing (visual input), which was associated with blood flow increases in the primary visual (striate) cortex (other simple visual stimuli also produce blood flow increases in this area), and modality-specific word-form processing, which was associated with blood flow increases in the extrastriate cortex. Subsequent experiments demonstrated that this latter area is also activated by words and pronounceable non-words, but not by consonant letter strings or false fonts.

In a separate but parallel comparison, the nouns were presented aurally instead of visually (Fig. 6.4). This resulted in blood flow increases in areas of the temporal cortex, where flow had not changed when the nouns were presented visually. However, in a subsequent experiment it was shown that blood flow increases could be elicited in these temporal cortical regions using visual word presentation if a pair of words was shown and the subjects were required to judge in silence whether the two words rhymed.

In the second level of comparison, the subjects were again presented a series of nouns, but this time they repeated the words aloud during the PET scan. The previous task in which the subjects passively viewed nouns served as the control task for comparison with the higher level "repeat words" task. Flow increased in the brain areas related to motor output and articulatory coding: the mouth area of the primary sensorimotor cortex, the supplemental motor area, and a portion of the insular cortex. (It was later demonstrated that blood flow increased in this insular area when subjects moved their mouth and tongue in the absence of visual word presentation or verbal output.) These same brain areas were activated whether the nouns were presented aurally or visually.

In the third and final level of comparison, subjects were asked to view the nouns and generate and state aloud a verb related to each noun. Whether the words were presented visually or aurally, blood flow increased in the inferior prefrontal cortex (PFC) and the dorsal portion of the anterior cingulate gyrus. This cingulate area was thought to participate in an anterior attention system engaged in selection for action, while the prefrontal area was thought to be involved in the process of semantic association.

Functional activation in disease states

A potentially powerful strategy for investigating the pathophysiology of psychiatric disorders involves dynamic imaging during cognitive tasks that involve the domains affected by the disorder. Differences in regional blood flow responses during cognitive or emotional tasks known to activate specific neural circuits may conceivably identify points within that circuit where dysfunction exists within a particular psychiatric illness. Moreover, scans acquired during activated states may identify abnormalities in regions where blood flow or metabolism appears normal in the resting state. Finally, scans acquired during the performance of a neuropsychological task may demonstrate that psychiatrically ill subjects employ aberrant neural circuits in the processing related to that task.

However, the design of experimental tasks for dynamic imaging paradigms involving psychiatrically ill subjects is complex, because any differences in stimulus and performance variables that exist between the experimental and control groups may be reflected by differences in the associated neurophysiology. For example, elementary stimulus features such as repetition rate have profound effects on blood flow responses. Somatosensory stimulation does not produce a measurable blood flow response in the cat somatosensory cortex until the stimulus frequency reaches 3 Hz.

An implication of these observations is that if stimulation frequencies differ between groups, the associated hemodynamic response is also likely to differ. For example, one series compared blood flow changes during performance of the Wisconsin Card Sort Task between control subjects and subjects with schizophrenia and found that the subjects with schizophrenia developed a blunted blood flow response in the dorsolateral prefrontal cortex while they were performing the task. However, the subjects with schizophrenia completed an average of only 1.5 categories during the scan, while the controls completed an average of 7.5 categories. Since the dorsolateral PFC is putatively involved in performing this task, the blood flow response likely differed between groups because the rate at which the stimulus reached the dorsolateral PFC was unequal, the behavioral output was dissimilar, or the cognitive processing within the dorsolateral PFC was abnormal in schizophrenia. Thus unless stimulus and response variables such as performance rate and accuracy are similar between experimental and control groups, blood flow response differences between groups may not necessarily signify regional dysfunction. Fortunately, fMRI technology provides the capability to image single trials, so that the image data can be analyzed on the basis of performance on different trial types (such as correct versus incorrect trials). Thus, examining brain activity only on correct trials, even when overall performance differences exist between psychiatrically ill and control groups, provides a method for addressing potential confounds related to behavioral performance.

Abnormalities of resting physiology in psychiatric disorders

Resting differences in blood flow or metabolism between psychiatrically ill and control subjects reflect a complex set of activations by the disease state. Regional metabolic differences may describe trait pathophysiological abnormalities associated with the genetic or environmental predisposition to a disorder, physiological state changes corresponding to symptoms (for example, hallucinations) or behaviors (such as obsessive thinking), or cytological changes that may cause or result from the illness or its manifestations (for example, the increased risk for alcohol abuse in bipolar disorder). Moreover, disparate states within a single diagnostic group may give varying functional patterns. For example, psychomotor agitation may have distinct functional anatomical correlates from psychomotor retardation, yet either may be present in major depressive disorder.

Another level of complexity relates to the nature of the metabolic signal. First, synaptic activity in the neuropil, rather than changes in the chemistry of cell bodies, accounts for nearly all of the metabolic changes observed during activation. Thus local changes in blood flow or metabolism in a specific region may occur either from increased interneuronal neurotransmission within that region or from increased afferent transmission from a projecting structure. Since local connections predominate in the cortex, blood flow and metabolic differences observed there are generally interpreted as reflecting local neuronal activity. In contrast, physiological changes in the basal ganglia or the thalamus are more likely to reflect afferent transmission originating from neurons in a distal structure.

Second, both excitatory and inhibitory transmission result in increased metabolic activity in the neuropil because both result in activation of energy-consuming, ion-pumping activity at the postsynaptic membrane. The differentiation between excitatory and inhibitory transmission in terms of local metabolism would presumably be reflected one synapse away, where the postsynaptic neuron makes its efferent synapses. However, such efferent activity may be diffusely distributed and may not be evident in the functional brain image.

Abnormalities in functional images can also be accounted for by differences in cell number. Tomographic methods provide physiological measurements per unit volume of intracranial contents, such that image data are affected by the inclusion of metabolically inactive cerebrospinal fluid (CSF) spaces resulting from atrophy or hypoplasia (known as the partial volume effect). The presence of atrophy or hypoplasia in some psychiatric illnesses creates difficulties in the interpretation of functional imaging data, since it is unclear whether observed differences in blood flow or metabolism result from true changes in these parameters, atrophy, or a combination of the two. Studies are beginning to address this problem using MRI quantitation of anatomical differences to correct physiological images for partial volume effects, although such techniques await validation.

Other issues in image analysis

Simple visual inspection of physiological images is generally not sensitive enough to detect the subtle abnormalities associated with psychiatric disorders, so comparisons of mean tracer uptake between psychiatric and control samples in specified regions are used to identify abnormalities. Deciding where to look in functional images is complicated, since an average PET slice is composed of several thousand volume elements (voxels) and modern tomographic instruments obtain 15–47 slices during a single scan. Dealing with comparisons across so many data points poses serious statistical problems in distinguishing true differences from differences arising by chance alone. One approach for reducing the number of statistical tests is to limit comparisons to a few regions-of-interest, in which the average value of all image voxels contained within a region-of-interest is compared between patients and controls.

To anatomically localize regional measurements within the relatively low resolution functional brain images, the primary blood flow or metabolic images are commonly transformed into a standardized stereotaxic space. These methods allow stereotaxic placement of regions-of-interest across subjects. Newer methods rely upon co-registration of PET and MRI images from the same subject, since anatomical detail is more easily seen in MRI images. Ultimately, methods under development that use anatomical information from the MRI scan to fluidly transform coregistered PET and MRI images into a standard three-dimensional space are expected to become the standard method for localization.

While the region-of-interest method is currently superior to other approaches for assessing differences in small structures (such as the amygdala), it reduces sensitivity for identifying abnormalities in the cortex in studies of psychiatric disorders, since the uncertain knowledge regarding the pathophysiology of these disorders and the limited information regarding the cortical areas involved in the production of psychiatric symptoms reduces the likelihood of preselecting regions-of-interest where abnormalities exist. A more sensitive approach for assessing cortical areas involves the use of statistical maps in which image voxels are computed as either unpaired t-values, for comparing the mean blood flow or metabolism of patient and control groups, or as paired t-values, for comparing mean differences across two distinct states in the same subject set (e.g., before and during a panic attack).

Another type of statistical image that is used to explore relationships between clinical ratings and regional physiology involves computation of correlational images (r-value

maps). These methods rely on the aforementioned transformations of primary tomographs into standardized stereotaxic space so images from different brains can be superimposed. Nevertheless, the generation of such statistical maps involves several thousand statistical comparisons (computations are performed for every image voxel), potentially leading to the statistical problem of obtaining differences by chance alone. Therefore conservative approaches confine the use of statistical maps to exploratory analyses in which areas of apparent significance in the statistical map generated from one subject set are used to generate candidate regions-of-interest, and the statistical probability that significant differences exist in such regions is tested in independent subject sets.

Neuroimaging studies of the major psychiatric disorders

Schizophrenia

Structural imaging
Neuromorphometric studies have consistently shown that individuals with schizophrenia have enlarged lateral and third ventricles, widened cortical sulci, and reduced temporal lobe structure size relative to healthy controls, although the magnitude of these abnormalities is subtle relative to that of the corresponding changes in dementia (Fig. 6.5). This ventricular enlargement is present even in patients suffering their first episode and correlates with negative symptomatology (apathy, anhedonia, avolition, paucity of speech), cognitive impairment, poor premorbid adjustment, persistent unemployment, poor response to antipsychotic medications, electroencephalogram abnormalities, and incidence of extrapyramidal side effects with antipsychotic drug treatment. In contrast, the ventricle-to-brain ratio is inversely correlated with psychotic symptoms. Ventricular enlargement does not correlate with the extent or duration of neuroleptic treatment, the use of electroconvulsive therapy (ECT), or the length of previous hospitalization.

The portions of the lateral ventricles that appear enlarged to the greatest extent are the temporal horns; enlargement in this region is evident even in new onset cases and has been confirmed in postmortem studies. This observation suggests that reduced tissue volume in the temporal lobe may account for enlargement of the ventricles. Consistent with this hypothesis, numerous studies have shown that temporal lobe volume is reduced in individuals with schizophrenia relative to healthy controls, particularly in the left hemisphere.

Investigators that have segmented gray and white matter have also reported that the volume of temporal lobe gray matter is decreased in schizophrenia. Within the temporal lobe, the most consistent findings are of reduced volume of the hippocampus, present even during the first episode.

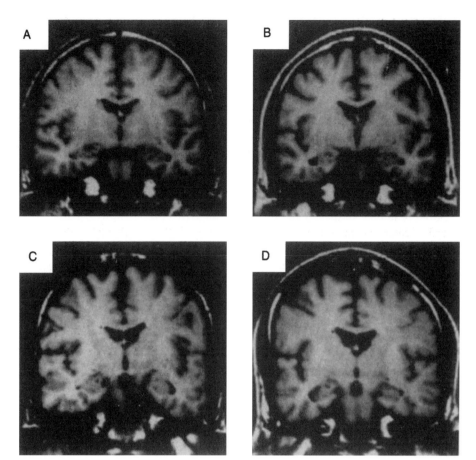

Fig. 6.5 MRI coronal views from two sets of monozygotic twins discordant for schizophrenia showing subtle enlargement of the lateral ventricles in the affected twins (B and D) as compared with their unaffected co-twins (A and C). Differences are apparent even when the affected twin had small ventricles. (From Suddath, RL, *et al.* (1990) *New Engl J Med* 399:791.)

Other regions of reduced volume in temporal lobe include the superior temporal gyrus and the parahippocampal gyrus. There are also reports of reduced amygdala volume, although this finding has not been confirmed by other studies. Postmortem neuropathological studies of schizophrenia have reported morphometric and cytoarchitectural abnormalities in some of these temporal lobe regions. The size reduction in the superior temporal gyrus, a putative auditory association area, correlates with the severity of auditory hallucinations, disordered thought flow, and reduced amplitude of the P300 component of the auditory event-related potential.

The size of the third ventricle is also consistently enlarged in subjects with schizophrenia relative to controls. This observation suggests that the tissue volume of structures lining the third ventricle, such as the thalamus and the midline forebrain limbic nuclei, may also be reduced in schizophrenia. Clinical correlates of the size of the third ventricle-to-brain ratio have been inconsistent, suggesting that third ventricle enlargement is present in a broader segment of patients with schizophrenia than lateral ventricle enlargement.

Studies of frontal lobe volume in schizophrenia have provided equivocal results, with one review suggesting that about 60% of studies find reduced frontal lobe volume in schizophrenia. However, the majority of these studies evaluated the volume of the entire frontal lobe rather than specific subregions. More recent studies have looked at specific subregions and provided evidence for reduced dorsolateral and orbitofrontal volumes, although additional research is needed to establish these findings. Several studies have also suggested that the width of the cortical sulci appears increased in schizophrenia as determined by semistructured qualitative ratings or quantitative measurements of sulcal or gyral width. Several of these studies have further reported that this sulcal widening is most pronounced in the PFC, a finding that is compatible with the results of postmortem studies indicating that neuronal organization is abnormal in parts of the prefrontal cortex in schizophrenia.

Changes in the volume of structures in the basal ganglia have also been reported in MRI studies of schizophrenia, with over 65% of studies reporting positive findings. Interestingly, most of the studies finding differences report increased basal ganglia volume (particularly caudate) among individuals with schizophrenia. However, previous antipsychotic drug exposure may play a critical role in increasing caudate volume, although this effect may be restricted to conventional neuroleptics and may not be seen with atypical neuroleptics that have relatively less inhibitory effects on dopamine D2 receptors. In studies of never-medicated individuals with schizophrenia, several groups have reported decreased rather than increased caudate volume.

A growing number of studies have also focused on the thalamus, although this structure has historically been difficult to segment with MRI because of reduced gray/white contrast. The majority of these studies (58%) report no differences between controls and patients. However, studies applying novel MRI imaging techniques specifically designed to image the thalamus are expected to yield more accurate results and are beginning to suggest evidence of reduced thalamic volume in schizophrenia.

Seven of ten CT studies reported that on qualitative inspection, cerebellar size is abnormally small in 5% to 17% of subjects with schizophrenia and in only 1% of controls. Consistent with the observation that reduced cerebellar size may exist in only a subset of subjects with schizophrenia, quantitative MRI studies have not consistently identified differences in the mean cerebellar volume when entire samples of schizophrenic and control subjects are compared, with approximately 70% of studies finding no quantitative differences between control and patients.

Resting blood flow and metabolism

Studies examining resting blood flow and metabolism in individuals with schizophrenia have provided mixed results. For example, several major reviews have concluded that "hypofrontality" (lower frontal/whole brain blood flow) among individuals with schizophrenia is not very robust when compared to controls and that patients and controls overlap to a considerable extent in meta-analyses. Nonetheless, there is some suggestion that individuals with negative symptoms may be more likely to show hypofrontality in resting blood flow.

One PET study demonstrated increased blood flow in the globus pallidus of subjects with schizophrenia who had never been treated with medications. A postmortem anatomical study reported that the volume of the pallidum is reduced in patients with schizophrenia, corroborating the potential importance of this structure in the pathophysiology of schizophrenia. Regional blood flow in a ventral striatal area located in the vicinity of the globus pallidus was shown to correlate with a "reality distortion" factor that reflected psychosis ratings.

Finally, metabolism in limbic structures such as the hippocampus and the anterior cingulate gyrus are reportedly reduced in schizophrenia. Psychosis ratings have been shown to correlate positively with blood flow in the left medial temporal cortex (in the vicinity of the hippocampus) and negatively with blood flow in the posterior cingulate gyrus in medicated subjects with chronic schizophrenia. Metabolism increases in parts of the temporal lobe following treatment, although it is unclear whether this change extends to the hippocampus.

Activation studies in schizophrenia

Many researchers have suggested that studies of cognitive and emotional activation are more likely to reveal important differences in functional brain activity in schizophrenia in comparison to resting blood flow studies. Consistent with this hypothesis, numerous studies have demonstrated changes in the activation of PFC, particularly dorsolateral PFC, in response to cognitive challenge among individuals with schizophrenia. The majority of these studies have used tasks thought to rely on the integrity of PFC, including measures of executive function such as the Wisconsin Card Sorting Task, The Tower of London, and verbal fluency, as well as measures of working memory (the ability to maintain and manipulate information over short periods of time).

In the majority of studies, individuals with schizophrenia have shown reduced prefrontal activation as compared to controls. Although patients with schizophrenia tend to perform worse than controls on these executive function and working memory tasks, the reduced task-related prefrontal activity appears to remain even after potential confounds associated with reduced performance and increased movement have been addressed. In a few studies, individuals with schizophrenia and/or their first degree relatives have shown increased dorsolateral prefrontal activation as compared to controls. Such results have been interpreted as evidence that the efficiency of neural processing is impaired in the prefrontal cortex. Findings of abnormal prefrontal cortex activity in response to cognitive challenge have been reported in never-medicated patients experiencing their first episode of schizophrenia as well as in medication-withdrawn individuals with chronic schizophrenia, and thus they do not appear to be explained by medication effects or illness chronicity. In some studies, the degree of reduced prefrontal activity in response to cognitive challenge has correlated with the severity of specific types of symptoms, such as disorganization (i.e., thought disorder, disorganized behavior), although other studies have been unable to replicate these results.

A growing number of studies have also found reductions in medial temporal lobe activity, including hippocampal activity, among individuals with schizophrenia. These results are consistent with numerous structural studies suggesting abnormalities in this region. The majority of these studies have used cognitive tasks designed to measure episodic memory (the ability to learn and retrieve new information), a cognitive domain thought to be particularly dependent on medial temporal lobe function, although a few studies have also found abnormal hippocampal activity in schizophrenia during working memory or executive function tasks. As described above, individuals with schizophrenia tend to perform worse than controls on episodic memory tasks, and more work is needed to determine the influence of behavioral performance on reduced task-related activity in medial temporal cortex in schizophrenia.

Although much of the functional neuroimaging literature

in schizophrenia has focused on deficits in prefrontal and temporal cortex, a growing number of studies suggest that patients also consistently demonstrate deficits in anterior cingulate cortex functions. Such anterior cingulate cortex disturbances have been found during the performance of both working memory and episodic memory tasks, as well as during the performance of verbal fluency tasks and response conflict tasks such as the Stroop task. In addition, several studies have noted disturbances in the functional activation of the thalamus in patients with schizophrenia during the performance of both working memory and episodic memory tasks.

Limitations of resting blood flow/metabolism and cognitive challenge studies

The interpretation of functional imaging data in schizophrenia, whether from resting studies or cognitive challenge studies, is potentially complicated by the neuromorphological abnormalities (such as enlarged ventricles, reduced hippocampal, and temporal lobe size) identified in structural imaging studies and the histopathological changes reported in postmortem studies. The former may produce partial volume effects that potentially influence, or even account for, the blood flow and metabolic decreases in the hippocampus and the temporal and frontal lobes.

The cytoarchitectural abnormalities include changes in the organization of neuronal layers in the hippocampus and reductions in the quantity of axonal processes in cortical layer II of the anterior cingulate gyrus. Such cytoarchitectural abnormalities may alter local synaptic activity and regional physiology, confounding the interpretation of functional imaging differences between schizophrenic and control subjects. Few studies have tried to address these issues by examining the relationship between structural abnormalities and functional activation disturbances in schizophrenia. Such studies have generally not found relationships between the volume of brain regions and functional brain activation in the same brain regions (though relationships have been found between decreased dorsolateral prefrontal cortex activity and both increased ventricular size and reduced hippocampal volume).

Neuroreceptor imaging in schizophrenia

Studies that have assessed dopamine D_2 receptor density in the striatum in unmedicated subjects with schizophrenia have produced conflicting results. Studies performed using PET and the tracer [11C]N-methylspiperone have found elevated D_2 density in some, though not all, patients with schizophrenia. In contrast, studies using PET and the tracer [11C]-raclopride or SPECT and [123I]-IBZM have not found significantly elevated D_2 receptor densities. In addition, a study using PET and [76Br]-bromospiperone found no differences between untreated patients and controls, and another using SPECT and [77Br]-bromospiperone found only a 10%

increase in the striatal uptake in subjects with schizophrenia relative to controls.

One explanation for the discrepancies is the dissimilarities in the specificity of these ligands, which have differential affinities for D_2, D_3, and D_4 receptors (all D_2 "family" receptors). For example, benzamide derivates such as raclopride bind to only D_2 and D_3 receptors, while butyrophenone derivatives such as spiperone bind to D_2, D_3, and D_4 receptors. However, recent research suggests that differential affinities for the D_4 receptor cannot explain discrepancies across studies, as the striatum contains too few D_4 relative to D_2 receptors to account for the magnitude of differences across studies. Another potential explanation is that endogenous dopamine concentrations affect displacement of benzamine and butyrophenone compounds differently, potentially contributing to the dissimilar results across studies.

This sensitivity of some dopamine D_2 receptor ligands to endogenous dopamine concentrations has been exploited to examine amphetamine-induced dopamine release in individuals with schizophrenia. In such studies, striatal D_2 receptor availability is measured prior to and after administration of intravenous amphetamine in unmedicated individuals with schizophrenia, using either SPECT and [123I]-IBZM or PET and [11C]-raclopride. Amphetamine induces dopamine release, which in turn leads to agonist-mediated receptor internalization, and consequent displacement of these radiotracers. These studies have consistently shown a larger amphetamine-induced decrease in tracer binding among individuals with schizophrenia as compared to controls, which is interpreted as reflecting a larger amphetamine-induced release of dopamine. Similar results have been found in medication-naive as well as medication-withdrawn patients with schizophrenia.

A few studies have also used PET radioligands to image D_1 receptor density in schizophrenia. The results of these studies disagree. One group found decreased densities of cortical D_1 receptors in the cingulate, prefrontal and temporal cortices. However, a more recent study found increased cortical D_1 receptor density in dorsolateral prefrontal cortex in individuals with schizophrenia. In this study, the elevation of dorsolateral prefrontal cortical D_1 receptor density strongly predicted poor working memory performance in the patients with schizophrenia. There were a number of methodological differences between these two studies, including their use of different radioligands, and further research is needed to elucidate alterations in D_1 receptor density and function in schizophrenia.

Magnetic resonance spectroscopy in schizophrenia

The most consistently reported finding from proton magnetic resonance spectroscopy studies of schizophrenia has been that N-acetylaspartate (NAA) is abnormally reduced in the hippocampus and frontal cortex. NAA is thought to measure neuronal integrity and reduced levels may reflect cell death, neuronal energetic compromise in cell bodies, and/or shrinkage or insult to axons. A few studies have found reduced NAA levels in both frontal and temporal lobes in unmedicated or never-medicated individuals with schizophrenia, but recent studies suggest that conventional antipsychotic drug treatment may influence NAA concentrations in individuals with schizophrenia.

The relationship between reduced NAA levels in frontal cortex and symptoms has not been consistent across studies, with some studies showing relationships to positive symptoms and others to negative symptoms. In addition, reduced NAA levels in frontal cortex have been associated with altered PFC activity in response to cognitive challenge in patients with schizophrenia.

Significance of neuroimaging abnormalities in schizophrenia

The most frequently cited explanation for the structural and functional alterations associated with schizophrenia is that they are neurodevelopmental in origin, reflecting some combination of genetic and environmental factors. Such explanations are consistent with the observation that many aspects of structural change (such as ventricular enlargement) and functional alterations are not correlated with age or illness chronicity and are demonstrable in patients suffering their first episode of the illness. Such results suggest that both structural and functional changes are present early in the disease course and change little over time (although some recent research challenges this latter assumption).

Postmortem studies of schizophrenia have noted a conspicuous absence of gliosis (an activation of neuroglia that accompanies neurodegenerative conditions), which argues against the presence of a neurodegenerative process. Postmortem studies have instead found regionally decreased tissue volume along with abnormal cytoarchitecture, supporting neurodevelopmental hypotheses for the etiology of schizophrenia.

It should also be noted that abnormalities affect multiple brain regions in schizophrenia and that lesions or dysfunction involving single structures are unlikely to explain either the entire disorder or specific symptoms. Schizophrenia instead appears to involve multiple and widespread brain circuits that support a variety of cognitive and emotional processes. Some researchers have thus suggested that the primary abnormality in schizophrenia is a disturbance in the connectivity between brain regions rather than disturbances intrinsic to any one region. The brain regions implicated in schizophrenia include the dorsolateral PFC, the medial temporal cortex, the anterior cingulate cortex, and anatomically related areas of the thalamus and basal ganglia. The anatomical connections among these regions form circuits that support cognitive processes such as working memory, episodic memory, language production, and behavioral in-

hibition, which are known to be impaired in schizophrenia. Understanding the functional connectivity of such brain regions in schizophrenia is being actively pursued using neuroimaging methodologies such as diffusion tensor imaging, a MRI technique that allows assessment of the integrity of white matter fiber tracts connecting brain regions, and multivariate analytic techniques that mathematically model the functional connectivity among brain regions during cognitive challenge.

Mood disorders

Mood disorders are particularly well suited for functional imaging studies because they appear to be associated with neurochemical changes but not with gross neuropathological changes (see Chapter 8) and their episodic nature and excellent response to treatment permit imaging in both symptomatic and asymptomatic states. Functional imaging studies may thus be capable of differentiating the physiological correlates of emotional symptoms from the pathophysiological changes that underlie the tendency to develop abnormal mood episodes. In addition, since the symptoms of mood disorders represent exaggerations or extensions of cognitive and emotional states that can be expressed by nondepressed subjects, the nature of blood flow or metabolic changes related to the depressed state can be explored by imaging normal subjects during experimentally induced sadness, anxiety, or sleep deprivation.

Mood disorder studies have largely been limited to depressed subjects because of the difficulties involved in scanning subjects in the manic state. The results of imaging studies of depression have appeared widely discrepant, with some studies reporting increases in PFC activity and others finding decreases or no differences in the PFC in depressed subjects relative to controls. However, some of these discrepancies appear related to methodological issues such as the depressive subtype selected, the presence of medication effects, and the location of the region-of-interest within the PFC.

Methodological issues in neuroimaging studies of mood disorders
Sample selection: the problem of heterogeneity
A major challenge facing imaging studies of mood disorders stems from the likelihood that the major depressive syndrome encompasses a heterogenous group of disorders (see Chapter 8). Besides the obvious clinical heterogeneity extant within affective disease, biological heterogeneity also exists. For example, neuroendocrine and neurochemical abnormalities are typically present in subgroups, but not entire samples, of depressed subjects. If major depression is associated with multiple pathophysiologic states, it is presumably associated with an assortment of functional brain images as well, and study results vary depending on the composition of the

subject sample. The imaging literature confirms this hypothesis, since subtyping depressed subjects has proven critical to reducing the variability of image data. Broad categories or subtypes that have been shown to have some neuroimaging findings that differ from each other include: (1) unipolar versus bipolar disorders; (2) "primary" depressive disorders versus depressive syndromes arising "secondary" to other psychiatric or medical disorders; and (3) late age-at-onset depression versus early age-at-onset depression (see Chapter 8).

Polarity of the subject sample

Bipolar disorder, in which both manic and depressive episodes occur, and unipolar depression (major depressive disorder), in which only depressive episodes occur, appear neurochemically, pharmacologically and, to some extent, genetically distinct. Unipolar and bipolar depressed subjects also differ in some of their respective structural and functional imaging correlates. For example, enlargement of the lateral and third ventricles has been consistently found in both young and elderly adults with bipolar disorder, but the ventricles appear normal in relatively young, non-delusional adults with unipolar depression. In addition, unipolar and bipolar depressed subjects appear physiologically distinct in parts of the dorsomedial, dorsolateral and ventral PFC and basal ganglia. Finally, morphometric studies show that major depressive disorder and bipolar disorder have similar gray matter reductions in the anterior cingulate cortex (ACC) ventral to the genu of the corpus callosum (that is, the subgenual ACC) but distinct volumetric abnormalities in the hippocampus and amygdala. In spite of such differences, many published studies have combined subjects with unipolar and bipolar depression without including separate comparisons based upon polarity. The results from such studies are consequently difficult to interpret.

Primary versus secondary depression

The results from studies of depressive syndromes that arise secondary to neurological disorders, drug withdrawal states, or other psychiatric disorders have in some cases differed from those reported for primary major depressive episodes arising in the absence of other psychiatric or general medical conditions. One group reported that in subjects with either Parkinson's disease or Huntington's disease, metabolism in the orbital cortex was decreased in depressed relative to non-depressed subjects with the same neurological disorder, a finding that was opposite in direction to the results from young subjects with primary depression. Another group confirmed this finding in depressed subjects with Parkinson's disease. In addition, this group found decreased blood flow in depressed relative to non-depressed patients with Parkinson's disease in a dorsal ACC region where blood flow decreases had also been identified in cog-

nitively impaired subjects with primary depression. Finally, in another study, prefrontal cortical activity did not differ between depressed and non-depressed subjects with basal ganglia infarctions.

These data suggest that results from functional imaging studies in secondary depressive syndromes are more heterogenous than those in primary depression, and may, in some cases, substantially differ between primary and secondary depressed subjects. This parallels the functional imaging findings in primary and secondary obsessive-compulsive syndromes, in which ventral prefrontal cortical metabolism is increased in the former, but decreased or unchanged in the latter (see below). Taken together, the neuroimaging results in primary and secondary depression support a neural model in which mood disorders are associated with dysfunctional interactions between multiple structures rather than increased or decreased activity in a single structure (Fig. 6.6; see also Fig. 8.1).

Confounding effects of medications in studies of depression

Most functional imaging studies in depression have been confounded by medication effects. Administration of antidepressant, antipsychotic or antianxiety drugs in the hours or days prior to scanning has been demonstrated to produce areas of decreased blood flow and metabolism in the PFC and limbic areas that are of interest in depression. It is thus unclear how reports of blood flow or metabolic decreases in medicated subjects can be interpreted if unmedicated baseline scans have not also been acquired.

Structural neuroimaging studies and correlation with relevant neuropathological data

Enlargement of cerebral ventricles

Similar to the findings in schizophrenia, CT and MRI investigations report abnormal lateral and third ventricle size in adults with bipolar disorder and in some subgroups with major depressive disorder (Fig. 6.7). In subjects with bipolar disorder, the magnitude of ventricular enlargement is similar to that found in subjects with schizophrenia. The increased ventricle-to-brain ratio in these studies has been reported to correlate with higher cortisol levels, hypothyroidism, CSF concentrations of the serotonin metabolite 5-HIAA, psychotic symptoms, lower premorbid functioning, and cognitive impairment.

Ventricular enlargement has generally not been identified in samples limited to relatively young, non-delusional subjects with unipolar depression or to older subjects with unipolar depression with an early age-of-onset. Ventricular enlargement implies that tissue hypoplasia or atrophy has occurred in regions surrounding the ventricles, although the specific regions accounting for ventricular enlargement in the mood disordered subgroups showing these findings remain under investigation.

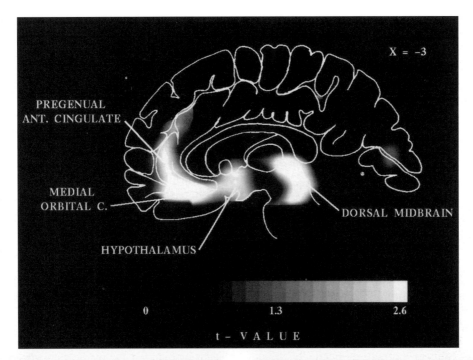

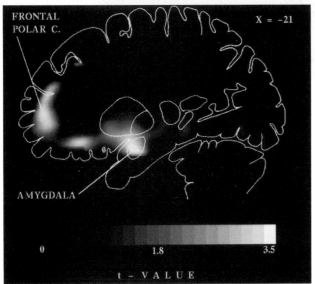

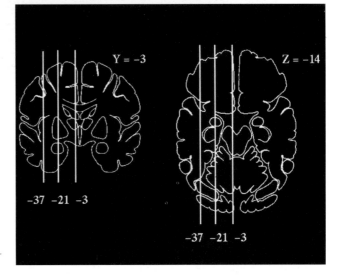

Fig. 6.6 Regional blood flow increases in subjects with unipolar depression who also meet criteria for familial pure depressive disease. The images shown are from an image of unpaired t-values, generated by subtracting composite images of mean blood flow from the depressed and control groups, and dividing the resulting difference image by the local variance. These statistical images were used to generate hypotheses regarding areas where regional activity may be abnormal in depression. The areas of significantly increased activity in depressed subjects relative to controls in the lateral orbital cortex (not shown), medial orbital cortex, the anterior insula (not shown), the pregenual anterior cingulate gyrus and the amygdala were subsequently confirmed using both regional blood flow and glucose metabolic image data from independent subject samples. Although no attempt was made to replicate the findings in the midbrain and hypothalamus because of the small size of these structures with respect to the spatial resolution of PET, both areas have been implicated in emotional expression and major depressive disorder by other types of information (see Chapter 8). The position of the two sagittal planes relative to the midline are indicated by the X coordinates, with negative X indicating left hemisphere. Anterior is toward the left. (Corresponding atlas outlines from Talairach, J and Tournoux, P (1988) *Co-Planar Stereotaxic Atlas of the Human Brain*, Stuttgart, Thieme.)

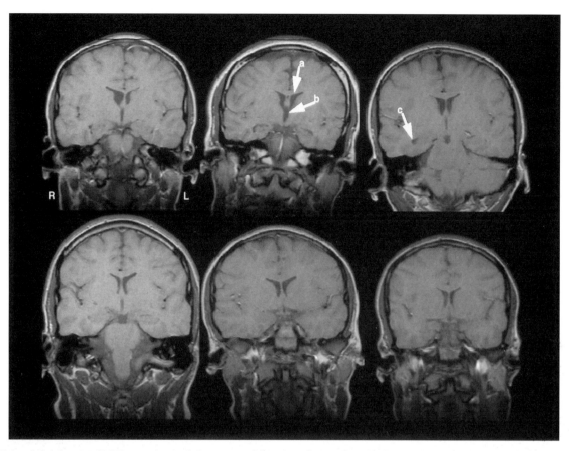

Fig. 6.7 T-1 weighted coronal MRI scans from adolescents with bipolar affective disorder (*top row*) compared with control subjects of similar ages (*bottom row*) demonstrating enlargement of the third ventricle (*b*), reversed asymmetry or prominence of the lateral ventricles (*a*), and the temporal horn of the lateral ventricles (*c*).

Frontal lobe structures

Although total cerebral and frontal lobe volumes have generally not differed between depressed and control samples, volumetric abnormalities of specific prefrontal cortical structures have been identified in many studies. The most prominent reductions have been identified within the subgenual ACC, where gray matter volume is decreased 20–40% in unipolar depressed subjects with familial pure depressive disease and subjects with familial bipolar disorder relative either to healthy controls or to mood-disordered subjects with no family history of mood disorders.

This finding has been confirmed by postmortem studies of clinically similar samples. Effective treatment with selective serotonin reuptake inhibitors did not alter the subgenual PFC *volume* in major depressive disorder, although this area appeared significantly larger in subjects with bipolar disorder who were chronically medicated with lithium or divalproex than in subjects with bipolar disorder who were either unmedicated or medicated with other agents. This finding is compatible with evidence that chronic administration of these mood stabilizers increases expression of the neuroprotective protein, Bcl-2, in the frontal cortex of experimental animals. The volume of the lateral orbital cortex has also been found to be reduced in both *in vivo* volumetric MRI studies and postmortem neuropathological studies of major depressive disorder.

Postmortem assessment of the subgenual ACC (the prelimbic portion of the anterior cingulate gyrus) demonstrated that this abnormal reduction in gray matter was associated with a *reduction* in glia, no equivalent loss of neurons, and increased neuronal density in major depressive disorder and bipolar disorder relative to healthy and schizophrenic control samples. In a tissue section that appeared to correspond to Brodmann area 24 cortex of the pregenual ACC, glial density was significantly reduced in layer VI in subjects with major depressive disorder or schizophrenia, but not in subjects with bipolar disorder (most of whom were receiving mood stabilizers which appear to exert neurotrophic/neuroprotective effects). The mean size of neurons was also reported to be reduced in the deep layers of subjects with major depressive disorder. These findings suggest that the volumetric abnormality in the subgenual PFC reflects a reduction of neuropil, the fibrous layers comprised of dendrites and axons that occupy most of the cortex volume.

Reductions in gray-matter volume and in the size of neurons and glia have also been reported in the dorsomedial/dorsal anterolateral PFC in major depressive disorder. Postmortem studies of major depressive disorder and bipolar disorder found abnormal reductions in the size of neurons and the density of glia in this region.

Temporal lobe structures

The volume of the entire temporal lobe has been reported to be decreased in subjects with bipolar disorder relative to healthy controls in some studies, but this finding has not been replicated by other studies of bipolar disorder and did not extend to major depressive disorder. Morphometric MRI studies of specific temporal lobe structures have more consistently reported significant reductions in hippocampal volume in major depressive disorder, with the magnitude of difference ranging from 8% to 19% relative to healthy controls. Some of these studies reported that the magnitude of the reduction in hippocampal volume was correlated with the total time spent depressed or number of depressive episodes. However, many groups have found no significant differences between samples with major depressive disorder and controls. The inconsistency in results may reflect methodological differences in the spatial resolution of the MRI images and pathophysiological heterogeneity encompassed within the criteria for major depressive disorder. For example, one study reported that hippocampal volume was abnormally decreased in depressed women who had a history of early-life trauma, but not in depressed women without early-life trauma or in women who had early-life trauma without depression.

Reductions in hippocampal volume were identified in two studies of bipolar disorder, but this finding has not been replicated by other studies. In postmortem studies of bipolar disorder, abnormal reductions in mRNA concentrations of synaptic proteins and in apical dendritic spines of pyramidal cells have been observed in the subicular and ventral CA1 subregions but not in most other hippocampal regions examined.

Two studies reported abnormalities of the hippocampal T1 MR signal in major depressive disorder. One observed that the T1 relaxation time was reduced in the hippocampus, but not in the entire temporal lobe, in subjects with unipolar depression relative to healthy controls, and another reported that elderly subjects with major depressive disorder have a higher number of areas showing low MR signal than age-matched controls in T1-weighted images. The significance of such abnormalities remains unclear.

There is conflicting literature regarding changes in the amygdala, with studies reporting that volume is abnormally increased, abnormally decreased, or unchanged from controls in both major depressive disorder and bipolar disorder. The extent to which the conflicting data in bipolar disorder are explained by medication effects remains unclear, since some mood stabilizers appear to exert neurotrophic/neuroprotective effects. Nevertheless, the reliability of amygdala volumetric data is limited by the ambiguity of some of this structure's boundaries in MRI images employed by extant studies (in which voxel size >1 mm^3). More recent studies that compared higher resolution MRI data (voxel size of 0.2 mm^3) obtained with higher field-strength magnets found that the amygdala volume is decreased in both the depressed and the remitted phase of major depressive disorder but is not significantly different in bipolar disorder, relative to healthy controls.

Basal ganglia

Some MRI studies reported that the volumes of structures in the basal ganglia are abnormally decreased in major depressive disorder. One study reported smaller putamen volumes in depressed subjects relative to controls, and two others found smaller caudate volumes in middle-aged or elderly depressed subjects relative to controls. One postmortem study reported that the volumes of both the caudate nuclei and the accumbens area were decreased in both major depressive disorder and bipolar disorder samples relative to controls. However, other recent MRI-based morphometric studies failed to find significant differences in caudate or lentiform nucleus (putamen plus globus pallidus) volumes between younger samples of subjects with unipolar depression and controls. In addition, MRI-based studies of bipolar disorder have not found significant differences in the volumes of basal ganglia structures with respect to controls. The factors accounting for the discrepant results across studies remain unclear.

Other cerebral structures

Morphometric studies of other brain structures in depression have produced less consistent results. One group reported that the thalamic volume was decreased in individuals with unipolar depression relative to controls, but another did not replicate this finding. Two studies of thalamic volume in bipolar disorder also reported conflicting results. Two MRI studies reported that vermal volume in the cerebellum is reduced in depressed subjects relative to controls, while a third did not.

Endocrine glands

Consistent with evidence that hypothalamic-pituitary-adrenal axis function is elevated in some subgroups of mood disorders, enlargement of the adrenal and pituitary glands has been reported in major depressive disorder. Between 30% and 50% of depressed subjects who underwent abdominal CT were judged to have enlarged adrenal glands; mean adrenal volumes have been reported to be 50–70% greater in depressed subjects than controls. One of these studies also showed that median adrenal volume of the depressed subjects decreased to approximately that of controls in a second scan acquired following remission. The results of these studies are potentially consistent with the finding that mean adrenal gland weight is abnormally increased in suicide victims. The cause of adrenal hypertrophy in major depressive disorder is putatively related to chronically elevated stimulation of the adrenal cortex by ACTH. Pituitary size was also reported to be enlarged in one MRI study of depression.

Abnormalities of corpus callosal volume in mood disorders

The genual subsection of the corpus callosum is reduced in volume in both depressed women and their high-risk, female offspring, studied between ages 10 and 14. These white-matter regions contain the transcallosal fibers that connect the orbital cortex, ACC, and dorsomedial/dorsal anterolateral PFC regions with their homologous cortices in the contralateral hemisphere. This result was evident in female offspring of mothers who suffered from major depressive disorder but not bipolar disorder. Insufficient numbers of males were studied to determine whether the abnormality extended to males. Of other corpus callosal regions studied, only the splenial sector differed between samples. This portion contains transcallosal fibers from the posterior cingulate cortex, a structure that is also implicated in major depressive disorder (see below).

Signal hyperintensities

Another type of neuromorphological abnormality in patients with mood disorders is manifested by signal hyperintensities in the deep white matter of T2-weighted MRI scans. These hyperintensities are seen in 25–50% of MRI scans in healthy nondemented elderly control subjects and in 5–10% of young healthy control subjects. In contrast, they appear in one-sixth to one-third of subjects with Type I bipolar disorder and in about two-thirds of elderly, unipolar depressed subjects with a late age-of-depression-onset (defined either as onset after age 55 or 60). The size of such white-matter hyperintensities is also increased in these samples with mood disorders compared with age-matched control groups (Fig. 6.8). Other disorders in which deep white-matter hyperintensities appear larger and more prevalent include multiple sclerosis, multi-infarct dementia, CNS infections and perinatal injuries. Thus the nature and etiology of these hyperintensities may differ across disease states, reflecting pathophysiologic changes in the white matter related to anoxia, ischemia, demyelination or immune disorders.

In elderly depressed subjects, the presence of hyperintensities in the basal ganglia and the deep and periventricular white matter correlates with a late age-of-depression-onset and with atherosclerotic risk factors. In such cases the signal hyperintensities predominantly localize to the striatum, thalamus, and deep white matter of the frontal lobes in sites corresponding to the distribution of penetrating arterioles of the lenticulostriate, thalamoperforate, and medullary arter-

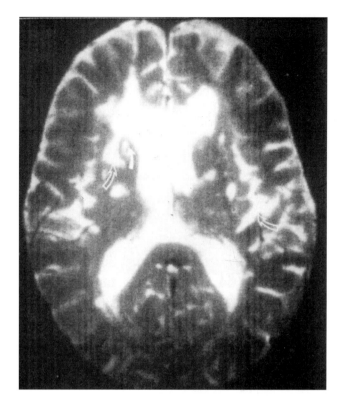

Fig. 6.8 Brain MRI, axial view through base of lateral ventricles showing large, confluent, deep white matter hyperintensities (*open arrows*) and hyperintensity in the right caudate head (*closed arrow*) in an elderly depressed patient. (Courtesy of Figiel, GS from Drevets, WC: *Brain Imaging in Psychiatry* in Sierles, FS (ed.) (1993) *Behavioral Science for Medical Students*, Baltimore, Williams and Wilkins.)

ies (Fig. 6.8). Postmortem assessments of the tissue containing such MRI signal hyperintensities demonstrate ischemia-related changes such as edema, dilated perivascular spaces, arteriosclerosis, and in the case of larger lesions, lacunar infarction. The presence of such abnormalities in late-onset, elderly depressed patients is associated with enlargement of the cerebral ventricles, which may reflect *ex vacuo* changes following ischemic damage. The presence of caudate hyperintensities or lacunae is associated with an elevated risk for the development of delirium during electroconvulsive or antidepressant drug therapy and extrapyramidal side effects during antipsychotic drug treatment. As discussed in Chapter 8, the anatomical locations where cerebral infarction has been associated with post-stroke depression are similar to the locations where signal hyperintensities are found in patients with late-onset depression (that is, in the left frontal lobes and the caudate). It is hypothesized that elderly depressed patients with a late age-of-onset acquire the mood disorder from an arteriosclerotic etiology, homologous to the case of post-stroke mood disorders.

In contrast to these observations in elderly depressed subjects, white-matter hyperintensities in young adult patients with bipolar disorder are not related to cerebrovascular risk factors, age, past treatment, or illness duration. Increased rates of MRI signal hyperintensities have been reported in one study of children and adolescents with bipolar disorder. The etiology of signal hyperintensities in these young subjects with bipolar disorder remains unclear, but it is likely to differ from that associated with late-onset depression.

Implications of structural abnormalities for functional imaging studies

The neuromorphometric abnormalities of ventricular enlargement in psychotic, elderly, or bipolar depressed patients, reduced frontal lobe size in bipolar or elderly depressed patients, and decreased temporal lobe size in subjects with bipolar disorder (see below) may produce partial volume effects in or adjacent to these structures. Thus, observed decreases in blood flow or metabolism in these areas in PET images from such subjects are difficult to interpret. Since studies evaluating young, non-delusional subjects with unipolar depression or subjects with unipolar depression characterized by young age-of-onset have generally failed to identify these neuromorphometric abnormalities, PET images from these groups have constituted the benchmark against which imaging findings in other depressive subtypes are compared. Nevertheless, preliminary evidence that even in young subjects with unipolar depression the amygdala, subgenual ACC, and parts of the PFC may be reduced in size indicate the importance of developing methods that correct PET measures for partial volume effects.

The deep white-matter and periventricular hyperintensities, caudate hyperintensities, and lacunar infarctions evident in the MRI images of elderly depressed patients present a greater problem for functional imaging studies. Since these hyperintensities appear to reflect arteriosclerotic/ischemic areas based upon perfusion imaging, postmortem histopathological assessment, and phosphorus-31 magnetic resonance spectroscopy evidence, they are presumably associated with reduced regional blood flow and metabolism on a cerebrovascular basis, irrespective of local synaptic activity. Consistent with the presence of ischemic/atherosclerotic changes, PET studies of elderly depressed subjects demonstrate diffuse areas of decreased blood flow and metabolism in the frontal cortex and other cortical and subcortical areas. (No attempt has been made in these studies to exclude subjects with MRI signal hyperintensities or lacunae.) Since corrections for the effects of these lesions in PET images are not possible, functional imaging studies that include elderly depressed subjects and report areas of decreased blood flow or metabolism with respect to controls can not be interpreted as reflecting differences in local neuronal activity, because the relationships between CBF, cerebral blood volume, oxygen extraction, and metabolism become altered in the presence of cerebrovascular disease. Nevertheless, studies using such patients as their own controls by imaging them before and after treatment may provide interpretable information. For example, one group showed that in elderly depressed patients imaged before and after either ECT or antidepressant drug therapy, successful treatment results in a *further decrement* in blood flow in the left prefrontal cortex. These findings converge with those from young unipolar depressed patients, in whom left prefrontal activity is elevated in the depressed phase relative to the remitted phase and decreases during effective treatment.

Functional imaging abnormalities in mood disorders

Prefrontal cortex (PFC)

The PFC comprises almost one-half of the human brain and contains numerous subdivisions based upon anatomical connectivity and cytoarchitectonic distinctions. The results of lesion analyses, electrophysiological, and functional imaging studies indicate that the PFC has myriad functional components, with distinct areas activated during language, attention, memory, motor planning, and emotion. The regions implicated in mood disorders are predominantly areas that have been shown to play roles in modulating emotional behavior.

The ACC situated ventral and anterior to the genu of the corpus callosum (termed "subgenual" and "pregenual," respectively) shows complex relationships between CBF, metabolism, and illness state, which appear to be explained by a left-lateralized reduction of the corresponding cortex, initially demonstrated by MRI-based morphometric measures and later by postmortem neuropathological studies of bipolar disorder and major depressive disorder. This reduction in volume exists early in the illness in familial bipolar disorder and major depressive disorder, but it may follow illness onset based upon preliminary evidence in twins discordant for major depressive disorder. One study reported that subgenual ACC metabolism correlated inversely with the number of lifetime depressive episodes.

Although baseline CBF and metabolism appear abnormally decreased in the subgenual ACC in PET images during major depressive episodes, computer simulations that correct PET data for the partial volume effect of reduced gray matter volume conclude the "actual" metabolic activity in the remaining subgenual PFC tissue is *increased* in depressed subjects relative to controls and decreases to normative levels during effective treatment. This hypothesis appears compatible with observations that effective antidepressant pharmacotherapy results in a *decrease* in metabolic activity in this region in major depressive disorder, that during depressive episodes metabolism shows a positive relationship with depression severity, and that blood flow increases in this region in healthy, non-depressed humans when sadness is induced via contemplation of sad thoughts or memories.

Some studies have reported that CBF and metabolism are increased in the pregenual ACC with major depressive disorder, while others reported abnormal reductions in activity. The variability of these results may have clinical relevance, as several studies report relationships between pregenual ACC activity and subsequent antidepressant treatment outcome. Depressed subjects who show increased flow or metabolism relative to controls prior to treatment have been reported to show positive clinical responses to both antidepressant drug treatment and total sleep deprivation, whereas subjects showing abnormally reduced metabolism at baseline had a poor treatment response. Similarly, a tomographic EEG analysis found that depressed subjects who ultimately showed the greatest clinical response to nortriptyline showed hyperactivity (higher theta activity) in the pregenual ACC at baseline, as compared to subjects showing poorer response. The effects of treatment on pregenual ACC flow and metabolism have also differed across studies, with activity decreasing in most PET studies, but increasing in some SPECT studies in post- relative to pre-treatment scans. The extent to which these discrepant findings are explained by differential effects across subregions of this area or between technical aspects of PET versus SPECT technology remains unclear.

It appears from animal studies that the cortex homologous to human subgenual ACC has extensive reciprocal connections with areas implicated in the expression of behavioral, autonomic and endocrine responses to threat, stress, or reward/nonreward, such as the orbital cortex, lateral hypothalamus, amygdala, accumbens, subiculum, ventral tegmentum, raphe, locus coeruleus, periaqueductal gray (PAG), and nucleus tractus solitarius (NTS). Humans with lesions that include subgenual PFC show abnormal autonomic responses to emotionally provocative stimuli and inability to experience emotion related to concepts that ordinarily evoke emotion. Rats with experimental lesions of prelimbic cortex also demonstrate altered autonomic, behavioral, and neuroendocrine responses to stress and fear conditioned stimuli. Glucocorticoid receptors exist in this region that when stimulated, reduced stress-related hypothalamic pituitary axis (HPA) activity. In rats, bilateral or *right*-lateralized lesions of the prelimbic and infralimbic cortex *attenuate* sympathetic autonomic responses, stress-induced corticosterone secretion, and gastric stress pathology during restraint stress or exposure to fear-conditioned stimuli. In contrast, *left*-sided lesions of this area *increase* sympathetic autonomic arousal and corticosterone responses to restraint stress. These data suggest that the right subgenual PFC facilitates expression of visceral responses during emotional processing, while the left subgenual PFC modulates such responses. The left-lateralized gray matter reduction of the ventral ACC in major depressive disorder and bipolar disorder may thus contribute to dysregulation of neuroendocrine and autonomic function in depression.

The pregenual ACC has anatomical connectivity similar to the subgenual ACC. The pregenual ACC shows elevated CBF during a greater variety of emotional conditions elicited in healthy controls or people with anxiety disorders. Electrical stimulation of this region elicits fear, panic or a sense of foreboding in humans and vocalization in experimental animals.

The pre- and subgenual ACC also appear to participate in evaluating the reward-related significance of stimuli. These areas send efferent projections to the ventral tegmental area (VTA) and substantia nigra, and they receive dense dopaminergic innervation from the VTA. In rats, electrical or glutamatergic stimulation of medial PFC areas that include prelimbic cortex elicits burst firing patterns from dopamine cells in the VTA and increases dopamine release in the accumbens. These phasic, burst firing patterns of dopamine neurons appear to encode information regarding stimuli that predict reward and deviations between such predictions and occurrence of reward. Ventral ACC dysfunction may thus conceivably contribute to disturbances of hedonic perception and motivated behavior in mood disorders. The extent of abnormal activity in the subgenual PFC may relate to switches between depression and mania, as subgenual PFC activity appears abnormally increased in manic subjects.

Dorsomedial/dorsal anterolateral PFC
Many studies reported abnormally decreased CBF and metabolism in areas of the dorsolateral and dorsomedial PFC in major depressive disorder. The dorsomedial region where flow and metabolism are decreased appears to include the dorsal ACC and an area rostral to the dorsal ACC involving cortex on the medial and lateral surface of the superior frontal gyrus (approximately corresponding to Brodmann area 9, and possibly 32). Postmortem studies of major depressive disorder and bipolar disorder have found abnormal reductions in the size of neurons and/or the density of glia in this portion of Brodmann area 9 that may be related to the reduction in metabolism in this region in the unmedicated depressed condition, as well as to the failure of antidepressant drug treatment to correct metabolism in these areas. It is noteworthy that remitted subjects with major depressive disorder who experience depressive relapse during tryptophan depletion have increased metabolic activity within these areas. This region would thus appear similar to other structures where histopathological and gray matter volume changes exist in depression insofar as they show increased glucose utilization in depressed relative to remitted conditions.

Blood flow normally increases in the vicinity of this dorsomedial/dorsal anterolateral PFC in healthy humans as they perform tasks that elicit emotional responses or require emotional evaluations. In healthy humans scanned during anxious anticipation of an electrical shock, CBF increases in this region to an extent that correlates inversely with changes in anxiety ratings and heart rate, suggesting that this region functions to attenuate emotional expression. In rats, lesions of the dorsomedial PFC result in exaggerated heart rate responses to fear-conditioned stimuli. Stimulation of these sites attenuates defensive behavior and cardiovascular responses evoked by amygdala stimulation, although the homolog to these areas in primates has not been established. In primates, the Brodmann area 9 cortex sends efferent projections to the lateral PAG and the dorsal hypothalamus through which it may modulate cardiovascular responses associated with emotional behavior. It is thus conceivable that dysfunction of the dorsomedial/dorsal anterolateral PFC may impair the ability to modulate emotional responses in mood disorders.

In contrast, the reduction in CBF in the dorsal ACC appears reversible with treatment, and has been associated with impaired mnemonic and attentional processing derived from neuropsychological test scores obtained near the time of scanning. This area has been implicated in selective attention during cognitive tasks, and hemodynamic activity decreases in this area in healthy subjects during anxious anticipation of a painful electrical shock. The reciprocal pattern of activation/deactivation in this region during cognitive versus emotional processing is hypothesized to relate to attentional impairments during depression.

Lateral orbital/ventrolateral PFC
In the lateral orbital cortex, ventrolateral PFC, and anterior insula, CBF and metabolism have been found to be abnormally increased in *unmedicated* subjects with primary major depressive disorder scanned while resting with eyes closed. The elevated activity in these areas appears mood-state dependent, and during treatment with somatic antidepressant therapies blood flow and metabolism decrease in these regions. The relationship between depression severity and physiological activity in the lateral orbital cortex/ventrolateral PFC is complex. While CBF and metabolism increase in these areas in the depressed relative to the remitted phase of major depressive disorder, the magnitude of these measures is inversely correlated with ratings of depressive ideation and severity. Moreover, while metabolic activity is abnormally increased in these areas in treatment-responsive, unipolar and bipolar depressed subjects, more severely ill or treatment refractory samples show CBF and metabolic values lower than or not different from those of controls. This inverse relationship between orbital cortex/ventrolateral PFC activity and ratings of depression severity also appears to extend to some other emotional states. For example, posterior orbital cortex flow also increases in subjects with obsessive-compulsive disorder or simple animal phobias during exposure to phobic stimuli and in healthy subjects during induced sadness, with the change in posterior orbital CBF correlating inversely with changes in obsessive thinking, anxiety, and sadness, respectively.

These data appear consistent with electrophysiological data and lesion analyses showing that parts of the orbital cortex participate in modulating behavioral and visceral responses associated with defensive, emotional, and reward-directed behavior as reinforcement contingencies change. These cells are thought to play roles in extinguishing unreinforced responses to aversive or appetitive stimuli via their anatomical projections to neurons in the amygdala, striatum, hippocampal subiculum, hypothalamus, periaqueductal gray, and other limbic and brainstem structures. The orbital cortex and amygdala send overlapping projections to each of these structures as well as to each other through which they appear to modulate each other's neural transmission.

Activation of the orbital cortex during depression may thus reflect endogenous attempts to attenuate emotional expression or interrupt unreinforced aversive thought and emotion. Consistent with this hypothesis, cerebrovascular lesions and tumors involving the frontal lobe increase the risk for developing major depression, with the orbital cortex being specifically implicated as the area where such lesions result in increased risk for depression. These observations also suggest that the reduction of CBF and metabolism in the orbital cortex and ventrolateral PFC during antidepressant drug treatment may not be a primary mechanism through which such agents ameliorate depressive symptoms. Instead, direct inhibition of pathological limbic activity in areas such as the amygdala and ventral ACC may modulate the pathophysiology associated with the production of depressive symptoms. The neurons in the orbital cortex may consequently "relax," as reflected by the return of metabolism to normal levels as antidepressant drug therapy attenuates the pathological limbic activity to which these neurons putatively respond.

The lateral orbital cortex also participates in integrating experiential stimuli with emotional salience and in associating reward-directed behavioral responses with the outcome of such responses, allowing redirection of behavior as reinforcement contingencies change. The lateral orbital cortex area implicated in major depressive disorder includes Brodmann area 47, which receives projections from sensory association cortices and shares extensive, reciprocal, anatomical connections with the amygdala, ACC, ventral striatum, hypothalamus, and other structures involved in the processing of rewarding stimuli and behavioral incentive. The abnormal reduction in gray matter in this area in major depressive disorder may thus conceivably contribute to the deficits in generating motivated behavior and reward salience that are experienced during depression.

Amygdala
Neurophysiological activity in the amygdala is altered in some depressive subgroups both at rest and during exposure to emotionally valenced stimuli. Basal CBF and metabolism

are elevated in mood-disordered subgroups who meet criteria for familial pure depressive disease, major depressive disorder-melancholic subtype, Type II bipolar disorder, nonpsychotic Type I bipolar disorder, or who prove responsive to sleep deprivation. In contrast, metabolism has not been found to be abnormal in subjects with unipolar depression who meet criteria for depression spectrum disease or who meet DSM criteria for major depressive disorder as the sole inclusion criterion, although the interpretation of the latter results was confounded by technical problems that reduced sensitivity for measuring amygdala activity.

The magnitude of the abnormal elevation of flow and metabolism in familial pure depressive disease ranges from 5% to 7% measured with state-of-the-art PET cameras. When corrected for spatial resolution effects, this difference would reflect an increase in the actual CBF and metabolism of about 50–70%. Such magnitudes are in the physiological range, as CBF increases ~50% in the rat amygdala during exposure to fear-conditioned stimuli as measured by tissue autoradiography. Metabolism in the amygdala decreases toward normative levels during antidepressant treatment that both attenuates depressive symptoms and prophylaxes against relapse.

One study reported that while metabolism in the amygdala was increased in depressed subjects compared to controls during wakefulness, the increase in metabolism occurring in the amygdaloid complex during rapid eye movement (REM) sleep was also greater in depressed subjects than controls. If confirmed in a larger sample, these data would imply that amygdala hypermetabolism exists in major depressive disorder even when conscious processing of stressors is dormant. Although it is conceivable that the elevated physiological activity in the amygdala associated with depression reflects an exaggerated response to the stress of scanning, the amygdala's normal hemodynamic response to stressors or threats rapidly habituates and would not be expected to persist as long as the period required for ^{18}F-deoxyglucose uptake during glucose metabolism imaging.

Functional imaging data acquired when subjects view emotionally valenced stimuli that normally activate the amygdala also demonstrate altered physiological responses in major depressive disorder. In the left amygdala, the hemodynamic response to viewing fearful faces is blunted in depressed children and depressed adults. This finding is consistent with the elevation of basal CBF and metabolism observed in the *left* amygdala in such cases, because tissue that is physiologically activated is expected to show an attenuation of further rises in the hemodynamic/metabolic signal in response to tasks that normally engage the same tissue. The duration of the response in the amygdala to emotionally valenced stimuli is also abnormal in depression. Another study found that although the initial CBF response in the amygdala to sad faces was similar in depressed subjects and controls, this response habituated during repeated exposures to the same stimuli in the controls but not in the depressed subjects over the imaging period. Another study reported that hemodynamic activity increased in the amygdala during exposure to negatively valenced words to a similar extent in depressed subjects and controls, but while the hemodynamic response rapidly fell to baseline in the controls, it remained elevated for >30 sec in the depressed sample.

The amygdala plays major roles in organizing other behavioral, neuroendocrine, and autonomic aspects of emotional/stress responses to experiential stimuli. These roles are potentially compatible with reports that CBF and metabolism in the amygdala correlate positively with ratings of depression severity that assess both emotional and neurovegetative aspects of the major depressive syndrome. For example, the amygdala facilitates stress-related corticotropin releasing hormone (CRH) release, and electrical stimulation of the amygdala in humans increases cortisol secretion, suggesting a mechanism through which excessive activity in the amygdala may participate in inducing the CRH and cortisol hypersecretion that is evident in major depressive disorder. In healthy controls, i.v. bolus administration of hydrocortisone is associated with elevated glucose utilization 90 min after injection. In PET studies of major depressive disorder and bipolar disorder, CBF and metabolism in the left amygdala correlates positively with stressed plasma cortisol secretion, which may reflect either the effect of activity in the amygdala on CRH secretion or the effect of cortisol on the function of the amygdala.

Abnormalities in anatomically-related limbic and subcortical structures

The ventrolateral, ventral anterior cingulate and orbital PFC and the amygdala share extensive interconnections with the mediodorsal nucleus of the thalamus, the ventral striatum and the medial caudate. CBF and metabolism are abnormally elevated in the medial thalamus and ventral striatum during the depressed phase of major depressive disorder and bipolar disorder and decrease during antidepressant pharmacotherapy. Some PET studies reported that CBF and metabolism in the caudate were abnormally reduced in major depressive disorder. These abnormalities may be specific to subtype, as psychomotor slowed or melancholic subjects show decreased activity in the dorsal caudate. One study, however, reported that metabolism was abnormally increased in major depressive disorder and decreased during both paroxetine treatment and interpersonal psychotherapy.

Several groups reported abnormally increased CBF in the posterior cingulate cortex in the unmedicated, depressed phase of major depressive disorder, and some have shown that posterior cingulate flow and metabolism decreased during antidepressant treatment. One laboratory specifically reported that the elevation of posterior cingulate flow in depressed subjects relative to controls correlated positively with anxiety ratings. Exposure to aversive stimuli of various types results in increased physiological activity in the posterior cingulate cortex. The posterior cingulate cortex appears to serve as a sensory association cortex and may participate in processing the affective salience of sensory stimuli. The posterior cingulate cortex sends a major anatomical projection to the pregenual ACC, through which it may relay such information into the limbic circuitry.

Abnormalities in other brain areas
Abnormally increased CBF has also been consistently reported in the medial cerebellum in major depressive disorder. Flow is increased in this region in experimentally induced states of anxiety or sadness in healthy subjects and in anxiety states elicited in subjects with anxiety disorders. Activation of this structure during depression and anxiety may conceivably reflect either the activation of established anatomical loops between the cortex and cerebellum or the role of the paleocerebellum in modulating autonomic function.

Regional CBF and metabolic abnormalities have been less consistently replicated in other structures. In the lateral temporal and inferior parietal cortex, some studies found reduced regional CBF and metabolism. Some of these areas have been implicated in processing sensory information. The significance of reduced activity in such areas in depression remains unclear.

Implications for anatomical circuits related to depression

Because alterations in regional CBF and metabolism predominantly reflect a summation of energy utilization associated with terminal field synaptic transmission, interpreting the regional abnormalities in depression involves consideration of anatomical connectivity. The glucose metabolism signal (to which CBF is tightly coupled) is dominated by the energy utilization associated with glutamatergic transmission. The functional and structural imaging data in primary depression converge with evidence from lesion analysis studies to implicate circuits involving parts of the PFC and mesiotemporal cortex along with anatomically-related areas of the striatum, pallidum, and thalamus in the pathophysiology of depression. The abnormally increased CBF and metabolism in the ventrolateral and orbital PFC, ventral ACC, amygdala, ventral striatum, and medial thalamus evident in individuals with unipolar depression more specifically implicate a limbic-thalamo-cortical circuit involving the amygdala, the mediodorsal nucleus of the thalamus and the orbital and medial PFC, and a limbic-striatal-pallidal-thalamic circuit involving related parts of the striatum and the ventral pallidum as well as components of the other circuit (Chapter 8, Fig. 8.2).

Nevertheless, it is unclear how increased synaptic trans-

mission through this circuit would ultimately affect cellular activity in a particular structure. For example, the morphological, histochemical, and electrophysiological evidence collectively indicate that while the reciprocal prefrontal-amygdalar projections are excitatory in nature, these connections appear to ultimately activate inhibitory interneurons that in turn lead to functional inhibition in the projected field of the amygdala (for PFC to amygdalar projections) or the medial PFC and ventrolateral PFC. The function of the PFC in modulating the amygdala may be impaired in mood disorders, based upon evidence from (1) *in vivo* fMRI data showing that abnormally sustained amygdala activity in response to aversive words or sad faces in major depressive disorder is associated with blunted activation of PFC areas and (2) postmortem studies of major depressive disorder and bipolar disorder showing volumetric and/or histopathological changes in the subgenual and pregenual ACC, lateral orbital cortex, dorsomedial/dorsal anterolateral PFC, hippocampal subiculum, amygdala, and ventral striatum.

The histopathological correlates of these abnormalities include a reduction in glial cells with no equivalent loss of neurons, loss of synaptic markers or proteins, elevated neuronal density, and reduced neuronal size; these findings suggest a reduction in neuropil. While the pathogenesis of these changes has not been established, it is notable that the dendritic arborization that forms the neuropil can undergo atrophy or "reshaping" in some limbic/paralimbic structures of the adult brain by sustained exposure to physiological elevations of glucocorticoid secretion in the presence of activation of excitatory amino acid (i.e., glutamatergic) neurotransmission in stress-responsive neural circuits. Notably, chronic antidepressant drug administration and repeated electroconvulsive shocks also desensitize NMDA-glutamatergic receptors in the rat frontal cortex and increase expression of neurotrophic and neuroprotective factors that may protect the cortex from continuing loss of neuropil. The reduction in metabolism in these regions during chronic antidepressant drug treatment may thus signal the attenuation of elevated glutamatergic transmission through this circuit.

Synaptic transmission through these circuits may differ across depressive subtypes, since the lesions involving the PFC (i.e., tumors or infarctions) and diseases of the basal ganglia (e.g., Parkinson's or Huntington's diseases) that are associated with higher rates of depression than other similarly debilitating conditions result in dysfunction at distinct points within these circuits and affect synaptic transmission in diverse ways (see Chapter 8). A common substrate in these cases may be the dysfunction of frontal-striatal modulation of limbic and visceral functions, as both the idiopathic, neuropathological changes evident in the orbital and medial PFC and ventral striatum in primary mood disorders (see above) and those found in neurodegenerative conditions that can induce depressive syndromes (e.g., Parkinson's disease, Huntington's disease, cerebrovascular disease) would be expected to alter function within these regions.

This model also has relevance for considering the pathophysiology of neuropsychiatric syndromes that occur comorbidly with major depression. For example, neuroimaging studies implicate the same neural circuits in the pathophysiology of obsessive-compulsive disorder, providing insights into the common coincidence of depressive and obsessional syndromes (see below). Notably the differences found in the ventral PFC between primary and secondary depression parallel the findings in primary and secondary obsessive-compulsive syndromes, in which metabolism in the ventral PFC is increased in the former but decreased or unchanged in the latter.

Imaging neuroreceptors and neurotransmitter synthesis in mood disorders

The development of neuroreceptor radioligands is providing expanding capabilities for non-invasive quantitation of *in vivo* receptor binding and dynamic neurotransmitter function. While this area is expected to become an increasingly common application for PET and SPECT technology, radioligands are available for relatively few receptor types. Partly because of this limitation, the studies conducted to date in mood-disordered samples have largely been limited to assessments of monoamine receptor systems.

Dopamine receptor imaging

In bipolar disorder, one study reported that the binding potential for the dopamine D_1 receptor radioligand, [^{11}C]-SCH-23990, was below the age-adjusted normal range in the frontal cortex in 9 of 10 subjects scanned in a variety of mood states. This finding awaits replication using D_1 receptor ligands that are more amenable to quantitation. Another study showed that psychotic subjects with bipolar disorder have increased striatal uptake of [^{11}C]- N-methylspiperone binding, a ligand for D_2-like dopamine receptor sites, relative to controls or non-psychotic subjects with bipolar disorder. The striatal D_2 binding in the psychotic subjects correlated positively with psychosis ratings in this study.

In major depressive disorder, two SPECT studies using ^{123}I-iodobenzamide (IBZM), a dopamine D_2 receptor ligand that is sensitive to endogenous dopamine concentrations, found increased striatal dopamine D2/D3 receptor availability during the depressed phase, which could potentially be explained by a reduction of endogenous dopamine release. A third SPECT study found a nonsignificant trend toward increased [^{123}I]-IBZM binding in depressed subjects relative to controls, which became significant in a subgroup who displayed overt psychomotor retardation. Interpretation of these data was confounded, however, by the presence of drug effects. Moreover, a PET study of the dopamine D2/D3 receptor radioligand [^{11}C]-raclopride did not replicate these results and found no difference either in baseline

dopamine D2/D3 receptor binding or in the magnitude of dextroamphetamine-induced dopamine release in unmedicated subjects with major depressive disorder.

Other preliminary PET data appear compatible with the hypothesis that dopamine release is reduced in major depressive disorder. One study found decreased dopamine transporter binding in depressed subjects relative to controls, which could potentially reflect a compensatory effect to reduced dopamine release. Another reported abnormally reduced uptake of the catecholamine precursor [^{11}C]L-DOPA and the serotonin precursor [^{11}C]5-hydroxytryptophan across the blood-brain barrier in major depressive disorder (although, the *regional* [^{11}C]5-hydroxytryptophan utilization was *increased* in depressed subjects relative to controls in a ventromedial PFC area that included pregenual ACC). If confirmed, these data would suggest that the rate of dopamine synthesis is reduced in major depressive disorder.

Serotonin receptor imaging

Within the serotonin system, the most robust findings have been that both pre- and post-synaptic serotonin type 1A (5-HT_{1A}) receptor binding potential is abnormally decreased in major depressive disorder. These studies have demonstrated a reduction in 5-HT_{1A} receptor binding potential in unmedicated depressed subjects relative to healthy controls in the raphe, hippocampus, amygdala, temporopolar cortex, insula, anterior and posterior cingulate cortex, and left orbital cortex/ventrolateral PFC using PET and [*carbonyl*-^{11}C]WAY-100635. The magnitudes of these differences have been similar to those found in postmortem studies of subjects with *primary* mood disorders or depressed, non-alcoholic suicide victims. These data were also compatible with the results of studies showing that unmedicated subjects with major depressive disorder have blunted hypothermic response and adrenocorticotropin (ACTH) and cortisol release in response to 5-HT_{1A} receptor agonist challenge. Imaging data acquired both pre- and post-paroxetine treatment did not find significant treatment-associated changes in 5-HT_{1A} receptor binding potential in any area. Preliminary data also suggest that post-synaptic 5-HT_{1A} receptor binding potential is abnormally decreased in bipolar disorder in a variety of neocortical regions.

Neuroimaging studies of other serotonin binding sites found less prominent differences in depression. Serotonin type 2A (5HT_{2A}) receptor imaging studies of depression have generally not identified significant differences in binding potential between depressed samples and controls when age effects were controlled. The abnormal reductions in serotonin transporter binding in the raphe and ventral PFC reported in depressed suicide victims post mortem have also been identified in a SPECT-beta-CIT study but not in a PET study using [^{11}C]-McN5652. Serotonin transporter binding in the striatum was reported to be increased in one study of major depressive disorder, but unchanged in another study.

Anxiety disorders

The nature of anxiety disorders permits the acquisition of scans within a single session in both a "resting condition" and a state in which the anxiety syndrome is elicited or exacerbated. Moreover, by scanning during repeated anxiety inductions in which patients typically develop the capacity to inhibit the fear response, functional imaging can be used to investigate the mechanisms of habituation. Finally, since psychiatrically healthy subjects can also experience anxiety, the anatomical correlates of experimentally induced anxiety can be compared in normal versus pathological anxiety.

Obsessive-compulsive disorder (OCD)

Structural imaging studies have reported conflicting findings in caudate size in subjects with obsessive-compulsive disorder. One study of adults with childhood-onset obsessive-compulsive disorder reported that the caudate volume is abnormally reduced, while another study of adults with obsessive-compulsive disorder found the right caudate volume is abnormally increased. Other investigators found no significant differences between obsessive-compulsive and control groups.

Most functional imaging studies of obsessive-compulsive disorder found increased blood flow and glucose metabolism in the orbital gyri bilaterally, which in most studies decreases toward normal during effective treatment with antidepressant drugs. Some studies also reported that metabolic activity is abnormally increased in the caudate and the anterior cingulate gyrus. During symptom provocation by exposure to relevant phobic stimuli (e.g., contact with soiled towels for patients with germ phobias), blood flow increases further in the orbital cortex, the caudate, and the anterior cingulate cortex. Thus the baseline metabolic changes may simply reflect the physiological concomitants of obsessive-compulsive symptoms and/or chronic anxiety. This observation is relevant to the interpretation of a study in which caudate metabolism decreased in obsessive-compulsive subjects during either pharmacological or behavioral treatment. This reduction in caudate metabolism was induced only by effective treatment with either modality (i.e., caudate metabolism was unchanged in nonresponders to either treatment), suggesting that it reflects a physiological correlate of symptom resolution rather than a primary physical effect of treatment.

An intriguing study of obsessive-compulsive disorder secondary to brain lesions described several cases of necrosis of the globus pallidus associated with induced obsessional symptoms. The PET images of these patients demonstrated decreased—rather than increased—metabolism in the ventral prefrontal cortex. This case resembles the literature in depression, where primary unipolar depression is associated with increases in ventral prefrontal blood flow or metabolism, but secondary depression induced by some basal ganglia disorders is associated with decreases in ventral prefrontal metabolism (see above).

The similarities between the imaging findings in primary obsessive-compulsive disorder and primary major depressive disorder in the ventral PFC illustrate a case where two distinct disorders may involve an overlapping neural circuit that potentially accounts for clinical features shared by both disorders. Obsessive-compulsive disorder and major depressive disorder are distinct in their course, prognosis, genetics, and neurochemical and neuroendocrine concomitants, and PET imaging data in some regions outside the ventral prefrontal cortex differ between major depressive disorder and obsessive-compulsive disorder. Nevertheless, substantial comorbidity exists between these disorders, as major depression is observed in about 70% of patients with obsessive-compulsive disorder, and pathological obsessions can arise in major depressive disorder. Moreover, pharmacological and neurosurgical interventions that ameliorate obsessive-compulsive disorder also effectively treat major depressive disorder. Finally, the clinical phenomenology of unipolar depression and obsessive-compulsive disorder is similar, as both conditions are characterized by persistent, intrusive, non-rewarding, or painful thoughts with an inability to switch to goal-oriented, rewarding cognitive-behavioral sets.

The neuroimaging literature provides insight into these clinical similarities by implicating the cortical-striatal-pallidal-thalamic circuitry in the pathophysiology of both disorders (see above). This circuitry generally appears to be involved in the organization of internally guided behavior toward a reward, switching of response strategies and habit formation. The cortical area of this circuit where activity is abnormally elevated in both obsessive-compulsive disorder and unipolar depression is the lateral orbital cortex, which as described above appears to participate in correcting behavioral responses that have become inappropriate as reinforcement contingencies change. Dysfunction within the cortical-striatal-pallidal-thalamic circuit that interferes with the role of the orbital cortex could conceivably underlie the inability to inhibit unrewarded thoughts and behaviors in both disorders.

Panic disorder

Structural MRI studies have not clearly established the existence of morphometric or morphological abnormalities in panic disorder. One study reported qualitative abnormalities of temporal lobe structure in panic disorder, although these findings have not been replicated. Another study reported that the volume of the entire temporal lobe was slightly reduced bilaterally in subjects with panic disorder relative to controls, although this finding essentially vanished when regional volumes were normalized to whole-brain volume.

Abnormalities of CBF and glucose metabolism have been reported in the vicinity of the hippocampus and parahippocampal gyrus in the baseline state in panic disorder, which is characterized by mild-to-moderate levels of chronic anxiety (termed "anticipatory anxiety"). In this state, Reiman *et al.* initially reported an abnormal resting asymmetry (left less than right) of blood flow and oxygen metabolism in a region-of-interest placed over the parahippocampal gyrus. Another study similarly found that glucose metabolism measured over the hippocampus/parahippocampal gyrus was asymmetric and concluded that this abnormality reflected an abnormal metabolic elevation on the right side. A third study also found abnormal metabolism in this vicinity, but with the opposite laterality (i.e., elevated metabolism in the left hippocampal/parahippocampal area), in lactate-sensitive subjects with panic disorder relative to healthy controls. In contrast, a fourth study reported that resting perfusion, measured using SPECT and 99mTc-HMPAO, was abnormally decreased in the hippocampus, bilaterally, in lactate-sensitive subjects with panic disorder relative to controls.

Each of these studies employed region-of-interest based approaches that were incapable of localizing the center-of-mass of the abnormality in this region. Reanalysis of some of these data using a voxel-by-voxel approach suggested that the abnormal radioactivity in the vicinity of the mesiotemporal cortex may actually reflect elevated metabolism in the adjacent midbrain. This midbrain region, which is in the vicinity of the PAG, has been implicated in lactate-induced panic, other acute anxiety states, and animal models of panic attacks.

Subjects with panic disorder have also been studied during panic elicited by a variety of chemical challenges. Panic attacks induced by intravenous sodium lactate infusion were associated with regional CBF increases in the anterior insula, medial cerebellum, and midbrain. Blood flow also increased in these regions in animal-phobic subjects during exposure to phobic stimuli and in healthy subjects during the threat of a painful electrical shock, suggesting that these CBF changes reflect neurophysiological correlates of fear processing in general. Consistent with this hypothesis, anxiety attacks induced in healthy humans using cholecysto-kinin-tetrapeptide (CCK-4) were also associated with CBF increases in the insular-amygdala region and the medial cerebellum.

Indirect evidence suggests that the neurophysiological responses in the PFC during panicogen challenge may differ between subjects with panic disorder and healthy controls. For example, panic attacks induced with CCK-4 were associated with CBF increases in the ACC in healthy humans, but flow did not significantly change in the ACC in subjects with panic disorder during lactate-induced panic. The ACC was also a region where flow significantly increased in healthy subjects but not in those with panic disorder during fenfluramine challenge. Finally, normalized medial frontal CBF reportedly increased in a study of healthy controls following yohimbine administration (after normalizing to remove effects on whole brain CBF), whereas relative prefrontal cortical flow was decreased in subjects with panic disorder relative to control subjects following yohimbine challenge.

Phobias

Phobic anxiety has been imaged in simple animal phobias by acquiring blood flow scans during exposures to the feared animal. During the initial fear-invoking exposure to the stimulus, flow increases in the lateral orbital/anterior insular cortex, bilaterally, the pregenual ACC, and the medial cerebellum (Fig. 6.9), areas where CBF also increases in other anxiety states (see above). During the development of habituation to phobic stimuli, the magnitude of the hemodynamic responses to the phobic stimulus diminished in the anterior insula and the medial cerebellum but increased in the left posterior orbital cortex in an area where flow had not changed during the exposures that preceded habituation (Fig. 6.10). The magnitude of the CBF increase in this latter region was inversely correlated with the corresponding changes in heart rate and anxiety ratings. As discussed above, the posterior orbital cortex was a site where CBF increased in subjects with obsessive-compulsive disorder during exposure to phobic stimuli, with the increase in flow being inversely correlated with obsessional ratings.

In social anxiety disorder, an imaging study employing an aversive conditioning paradigm (in which the unconditioned stimulus was an aversive odor and the conditioned stimulus was a picture of a human face) showed that hemodynamic activity decreased in the amygdala and the hippocampus during presentations of the conditioned stimulus in healthy controls but increased in subjects with social phobia. Interpretation of these data was confounded by the problem that both human faces and aversively conditioned stimuli normally activate the amygdala, so it remained unclear which of the stimuli produced abnormal responses in social phobia. Nevertheless, these data appear conceptually intriguing given the role of hippocampal-amygdalar projections in mediating contextual fear and the possibility that deficits in the transmission of information regarding context may be involved in the pathogenesis of phobias.

Post-traumatic stress disorder (PTSD)

Structural MRI studies of PTSD have identified subtle reductions in the volume of the hippocampus in PTSD samples relative to healthy or traumatized, non-PTSD control samples. Although limitations existed in these studies in the matching of alcohol use/abuse in the PTSD and control samples, the reductions in hippocampal volume did not correlate with the extent of alcohol exposure in the PTSD samples, and no volumetric differences were found between PTSD and control samples in the amygdala, entire temporal lobe, caudate, whole brain, or lateral ventricles. While the magnitude of the reduction in hippocampal volume only ranged

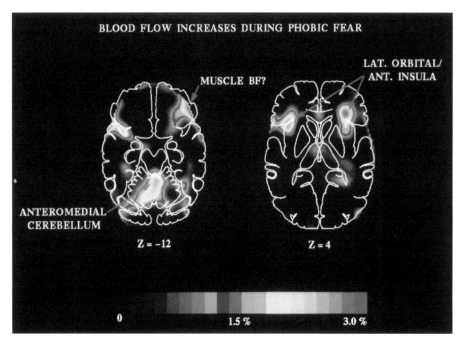

Fig. 6.9 Regional blood flow increases in the lateral orbital/anterior insular cortex bilaterally and the anteromedial cerebellum during phobic anxiety. Blood flow also increases in these areas in subjects with panic disorder during a lactate-induced panic attack and in psychiatrically healthy humans during anxious anticipation of a painful electrical shock. The image shown is a composite image depicting the average changes in blood flow in the fearful condition relative to the nonfearful control condition from a group of subjects with simple animal phobias. Phobic anxiety was elicited by exposing subjects to a relevant phobic stimulus (either a snake or a tarantula). The area of increased blood flow marked "muscle bf" has its center-of-mass located outside the brain over the temporalis/masseter muscles, where teeth clenching also produces increases in blood flow. This response presumably reflects increased flow in the facial muscles during anxiety, which is commonly seen in PET studies that involve anxiety induction. Only the medial edge of the blurred representation of this muscle blood flow change is evident in this image section, which has been templated to exclude pixels outside the brain boundary. The subjects' left is on left side of the image, and the anterior aspect is toward the top. The bar indicates the percentage of change in regional blood flow from the anxious condition relative to the control condition. The Z coordinate provides the position (in mm) of each horizontal image plane relative to a plane containing the anterior and posterior commissures, with positive indicating dorsal and negative, ventral. (From Drevets, WC (1995) *et al. J Cereb Blood Flow Metab* 15:S856.)

from 5% to 12% in the PTSD samples relative to trauma-matched controls, these abnormalities were associated with short-term memory deficits in some studies. It remains unclear whether the difference in hippocampal volume may reflect a result of the chronic stress associated with PTSD (e.g., resulting from sustained exposure to elevated glucocorticoid concentrations) or a biological antecedent that may confer risk for developing PTSD.

The design of many functional imaging studies of PTSD has been guided by hypotheses that this condition involves the emotional-learning circuitry associated with the amygdala, since the traumatic event constitutes a fear-conditioning experience and subsequent exposure to sensory, contextual, or mnemonic stimuli that recall aspects of the event elicits psychological distress and sympathetic arousal. Compatible with this expectation, some studies demonstrated activation of the amygdala when subjects with PTSD listened to auditory scripts describing the trau-matic event or recordings of combat sounds, or internally generated imagery related to the traumatic event in the absence of sensory cues. However, other studies found no significant changes in CBF in the amygdala as subjects with PTSD listened to scripts describing the traumatic event or viewed trauma-related pictures, and studies comparing CBF responses to trauma-related stimuli have not shown significant differences between subjects with PTSD and trauma-matched, non-PTSD controls in the amygdala.

The extent to which these negative findings reflect limitations in statistical sensitivity or temporal resolution of PET must be addressed in provocation studies involving larger subject samples and employing fMRI, instead of PET. Notably a preliminary fMRI study found exaggerated hemodynamic changes in the amygdala in subjects with PTSD relative to trauma-matched, non-PTSD controls during exposure to pictures of fearful faces presented using a backward masking technique. If replicated, this finding may

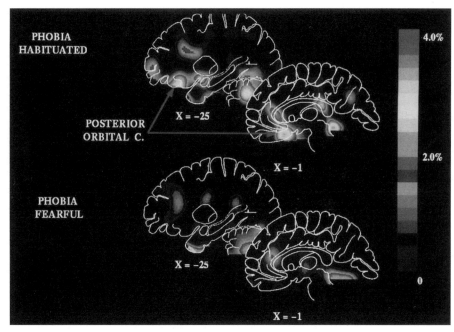

Fig. 6.10 Habituation to a phobic stimulus was accompanied by the development of a blood flow response in the posteromedial orbital cortex during repeated exposure to a phobic stimulus (phobia habituated). The magnitude of the blood flow change in this region correlated inversely with the accompanying changes in heart rate and anxiety ratings. In contrast, blood flow did not change in this area in the same subjects scanned during initial exposures to the same animal (phobia fearful). The images shown are from the study described in Fig. 6.9, with the habituated state referring to scans acquired during the fourth or fifth exposures to the animal, when a markedly attenuated anxiety response was obtained relative to the initial exposures. Regional blood flow changes during the *initial* exposures are reflected by the phobia fearful image slices here and by the image sections in Fig. 6.9. In PET studies involving normal subjects and obsessive-compulsive subjects exposed to anxiety-provoking stimuli, blood flow increases in the posteromedial cortex during the initial exposure to anxiogenic stimuli, with the magnitude of the blood flow rise correlating inversely with symptom ratings. This inverse correlation is consistent with evidence from electrophysiologic and lesion analysis studies suggesting that the posteromedial orbital cortex functions to inhibit or modulate non-reinforced anxiety responses. Phobic subjects fail to activate this region until they have undergone repeated exposure to the phobic stimulus (as applied during the process of systematic desensitization—the treatment of choice for simple phobia). Following the development of habituation, this region is successfully activated, and possibly related to this neurophysiological change, the anxiety response to the non-reinforced stimulus can be inhibited. Anterior is toward the left. The bar indicates the percent change in regional blood flow in the anxious minus the control condition. The X coordinate provides the position (in mm) of each sagittal image plane relative to the midline, with negative X indicating left. (From Drevets, *et al.*, 1995.)

suggest that the emotional dysregulation associated with PTSD may involve amygdalar responses to emotional stimuli of various types.

Other limbic and paralimbic cortical structures have also been implicated in provocation studies of PTSD. In both subjects with PTSD and trauma-matched, non-PTSD controls, CBF increases in the posterior orbital cortex, anterior insula, and temporopolar cortex during exposure to trauma-related stimuli, but these changes have generally not differentiated PTSD and control samples. In contrast, the pattern of CBF changes elicited in the medial PFC by traumatic stimuli does appear to differ between subjects with PTSD and controls. During exposure to trauma-related sensory stimuli, flow reportedly decreased in the left but increased in the right pregenual ACC in PTSD, potentially consistent with the evidence reviewed above that the role of the medial PFC in emotional behavior is lateralized in experimental animals. However, CBF in the right pregenual ACC increased significantly more in non-PTSD, trauma-matched controls than in subjects with PTSD. Moreover, in the infralimbic cortex, CBF decreased in samples with combat-related PTSD but increased in combat-matched, non-PTSD controls during exposure to combat-related visual and auditory stimuli.

The infralimbic cortex has been shown to play a major role in extinguishing fear-conditioned responses in rodents. If this finding extends to humans, then the observation that subjects with PTSD fail to activate these structures to a similar extent as traumatized, non-PTSD controls during exposure to traumatic cues suggests that neural processes mediating extinction to trauma-related stimuli may be impaired in PTSD. Compatible with this hypothesis, PTSD samples have been shown to acquire *de novo* conditioned responses more readily and extinguish them more slowly than control samples. Such a deficit could conceivably be related to the vulnerability to developing PTSD, since PTSD occurs in only 5–20% of individuals exposed to similar traumatic events.

Cocaine dependence

Acute administration of cocaine produces a decrease in cerebral blood flow, particularly in the frontal cortex. Other euphoriants (e.g., alcohol) produce similar effects acutely. In cocaine-dependent subjects, PET and SPECT studies reveal patchy perfusion defects in multiple areas of the cortex and the basal ganglia that persist for several weeks following cessation of cocaine use. These defects are more likely to be apparent in subjects dependent upon both cocaine and alcohol than in subjects dependent upon cocaine alone. In the areas where these perfusion defects are found, local blood flow decreases further during acute cocaine administration.

Neuroreceptor imaging has been used to assess the effects of chronic cocaine abuse on postsynaptic dopamine receptors and dopamine reuptake sites. PET studies demonstrate that chronic cocaine use results in downregulation of D_2 receptor density in the striatum for up to one month following cessation of cocaine use, consistent with evidence obtained in experimental animals. In cocaine users imaged beyond one month of abstinence, ^{18}F-N-methylspiroperidol uptake in the striatum does not differ with respect to controls, suggesting that the density of postsynaptic dopamine receptors recovers from the effects of cocaine after a drug-free interval. SPECT imaging of the dopamine transporter using iodinated β-CIT, a cocaine analog, shows abnormally increased density of these sites in cocaine-dependent subjects, consistent with postmortem studies in cocaine abusers dying of overdose. Taken together, these findings suggest that chronic use of cocaine, which binds to dopamine transporter sites and blocks dopamine reuptake, results in downregulation of postsynaptic D_2 sites and upregulation of dopamine transporter sites. In the absence of repeated cocaine exposure, this state may produce a functional dopaminergic deficiency in the reward-related mesolimbic dopamine system, manifested by depressed mood, anhedonia, and cocaine craving.

Other neuropsychiatric disorders

Tourette's syndrome

MRI studies of adults and children with Tourette's syndrome have reported decreased volume of the left basal ganglia and loss of the normal asymmetry between right and left basal ganglia structures with respect to controls. The basal ganglia have been implicated in the pathophysiology of this syndrome by other types of information. In addition to the motor and vocal tics that are the hallmark of Tourette's

syndrome, a high proportion of patients with this disorder manifest obsessions and compulsions.

In contrast to the functional imaging findings in primary obsessive-compulsive disorder, the PET images of patients with Tourette's syndrome show decreased metabolism in the ventral prefrontal cortex and the caudate, providing another example in which the functional anatomy differs between a primary psychiatric disorder and a basal ganglia disorder that induces a clinically similar neuropsychiatric syndrome. The propensity of dysfunction in neural circuits formed by the basal ganglia, the thalamus and the prefrontal cortex for maintaining pathological cognitive and/or behavioral responses, manifested clinically by obsessive thoughts and compulsive behaviors, is discussed above.

Attention deficit hyperactivity disorder (ADHD)

Three MRI studies of children with ADHD have reported abnormal reductions in the size of the corpus callosum, which in one study correlated with classroom ratings of hyperactivity. Abnormal caudate asymmetry has also been reported in children with ADHD, and one group found that children with ADHD fail to demonstrate the normal developmental decrement in caudate volume over the preadolescent and adolescent years. A preliminary PET imaging study of ^{18}F-Dopa uptake also implicated the striatum in ADHD, finding abnormally reduced uptake in the putamen. The potential importance of this finding is highlighted by the beneficial effects of agents that enhance dopamine function (e.g., methylphenidate) in treating ADHD.

Autism

In a majority of subjects with idiopathic autism the area of the cerebellar vermis has been found to be abnormally reduced in MRI images, compatible with postmortem evidence that the numbers of Purkinje and granule cells are abnormally reduced in the cerebellum in autism. However, MRI studies have also suggested that a minority of autistic subjects have abnormal enlargement of the cerebellar vermis. Reduced parietal lobe size and increased incidence of developmental cortical malformations such as polymicrogyria, macrogyria, or schizencephaly have also been reported in autism.

Annotated bibliography

Charney, DS and Drevets, WC: The neurobiological basis of anxiety disorders, in Davis K, Charney, DS, Coyle J, and Nemeroff, CB (eds) (2002) *Psychopharmacology: The Fifth Generation of Progress*, New York, Lippincott, Williams & Wilkins, Chapter 63, pp. 901–930.
Provides an overview of neuroimaging abnormalities in anxiety disorders, together with the relevant neurobiology.

Drevets, WC, Gadde, KM, and Krishnan, KRR: Neuroimaging studies of mood disorders, in Charney, DS, Nestler, EJ, and Bunney, BJ (eds) (2004) *The Neurobiological Foundation of Mental Illness*, 2nd Edition, New York, Oxford University Press.
This review provides a detailed, fully referenced review of the in vivo neuroimaging and postmortem neuropathological abnormalities that have been identified in mood disorders.

Liddle, P and Pantelis, C: Brain imaging in schizophrenia, in (2003) Hirsch, SR and Weinberger, D (eds) *Schizophrenia*, Malden, MA, Blackwell Press.
Reviews investigations of structural abnormalities and both resting and functional activation studies in schizophrenia.

Moonen, CTW and Bandettini, PA (1999) *Functional MRI*, New York, Springer, Inc.

This book provides a collection of reviews that describe the physical principles underlying fMRI technology and discuss the strengths and limitations of its application in human brain mapping.

Raichle, ME. Circulatory and metabolic correlates of brain function in normal humans, in (1987) Brookhart, JM and Mountcastle, VB (ed.) *Handbook of Physiology Section I: The nervous system Vol. V: Higher functions of the brain*, Bethesda MD, American Physiological Society, pp. 643–674.
An overview of functional imaging that critically assesses the modalities available for blood flow and metabolism imaging and discusses constraints on the design and interpretation of brain mapping experiments that relate to the nature of these physiological signals.

CHAPTER 7

Referral of Patients: Mental Health, Family, and Community Resources

Mark C. Johnson, MD, Katrin Tobben, MSW, LCSW, and Barry A. Hong, PhD

Introduction

Just as gastric distress and chest pain do not usually present first to the gastroenterologist and cardiologist, so emotional and mental distress do not usually present first to the psychiatrist or other mental health specialist. Findings from the Epidemiologic Catchment Area Study, a comprehensive survey of psychiatric disorders, demonstrate that it is primary care physicians who are the front line of the mental health system in the United States. This means the non-psychiatric physician plays a key role in early intervention—whether of transient depression, for example, or in suspecting the prodrome for schizophrenia. Such efforts are fueled by evidence that the course of schizophrenia is improved and lifetime disability decreased by early intervention. Early intervention is possible only with the assistance and recognition of non-psychiatric physicians and other community professionals.

Once diagnosed and in treatment, patients with schizophrenia, bipolar disorder or major depressive disorder can often be managed by the primary care physician. Successful management requires utilizing a variety of mental health professionals in consultative and adjunctive roles, comparable to the use of other adjunctive therapies, such as physical therapy and nutrition consults, in other equally treatable non-psychiatric conditions. The professionals that may be consulted include the psychiatrist, psychologist, social worker, mental health case manager, and pastoral counselor. Obtaining maximum recovery for the patient with a mental health diagnosis is a satisfying and rewarding aspect of health care.

Role of the primary care physician

Recent studies of depression in general medical practices es-

timate depressive symptoms in 41% of medical patients studied over six months. In epidemiological investigations, almost 10% of the population had significant depressive symptoms and 6% had general anxiety disorder (GAD) at some time in their lives.

The first task faced by the primary care physician is diagnosis (see also Chapters 2 and 3). This is made more difficult by the fact that patients rarely volunteer the complete story of their psychiatric problems. It is common for people to have complex histories involving more than one psychiatric disorder or comorbid condition. Without a thorough history it is easy to obtain an account of only one disorder. For instance, patients who are depressed may tell of their depressive symptoms but not discuss their phobias, obsessions, or excessive drinking. Disruptions with work and family relationships may also go unmentioned by the patient and unnoticed by the doctor even when a psychiatric illness has been identified. It is necessary to take a complete history of academic, occupational, and social functioning to supplement the patient's spontaneous account. Only in this way can accurate diagnosis of the illness be made and its complexities and full impact on the patient and family be understood. This thorough and complete history forms the basis for informed decisions about which patients to treat, which to refer to a psychiatrist, and what other kinds of referrals to arrange in order to support the patient and family in their ongoing health care needs.

Families should be actively engaged and carefully listened to. Their contribution to ancillary initial and interim history plays an important role in ongoing treatment. They can also help determine which interventions and lifestyle adjustments are feasible within their particular family. The majority of people who are chronically disabled by mental illness are actively involved with their families, often at great financial and personal cost to the family, making family involvement in care crucial to success. Even patients being discharged from the hospital may be far from well and in need of care by friends and family to avoid rehospitalization.

Which psychiatric patients are treated by primary care physicians?

The vast majority of people with mental distress who receive medical treatment are routinely treated in the primary care office and are not referred to other specialists. Selecting those who should be referred is related to the primary care physician's comfort in treating particular psychiatric disorders and is a function of time, experience, and perception.

Time is precious. Is it more effective to invest it now as opposed to later? If so, how? Is it more effective to get a consult? Is it appropriate to transfer care? Will investing more time now result in benefit to other patients with similar problems? Often the best primary care use of the mental health professional is to gain knowledge now, which can also be used later. Arranging a consult with a clear plan to take the patient back after the condition has stabilized is one way to maximize efficient use of time in both the present case and future situations. It is a valuable way to gain experience in dealing with particular recurring diagnoses and treatment complications.

A significant issue in making referrals is the number of mental health professionals in the community and the ability to get a patient a timely appointment. The primary care physician needs to know psychiatrists and other mental health specialists in order to have confidence that proper treatment and collaboration will occur. Where there is a shortage of psychiatric resources it may be beneficial to arrange regular psychiatric teaching rounds and case studies under the auspices of a local hospital or county medical society.

Primary care physicians routinely treat patients who have symptoms of depression and anxiety, obsessions and compulsions, and complaints of physical symptoms in the absence of objective findings. On occasion, symptoms do not improve, multiple psychotropic medications are indicated, or more time is needed to attend to an array of problems. For these and similar situations it is important to be knowledgeable about resources for consults and referrals. Additionally, maintaining current data-based knowledge about newer psychiatric medicines is helpful. For instance, using the new-generation antidepressants in place of benzodiazepines in the treatment of general anxiety disorder, panic attacks, and phobias greatly simplifies the task of treating those disorders by removing the risk of addiction, drug-seeking behavior, and the withdrawal syndrome often confused with the very disorder being treated. A greater understanding of bipolar disorder and range of effective medications has resulted in many cases previously treated as "nerves," with poor to modest results and lingering illness, now being treated quite

successfully with non-addictive anticonvulsants that have mood-stabilizing properties, such as, for example, valproate, lamotrigine, carbamazepine, and oxcarbamazepine. These might be familiar medications to the primary care physician, who may have used them in treating seizure disorders. Likewise, in the past it was not unusual to refer the patient with depression who was considered a treatment failure after only one antidepressant had been tried. New-generation antidepressants have a better correlation between starting dose and therapeutic dose, which increases the potential for the front-line treatment of depression to be successful, if the patient is maintained on the antidepressant for an adequate length of time. When a given dose does not provide full relief, improved side effect profiles allow the non-psychiatric physician greater latitude in attempting dosage increases toward the maximum recommended dose, in order to obtain a full therapeutic effect.

RESOURCES

- Community Mental Health Centers have information on community support services for the mentally ill and their families.
- The social work department of the local hospital.
- The National Organization for the Mentally Ill (NAMI)
  - National helpline: 1–800–950–6264
  - Website: www.nami.org
- Depression and Bipolar Support Alliance
  - National helpline: 1–800–826–3632
  - Website: www.dbsalliance.org
- Substance Abuse and Mental Health Services Administration (SAMHSA)
  - Website: www.mentalhealth.org
- Alcoholics Anonymous (AA), Narcotics Anonymous (NA), and similar 12-step programs, are listed in the local phone book.

Psychiatric consultation

Psychiatric expertise can and often should be brought to bear in making or confirming a diagnosis once a psychiatric disorder is suspected. It is particularly useful in initiating, recommending, adjusting, or affirming treatment when the illness presents with complex phenomenology, including multiple social and personality problems.

The most useful consultation is one that involves direct physician-to-physician communication before and particularly after the consultation. In making the referral the need for follow-up communication should be indicated. Though traditional approaches to confidentiality may mitigate against sharing a full psychiatric evaluation, it is still quite reasonable to at least provide a brief letter indicating diagnosis, treatment options, and willingness to have a brief discussion of the case.

In many cases, the greatest value to the primary care physician of the psychiatric consultation, whether brief or extended, may well be the continuing education process that can result from ongoing collaboration with a particular specialist. This helps in targeting early intervention—invaluable to the patient and family. It also enables successful ongoing medication management and can smooth interactions with mental health professionals of various backgrounds who help provide the other treatments and services that are part of effective mental health care.

Preparing for a mental health referral

The referring physician, the mental health professional receiving the referral, and the patient all need preparation for a successful referral to occur.

Many patients are reluctant to ask for direct help with emotional problems or to begin treatment with a mental health professional. The primary care physician can do much to facilitate a successful mental health referral by assuming the appropriate attitude and behavior. First, the referring physician can reassure the patient that mental health and physical health are equally important to wellbeing. Second, the purpose and goals for the referral should be made clear to the patient and to the mental health professional. Like any good consultation or referral, a clear question or two will bring focus to the process. If the primary care physician is requesting advice or guidance from a mental health professional, it is important that they be understood by everyone involved to avoid confusion about roles and continuity of care. Even general questions can be useful. Should the patient be referred to a psychiatrist or to a non-medical therapist? Will this couple benefit from marital therapy? Is this grief reaction normal or abnormal? Who could best provide counseling for this normal, but very intense, grief reaction?

In other situations, the primary care physician and the patient request formal assessment and, if indicated, treatment by a mental health professional. The mental health professional informs the primary care physician when the patient has been seen and that treatment will or will not begin. It is possible that a primary care physician's initial diagnosis may be modified or clarified; for example, a person judged to be "depressed" by the primary physician might fall short of the psychiatric criteria for major depressive illness but fulfill criteria for dysthymic disorder. Although confidentiality is respected, it is customary for psychiatrists and other mental health professionals to acknowledge that they have evaluated patients referred to them and to provide general feedback to the referring physician. Patients should clearly understand these different types of referrals and the feedback that will be provided, so they can have full confidence in all the professionals comprising their treatment team.

Mental health professionals

Credentials and training

In order to choose the referral that will be most beneficial to the patient, the primary care physician must be informed about the different types of mental health professionals available in the community and know what to expect from them. Referrals are often limited to a narrow range of professional acquaintances or by the patient's preference or bias (for example, the patient may say, "I'm not crazy," or "I won't take a drug that will affect my mind"). Many different mental health professionals are competent to provide psychotherapy and may further subspecialize with regard to type of psychotherapy or diagnosis treated.

In this section, the various types of professionals are described in brief, and their unique mental health training and skills are noted.

Psychiatrists are licensed physicians, either doctors of medicine or osteopathy (MDs or DOs), whose expertise is the assessment and treatment of the whole range of psychiatric problems, particularly the most acute and severe psychiatric problems that might necessitate hospitalization. Psychiatrists are also experts in differentiating psychiatric disorders that may in fact present as non-psychiatric illness. Formal psychiatric subspecialties include child and adolescent psychiatry, geriatric psychiatry, addiction psychiatry, forensic psychiatry, and psychosomatic medicine. Psychiatrists admit patients to hospitals, perform physical examinations, order laboratory tests, prescribe medication as indicated, and may undertake counseling and psychotherapy as well. Psychiatrists have completed medical school, a year of rotating or general residency, and a three-year residency program in psychiatry. Subspecialties require at least a year of additional training.

Psychologists are licensed providers of psychological services. They are generally trained at a doctoral level and have received a doctor of philosophy (PhD) degree from a university or a doctor of psychology (PsyD) degree from a professional school of psychology. Not all psychologists with doctoral training are eligible to provide psychological services. Psychologists who are clinically trained take additional clinical practicum courses in graduate school to prepare to become providers of psychological services, and they complete a year-long internship as part of their PhD training. They provide psychological services in hospitals and medical centers as hospital-based providers and as independent practitioners in the community. In hospitals they may be part of a psychological consultation service as well as offer screening and pre- and post-procedure support to various medical services (e.g., renal transplant, bone marrow transplant, oncology, etc.).

Training in psychology covers a wide range of psychological schools and theories, making many psychologists skilled in more than one modality of psychotherapy and in treating various diagnoses. All states require psychologists to be licensed to practice. In addition, psychologists perform cognitive and neurological assessments. Most clinical psychologists assess cognitive function by means of tests and a clinical interview.

Neuropsychology is a subspecialty of psychology for which psychologists take advanced training in brain physiology-behavior relationships beyond the usual training of most clinical psychologists. *Neuropsychologists* work with other psychologists, psychiatrists, and neurologists to assess cognitive problems, including dementia and memory, attention, learning, and biologically based communication disorders. In some communities, cognitive and neuropsychological assessment is available on a sliding scale basis through the clinical psychology departments of local universities.

Social workers, who have completed two years of postgraduate training for the master of social work (MSW) degree, are licensed in all states to provide social work services in agencies, hospitals, and independent practice. Because of their training in human service administration, community organization, and direct client services, social workers often direct or work in community organizations for the mentally ill or emotionally disturbed. Medical social workers in hospitals coordinate human and financial resources. They often provide brief individual, couple, and family counseling to all types of patients — medical, surgical and psychiatric — as the need arises. Psychiatric social workers have generally received specialized mental health training during social work school. It is also not uncommon for psychiatric social workers to have completed advanced training in psychotherapy beyond the MSW degree.

Nurses have an increasing role in the treatment of psychiatric patients beyond their hospital roles. Many registered nurses focus on psychiatric nursing without extra formal training. Specialty training beyond the Bachelor of Science is available to qualify as advanced practice psychiatric nurses or clinical nurse specialists in psychiatry. These nurses can work with psychiatrists in the initial medical and psychiatric assessments of patients, and in some states they can prescribe medication under physician supervision.

Marriage and family therapists constitute another set of mental health specialists. Generally individuals, couples, or families who have communication or role problems are candidates for this type of therapy. The "patient" is usually the couple or the family unit, although it is common for there to be a designated patient, typically the family member whose behavior raised the need for outside help. Assessment often includes the use of genograms and family maps. These are used to help trace the themes of family and couples therapy. Many different professionals are trained in marriage and/or family therapy in their degree programs and practicum placements. Psychologists, social workers, psychiatrists, pastoral counselors, and clergy may all engage in marital and family therapy. There are also specific formal training programs in marital and family therapy that provide a specialty level of preparation. Many states license graduates of those programs as MFTs (marriage and family therapists). Because of the breadth and depth of marriage and family therapy training and the experience required for clinical membership in the American Association of Marriage and Family Therapists (AAMFT), therapists who are clinical members, regardless of degree program, often include their professional membership as a credential to indicate their extensive training in that specific field.

Pastoral counselors are available for helping with emotional and spiritual distress. In the highly religious patient, it can be difficult to distinguish normal religious belief and practice from religiously expressed psychopathology, e.g., "trust in God" from hyper-religiosity — "God says no one else has ever done it before and I have to do it to prove my trust." More than one mental health professional has misinterpreted orthodox religious belief and practice for illness, resulting in misdiagnosis in some cases, and so failed to take advantage of a patient strength that could be used in learning to handle and recover from illness. Many clergy have training and experience in counseling and are members of the American Association of Pastoral Counselors (AAPC), a national organization that certifies religious counselors. In addition, some clergy are licensed as professional counselors or social workers.

Mental health case managers are essential in helping patients and families access resources and improve daily life. They are routinely employed by health care systems, clinics, hospitals, and outpatient facilities to work with the severely ill, whose level of dysfunction can overwhelm families, friends, and patients themselves. Case managers often attend office visits with the patient and can provide valuable descriptions of patient behaviors, difficulties, and successes that have occurred since the last office visit. Case managers come from a wide variety of academic backgrounds and degrees and often receive most of their training on the job. The assistance of a case manager is often an important ingredient for keeping a patient in the community and out of the hospital. The case manager is a key team member in the psychosocial rehabilitation of the severely ill patient and should be utilized by the physician seeking maximal patient recovery.

Professional counselors provide assessment and treatment for individuals, couples, and families who have problems in living, especially in the areas of life development, career decisions, and personal problems. Professional counselors generally are not considered trained to make psychiatric diagnoses. Often, individuals with backgrounds in education, religion, and substance abuse gain advanced training as professional counselors. Most states license the activities of professional counselors, who are generally referred to as licensed professional counselors (LPCs).

Locating mental health professionals and resources

When a physician is not familiar with specific local mental health resources or practices in an area with few mental health specialists, the county social work department and social workers at local hospitals are important resources. The hospital social worker knows about other local resources and should be aware of "out-of-the-area" sources of help, including statewide mental health consumer telephone helplines and programs. Mental health associations can provide information about providers, community agencies, and counseling programs with sliding fee scales. Physicians should make themselves aware of local mental health resources and keep that knowledge current. Making an initial non-crisis contact with a psychiatrist will help obtain and maintain access, which will be very useful later when crises occur.

Community mental health centers

Community mental health centers are staffed by multidisciplinary mental health professionals, including psychiatrists, and typically serve specific geographical areas. In addition to acute and chronic care, these centers provide community education and consultation and encourage collaboration with primary care physicians.

Community mental health centers usually receive state and/or federal funding to provide services for people of low income living in the area, but they may also provide services without geographic restriction to patients with traditional insurance or other means of payment. They are a ready source of case management services. Once a case manager is assigned, the patient and family can expect regular calls and scheduled visits based on the "level of care" assigned to the patient. Some centers provide psychotherapy; others limit their services to case management. These centers may be a physician's only resource for the underinsured or non-insured patient.

Employee assistance programs (EAPs)

These are programs established for businesses, companies, and industry as a resource for their employees. EAPs are commonly used to provide stigma-free help with stress, personal, and family problems that might overwhelm an employee. The goal is to provide a low-barrier, easy-access means of avoiding or minimizing illness. In these programs, mental health professionals, typically MSWs, LPCs and MFTs, work with individual employees and their families to resolve crises and serve as the intermediary for a mental health referral if ongoing treatment is needed. In many instances, an EAP counselor sees an individual for a brief assessment and makes a referral immediately. In other cases, the EAP counselor sees an employee for brief psychotherapy, usually six sessions or less.

For a person who works for a company that provides this resource, the EAP is often a good starting point for a mental health referral and may be a required step to obtaining a referral. The EAP counselor is generally aware of community resources and familiar with the mental health benefits in the employee's insurance coverage. Because of the relationship of an EAP counselor to an employee's company, sometimes employees are reluctant to use these services out of fear of compromised confidentiality. In these cases, respecting the patient's wishes, the physician may make a direct referral, bypassing the EAP.

The role of families

The effects of chronic mental illness on the family can be profound. Families reorganize their lives around the illness, deal with unusual, sometimes violent behaviors, and, in the extreme, interact with hospitals, police, and the legal system. Even the most willing families may pay a tremendous emotional and financial toll in caring for the chronically ill family member, especially if their loved one's emotional and mental distress is unrelenting. Mental illness disrupts family life by altering normal family roles. For example, when schizophrenia appears in adolescence it disrupts normal growth and development, creating a perpetual adolescent with all the age-related difficulties and without a foreseeable end. A great deal of sadness and grief is often felt and expressed about the lost potential of this child with debilitating mental illness. "John will never work, marry or have children." Family members may feel cheated that they may never be a "normal" family.

These families may become isolated from friends and extended family. Whether this happens as the result of embarrassment or simply through the stress and drain on energy that results from living in an unpredictable state of crisis, it means that families often lose the normal social support they find with other difficult situations.

With research increasingly demonstrating a biological cause of mental illness, it is easier for parents to accept that the illness is not their "fault." The physician should remain aware, however, that parental guilt is not always responsive to facts. It may take not only repeated assurance but counseling to handle the grief of lost dreams and hopes and enable the parents and the spouse to cope successfully with their loved one's mental illness.

Marital relationships may be disrupted with a real loss of partnership when one spouse is incapacitated by illness. If the incapacity is severe or prolonged, the healthy spouse often assumes a parental role toward the dependent spouse. This means a loss of previous intimacy and companionship as well as becoming a witness to the suffering of the loved one who is ill. Spouses may have to bear the primary responsibility of raising children alone and take on additional household and family management duties. Shame, embarrassment, feelings of inadequacy, and sheer fatigue contribute to increasing isolation of the healthy spouse. When someone going through depression or another mental illness is married, patience, flexibility, and help are needed for both spouses.

Children who grow up with a parent or sibling who is mentally ill may feel short-changed by the loss of a "normal" childhood. Whereas some children do well and even thrive under the chaos, studies have shown increased incidence of anxiety and depression in adult life. A child's reaction varies according to the severity and chronicity of the illness and the general level of stress and chaos at home. Mental illness has been compared to "a death in the family, which is complicated by stigma, the cyclical nature of the illness, and the continuing physical presence of the bereaved."

What do families need?

Families need information about the illness and its treatment. As the primary caregivers, family members must understand the diagnosis and treatment plan. They have often been excluded from receiving information because of confidentiality issues. They need to know the diagnosis, the prescribed medications and the reasons for their use, potential side effects, and the expected response curve and variants of it. They also benefit from learning behavioral management techniques to use in caring for their loved ones.

Families should be included in treatment planning and viewed as partners in the treatment process. They are experts in their own right, with valuable past and present knowledge of their family member to share with the professional caregiver. It is important to recognize that even though the family may be healthy apart from the impact of mental illness, any family can show strain, have difficulty coping in stressful circumstances, and need some help of its own. Families need to know techniques for managing the symptoms of psychiatric illness, especially how to handle difficult behaviors, such as the positive and negative symptoms of schizophrenia, aggressive behavior, and suicidal or self-destructive behavior. They also need to learn coping strategies for managing poor hygiene, social withdrawal, and

refusal to cooperate with treatment and where to set healthy boundaries and limits.

A family can often make changes in the environment that favorably impact the treatment of the illness. For instance, people with schizophrenia do better in a calm environment than in one where there are high levels of expressed emotions.

Family members may need permission and encouragement to take care of their own needs. It is not unusual to find them neglecting themselves out of guilt over the illness or sorrow for the loved one suffering from it. They may suffer from a variety of stress-induced complaints. Families benefit from maintaining a social life, regular exercise, good nutrition, and proactive stress management.

Planning for the future should address the situation where the patient who is cared for by parents will outlive the parents. There are differences of opinion about whether adult children should continue to live at home, given the impact on the family and the usual result of stifled independence. It is much more difficult to learn to live independently in later years after being sheltered for an entire lifetime. It is generally felt that the move to independent living is smoother while the parents are still alive and in good enough health to be actively involved in the transition.

Where can families find what they need?

Often a family's introduction to resources for ongoing assistance occurs when their relative is hospitalized. The psychiatric social worker at the hospital is a source of information about resources and support services in the community. Many hospitals also offer education groups or seminars that address issues facing the family.

Another source of support is the National Alliance for the Mentally Ill (NAMI), founded in 1979. This organization is a proponent of the disease model of mental illness rather than a psychological theory of origins. It lobbies for improved funding for medical research and advocates for better services for the mentally ill. One of NAMI's guiding principles is that the best help is self-help. Its roughly 1200 chapters are perhaps best known for the education and support they provide through family-led support groups and consumer-oriented educational programs.

Adjunctive care—case management

Most people who are treated for psychiatric disorders, especially those whose treatments are followed by primary care physicians, are not chronically disabled by their illnesses. Though major depression, the various anxiety disorders, and alcoholism are recurrent or even chronic, these common illnesses usually can be managed well enough to keep the periods of disability brief.

A minority of psychiatric patients have such severe brain

dysfunction that they are disabled for long periods and require a comprehensive system of support services, including stable housing, financial support, access to general and specialized health care, medications, structured daily activities, structure for daily routines, and ways to meet unexpected crises and needs. With the advent of new-generation antipsychotics with improved symptom-response and side-effect profile, medications may be managed by primary care physicians with occasional consultation from psychiatrists for hospitalization, exacerbations of symptoms, and routine reassessment of treatment options. Case management provides the adjunctive care needed to enable both primary care physicians and psychiatrists to be successful members of the treatment team. Knowing how to interact with, listen attentively to, and direct case managers effectively is a valuable skill needed in order to make good use of this particular adjunctive treatment modality.

Mental health case managers

Many publicly funded programs for people disabled by chronic psychiatric disorders provide case managers, community support workers, and other support individuals. These individuals are paid to take care of many of the day-to-day details necessary to help an emotionally and mentally distressed person enjoy life, live interdependently in the community, and minimize hospitalization. Case management services can be provided in a variety of locations (office, home, school, worksite, etc.), include help with transportation, and can be much less expensive than private duty nursing. This is an invaluable service to patients who live independently in houses or apartments.

Case managers can identify other programs and services for which patients (called clients by most mental health case managers) may be eligible and assist with negotiating the administrative maze of admission to those programs. Frequently, they are the first ones to be contacted when their clients are in crisis and often can avert a hospitalization with a temporary increase in their services.

Mentally ill people who need more supervision in order to function in the community may receive it from community support workers trained at the bachelor's level rather than from MSWs. Intensive community support services may stipulate at least weekly, but sometimes daily, contact with a client in either the client's home or elsewhere in the community. The worker may assist with chores, such as grocery shopping and laundry, give reminders about personal hygiene, make sure their clients have obtained all their prescribed medications (including both psychiatric and non-psychiatric medications), and provide transportation to appointments with physicians of all specialties. They may help manage finances, pay bills, organize an apartment, and help their clients develop a support system that promotes increased responsibility in managing their daily lives. In short, case managers and community support workers act much like surrogate family members.

PEARLS & PERILS

Contact the case manager for:
1 Missed appointments.
2 Potential for hospitalization, hospital admission, or hospital discharge.
3 Any change in current condition that requires a change in the frequency of appointments.
4 Any unusual incident or significant treatment changes:
  • Death or serious injury
  • Reasonable cause to believe there has been neglect or physical or sexual abuse
  • Any unusual incident requiring a significant response or intervention
  • Behavioral crises including:
    • Problematic or disruptive behaviors
    • Under the influence of alcohol or drugs
    • Harassment and threats
    • Suicide attempts
    • Assault
    • Arrest
  • Medical emergencies
  • Newly diagnosed serious illnesses
  • Involuntary commitment
These are events for which timely communication between all members of the treatment team (psychiatrists, primary care physicians, psychologists, social workers, pastoral counselors, etc.) is useful, both in managing the current crisis and in preparing for recovery.

Housing

A number of mentally ill people are able to live in their own homes or apartments with little supervision or assistance. As already noted, case managers or family members may help with transportation and appointment reminders. However, even with support services, some people are unable to handle their business affairs, meals, and medications and need to live in a more supervised setting. Community programs such as group homes, halfway houses, boarding homes, residential care facilities, or sheltered care facilities are examples of such settings. These services vary, even among facilities of the same type. Most facilities provide meals and dispense medications to the residents. Some homes offer regularly scheduled activities and field trips; others provide little stimulation other than television. These homes are almost never locked facilities, so residents are free to come and go within the limits of the house rules. For many patients who are mentally ill, even the least structured of these homes may still provide more structure than they would otherwise have. Many patients, despite the recommendations of the psychiatrist, family, and community social worker, refuse to live in a group setting. They offer many reasons, such as not wanting to share a room with another resident, not agreeing with the rules (such as curfew) or disliking the food.

Another housing option is the supervised apartment. Case-management systems provide weekly to daily contact and even live-in attendants whose job it is to make sure the patient's needs are being met living alone rather than in a group home. Many people prefer to live in subsidized apartments, where they are often mixed in with the elderly and people who are physically disabled. Obviously, a case manager can be especially helpful in locating the best housing for a particular person, which involves knowing which kind of housing is clinically indicated, what kind a patient will accept, and what funds are available to pay for it.

Many patients live with their families who provide most of their care. Family members handle such basic skills as personal hygiene, meal preparation, money management, and making sure the patient takes medication as prescribed. However, many times it is in the best interests of the patient and the family for the person who is mentally ill to live elsewhere. This is especially important in promoting independent functioning, as it is with all children and parents.

Financial support

People with a serious mental illness are usually eligible for disability payments as well as state and federally funded health care. If they worked before becoming ill, they may have enough work credits to be eligible for Social Security Disability (SSD) payments. After two years of receiving SSD benefits, they are eligible for Medicare, regardless of age.

Disabled people with no work history and no or low income may be eligible for Supplemental Security Income (SSI), which provides a monthly stipend. Financial eligibility and stipend size vary from state to state and may include consideration of the total household income instead of just the income of the person who is mentally ill. It typically takes 12 months of impairment to qualify for disability stipends. It is possible to have both SSD and SSI, and it is possible to have both Medicare and Medicaid.

Guardians and payees

Unless they have been judged in need of a guardian, people who are mentally ill can make their own decisions, even if these decisions are unwise in the opinion of family or mental health professionals. They can decide where they will live, how they will spend their time, and whether they will take their medication. Because their judgment may be impaired by the illness itself, this can be a source of great frustration for families, friends, and health care professionals. Even without a guardian, a "payee" (who does not have to be a family member) can be appointed when a patient's judgment is consistently impaired. The "payee" takes over any income and determines how it is spent.

Access to general health care

Finances and insurance strongly influence where psychiatric treatment and general health care are obtained. Many psychiatrists accept Medicare, with the patient responsible for the copayment. In many states the number of physicians who accept Medicaid is often limited, and these "Medicaid-only patients" must use the state's publicly funded mental health system. "Private" insurance and managed care plans often set a different reimbursement percentage for outpatient psychiatric care than for other medical care. For example, an insurance policy may cover 80% of the cost of a primary care office visit pay but only 50% of the charges for mental health treatment.

Medication cost
Many psychiatric drugs are extremely expensive, especially when they are new on the market. An example is clozapine, before it became available as a generic. Early cost estimates were $9000 per year for the medication and the required weekly CBCs, more than the annual income of some patients who needed it. The brand name drug eventually became available on state Medicaid formularies and today is available in generic form. The medication samples and coupons made available to physicians by pharmaceutical companies are often the main supply of medication to the uninsured patient. Fortunately, most companies offer patient assistance programs to provide free medications for people with low or no income. Specific information about these programs can be obtained by calling the manufacturer's customer service line found in the Physicians Desk Reference or at the www.PDR.net internet address.

Medication compliance
Complying with a complex medication regimen correctly is no easy task for the patient with cognitive or mood impairment. Someone to help oversee the filling of weekly pillboxes can greatly improve this aspect of medication compliance. Many manufacturers of antipsychotic medication have special telephone services to help patients remember to take medications and keep appointments. Information regarding these services can be obtained through the individual sponsoring pharmaceutical company.

Patients on psychotropics feel the same reluctance to take medication that other patients do. In addition, some may also think that taking a psychiatric medication is a confirmation that they "must be crazy." Such perceptions are enhanced by the illness itself, which often robs patients of insight into the need for medications. Even if patients do not resist taking medications, their altered cognitive function may interfere with their ability to take them consistently. Simplifying the medication regime to once or twice a day greatly enhances the likelihood of medication compliance. Unfortunately, just as with patients on antibiotics, once they begin to feel better, it is not uncommon for patients to stop taking their medications despite the possibility or presence of a lifelong illness.

Vocational training

Many patients are able to hold full or part-time jobs. The ability to work is a badge of normality and self-reliance. Many people see employment as the mark of success, even if they have a minimum-wage job without health insurance benefits. Contributing to others is a common human need, whether as a volunteer or employee. The importance of a job to the person with mental illness must not be overlooked despite the obstacles to successful employment.

State-funded vocational rehabilitation programs can provide job training and continuing education for qualified applicants. Other private programs under the umbrella of psychosocial rehabilitation provide job training as well.

Day programs

The negative symptoms of schizophrenia and the apathy associated with chronic depression interfere with motivation and the desire for normal social interaction. Structured use of time is an important part of treatment in these cases. Even the person who is unable to work will benefit from having a place to be at a specified time and activities to engage in once there. There are a wide variety of day programs, which vary in their activities, purpose, and eligibility requirements.

The "clubhouse" model is a particularly popular approach to day programs. These are run by clubhouse members who are patients themselves. Specific work groups and tasks teach responsibility and work skills. Additional "clubhouse" programs may include job training and supported housing. The clubhouse goal is to maximize the functioning in the community of people who are chronically ill.

Adult day care allows the elderly patient who requires supervision to continue living at home. Day care centers offer activities that provide stimulation, nutrition, and socialization. Many take care of personal hygiene and provide other basic types of care as well.

Partial hospitalization is mostly used for short-term crisis intervention whether in an attempt to avoid hospitalization by rapidly halting decompensation or as a transition back into the community after hospitalization.

Other resources

Transportation can be problematic for any of the previously mentioned programs when transportation services are not included in the program. Case managers can often provide transportation or cab vouchers for patient trips, including those to the primary care office, laboratory, and hospital.

Volunteer work is available to some people who are mentally ill even if they cannot hold paying jobs. The volunteer job helps promote a sense of self-worth and may teach skills that lead to successful employment. The local United Way chapter or Mental Health Association may be a helpful source of information regarding volunteer opportunities. Support groups run by volunteers supplement formal treatment programs. They focus on coping skills needed for dealing with a specific problem or illness, and they have application to a much wider variety of people than the chronically ill or disabled population. Psychoeducational groups have wide use in medicine with application for cancer, stroke, Parkinson's disease, asthma, depression, obsessive-compulsive disorder, and Alzheimer's disease.

National organizations formed around a particular illness or disease provide education, research funding, and support through chapters in the local community. These include the Mental Health Association (MHA), the Alzheimer's Association, the National Association for the Mentally Ill (NAMI), and the Depressive and Bipolar Support Alliance. Women's shelters are often available for women who are living in violent or otherwise abusive situations. They may have local, state, religious, or community sponsorship. For people who at times need a "listening ear," mental health hotlines, life-crisis phone services, and suicide prevention hotlines are valuable resources.

Comorbidity

High rates of comorbidity with drug and alcohol dependence further complicate diagnosis and recovery, as in some cases the substance use appears to be a "self-medicating" attempt to treat feelings and symptoms. Regardless of the reason for their use, drugs and alcohol interfere with treatment and recovery as well as with necessary and normal aspects of life such as maintaining a home, friends, and employment.

Special referral situations

Risk of suicide or homicide

Suicidal and homicidal behavior and communications should always be treated seriously by any physician. The referral of care to a psychiatrist is almost always indicated in those cases. A physician should never consider a suicide threat "just" a call for help or conclude that people who speak about suicide won't follow through and commit the act. A verbal agreement or contract with the patient not to commit suicide is not an effective way to deal with such threats. In the case of suicidal and homicidal patients, the physician should ask whether the patient has intent, a plan, and the means to execute the plan. It is not uncommon for individuals to surrender pills, knives, guns, and other items to a relative, case manager, nurse, or physician when asked to do so. Furthermore, in the case of a threatened suicide or homicide, health care providers are ethically obliged to intervene to protect lives. There is a legal "duty to warn" the intended victims of homicidal threat as well as to notify the police regarding the threat. This is a genuine means of attempting to protect lives and reduce harm from a homicidal person, affirmed by *Tarasoff vs University of California* (1976).

Referral of the patient to an emergency room of a hospital with a psychiatric division is usually necessary when there is a risk of a patient harming themselves or others. It is often helpful to enlist the help and support of a family member or friend. In some cases the family may be needed to transport the patient to a psychiatric treatment facility and to attest to suicidal risk in case involuntary hospitalization is necessary. Patients whom the physician in good faith believes to be of danger to themselves or others can also be transferred to a hospital by ambulance.

Involuntary hospitalization

Procedures for involuntary psychiatric evaluation and admission differ from state to state. Generally, individuals must be judged an imminent danger to themselves or others. The court allows individuals to be involuntarily evaluated for a specific time if the request has been made by a physician, mental health professional, or a state-appointed evaluator. Cooperation of relatives is essential when they are the only ones who can give direct evidence of the threatening or troublesome behavior.

It should be noted that a person can refuse treatment even if hospitalized under court order. A court must separately specify an order for involuntary treatment. Health care power-of-attorney often does not apply to psychiatric treatment. In some states, alcohol and drug abuse may be excluded altogether from involuntary procedures.

Abuse and neglect

When neglect or abuse of a child or an elderly or disabled person is suspected, health care professionals are mandated to report it to the authorities. This is usually accomplished with a call to a state-run hot line that initiates an investigation. The call needs to be fully documented in the medical record. In cases of other abused adults, there is no legal mandate to report abuse. Some victims continue to remain in abusive relationships, covering up or minimizing what was done to them. Probably the largest group is battered women, who come to medical facilities for treatment of physical injuries, depression, or anxiety. However, after treatment they often choose to return to their abusers. They are sometimes receptive to referrals to organizations that provide services for abused women with specially trained counselors (usually women) through individual and group therapy. Shelters can help with safety planning, legal action, and temporary placement for at-risk women and their children in undisclosed locations.

Disability assessments for mental illness

Psychologists and psychiatrists perform assessments of the degree of mental disability. To be considered disabled, an individual must have a chronic psychiatric problem with impaired ability to work and keep a job; merely having a psychiatric disorder does not qualify an individual for a psychiatric disability. Even if an acute problem has a significant duration and great severity, the psychiatric illness might not meet the definition of a chronic mental health condition and automatically qualify the patient as disabled. The impact of being declared disabled is often greater than the stigma of a psychiatric disorder. For many, disability means one is not a productive member of society. For that reason some patients seek to return to work as the psychiatric illness improves. They may need help to successfully accomplish the financial balancing act of increasing income while going off "disability" (one of the challenges of the disability stipend).

There are a number of ways Social Security currently helps facilitate a return to the work force. When earned income from a job exceeds a certain dollar amount, disability payments begin to be reduced in proportion to increased earnings until "adequate" income is achieved and the payments stop altogether. A common weak link in the process is a lack of provision for health care expenses not provided by the employer, but necessary to remain well. To reduce fear of failure and encourage reentry into the labor force, Social Security has made provisions for automatic reinstatement of full benefits (including Medicare) for a period of five years after an individual's payments stop in the event that the person becomes disabled again. This is not a well-known fact and many people shy away from work for fear of losing these benefits, unaware there is this "safety net" to the attempt to work again.

Alcohol and drug abuse treatment

Primary care physicians are often the first professionals to make a referral to self-help organizations such as Alcoholics Anonymous (AA) and Narcotics Anonymous (NA). These programs are not medical, but they are administered by people who are themselves recovering alcohol or drug abusers.

Formal licensed treatment programs for chemical dependence are staffed by physicians who may or may not be psychiatrists. The physician's level of involvement varies from program to program. Most of the treatment, including individual, group, and family therapy, is carried out by nonmedical therapists. In fact, many of the counselors do not have academic degrees. The practice of inpatient hospital treatment programs lasting several weeks (28 days) has been replaced with short periods of detoxification (3–4 days) followed by a day treatment program or outpatient treatment with follow-up sessions for longer intervals. Residential chemical dependency (CD) treatment programs still can be found, although the waiting list can be considerable. There are also private residential CD programs, but they are expensive without insurance coverage.

Some programs do not cooperate well with physicians and can be misinformed regarding, or hostile to, the medical model of psychiatric disorder. Such programs may advise against the use of any drugs for the treatment of psychiatric disorders and view any medication as antithetical to treatment. Fortunately this view is less common than in the past. A referral to a program with this philosophy could prove disastrous for patients who are severely mentally ill and whose health may depend on being maintained on medications. Many programs will allow psychiatric medications in general but not allow medications that are potentially addictive. Because of the varying nature of different programs and their advantages and disadvantages for different individuals, the primary care physician might best serve patients by using intermediate referral sources. The physician should find knowledgeable colleagues who can give advice about the bewildering array of treatment programs available nearby.

Unfortunately, one treatment modality alone may not be adequate, although many programs do not provide comprehensive help. For example, an alcoholic patient may need the help of AA, an outpatient day program, and an individual therapist. Treatments in this area need to be individually tailored. Positive outcomes often occur only after several attempts at treatment have failed. As with most treatments, psychological or medical, outcome is related to the level of motivation by the patient. Individuals with jobs and good family support maintain higher and longer levels of motivation with better treatment outcomes.

Pain control and management

Pain management programs should be administered by multidisciplinary treatment teams. Neurologists and anesthesiologists often manage the diagnosis and treatment of acute and chronic pain. Psychiatrists and psychologists evaluate the personality variables and psychiatric symptoms associated with functional pain. These evaluations may be useful in determining how aggressively a biological cause of pain should be sought and how to assist the patient in managing chronic pain. In programs for chronic pain patients are taught to live with their pain levels and are encouraged to resume as much of their normal activity as possible. Treatment programs measure progress in regaining strength, activities, and self-control and do not measure pain per se, as the target is learning to live with a certain level of it, rather than focusing on it.

Specific behavioral medicine interventions

Problems such as stress, smoking, sleep disturbance, weight control, shyness, and phobias are often treated by clinical psychologists. These symptoms occur in psychiatric illness, in medical illness, or as isolated complaints. Patients with these behavioral problems are treated in individual or in group sessions. Most clinicians working in these areas use psychological approaches that emphasize behavioral, cognitive, and skill-training procedures. Anxiety-reducing medicines may or may not be used. When patients are treated in group sessions, treatment may resemble an educational class more than traditional group therapy. The goal of treatment is to enable patients to be more functional and to exercise greater control of their thinking, emotions, and behavior.

Behavioral clinicians and treatment programs are found in hospitals, in managed care settings, and in some colleges and universities. Clinical psychologists in private practice are trained to provide these treatments as well. In some communities, the clinical psychological service center or the clinic of the university psychology department provides for these services on a sliding scale basis. In these centers, advanced doctoral students provide assessment and treatment under the supervision of clinical psychology supervisors and professors.

> ### Points to remember
>
> - Once diagnosed correctly, diligent management of symptoms through medication, regular follow-up appointments with a physician, and use of community-based support services leads to the greatest improvement in functioning.
> - Stigma and lack of knowledge about mental illness often lead to shame, embarrassment, and ultimately social isolation. People break out of that pattern by working together with professionals, family members, and friends.
>
> **PEARLS & PERILS**

Annotated bibliography

Depression Guideline Panel (1993) *Clinical Practice Guideline No. 5: depression in primary care*, vol 1: *Detection and diagnosis*; vol 2: *Treatment of major depression*, Agency for Health Care Policy and Research Publication 93–0550, Rockville, Md., U.S. Department of Health and Human Services, Public Health Service.
Volume 1 provides a general overview of mood disorders, including guidelines for detecting comorbid psychiatric and medical disorders. Screening instruments and psychological tests are also discussed. Volume 2 provides a thoughtful and critical review of all the current treatments for depression.

Lefley, HP and Wasow, M (eds) (1994) *Helping Families Cope With Mental Illness*, Langhorne, Penn., Harwood Academic Publishers.

This book offers detailed information about the impact of mental illness on the family and about what families need from professionals. There is also useful information for professionals interested in implementing family education and support programs.

Mueser, KT and Gingerich, S (1994) *Coping With Schizophrenia,* Oakland, Calif., New Harbinger Publications.

This is an extremely useful book for families with members who are schizophrenic. It is written in everyday language and contains practical information about community resources and about ways of dealing with symptoms and behaviors stemming from the illness. It also offers suggestions about how to meet families' needs.

SECTION 2

Psychopathology

Keith E. Isenberg, MD

CHAPTER 8

Depression, Mania, and Related Disorders

Wayne C. Drevets, MD and Richard D. Todd, PhD, MD

Introduction

The World Health Organization ranks depression as one of the top three health conditions in terms of burden of disease. This chapter discusses the diagnosis and treatment of major depressive disorder, dysthymic disorder, bipolar disorder (manic-depressive illness), and cyclothymic disorder. In addition, an overview of current knowledge regarding the etiology and natural history of these disorders is presented. Though these disorders occur in children and young adolescents, our comments are generally limited to older adolescents and adults.

Phenomenology of mood disorders

Major depressive disorder rivals hypertension as the most frequently encountered illness in primary health care. Nevertheless, this and the other mood disorders remain among the most poorly understood human diseases. Factors that have hindered elucidation of the pathophysiology of these illnesses include the dearth of gross neuropathological changes associated with primary mood disorders, the lack of satisfactory non-human animal models, the limitations in studying human brain function *in vivo*, and the complexity of studying interactions between psychosocial stressors and biological predisposition. Moreover, while scientific investigation has demonstrated that mood disorders are associated with genetic, neurochemical, neuroendocrine, and neurophysiological factors, biological markers have lacked the sensitivity and specificity needed to distinguish illness subtypes from one another or from normative states, preventing the nosology of mood disorders from advancing beyond the syndromic level.

Because of this limitation, the syndromes identified as individual mood disorders do not reflect discrete disease entities but rather are presumed to encompass diverse groups of neuropsychiatric disorders. Heterogeneity is manifested by the ranges of behavioral signs (e.g., from psychomotor retardation to agitation), symptoms (e.g., from insomnia to hypersomnolence), and biochemical abnormalities found within the same syndrome (e.g., from abnormally low (in nonpsychotic depression) to high (in psychotic depression) cerebrospinal fluid levels of homovanillic acid). Moreover, some, but not all, patients present with phenomenologically distinct states over the illness course, suffering manic as well as depressive syndromes. Diverse biological antecedents appear capable of inducing mood disorders, as depressive or manic syndromes can be produced by dissimilar neurological disorders, endocrine disturbances, or pharmacological agents. Major depressive episodes can also occur in the absence of medical or psychosocial stressors as "primary," familial, idiopathic disorders or may arise secondary to other psychiatric disorders in which neuropathological changes have been identified (e.g., schizophrenia). Finally, some cases of mood disorders appear to have been initiated and maintained by psychosocial precipitants. Thus, while pathophysiologic correlates of mood disorder subtypes have not been established, mood disorders include a group of conditions stemming from a variety of genetic, neuropathological or psychosocial factors working alone or in concert with one another.

The clinical heterogeneity within mood syndromes has enabled the coexistence of both psychological and biological theories regarding the etiology and treatment of mood disorders. For example, Sigmund Freud studied mildly ill, nonhospitalized patients and concluded that depression was rooted in a psychological reaction to the loss of a highly-valued "love object," highlighting the similarities between depression and bereavement. More recently, competing hypotheses have arisen from behaviorist roots, which hold that depression results from thought patterns in which life events, social interactions, and self-perceptions are habitually viewed negatively, resulting in a lowered mood. The proponents of these "cognitive-behavioral" theories have also primarily relied upon studies in less severely depressed outpatients. In contrast, the medical model approach adopted by much of the psychiatric research community emanates from the work of Emil Kraepelin, who described the symptoms of syndromes observed in severely ill, hospitalized patients. Kraepelin coined the term "manic-depressive psychosis" to encompass both bipolar and unipolar mood disorders and insisted that the cause of such disorders was "innate" and independent of social and psychological forces.

Psychological theories follow logically from simple observations that mood is normally affected by social, medical, psychological, and spiritual/religious factors, leading to the assumption that mood disorders constitute reactions to psychosocial or medical stressors. Differing from a normally reactive low mood, however, the major depressive syndrome does not simply arise in response to medical or psychosocial stressors and, in most cases, the role that adverse life events play in precipitating pathological mood episodes remains unclear. Furthermore, mood disorders persist for protracted periods of time, are not alleviated by positive life events, reach extremes in magnitude such that function is impaired, and can be ameliorated and prevented by somatic treatments that do not affect mood states in subjects without mood disorders.

The extant scientific data support biological rather than psychosocial hypotheses regarding the pathogenesis of severe mood disorders. These data suggest that mood disorders constitute diseases that affect brain circuits which modulate the set point and stability of emotion. The ultimate resolution of disagreements regarding the nature of mood disorders is expected to depend upon elucidation of the pathophysiological correlates and the molecular genetics of the familial forms of mood disorders. Nevertheless, in view of the clinical heterogeneity represented within the mood disorders, it should not be anticipated that every case would fall into such categories, as some patients with mild or atypical forms of the major depressive syndrome may elude biologically-based classifications.

Classification

In the progression of disease nosology from the levels of symptom to syndrome to pathophysiology to etiology (e.g., symptom: moodiness and forgetfulness; syndrome: "general paresis;" pathophysiology: "pachymeningitis hemorrhagica," diffuse neuronal degeneration, and neuroglial proliferation; etiology: infectious involvement of the brain with *Treponema pallidum* [neurosyphilis]), psychiatric diagnosis largely remains at the syndromatic level. To differentiate mood disorders from feelings of sadness, despondency, or elation, which occur normally in reaction to life circumstances, diagnostic criteria based upon clusters of clinical symptoms and behavioral signs are used. While such criteria are susceptible to subjective interpretation by both the patient and the examiner, the diagnosis of major depressive disorder (MDD) or bipolar disorder using this system has high interrater reliability and diagnostic stability across time. For example, about 84% of people with unipolar depression retain the diagnosis of MDD after several years of follow-up. Moreover, most cases for whom the diagnosis ultimately changes receive another mood disorder diagnosis, as about 10% of cases initially diagnosed as MDD convert to a diagnosis of bipolar disorder as a result of the subsequent development of mania. In either of these mood disorders, the diagnostic criteria for a major depressive episode are useful for demarcating a pathological mood state likely to respond to somatic antidepressant treatment.

Biological markers with adequate sensitivity and specificity to establish a mood disorder diagnosis are not available. While laboratory analyses such as the "dexamethasone suppression test" and sleep EEG studies can be confirmatory in ambiguous cases, a negative result does not reliably exclude and a positive result does not delimit the diagnosis of a mood disorder. Laboratory analyses, electroencephalographic (EEG) studies, neuroimaging results and neuropsychological testing are instead used largely to exclude general medical or neurological illnesses that can present with depressive symptoms (Chapter 27).

The absence of biological markers for disease can lead to diagnostic uncertainty when the severity of illness is mild, and the threshold for assigning a diagnosis and recommending treatment can be ambiguous. However, most patients who seek treatment from a physician are experiencing symptoms of moderate-to-severe intensity, and the diagnosis in these cases is relatively straightforward. When the diagnosis remains questionable, a family history of mood disorders weights the decision toward a positive diagnosis, since mood disorders follow a familial pattern of transmission.

The current diagnostic criteria for mood disorders are compiled in the *Diagnostic and Statistical Manual of Mental Disorders* (DSM-IV). The symptom constellations fundamental to this classification are the major depressive episode as a pathological mood state characterized by dysphoric mood, the manic episode as a pathological mood state characterized by euphoric mood, and the hypomanic episode as a mild form of mania. The diagnostic framework built upon these syndromes identifies major depressive disorder as single or recurrent depressive episodes (also called "unipolar depression"), bipolar disorder (classically "manic-depressive illness") as a course in which manic episodes occur with or without depressive episodes, dysthymic disorder as a chronic subsyndromal depressive episode, and cyclothymic disorder as a milder expression of bipolar disorder.

The DSM-IV criteria for mood disorders are based upon refinements of the criteria developed in natural history studies at Washington University by Eli Robins, MD, Samuel Guze, MD, and George Winokur, MD. The older term "affective disorders" has been replaced in the DSM-IV by the term "mood disorders." Affect is the mood state inferred by the clinician from the patient's appearance, behavior, and verbally communicated emotional state, while mood indicates the subjective emotional state described by the patient. A feature of the Washington University criteria that was not adopted by DSM-IV, but is applied and discussed herein, is the distinction between "primary" and "secondary" mood disorders. This concept is useful for both clinical and research approaches to mood disorders, just as this dichotomy has proven useful in other areas of medicine.

Major depressive disorder and dysthymic disorder

Diagnostic criteria

The diagnosis of MDD is based upon the presence of a major depressive episode (Box 8.1) and the absence of other medical or major psychiatric illnesses that might be associated with it, e.g., Parkinson's disease or schizophrenia (Box 8.2 and Table 8.1). The major depressive episode consists of a pathologic disturbance of mood and affect in which a persistent negative emotional state has been present for at least two weeks. Emotional changes alone do not warrant the diagnosis; they must be accompanied by changes in energy, sleep, appetite, activity, and cognition (Box 8.1).

Dysthymic disorder is characterized by chronic, persistent depressive symptoms of at least two years duration (Box 8.3). Too few depressive symptoms are present to warrant the diagnosis of MDD (i.e., dysthymia is a "subsyndromal" depressive syndrome), and the depressed mood is less severe than that associated with MDD. Dysthymia is a heterogenous condition. Some people with dysthymia have a long history of being unhappy, classically termed "depressive neurosis," and such patients typically respond poorly to antidepressant treatment. Others appear to have a mild form of MDD and may later develop full criteria for a major depressive episode. This latter group generally proves responsive to antidepressant pharmacotherapy.

Box 8.1 A major depressive episode

A. Five (or more) of the following symptoms have been present during the same two-week period and represent a change from previous functioning; at least one of the symptoms is either (1) depressed mood or (2) loss of interest or pleasure. **Note**: Do not include symptoms that are clearly due to a general medical condition, or mood-incongruent delusions or hallucinations.

1 Depressed mood most of the day, nearly every day, as indicated by either subjective report (e.g., feels sad or empty) or observation made by others (e.g., appears tearful). **Note**: In children and adolescents, can be irritable mood.

2 Markedly diminished interest or pleasure in all, or almost all, activities most of the day, nearly every day (as indicated by either subjective account or observation made by others).

3 Significant weight loss when not dieting or weight gain (e.g., a change of more than 5% of body weight in a month), or decrease or increase in appetite nearly every day. **Note**: In children, consider failure to make expected weight gains.

4 Insomnia or hypersomnia nearly every day.

5 Psychomotor agitation or retardation nearly every day (observable by others, not merely subjective feelings of restlessness or being slowed down).

6 Fatigue or loss of energy nearly every day.

7 Feelings of worthlessness or excessive or inappropriate guilt (which may be delusional) nearly every day (not merely self-reproach or guilt about being sick).

8 Diminished ability to think or concentrate, or indecisiveness, nearly every day (either by subjective account or as observed by others).

9 Recurrent thoughts of death (not just fear of dying), recurrent suicidal ideation without a specific plan, or a suicide attempt or a specific plan for committing suicide.

B. The symptoms do not meet criteria for a mixed episode.

C. The symptoms cause clinically significant distress or impairment in social, occupational, or other important areas of functioning.

D. The symptoms are not due to the direct physiological effects of a substance (e.g., a drug of abuse, a medication) or a general medical condition (e.g., hypothyroidism).

E. The symptoms are not better accounted for by bereavement, i.e., after the loss of a loved one, the symptoms persist for longer than two months or are characterized by marked functional impairment, morbid preoccupation with worthlessness, suicidal ideation, psychotic symptoms, or psychomotor retardation.

From American Psychiatric Association (2000) Diagnostic and Statistical Manual of Mental Disorders, 4th Edition, Text Revision, Washington, D.C., American Psychiatric Association.

DIAGNOSTIC CRITERIA

Box 8.2 Major depressive disorder*

- Presence of major depressive episode(s) (see Box 8.1).
- The major depressive episodes are not better accounted for by schizoaffective disorder and are not superimposed on schizophrenia, schizophreniform disorder, delusional disorder, or psychotic disorder not otherwise specified.
- There has never been a manic episode (see Box 8.6), a mixed episode, or a hypomanic episode (Box 8.7).

* The illness course is specified as either single episode or recurrent.

Adapted from American Psychiatric Association (2000) Diagnostic and Statistical Manual of Mental Disorders, 4th Edition, Text Revision, Washington, D.C., American Psychiatric Association.

DIAGNOSTIC CRITERIA

Table 8.1 Major depressive disorder

DIAGNOSIS

Discriminating feature

1 Pervasive depressed mood or loss of interest or pleasure present >2 weeks, which constitutes a change from previous functioning.

Consistent features

1 Episodic course.
2 Fatigue or loss of energy.
3 Change in sleep pattern, appetite, libido.
4 Anxiety, worrying, or tension.
5 Recurrent negative thoughts of guilt, self-reproach, death, or suicide.
6 Improvement during somatic antidepressant treatment.
7 Irritability.
8 Impaired concentration.
9 Diminished involvement in social and other motor activities.
10 Apathy, amotivation.

Variable features

1 Suicide risk.
2 Psychotic or obsessional features.
3 Panic attacks.
4 Psychomotor retardation or agitation.
5 Comorbid substance abuse.
6 Family history of mood disorder.
7 Anorexia with weight loss.
8 Hyperphagia with weight gain.
9 Increased somatic complaints.
10 Mood no longer reactive to positive events.

Box 8.3 Dysthymic disorder

DIAGNOSTIC CRITERIA

A. Depressed mood for most of the day, for more days than not, as indicated either by subjective account or observation by others, for at least two years. **Note:** In children and adolescents, mood can be irritable and duration must be at least one year.

B. Presence, while depressed, of two (or more) of the following:
 1 poor appetite or overeating
 2 insomnia or hypersomnia
 3 low energy or fatigue
 4 low self-esteem
 5 poor concentration or difficulty making decisions
 6 feelings of hopelessness.

C. During the two-year period (one year for children or adolescents) of the disturbance, the person has never been without the symptoms in Criteria A and B for more than two months at a time.

D. No major depressive episode (Box 8.1) has been present during the first two years of the disturbance (one year for children and adolescents), i.e., the disturbance is not better accounted for by chronic major depressive disorder, or major depressive disorder, in partial remission. **Note:** There may have been a previous major depressive episode provided there was a full remission (no significant signs or symptoms for two months) before development of the dysthymic disorder. In addition, after the initial two years (one year in children or adolescents) of dysthymic disorder, there may be superimposed episodes of major depressive disorder, in which case both diagnoses may be given when the criteria are met for a major depressive episode.

E. There has never been a manic episode (Box 8.5), a mixed episode, or a hypomanic episode (Box 8.6), and criteria have never been met for cyclothymic disorder (Box 8.8).

F. The disturbance does not occur exclusively during the course of a chronic psychotic disorder, such as schizophrenia or delusional disorder.

G. The symptoms are not due to the direct physiological effects of a substance (e.g., a drug of abuse, a medication) or a general medical condition (e.g., hypothyroidism).

H. The symptoms cause clinically significant distress or impairment in social, occupational, or other important areas of functioning.

From American Psychiatric Association: Diagnostic and Statistical Manual of Mental Disorders, 4th Edition, Text Revision, Washington, D.C., 2000, American Psychiatric Association.

KEY CLINICAL QUESTIONS AND WHAT THEY CAN UNLOCK

- *How do I screen for depression?*

  Several approaches can be taken to screening for depression, and each practitioner is encouraged to develop the approach or mix of approaches that best suits a specific practice. One strategy that can be useful is to ask patients about persistent (more than two weeks) low mood and loss of interest in activities. These symptoms are considered critical to the diagnosis of depression, and most depressed patients endorse one or the other, if not both. Positive responses should be followed by questions about the remaining symptoms of depression. Another approach is to ask about symptoms of depression when examining patients with chronic medical illness, focusing a thorough examination for depression on patients who have complaints that are disproportionate to findings. The risk of depression in patients with chronic illness is increased 3–5 times. The practitioner has to decide how to count symptoms towards depression for these patients—inclusive, exclusive, or neutral—because chronic illnesses are often associated with symptoms such as fatigue and insomnia independent of the presence of depression. An inclusive approach to symptomatology (counting all endorsements of depressive symptoms towards the diagnosis of depression) may overdiagnose depression and expose patients to risks of treatment needlessly. An exclusive approach (attributing some symptoms like fatigue to the medical illness) may deny treatment to patients who would benefit from it. A neutral approach (make an attribution judgment, depression or chronic medical illness) is difficult to execute because of a lack of rules about making the judgment. Whatever approach is used, close follow-up and reassessment is recommended.

- *How long should prophylactic medication treatment for depression be sustained?*

  The successful treatment of the first episode of depression should be followed by at least six months of pharmacotherapy, probably longer if the episode was severe or associated with psychosis. More than three episodes of depression is an indication for indefinite treatment, and the issue may become one of identifying the "best" treatment.

Clinical picture

The clinical presentation is variable, and the chief complaint may reflect an assortment of somatic, emotional, or neuropsychological symptoms. Since mood disorders follow an episodic course, a salient feature of mood syndromes is that the current symptoms constitute a clear deviation from the patient's usual mood, activity, and level of functioning. It can be helpful to have patients compare their current mood, desire to socialize, sleep pattern, libido, and concentration to their own baseline with questions such as, "Do you still enjoy _____?", filling in the blank with items such as seeing grandchildren or engaging in hobbies, work, or sex. Nevertheless, episodes of depression may persist for several years, and some patients find it difficult to estimate their "normal baseline."

Emotional manifestations

The emotional experience during a major depressive episode is marked by the intrusion of negative emotions and the absence of positive emotions. Since the pathophysiology of MDD remains obscure, the lay term "depression" has been applied to the group of neuropsychiatric disorders encompassed by this syndrome. Nevertheless, some patients meeting criteria for MDD do not endorse feeling sad or depressed. An equally common emotional change is a pervasive loss of interest or pleasure in activities that previously produced positive emotion. For example, the enjoyment derived from interpersonal relationships, church activities, work, hobbies, food, or sex vanishes. This inability to experience pleasure is called anhedonia.

Patients with MDD also may experience anxiety, irritability, or despondence. Anxiety may be manifested as anxious mood, fear, worry, or motor tension, which may dominate the clinical picture. A minority of patients manifest panic attacks, obsessions, compulsions, or phobias. In primary MDD, anxiety symptoms are usually limited to the duration of the depressive episode and resolve during effective antidepressant pharmacotherapy. Irritability can be most troublesome for family members and may consequently serve as the presenting complaint of patients sent for treatment by their families. Female patients with MDD often experience increased irritability and dysphoria during the one- to two-week period prior to menses, leading some to complain of having "premenstrual syndrome." Patients may also describe feeling discouraged, worthless, or hopeless. Some report that simple emotional descriptors do not adequately characterize the mood phenomena, using terms such as "psychic pain" or "emotional deadness" instead.

Diurnal variation of the mood disturbance is relatively specific to mood disorders. This is usually manifested by severely depressed mood and anergia upon awakening that persists throughout the morning, but then progressively diminishes during the afternoon and evening. A reversal of this pattern can also occur in which evening is the period when depressive symptoms are worse.

Neurovegetative manifestations

The neurovegetative features of the major depressive episode are as critical to the diagnosis of mood disorders as the emotional components. They facilitate distinctions between a major depressive episode and a "normal" low mood that is reactive to life situations. In many cases, changes in sleep, energy, or appetite precede the changes in emotion. The neurovegetative features can thus serve as harbingers of a recurrence in patients with a history of MDD.

The most common symptom associated with a major depressive episode is anergia, described as a loss of energy or easy fatigability (Table 8.2). This symptom may constitute the chief complaint. Anergia is a common reason for depressed patients to consult physicians, highlighting the need for clinicians to be alert to physical symptoms as presenting complaints for MDD.

Sleep disturbances are also commonly present. These include initial insomnia (difficulty falling asleep), middle insomnia (awakening during the night with difficulty returning to sleep), terminal insomnia (awakening early in the morning with inability to return to sleep), or hypersomnia (excessive sleeping). Sleep changes may also serve as the presenting complaint for MDD. Young adults or adolescents are more likely to experience initial insomnia while terminal insomnia is more common in elderly patients.

Alterations in appetite and weight are also common symptoms. Anorexia and weight loss can be observed in depressed patients of any age, but are particularly prominent in elderly patients. Reduced oral intake during a major depressive episode may lead to dehydration and malnutrition in depressed elders, contributing to the morbidity associated with geriatric depression. In addition, hyperphagia with weight gain can be observed in younger patients. Dramatic weight fluctuations without other medical explanation should lead the clinician to inquire about other depressive symptoms.

Finally, loss of libido and other types of sexual dysfunction are common. It is unclear whether these symptoms reflect pathophysiological involvement of hypothalamic or neuroendocrine function or simply indicate another manifestation of anhedonia. The former explanation is suggested by observations that reduced libido may be the most persistent depressive symptom during treatment, continuing even after mood, hedonia, and self-esteem have returned to baseline. Moreover, some antidepressant drugs produce sexual dysfunction as side effects, necessitating monitoring for the development of new sexual problems during treatment. Disturbances of sexual function contribute to the strain that mood disorders place upon marital relationships.

Psychological manifestations

Disturbances of thought content, self-perception, and assessment of one's current and future circumstances also accompany depressive episodes. Negative thoughts intrude upon the conscious thought processes and reverberate to the extent that the ability to inhibit such thoughts seems impaired. In severely depressed patients, psychotherapeutic

TABLE 8.2

Symptoms of index major depressive episode

Symptoms*	No. and percentage of patients (n = 100)
Reduced energy level	97
Impaired concentration	84
Anorexia	80
Initial insomnia	77
Loss of interest	77
Difficulty starting activities	76
Worry more than usual	69
Subjective agitation	67
Slowed thinking	67
Difficulty with decision making	67
Terminal insomnia	65
Suicide ideation or plans	63
Weight loss	61
Tearfulness	61
Movements slowed (subjective perception)	60
Increased irritability	60
Feels will never get well	56
Diurnal variation	46
Difficulty finishing activities once started	46
Prominent self-pity	45
Inability to cry	44
Constipation	43
Impaired expression of emotions	42
Ruminations of worthlessness	38
Decreased libido	36
Anxiety attacks	36
Difficulty doing activities once started	35
Ruminations of guilt	32
Complains more than usual	28
Any type of delusion	27
Phobias during depression only	27
Multiple somatic symptoms during depression only	25
Communication of suicidal ideas, plans, or attempts	22
Place major blame for illness on others	19
At least one depressive delusion	16
Death wishes without suicidal ideation	16
Suicide attempts	15
Other delusions	14
Obsessions during depression only	14
Depersonalization and derealization	13
Ruminations of sinfulness	12

Source: Adapted from Baker *et al.* (1971) as reprinted by permission from Winokur G. in Winokur and Clayton (1994) *The Medical Basis of Psychiatry*.

* The inclusion criteria for this study required that subjects had reported a mood change that they described as *either* feeling depressed, blue, sad, low, discouraged, or that the future looked gloomy. The proportion of subjects endorsing each of these individual symptoms was not addressed, however.

attempts are unsuccessful at alleviating thoughts of guilt, death, suicide, or hopelessness, highlighting their obsessional or, at times, delusional nature. Ruminative ideation resolves relatively abruptly once a successful response to an antidepressant drug or electroconvulsive therapy (ECT) is achieved, which suggests that abnormal brain processes underlie and maintain such symptoms.

The most dramatic disturbance of the thought content is preoccupation with death or suicide. Suicidal thoughts are common in patients with MDD (Table 8.2), and their appearance in patients with MDD should be taken seriously (see Chapter 29). Thoughts of death and suicide are often described as intrusive and difficult to interrupt. They are generally accompanied by a desire for death and the idea that death alone will provide relief from the depressive episode. The poor insight of depressed patients contemplating suicide is illustrated by their conviction that family members, including spouses and small children, will be "better off" without them. The determination of some depressed patients to commit suicide and the violent means which they sometimes select bear testimony to the great suffering associated with MDD.

Tips for detecting and managing depression

PEARLS & PERILS

- The predominant emotional change associated with major depressive episodes may not be depressed mood but may instead be anxiety or pervasive loss of interest or pleasure.
- The most common symptom associated with major depressive episodes is not an emotional symptom but rather a physical symptom: namely, fatigue or anergia.
- Major depressive episodes are associated with a significant risk of suicide, and patients suspected of suffering from a mood disorder should be asked if they are contemplating suicide.
- Patients who meet criteria for a major depressive episode usually benefit from antidepressant pharmacotherapy.

Other prominent distortions of thought content involve self-deprecatory ideation and hopelessness. Incessant ruminations on past failures or perceived shortcomings may occupy a majority of the thought stream. Many patients describe awakening during the night to thoughts of self-reproach. In concert with such thoughts, self-confidence deteriorates and patients feel unable to handle the conflicts or challenges at work or home that they have previously mastered. A sudden decrement in self-esteem is a usual concomitant of the depressive episode and can provide an important clue to its presence. Hopelessness regarding the future may

develop in spite of evidence that the patient's social, economic, or medical status has not changed and, to the examiner or the family, appears positive. Hopelessness is reportedly associated with an elevated risk for suicide during a depressive episode.

Ruminations of guilt may achieve a delusional level. For example, patients may develop the belief that they have committed the "unpardonable sin" or have "lost their salvation," ideas that arrive with the onset of the depressive episode and depart with its remission. Patients may also describe persistent guilt regarding seemingly minor offenses they perceive having committed during interpersonal interactions. In many cases these involve statements made years earlier that have been forgotten by the recipient and are not contemplated by the patient outside the context of a depressive episode. Finally, pathological guilt may target behaviors or events that the patient has not normally associated with guilt in the past.

Psychotic features such as delusions or auditory hallucinations are present in up to 20% of patients with a depressive episode and occur most commonly in elderly patients or patients who are in the depressed phase of bipolar disorder. Depressive delusions are usually "mood congruent," in that they involve typical depressive themes of personal inadequacy, guilt, disease, death, nihilism or deserved punishment. Delusions in the setting of a major depressive episode have important treatment implications, with the most effective treatments being either ECT or a combination of an antidepressant drug and an antipsychotic drug. In addition, while a diagnosis of MDD is associated with a decreased risk for violence relative to the base rate for the population, when patients with MDD commit violent acts against other people, they are often responding to persecutory or nihilistic delusions. Auditory hallucinations are less common in MDD and usually convey persecutory content. Visual, tactile or olfactory hallucinations are exceedingly rare in mood disorders, and their presence should prompt a search for metabolic, toxic, or neurological disturbances.

Psychosomatic symptoms

Depressed patients often complain of headaches, pains, gastrointestinal disturbances, or cardiovascular symptoms. Headache is present in the majority of cases, and when associated with a depressive episode, it resolves along with the other depressive symptoms. Headaches may be related to increased contraction of the head and neck musculature. For example, psychophysiological studies demonstrate that the frontalis muscles have greater electromyographic activity in resting patients with depression than non-depressed subjects who are intentionally contracting their facial muscles. Gastrointestinal complaints are also common and include functional ("irritable") bowel syndrome, constipation, and abdominal pain (possibly reflecting a heightened sensitivity to visceral sensation). When medical workup for somatic complaints has proven negative, the alert clinician should attempt to elicit other criteria for major depression.

Psychomotor manifestations

Psychomotor agitation and retardation are striking clinical features of severe depressive episodes. Agitation presents more commonly in elderly depressed patients and retardation in younger patients with bipolar depression. In over one-half of cases, the psychomotor activity is not disturbed, so a relatively normal appearance does not rule out MDD. Agitation is evident in about 30% of patients hospitalized for depression. When present, it may dominate the clinical presentation, as patients pace, wring their hands, or incessantly complain of worries and nervousness. Such patients may repeatedly bemoan their fate, ask for reassurance, or beg for help, yet they cannot be consoled. Psychomotor retardation is observed in about 20% of hospitalized patients as a decrease in the rate and the amount of movement and speech or as latency in the onset of speech. The slowing can sometimes be elicited by having patients perform simple motor tasks. In outpatients, psychomotor retardation is less commonly evident on the mental status examination, but may nevertheless be described by the patient as a sense that the rate of their thought flow has slowed.

Neuropsychological manifestations

Depressed patients often complain vociferously of impairments in concentration, memory, or ability to make decisions. In many cases, however, employers, family members, and friends are unaware of any deficits in thinking or performance. In other cases, school or work performance deteriorates, reflecting the combined impact of diminished motivation, preoccupation with obsessive ruminations, severe anxiety, or insomnia, as well as impaired concentration. Occasionally, the lack of effort and motivation on the part of the patient during the mental status examination may give the appearance that memory is impaired. This presentation has been referred to as "pseudodementia" or "dementia of depression," in which manifestations of the memory impairment resolve with effective antidepressant treatment (see Chapter 26). Core signs of dementia, such as aphasia, anomia, acalculia, agraphia, or apraxia, are not associated with primary mood disorders, and their presence suggests that if the depressive syndrome is present, it has occurred in the setting of a neurological disorder.

Studies employing neuropsychological tests that assess specific aspects of attention, memory, or sensory processing have demonstrated wide ranging, but clinically subtle, cognitive deficits in depression and mania. These include deficits in early information processing, recollection memory and planning, biases in attention to and perception of affectively valenced information, and abnormal responses to negative feedback. Some residual deficits are also evident in a proportion of remitted subjects, even when controlling for mood.

QUOTATION OF A DEPRESSED PHYSICIAN

Firstly, it is very unpleasant: depressive illness is probably more unpleasant than any disease except rabies. There is constant mental pain and often psychogenic physical pain too. If one tries to get such a patient to titrate other pains against the pain of his depression one tends to end up with a description that would raise eyebrows even in a medieval torture chamber.

Naturally, many of these patients commit suicide. They may not hope to get to heaven but they know they are leaving hell. Secondly, the patient is isolated from family and friends, because the depression itself reduces his affection for others and he may well have ideas that he is unworthy of their love or even that his friendship may harm them. Thirdly, he is rejected by others because they cannot stand the sight of his suffering.

There is a limit to sympathy. Even psychiatrists have protective mechanisms for dealing with such cases: the consultant may refer the patient to an outpatient clinic; he may allow too brief a consultation to elicit the extent of the patient's suffering; he may, on the grounds that the depression has not responded to treatment, alter his diagnosis to one of personality disorder—comforting, because of the strange but widespread belief that patients with personality disorders do not suffer.

Fourthly, and finally, the patient tends to do a great cover-up. Because of his outward depression he is socially unacceptable, and because of his inward depression he feels even more socially unacceptable than he really is. He does not, therefore, tell others how bad he feels.

Most depressives, even severe ones, can cope with routine work—initiative and leadership are what they lack. Nevertheless, many of them can continue working, functioning at a fairly low level, and their deficiencies are often covered up by colleagues. Provided some minimal degree of social and vocational functioning is present, the world leaves the depressive alone and he battles on for the sake of his god or his children, or for some reason which makes his personal torment preferable to death.

Reprinted with permission from Goodwin and Guze, *Psychiatric Diagnosis*, 1989.

QUOTATION OF A DEPRESSED PATIENT

"Now that I've had both depression and cancer, I'd have to say the cancer has been easier to deal with. Cancer is something tangible that you can understand and describe to other people. With major depression you suffer horribly, but you can neither comprehend why you feel the way you do nor communicate your suffering to others. When you talk about the pain of major depression with others it makes no sense to them." —*stated by a patient following successful treatment of her depression with doxepin, prior to her death from breast cancer.*

Impairment of insight and judgment

Insight may be impaired to the point that patients deny that they are ill or that their illness is treatable. Even patients who have experienced excellent antidepressant treatment responses during previous episodes may maintain that only death will relieve their suffering. Patients may also cry profusely or discuss suicide plans with the physician yet deny feeling depressed or being ill. Such cases require intervention by the family and the clinician to initiate and complete treatment.

Impaired insight can result in poor judgment, and depressed patients may attempt to change jobs, discontinue school or seek divorce because they think that such a change will relieve their symptoms. It is generally prudent for the clinician to advise against making such changes until the depressive episode has been effectively treated. Other examples of failures in judgment include the propensity of some patients to act upon depressive delusions or to self-medicate with illicit drugs or alcohol.

Alcohol and illicit drug use

Some patients increase alcohol use during depressive episodes, describing a desire to self-medicate for their anxiety, insomnia, or dysphoria. Others decrease alcohol use after experiencing a worsening of such symptoms or an increase in suicidal behavior related to alcohol consumption. The former group generally admits that any relief obtained from alcohol is short-lived and is usually succeeded by an exacerbation of the depressive symptoms. New onset of alcohol abuse, particularly after age 40, should prompt a careful evaluation for signs and symptoms of a mood disorder.

Illicit drugs are also employed to alleviate depressive symptoms. Marijuana, cocaine, and ecstasy are common agents abused by patients with mood disorders. Cocaine can produce depressed mood as a withdrawal symptom, making the differential diagnosis between cocaine dependence with secondary depression versus primary depression with secondary cocaine abuse difficult.

Diagnostic subtypes

In an attempt to address the clinical heterogeneity of MDD, depressive syndromes have been subdivided in numerous classification schemes. DSM-IV recognizes melancholic and seasonal subtypes of MDD. The other subtypes described below have proven to be useful in selecting subject samples for mood disorders research and have noteworthy clinical implications as well.

Melancholic type

The DSM-IV criteria for melancholic subtype are thought to identify a more severe form of MDD (Box 8.4). These criteria emphasize nonreactive mood, pervasive anhedonia, promi-

nent neurovegetative symptoms, psychomotor signs, and freedom from characterological disturbances. A substantial body of evidence suggests that this cluster of signs and symptoms predicts a good outcome in response to ECT or antidepressant drug treatment.

Box 8.4 Melancholic features specifier

DIAGNOSTIC CRITERIA

Specify if:
With melancholic features (can be applied to the current or most recent major depressive episode in major depressive disorder and to a major depressive episode in bipolar I or bipolar II disorder only if it is the most recent type of mood episode).

A. Either of the following, occurring during the most severe period of the current episode:
 1 loss of pleasure in all, or almost all, activities
 2 lack of reactivity to usually pleasurable stimuli (does not feel much better, even temporarily, when something good happens).

B. Three (or more) of the following:
 1 distinct quality of depressed mood (i.e., the depressed mood is experienced as distinctly different from the kind of feeling experienced after the death of a loved one)
 2 depression regularly worse in the morning
 3 early morning awakening (at least two hours before usual time of awakening)
 4 marked psychomotor retardation or agitation
 5 significant anorexia or weight loss
 6 excessive or inappropriate guilt.

From American Psychiatric Association (2000) Diagnostic and Statistical Manual of Mental Disorders, 4th Edition, Text Revision, Washington, D.C., American Psychiatric Association.

Seasonal depression

The course of depressive episodes exhibits a seasonal pattern in some cases, with depression onset occurring in fall and winter and symptom remission ensuing in the spring. Seasonal depression may be more common in northern geographical locations (e.g., Scandinavia, Canada, and the New England or Pacific Northwestern states), suggesting that it is more prevalent at latitudes where the period of sunlight exposure substantially shortens during winter. Up to one-half of such patients have bipolar disorder. Winter seasonal depression may respond to phototherapy.

Primary versus secondary mood disorders

A mood disorder is considered primary when the pathological mood episode arises in the absence of other psychiatric disorders or chronic debilitating medical disorders that might be associated with it. In contrast, a major depressive episode is considered secondary to another psychiatric disorder if the first depressive episode historically ensued after the onset of the other disorder. Similarly, if the first major depressive episode ensues after the onset of a major medical illness it can be considered secondary. This does not necessarily signify that the depression is etiologically related to the other disorder. The concept of "comorbidity" also attempts to characterize multiple, concomitant psychiatric syndromes, but such knowledge is less useful without the hierarchical information provided by the primary versus secondary distinction.

Whether a depressive episode is primary or secondary to another illness holds prognostic and therapeutic implications. As discussed below, treatment selection is generally directed toward the primary, rather than the secondary disorder. In addition, whereas primary mood disorders are often associated with a return to the premorbid baseline (i.e., relative normalcy) between episodes, many secondary depressions are not, since the pre-existing primary disorder is often a chronic illness (e.g., schizophrenia or obsessive-compulsive disorder). Furthermore, the risk of suicide is significantly higher in primary MDD than in secondary depression, with the exception of depression secondary to alcoholism, which also carries a high risk for suicide. Finally, the sleep EEG, neuroendocrine and neuroimaging abnormalities found in patients with MDD or bipolar disorder are usually not found in patients with secondary depression.

Classification of primary unipolar depression using family history

A classification that has proven useful in selecting relatively homogenous samples of patients with unipolar depression for neuroimaging studies identifies three subtypes based upon family history. Familial pure depressive disease (FPDD) is defined as primary unipolar depression in an individual who has a parent, sibling or offspring with primary unipolar depression but no family history of alcoholism, antisocial personality disorder or mania. Depressive spectrum disease (DSD) is unipolar depression in a patient who has a first-degree relative with alcoholism or antisocial personality disorder. Sporadic depressive disease is unipolar depression in a subject who has no first-degree relatives with a history of depression, alcoholism, or antisocial personality disorder. FPDD has been associated with abnormal dexamethasone suppression test results in 70–85% of cases, regional cerebral blood flow abnormalities in limbic-cortical-thalamic circuits in 75–90% of cases, and preferential responsiveness to ECT (see the related section in this chapter).

In contrast, subjects with DSD are less likely to demonstrate abnormal neuroendocrine, sleep EEG, or neuroimaging results. Patients with DSD are more likely to have life events that provoke a depressive episode or a history of personality difficulties along with a stormy social history (i.e., multiple marital and social problems) that culminate in

a depressive episode. Moreover, as a consequence of having family members with alcoholism or sociopathy, they are more likely to have been exposed to psychosocial traumas such as childhood abuse and may need referral for psychotherapy to address the sequelae of such events. The specificity of this taxonomy is limited by the high prevalence of alcoholism, as some severely depressed, melancholic patients who otherwise resemble subjects with FPDD are assigned to the DSD category because they have a relative with alcoholism.

Late-onset depression

As the age of depression onset increases, the degree of familial aggregation of depression decreases, implying that genetic risk factors become less important and acquired factors more important in late-onset depression. Insight into the nature of these acquired factors has been provided by magnetic resonance imaging (MRI) evidence that signal hyperintensities appear in the frontal lobe, the caudate, and the white matter adjacent to these structures in 70–80% of subjects with depression onset after age 60. Postmortem and magnetic resonance spectroscopy data have demonstrated that these signal hyperintensities probably reflect arteriosclerotic/ischemic lesions, and the occurrence of such abnormalities in depressed patients correlates with both atherosclerotic risk factors and age.

As expected in the presence of such lesions, PET images from elderly patients with depression show decreased blood flow in diffuse areas of the frontal lobe, which decreases further with treatment (Chapter 6). The cerebral ventricles are also enlarged in patients with depression onset after age 60 (an abnormality that persists after successful treatment), which may reflect *ex vacuo* changes following ischemic damage. It is noteworthy that the anatomical locations where signal hyperintensities have been found in subjects with late-onset depression are similar to locations where cerebrovascular infarction has been associated with an elevated risk for the development of post-stroke depression, namely the frontal lobes (especially the orbitofrontal region) and the caudate. Therefore, it is thought that patients with late-onset depression who have such MRI abnormalities constitute a subgroup acquiring a mood disorder secondary to arteriosclerotic damage in the emotional circuitry, homologous to the case of post-stroke mood disorders.

A late age-of-depression onset carries several clinical implications. Patients with late-onset depression commonly have neuropsychological impairments that persist after depressive symptoms have remitted. They tend to have a single, chronic episode and are less likely to have recurrent episodes following symptom remission. Finally, they are less likely to respond completely to antidepressant drug treatment and prove more susceptible to the development of delirium during treatment with ECT or tricyclic antidepressant agents.

Prevalence and natural history

Age of onset

The onset of MDD can occur throughout the life span, although the first depressive episode usually occurs after puberty. The median age of onset is about 34 years. About 20% of patients experience illness onset during the teenage years. As described previously, depression onset after age 55–60 is associated with a distinct set of risk factors, clinical course, neuroimaging abnormalities, and treatment responsiveness as compared with early-onset illness.

The median age of onset has been decreasing and the lifetime risk of MDD has been increasing in cohorts of individuals born more recently. The reasons for these secular trends are unclear, but they do not appear to be accounted for by changes in diagnostic methods. Similar changes in the age of onset and lifetime prevalence of MDD have been observed worldwide.

Epidemiology

The limitations in establishing diagnoses have contributed to substantial variability across epidemiological studies. In a large population-based study, the lifetime prevalence (i.e., the proportion of people in a population who had experienced a disorder up to the time of assessment) for a major depressive episode varied between 3.7% and 6.7% over three catchment areas in the United States. The lifetime prevalence for dysthymia varied between 2.1% and 3.8%. Other studies reported higher lifetime prevalence rates of MDD, ranging from 8.1% in an Iowa study to 18% in a Connecticut study. The prevalence rates reported from other countries have generally fallen within this same range.

Reported annual incidence figures for MDD vary widely, ranging from 247 to 7,800 cases per 100,000 per year. In one series, 82 to 201 males and 320 to 500 females per 100,000 per year began receiving antidepressant treatment. This gender difference is not limited to the population seeking treatment, since all studies of unipolar depression show that females are about twice as likely to be affected as males, including those studies that identify both treated and untreated cases.

In the otherwise healthy elderly population, it remains controversial whether the point prevalence of MDD differs from that found in the general population. However, the point prevalence of MDD is clearly higher in special elderly populations, rising to 13% in elderly patients with concomitant medical illnesses admitted to acute care facilities and to 20% in elderly people free of cognitive impairment who are confined to long-term care facilities. Psychosocial and physiological stressors are increased in these subgroups, and the higher prevalence of mood disorders in these populations is likely to have a multifactorial explanation. (See sections on bereavement, mood disorders induced by medical disorders, and late-onset depression.) The management of geriatric depression is often complicated by treatment resistance, intercurrent medical disorders, psychotic features, and increased disability, which can necessitate relatively protracted periods of intensive treatment. Related in part to such issues, this age group occupies a disproportionately high percentage of the inpatient beds devoted to the treatment of depression.

Family clustering

A number of studies have examined the risk to relatives of depressed patients of developing mood disorders or other psychiatric problems. As discussed previously, MDD is often comorbid with alcoholism or anxiety disorders. The lifetime risk of a first-degree relative developing depression is about 30% (2–10 times the risk in the general population). The risk for a first-degree relative developing bipolar disorder is about 1% (about the same as in the general population). Earlier age of onset of MDD is associated with higher rates of both unipolar and bipolar illness in relatives. This familial clustering is thought to represent the contribution of genetic elements to liability for developing illness.

The risk of alcoholism and anxiety disorders in the relatives of depressed patients is 10–20%. Relatives of patients with early-onset depression are at an even higher risk for developing alcoholism. Controversy exists regarding the explanation for the increased prevalence of substance abuse and anxiety disorders in the relatives of depressed adults. Current data support the independent transmission of alcoholism and depression in families but indicate a complex interaction between depression and anxiety disorders.

Course

The usual course of MDD consists of recurrent depressive episodes that are separated by a return toward the premorbid baseline (i.e., feeling "back to normal"). Single episode cases are seen, but when followed over periods of 15 or more years, most individuals have at least one recurrence. Following an initial episode, the average number of episodes over the next 20 years is five or six. Following either spontaneous remission or discontinuation of antidepressant drug treatment, about 35% of patients experience recurrence of the depressive syndrome within one year. When only those patients who have had three or more prior episodes are considered, relapse occurs more rapidly, with 40% having relapsed by 15 weeks. Thus, the clinician should always warn recovered patients and their families that additional episodes are likely and educate them regarding early warning signs of recurrence. Periodic follow-up is generally indicated.

Treatment clearly affects some aspects of the natural history of MDD. In studies performed prior to the use of antidepressant drug treatment, the average length of depressive episodes ranged from 6 to 13 months and only 50% of patients had recovered at one-year follow- up. At three- to five-year follow-up, 70% of untreated depressed patients had recovered; at 15-year follow-up, 85% had recovered. Thus, chronicity of depressive episodes generally does not continue indefinitely. With antidepressant treatment, the duration of depressive episodes is shortened and chronicity is less of a problem. One study showed that, with treatment, 63% of depressed patients had recovered at four months. Eighty percent of patients who were chronically depressed for two years recovered in the ensuing three years with treatment. Between episodes patients may report a complete return to normalcy or simply a lessening in the severity of residual depressive symptoms. In either case, the level of functioning usually improves in unipolar patients between episodes. Nevertheless, up to 20% of patients with unipolar depression develop a chronic illness that is difficult to treat.

Ten to fifteen percent of patients who initially present with a depressive episode eventually develop a manic episode. The risk factors for converting to a bipolar course include family history of bipolar disorder, psychotic features accompanying the depressive episode, and earlier age of onset. Patients with such risk factors should be warned about the risk for developing mania during treatment with antidepressant drugs.

Complications

Primary MDD carries a substantial risk of suicide (Chapter 29). A major depressive episode is the most significant precursor of suicide and has been associated with about one-half of completed suicides. Mortality from other causes is also elevated in patients with mood disorders. For example, MDD is associated with excessive mortality resulting from accidental death, which may in part reflect suicides that cannot clearly be established. Moreover, the risk of cardiovascular mortality is doubled in depressed versus nondepressed patients who have been approximately matched for atherosclerotic risk factors or heart disease. This observation could relate to decreased medical compliance when depressed or to the autonomic changes associated with MDD. Depression may also result in reduced oral intake, resulting in dehydration or malnutrition. In addition, depression is associated with diminished physical activity. Such problems may predispose patients to medical complications such as falls, hip fractures, or pulmonary embolism.

Depressive episodes are accompanied by substantial suffering, disability, and social impairment. Most aspects of life are adversely affected by the reduced interest, energy and motivation, the incessant preoccupation with negative ideation and the impaired concentration associated with a depressive episode. As a result, major depressive episodes can lead to job loss, scholastic failure, divorce, and social isolation.

Differential diagnosis

Bereavement

The "normal" emotional state that most closely resembles a major depressive episode is acute bereavement. Since up to one-third of people who lose their spouse would meet criteria for a major depressive episode within three months of their spouse's death, the recent death of a loved one is considered an exclusion criterion for the diagnosis of MDD (Box 8.1). Bereavement is less persistent than major depression and is generally associated with fewer depressive symptoms. MDD differs from bereavement in that the depressive episodes may appear in the absence of precipitants, respond to antidepressant drug treatment, follow an episodic course, appear comorbidly with other psychopathological signs (e.g., mania, psychosis, obsessions, compulsions, suicide, or pathological guilt), and be associated with neurochemical and neuroendocrine abnormalities (e.g., nonsuppression of cortisol release following dexamethasone administration is common in depression but not bereavement).

Although DSM-IV permits the presence of acute bereavement to exclude a diagnosis of MDD for only two months (Box 8.1), grieving patients are generally not treated with antidepressant therapy unless they fulfill criteria of a major depressive episode more than 6–12 months after losing their loved one, because somatic antidepressant treatments do not significantly alter the emotional state associated with uncomplicated grief. Suicidal ideation or delusional guilt is rare in bereavement but, when present, indicates a need for more aggressive treatment. Bereaved people meeting criteria for a major depressive episode beyond one year ("complicated bereavement") likely have had a psychiatric disorder preceding their loved one's death.

Secondary depression

Psychiatric disorders commonly associated with secondary depression are schizophrenia, obsessive-compulsive disorder, panic disorder, post-traumatic stress disorder, social anxiety disorder, generalized anxiety disorder, somatization disorder, substance abuse/dependence, or personality disorders (e.g., antisocial personality disorder). The application of the label "secondary" also encompasses major depression associated with debilitating medical illnesses (e.g., chronic pain syndromes or paraplegia from long neuronal track damage). The psychiatric disorders commonly associated with secondary depression that hold particular implications for treatment are discussed below.

Obsessive-compulsive disorder (OCD)
About one-half of patients with OCD develop major depressive episodes (Chapter 10). The antidepressant drugs that

potently inhibit serotonin reuptake (i.e., clomipramine, fluoxetine, fluvoxamine, sertraline, and paroxetine) are significantly more effective for OCD than those that do not, making them the agents of choice for secondary depression in patients with OCD. These antidepressant agents may also be relatively more effective for primary MDD with secondary obsessions.

Panic disorder

About one-half of patients with panic disorder develop major depressive episodes following the onset of panic disorder (see Chapter 9). Since about one-third of patients with primary MDD develop panic attacks following onset of the mood disorder, the determination of whether a patient has primary depression with secondary panic disorder or primary panic disorder with secondary depression can be difficult. The family history is instructive, since relatives with mood disorders predominate in the former case and relatives with anxiety disorders in the latter. In addition, primary panic disorder usually has an onset prior to age 40. The onset of panic attacks after this age in a depressed patient usually indicates that the mood disorder is primary.

The diagnostic dilemma between primary panic disorder versus primary MDD does not necessarily translate into a problem with treatment selection as long as effective antidepressant dosages of an antidepressant drug are prescribed. In addition to their antidepressant effects, antidepressant drugs exert prophylactic effects against panic attacks. A benzodiazepine such as alprazolam can be added to the antidepressant on a "take-as-needed" basis for acute management of panic attacks. This is especially useful early in treatment, since the antipanic effect of antidepressant drugs does not appear until the third week of treatment. While benzodiazepines can be effective monotherapy for primary panic disorder with secondary depression, they are generally not sufficiently effective for managing primary MDD with secondary panic disorder.

Schizophrenia

At least one-half of patients with schizophrenia develop major depressive episodes (Chapter 13). Since delusions and hallucinations can also occur in primary mood disorders, a diagnostic dilemma can exist between primary MDD with psychotic features and schizophrenia with secondary depression. The diagnosis usually becomes clear with longitudinal follow-up. The diagnosis is more likely to be MDD with psychotic features if remission of delusions or hallucinations is maintained following discontinuation of the antipsychotic drug or if the illness course is episodic rather than chronic. Schizophrenia, in contrast, is typically accompanied by progressive social deterioration and "negative" symptoms (e.g., impoverished speech and thought content, blunting of affect and personality, loss of initiative, and apathy). Finally, the family history provides diagnostic clues, since MDD with

psychotic features typically occurs in patients who have relatives with mood disorders.

Initial management of either MDD with psychotic features or schizophrenia with secondary depression usually involves combined treatment with an antipsychotic drug and an antidepressant drug, although addition of the antidepressant drug is usually minimally effective for depressive symptoms associated with schizophrenia.

Somatization disorder

Patients with somatization disorder (Chapter 17) complain as dramatically of depressive and anxiety symptoms as they do of somatic symptoms. They tend to score highly on depression rating scales because they endorse most symptoms. Their affect, however, is usually not appropriate to the severity level indicated by their complaints. While they describe suicidal thoughts and intense dysphoria they may smile, jest or demonstrate "la belle indifférence." They often report resolution of their depressive complaints after only a few days of follow-up—before treatments are expected to be effective.

Patients with primary MDD can also develop somatic complaints that are not explained by the medical evaluation. These complaints seldom spread throughout the entire review-of-systems as they do for patients with somatization disorder. In addition, conversion symptoms (unexplained neurological symptoms) are uncommon in primary mood disorders. Finally, in patients with primary MDD the unexplained somatic complaints have generally not been present outside of the historical context of a depressive episode and resolve completely with effective antidepressant treatment. In contrast, patients with somatization disorder have long histories of unexplained somatic complaints dating to adolescence or early adulthood that have been present even in the absence of secondary depression.

Alcohol dependence

Patients with primary alcoholism may develop secondary depression. The differential diagnosis in this case includes primary MDD with secondary alcohol dependence, because some depressed patients increase their drinking behavior during episodes of illness (see above). In either case, a major goal of treatment involves discontinuation of the alcohol use. Antidepressant drugs may benefit primary MDD or secondary depression, and the newer generation agents that are nonlethal in overdose and not potently sedating are preferable.

Alcohol may produce depressive symptoms by direct and withdrawal effects. During intoxication, mood can become labile or dysphoric, judgment is impaired and patients become disinhibited and impulsive. Patients may present to the emergency room in this condition following a suicide attempt or complaining of suicidal intention. While intoxicated they may endorse criteria for the major depressive syndrome. When reinterviewed during sobriety, many of these patients deny any further suicidal ideation or death wish and neither demonstrate nor endorse the emotional and neurovegetative manifestations of a depressive syndrome. Depressive symptoms associated with alcohol withdrawal commonly last two weeks or more.

Cocaine/amphetamine dependence

Depressed mood and anhedonia are observed during the first few weeks or months following withdrawal from cocaine or amphetamine dependence. These agents block reuptake or facilitate release, respectively, of dopamine in the mesolimbic dopaminergic projections that are thought to subserve a "reward-related system" in the brain. During repeated exposure to cocaine, the postsynaptic dopamine receptors in the mesolimbic system become desensitized. It is thought that this subsensitive receptor state may be associated with anhedonia once dopamine transmission is no longer being facilitated by cocaine. These emotional symptoms generally resolve within one week to several months, which is postulated to reflect the restoration of dopamine receptor sensitivity toward the pre-cocaine baseline. Depressed mood and anhedonia may increase risk for relapse during cocaine withdrawal and may be reduced by antidepressant drug treatment (although antidepressant treatment does not appear to substantially alter the relapse rate of cocaine dependence).

Depressive disorders induced by pharmacologic agents or medical disorders

DSM-IV includes a category of "mood disorders due to ___" (where the clinician fills in the blank for a medical disorder) when a mood syndrome, "[based upon] the history, physical examination, or laboratory findings, is the direct physiological consequence of a general medical condition" and is not better accounted for by an "adjustment disorder with depressed mood in response to the stress of having a general medical condition." The latter term, "adjustment disorder," is applied to depressive symptoms that do not meet criteria for MDD but are felt to constitute maladaptive psychological responses to the disability, pain, or terminal nature of a medical disorder (DSM-IV). Ideally, the determination that a secondary major depressive syndrome arises as a pathophysiological consequence of the primary condition is based upon studies establishing an increased risk for the development of the major depressive syndrome when that primary condition is compared with control conditions that are matched for disability, suffering, and prognosis (Chapter 27). Such studies are difficult to accomplish.

Conceptually, the term "mood disorders due to ___" is applied to specific conditions that are thought to induce depressive or manic episodes through their neuropathological or neurochemical effects on the neural systems that subserve emotional processing and modulation. For example, Parkinson's disease is associated with a two- to four-fold increase in the risk for the depressive syndrome compared with quadriplegia resulting from long track damage, and a four- to eight-fold increase in the risk when compared with severe degenerative arthritis. In Parkinson's disease the degeneration of mesolimbic (in addition to nigrostriatal) dopaminergic projections is thought to affect central reward-related and mood/anxiety systems. Although many patients with chronically debilitating medical conditions also have clinically significant depression, it is probably best not to consider the diagnosis as "mood disorders due to" the chronically debilitating medical illness unless it has been established that there is a direct physiologic mechanism whereby the medical disorder actually causes the depression such as described above for Parkinson's disease. Sometimes it may be difficult to know whether there is a direct causal relationship. For example, diabetes mellitus may produce diffuse changes in small vessels or neurons in the limbic system. If the patient with diabetes is depressed, is this depression a direct result of the diabetes?

In summary, the distinction between induced mood syndromes and secondary depressive syndromes remains nebulous since the pathophysiology of these conditions is not understood. At present, the uncertainty regarding the neural substrates of human emotion and of primary mood disorders permits only hypotheses and not clear pathophysiological links between medical disorders and induced mood syndromes. Since current knowledge does not permit reliable distinctions between mood disturbances that are physiological responses from those that are psychological responses to a medical stressor, some advocate grouping depressive syndromes arising in the setting of any medical condition under the general category of "secondary" mood disorders.

The medical diseases that can putatively induce depressive syndromes based upon their increased risk of being associated with depressive episodes relative to similarly debilitating conditions include endocrine disturbances (e.g., hypothyroidism or Cushing's syndrome); degenerative basal ganglia disorders (e.g., Parkinson's, Huntington's or Wilson's diseases); epileptic foci involving the temporal lobe; and structural lesions (tumors, infarcts or injury) involving the striatum, the frontal lobe, or the mesiotemporal cortex (Chapter 27). The association between these diseases and pathological mood syndromes holds implications for the pathophysiology of the primary mood disorders, as discussed below. For example, in Huntington's disease and Parkinson's disease, the major depressive syndrome often arises prior to motor manifestations and prior to the patient having knowledge of their risk for the disease. The striatal neuronal degeneration occurring in this early period of Huntington's disease and the dopaminergic cell death occurring in Parkinson's disease may thus provide important insights into the pathophysiology of the primary mood disorders, which are also associated with striatal abnormalities in neuroimaging studies (see Chapter 6).

The DSM-IV category for mood effects related to pharmacologic agents is "substance-induced mood disorder," with specification added as to whether the major depressive syndrome appears to be associated with the direct effects of the drug or with its withdrawal effects. The former category largely consists of agents that putatively induce neuroendocrine or biochemical abnormalities similar to those found in the primary idiopathic mood disorders. Examples include corticosteroids (e.g., prednisone) and catecholamine depleting agents (e.g., reserpine). Mild to moderate depressive symptoms have also been reported by some women while taking oral contraceptive agents. No clear mechanism is evident for other medications that are associated with an increased risk for developing depressive episodes, such as cimetidine. The drug withdrawal states associated with depressive symptoms include withdrawal from sedative-hypnotic agents (e.g., barbiturates and alcohol) or psychostimulants (e.g., cocaine or amphetamine).

The bipolar disorders and cyclothymic disorder

Bipolar disorder (or manic-depressive illness) is often a severe, chronic illness characterized by periods of depression and elation. If untreated, patients suffer prolonged distress and impairment. Manic and depressed phases are both associated with significant morbidity and mortality. Cyclothymia represents a clinically milder but distinct disorder. In contrast to dysthymic disorder (a chronic subsyndromal depressive episode), cyclothymia includes alternations between subsyndromal manic and depressive episodes. For the majority of bipolar disorder patients, effective treatments exist. However, even with optimal treatment most patients need some level of long-term medical care. Because of the variable presentation, course, and severity of these relatively common disorders, suspected cases of bipolar disorder should have comprehensive psychiatric evaluations for diagnosis and initial treatment planning.

Diagnostic criteria

Bipolar disorder is defined by the presence of a manic episode alone or by a hypomanic episode with a history of one or more depressive episodes (Boxes 8.5–8.7, Table 8.3). As defined in DSM-IV, a manic episode represents a distinct period of abnormally and persistently elevated, expansive, or irritable mood lasting at least one week in duration. During mania, patients experience psychomotor restlessness, an inflated sense of self-esteem or grandiosity, a decreased need for sleep, a sense that their thoughts are racing, and pressured speech. Distractibility is common and the flow of speech demonstrates rapid changes in thought content ("flight of ideas"). Individuals often show an increased interest in or an excessive involvement in pleasurable activities

(e.g., sexual indiscretions) or activities of questionable judgment (e.g., spending sprees). Psychotic features such as paranoia or delusions may be present. The disturbance in mood must be severe enough to cause impairment in occupational or social functioning and cannot be directly due to the effects of a pharmacological substance or a medical condition (e.g., stroke or hyperthyroidism).

Box 8.6 A manic episode

A. A distinct period of abnormally and persistently elevated, expansive, or irritable mood, lasting at least one week (or any duration if hospitalization is necessary).

B. During the period of mood disturbance, three (or more) of the following symptoms have persisted (four if the mood is only irritable) and have been present to a significant degree:
   1. inflated self-esteem or grandiosity
   2. decreased need for sleep (e.g., feels rested after only three hours of sleep)
   3. more talkative than usual or pressure to keep talking
   4. flight of ideas or subjective experience that thoughts are racing
   5. distractibility (i.e., attention too easily drawn to unimportant or irrelevant external stimuli)
   6. increase in goal-directed activity (either socially, at work or school, or sexually) or psychomotor agitation
   7. excessive involvement in pleasurable activities that have a high potential for painful consequences (e.g., engaging in unrestrained buying sprees, sexual indiscretions, or foolish business investments).

C. The symptoms do not meet criteria for a mixed episode.

D. The mood disturbance is sufficiently severe to cause marked impairment in occupational functioning or in usual social activities or relationships with others, or to necessitate hospitalization to prevent harm to self or others, or there are psychotic features.

E. The symptoms are not due to the direct physiological effects of a substance (e.g., a drug of abuse, a medication, or other treatment) or a general medical condition (e.g., hyperthyroidism).

Note: Manic-like episodes that are clearly caused by somatic antidepressant treatment (e.g., medication, electroconvulsive therapy, light therapy) should not count toward a diagnosis of bipolar I disorder.

From American Psychiatric Association (2000) Diagnostic and Statistical Manual of Mental Disorders, 4th Edition, Text Revision, Washington, D.C., American Psychiatric Association.

DIAGNOSTIC CRITERIA

Box 8.6 A hypomanic episode

A. A distinct period of persistently elevated, expansive, or irritable mood, lasting throughout at least four days, that is clearly different from the usual nondepressed mood.

B. During the period of mood disturbance, three (or more) of the following symptoms have persisted (four if the mood is only irritable) and have been present to a significant degree:
1 inflated self-esteem or grandiosity
2 decreased need for sleep (e.g., feels rested after only three hours of sleep)
3 more talkative than usual or pressure to keep talking
4 flight of ideas or subjective experience that thoughts are racing
5 distractibility (i.e., attention too easily drawn to unimportant or irrelevant external stimuli)
6 increase in goal-directed activity (either socially, at work or school, or sexually) or psychomotor agitation
7 excessive involvement in pleasurable activities that have a high potential for painful consequences (e.g., the person engages in unrestrained buying sprees, sexual indiscretions, or foolish business investments).

C. The episode is associated with an unequivocal change in functioning that is uncharacteristic of the person when not symptomatic.

D. The disturbance in mood and the change in functioning are observable by others.

E. The episode is not severe enough to cause marked impairment in social or occupational functioning, or to necessitate hospitalization, and there are no psychotic features.

F. The symptoms are not due to the direct physiological effects of a substance (e.g., a drug of abuse, a medication, or other treatment) or a general medical condition (e.g., hyperthyroidism).

Note: Hypomanic-like episodes that are clearly caused by somatic antidepressant treatment (e.g., medication, electroconvulsive therapy, light therapy) should not count toward a diagnosis of bipolar II disorder.

From American Psychiatric Association (2000) Diagnostic and Statistical Manual of Mental Disorders, 4th Edition, Text Revision, Washington, D.C., American Psychiatric Association.

Box 8.7 Bipolar disorders (Type I)

Bipolar I disorder, single manic episode
A. Presence of only one manic episode (Box 8.5) and no past major depressive episodes.
B. The manic episode is not better accounted for by schizoaffective disorder and is not superimposed on schizophrenia, schizophreniform disorder, delusional disorder, or psychotic disorder not otherwise specified.

Bipolar I disorder, most recent episode hypomanic
A. Currently (or most recently) in a hypomanic episode (Box 8.6).
B. There has previously been at least one manic episode (Box 8.5) or mixed episode.
C. The mood symptoms cause clinically significant distress or impairment in social, occupational, or other important areas of functioning.
D. The mood episodes in criteria A and B are not better accounted for by schizoaffective disorder and are not superimposed on schizophrenia, schizophreniform disorder, delusional disorder, or psychotic disorder not otherwise specified.

Bipolar I disorder, most recent episode manic
A. Currently (or most recently) in a manic episode (Box 8.5).
B. There has previously been at least one major depressive episode (Box 8.1), manic episode (Box 8.5), or mixed episode.
C. Same exclusion criterion as D above.

Bipolar I disorder, most recent episode depressed
A. Currently (or most recently) in a major depressive episode (Box 8.1).
B. There has previously been at least one manic episode (Box 8.5) or mixed episode.
C. Same exclusion criterion as D above.
Note: The bipolar II disorder diagnoses are comparable, with these inclusion criteria requiring the presence of a hypomanic episode (Box 8.6) rather than a manic episode (Box 8.5) in a subject who has never experienced a manic episode.
Adapted from American Psychiatric Association (2000) Diagnostic and Statistical Manual of Mental Disorders, 4th Edition, Text Revision (DSM-IV-TR), Washington, D.C., American Psychiatric Association.

The criteria for a hypomanic episode are similar to those of a manic episode except that the disturbance of mood is not severe enough to cause marked impairment in occupational or social functioning. In addition, no psychotic features are present. Hypomania is characterized by a distinct period of persistently elevated or irritable mood lasting at least four days that is different from the individual's usual mental state. During the mood disturbance there is persistent inflated self-esteem or grandiosity, decreased need for sleep, increased talkativeness, flight of ideas, or racing thoughts. Distractibility, increased goal-oriented activity, and excessive involvement in pleasurable activities are common. As with mania, symptoms cannot be due to the effects of medications, substances of abuse, or general medical conditions.

Bipolar disorder is usually divided into two forms, I and II. The diagnosis of bipolar I disorder requires a manic episode.

Table 8.3 Bipolar disorder, manic or hypomanic phase

Discriminating feature

1 Distinct period of abnormally and persistently elevated, expansive, or irritable mood, lasting ≥ one week.

Consistent features

1 Episodic course.
2 Labile mood and affect.
3 Elevated self-esteem, grandiosity.
4 Elevated psychomotor activity: agitation, restlessness, increased energy, racing thoughts.
5 Speech faster, louder, or more voluminous.
6 Insomnia with decreased subjective need for sleep.
7 Family history of mood disorder.
8 Distractibility (i.e., attention too easily drawn to unimportant or irrelevant external stimuli).
9 Increased involvement in goal-directed or pleasurable activities.
10 Impaired insight and judgment.

Variable features

1 Threatening speech or behavior.
2 Auditory hallucinations, persecutory or grandiose delusions (consistent in mania).
3 Comorbid substance abuse.
4 Excessive religiosity above usual baseline and outside religious group norms.
5 Catatonic features.

Box 8.8 Cyclothymic disorder

A. For at least two years, the presence of numerous periods with hypomanic symptoms (Box 8.7) and numerous periods with depressive symptoms that do not meet criteria for a major depressive episode. **Note:** In children and adolescents, the duration must be at least one year.

B. During the above two-year period (one year in children and adolescents), the person has not been without the symptoms in criterion A for more than two months at a time.

C. No major depressive episode (Box 8.1), manic episode (Box 8.6), or mixed episode has been present during the first two years of the disturbance.
Note: After the initial two years (one year in children and adolescents) of cyclothymic disorder, there may be superimposed manic or mixed episodes (in which case both bipolar I disorder and cyclothymic disorder may be diagnosed) or major depressive episodes (in which case both bipolar II disorder and cyclothymic disorder may be diagnosed).

D. The symptoms in criterion A are not better accounted for by schizoaffective disorder and are not superimposed on schizophrenia, schizophreniform disorder, delusional disorder, or psychotic disorder not otherwise specified.

E. The symptoms are not due to the direct physiological effects of a substance (e.g., a drug of abuse, a medication) or a general medical condition (e.g., hyperthyroidism).

F. The symptoms cause clinically significant distress or impairment in social, occupational, or other important areas of functioning.

From American Psychiatric Association (2000) Diagnostic and Statistical Manual of Mental Disorders, 4th Edition, Text Revision, Washington, D.C., American Psychiatric Association.

The individual may also have experienced depressive episodes or mixed episodes of manic and depressive symptoms in the past. The diagnosis of bipolar II disorder requires at least two prior major depressive episodes and a hypomanic episode. Once an individual qualifies for the diagnosis of bipolar I or bipolar II disorder, the diagnosis during subsequent mood episodes continues to be bipolar disorder, with the most recent episode being described as depressed or manic.

In contrast to bipolar disorders, cyclothymic disorder (Box 8.8) is characterized by numerous fluctuating periods of hypomanic and depressive symptoms that occur for at least two years (one year for adolescents). None of these episodes of either hypomanic or depressive symptoms meet the full criteria for a manic or hypomanic episode or a major depressive episode. Cyclothymia is a chronic disorder that often progresses to the development of bipolar I or bipolar II disorder.

Clinical picture

The emotional, neurovegetative, psychological, psychosomatic, psychomotor, and neuropsychological manifestations of the depressed phase of the bipolar disorders are the same as those described previously for major depressive disorder. The manic or hypomanic phases of bipolar disorder, however, possess a unique constellation of features.

Emotional manifestations

As described in the diagnostic criteria of DSM-IV, a principal feature of the manic or hypomanic state is a distinct change in mood state characterized by a persistently elevated, expansive, or irritable mood. Individuals do not describe themselves as having a problem, but as feeling "better than ever" or being full of energy and drive. Patients often describe feeling powerful or indestructible. Family members or acquaintances portray them as being more active, upbeat, euphoric or irritable than usual and not recognizing normal social boundaries. In contrast to depressive disorders where the primary feeling is one of either sadness or anhedonia, individuals in manic or hypomanic states often feel elated and are overly optimistic.

The primary distinction between the emotional disturbances of individuals who are manic, hypomanic or cyclothymic is one of degree. In a manic state the mood disturbances result in marked impairment of occupational or social functioning, whereas in hypomanic or cyclothymic states euphoria does not cause significant impairment. As in the major depressive syndrome, irritability is often present. However, in contrast to the irritability noted in depression, irritability in manic syndromes is associated with increased energy and motivation, and feelings that others are inhibiting the individual's progress or recognition.

I was well on my way to madness; it was 1974, and I was 28 years old. Within three months I was manic beyond recognition and just beginning a long, costly personal war against a medication that I would, in a few years' time, be strongly encouraging others to take. My illness, and my struggles against the drug that ultimately saved my life and restored my sanity, had been years in the making.

From Kay Redfield Jamison (1995) *An Unquiet Mind*, Alfred A. Knopf.

I'll admit it: there's a great deal of pleasure to mental illness, especially to the mania associated with manic depression. It's an emotional state similar to Oz, full of excitement, color, noise, and speed—an overload of sensory stimulation—whereas the sane state of Kansas is plain and simple, black and white, boring and flat.

From Andy Behrman (2002) *Electroboy*, Random House.

Neurovegetative manifestations

In major depressive disorder the most common neurovegetative symptoms are fatigability and loss of energy. The reverse is true for mania. Individuals generally describe needing only a few hours of sleep a night or do not sleep at all for several days. They have more energy and drive than usual. Alterations in appetite and weight are less predictable than in major depressive disorder, although weight loss is common in manic states secondary to increased activity levels. Such overactivity and weight loss in the elderly can contribute to a marked worsening of other medical conditions or lead to malnutrition. Also in contrast to the depressive syndromes, manic or hypomanic individuals often describe increased libido and increased enjoyment of pleasurable activities. This often involves increased interest, if not outright promiscuity, in sexual activities. These behaviors can put the individual at increased risk for sexually transmitted diseases and for legal difficulties.

Psychosomatic symptoms

Whereas psychosomatic symptoms are common in depressed individuals, most manic or hypomanic individuals describe themselves as having no physical complaints or problems.

Psychomotor manifestations

Psychomotor agitation is very common in manic and hypomanic states. Patients have increased motoric activity, pacing, tapping behaviors, etc. Psychomotor retardation is uncommon, though it can be associated with manic catatonic states in which there may be immobility. Such catatonic states, which may involve excessive motor activity or immobility, can be life threatening due to the decreased intake of food and fluids and must be aggressively treated with hospitalization.

Neuropsychological manifestations

Most manic or hypomanic patients feel that their concentration, memory, and ability to make decisions are markedly improved. These self-observations are often belied by their inappropriate and self-destructive behaviors. Although work and school performance may improve and productivity may increase in the initial stages of a manic episode, as the manic state worsens, work and school performance deteriorates. In contrast to the lack of motivation experienced in depression, deteriorated work and school performance during manic states typically results from the loss of normal social boundaries and judgment. In severe manic states, patients may appear as if they have schizophrenia because of their disorganization of thought and the presence of delusions and auditory hallucinations. During manic episodes, patients also describe a sensation of racing thoughts, which interferes with their ability to organize activities. This is clinically apparent as pressured or rapid speech or as frequent, tangential shifts in the topic of conversation ("flight of ideas").

Impairment of insight and judgment

A classic manifestation of manic states is the loss of economic and social judgment. Many patients engage in spending sprees or convince other individuals that they have large resources while buying far beyond their means. In untreated manic states, individuals may ruin their family's financial position. In addition, there is a clear lack of social judgment and inhibition, which may result in spousal or child physical abuse or other violent behavior. Violent behavior is more common in the presence of psychotic symptoms. As discussed previously, poor judgment with respect to sexual contacts may place the individual at risk for sexually transmitted diseases or pregnancy.

Alcohol and illicit drug use

Patients in manic or hypomanic states commonly abuse alcohol or other substances. This may represent attempts to self-medicate or potentiate euphoria with alcohol or drugs of abuse, or it may reflect increased engagement in pleasurable activities along with diminished judgment. In today's culture, patients most commonly abuse alcohol, cocaine, amphetamines (or related stimulants), marijuana, and sedative-hypnotics. At times, it becomes difficult to distinguish a manic episode from drug-induced or drug withdrawal-related behaviors.

Prevalence and natural history

Age of onset

The average age of onset has been reported to be in the early 20s, with at least 20% of cases arising in adolescence. However, the age of onset is often obscure because patients with bipolar disorder may suffer symptoms for several years prior to formal diagnosis. Moreover, they typically suffer one or more depressive episodes prior to the first manic or hypomanic episode. Hence, these individuals receive a formal diagnosis at a later age although their true onset of illness was earlier. In addition, studies of children and young adolescents have suggested that the frequency of bipolar disorder with early onset has been underestimated. Moreover, as for MDD, there is evidence that the age of onset of bipolar disorder is decreasing among more recently born individuals. In contrast to MDD, onset of bipolar disorder after 40 years of age is rare and should prompt a full medical evaluation.

Much less is known about the age of onset distribution for cyclothymia. Many well-documented cases of cyclothymia developed several years prior to the onset of clear-cut bipolar disorder.

Epidemiology

The prevalence of the bipolar disorders is between 1.5% and 3% of the general population. Based upon community samples, the lifetime prevalence is approximately 0.8% for bipolar I disorder, 0.5% for bipolar II disorder, and 0.5% for cyclothymic disorder. Unlike MDD, the prevalence of these disorders is the same for men and women. Also in contrast to MDD, there is little evidence that the prevalence of the bipolar disorders is changing. No association with race, ethnic group or socioeconomic class of the parents has been identified, although affected individuals often drop in social class after disease onset. Although the bipolar disorders are much less common than MDD per se, the marked degree of personal and familial morbidity and mortality associated with these disorders makes them important public health problems.

Familial clustering

As with MDD, the bipolar disorders cluster in families. For bipolar I disorder, the risk among first-degree relatives is 6–7% for bipolar I disorder, 2–5% for bipolar II disorder, and 25–35% for MDD. In contrast, first-degree relatives of bipolar II patients are at significantly increased risk for developing bipolar II disorder and MDD, but not for developing bipolar I disorder. For early onset cases of bipolar I or II disorder, the number of relatives with mood disorders is especially high. Cyclothymic disorder has been less well studied, but the prevalence of bipolar disorders and MDD among first-degree relatives of patients with cyclothymic disorder also appears increased.

For all of these mood disorders, the familial risk for substance abuse disorders (especially alcoholism) is elevated. Hence, the diagnosis of a patient with bipolar disorder identifies a family with markedly increased risk for both affective disorders and substance abuse disorders. It is prudent to screen family members for these conditions.

Course

Patients with bipolar disorders commonly experience several major depressive episodes prior to their first manic or hypomanic episode. Early in the illness course, episodes of depression or mania are often separated by relatively long periods of normal behavior, but without treatment, subsequent episodes become increasingly frequent. Untreated manic or depressive episodes typically last several months. With treatment, however, both manic and depressed episodes decrease in length and severity.

The course of the bipolar disorders shows marked variability both within and between individuals. For 10–15% of patients with bipolar I or II disorder, the frequency of episodes increases over time to four or more per year. This "rapid cycling" form carries a relatively poor prognosis, as such patients are less responsive to treatment and suffer greater social and occupational morbidity and higher suicide rates. Some patients develop episodes that have prominent features of both mania and depression. These "mixed episodes" may confuse physicians regarding response to treatment. Psychotic symptoms may develop during any manic episode, but once present, subsequent manic episodes are more likely to be accompanied by psychotic features. Approximately 20–30% of patients with bipolar I disorder and 15–20% of patients with bipolar II disorder do not experience total recovery between episodes. These patients manifest continued mood lability, irritability, and occupational and social impairment.

The course of cyclothymic disorder is chronic by definition (Box 8.8). Twenty to fifty percent of patients with cyclothymic disorder progress over the next few years to bipolar disorder.

Complications

Bipolar disorder, like primary MDD, carries an increased risk of suicide and accidental death. Suicides are more common during depressed or mixed manic/depressive episodes and while intoxicated. Accidental injury and death are more common in manic and hypomanic states as a result of poor judgment and increased risk-taking behavior. In the elderly, mania is associated with increased medical morbidity due to malnutrition and exhaustion states that result from increased activity and decreased sleep. Manic episodes in patients with atherosclerotic vascular disease or other serious medical problems are particularly likely to increase mortality and morbidity.

Mania, hypomania, and cyclothymia are all associated with marked occupational, scholastic, and social impairment. The risks for substance abuse, divorce, spousal abuse, child physical abuse, truancy, school failure, job loss, and financial distress are markedly increased in untreated mania. While individuals in hypomanic episodes can become more creative and productive, irritability and difficulties getting along with family or peers may result in frequent job changes or divorce. The morbidity associated with depressive episodes is similar to that as previously described for MDD. Individuals with mixed manic/depressive episodes appear to have the highest psychosocial morbidity.

Differential diagnosis of the bipolar disorders

The differential diagnosis of the bipolar disorders is dependent on the phase of illness. The depressed phase of bipolar I or bipolar II disorder must be distinguished from that of MDD. This differential is critical, since the treatment implications for depressive episodes with or without a history of mania differ. The depressed phase of bipolar disorder must also be distinguished from depressive syndromes induced by general medical conditions or pharmacological substances. Substance-induced depressive disorders can be particularly difficult to distinguish from depressive episodes with a history of mania when only cross-sectional information is available. In these cases, the identity of the drug ingested may suggest a substance-induced mood disturbance. Agents that can produce such syndromes include alcohol, cocaine, barbiturates, and corticosteroids.

When the manic phase of bipolar I disorder is accompanied by psychotic features, it must be distinguished from other psychotic disorders, such as schizoaffective disorder and schizophrenia. These disorders can all present with irritability, grandiosity, hallucinations, delusions or paranoia. Marked changes in mood and a history of prior manic and depressive episodes are more typical of bipolar disorder. In contrast, the other psychotic disorders are characterized by primary disturbances in perception that exist, at least for significant periods of time, in the absence of changes in mood. In addition, the family histories usually differ between bipolar and psychotic disorders, as discussed previously. The distinction of mania from schizophrenia or schizoaffective disorder can prove especially difficult in adolescents or in cases where the past psychiatric and family histories are unavailable.

Manic-like or hypomanic-like episodes may also be associated with general medical conditions or with substance abuse. For example, hyperthyroidism may result in an agitated state clinically indistinguishable from mania. Mania has also been reported following stroke or traumatic injury, and it may arise rarely in patients with Huntington's disease or cerebral tumors (Chapter 27). Manic-like or hypomanic-like symptoms are often associated with intoxication or withdrawal from a variety of illicit drugs (e.g., cocaine, phencyclidine, or amphetamine). Manic-like episodes may also be precipitated by antidepressants.

KEY CLINICAL QUESTIONS AND WHAT THEY CAN UNLOCK

- *How can I distinguish acute mania from schizophrenia?*
  When seeing an individual for the first time, it can be difficult to distinguish mania of psychotic proportions from an acute schizophrenic episode, especially in the absence of a clear history or medical records. The physician should ask the patient and, with permission, significant others about the symptoms listed in Boxes 8.6 and 8.9. Although this diagnostic distinction may not be critical for acute treatment because treatment would most likely involve the use of atypical antipsychotic medications independent of the diagnosis, distinguishing mania from schizophrenia is important for the initiation of longer-term treatment plans and education. In general, a family history of a close relative with schizophrenia or bipolar disorder should tip the clinician toward making a similar diagnosis. The presence of a recent history of grandiose or elated behavior would suggest a diagnosis of mania while the absence of such changes in mood would suggest the diagnosis of schizophrenia.

- *Can I treat the depressed phase of bipolar disorder with an antidepressant alone?*
  The main problem with treating the depressed phase of bipolar disorder with an antidepressant alone is the potential of all current antidepressants to precipitate a switch to a manic episode. Hence, one would want to use monotherapy only in exceptional cases. As a general practice, if an antidepressant is going to be used, it is better to start the antidepressant after therapeutic levels of a mood stabilizer, such as lithium or valproate, have been established. Because the time course of response to antidepressant action is on the order of weeks, starting a mood stabilizer concomitantly or before the antidepressant will not substantially delay the effects of the antidepressant treatment.

- *How long should prophylactic medication treatment for bipolar disorder be sustained?*
  Mood disorders tend to recur and persistent pharmacotherapy reduces the risk of recurrence. Most patients with bipolar disorder require indefinite

treatment, and the task of long-term management may be to encourage compliance, to manage side effects and toxicity, and to keep treatment regimens as simple as possible.

- *What is an effective role for the nonpsychiatric physician in the management of bipolar disorder?*

  In the past, psychiatrists have managed the treatment of most patients with bipolar disorder. The diagnosis can be difficult to make, and medications like lithium may require the expertise of the specialist because of narrow therapeutic indices and poor patient tolerance. Coordination of care between psychiatrists and nonpsychiatrists can minimize the risk of drug interactions (e.g., lithium and angiotensin converting enzyme inhibitors) and effectively manage complications of the illness (alcohol/drug disorders, divorce) and treatment (obesity from antipsychotics). Recognition of milder cases (e.g., hypomania), availability of therapeutic agents with relatively uncomplicated side-effect profiles (second generation antipsychotics—risperidone, quetiapine and olanzapine are indicated for mania), and unavailability of psychiatric referral resources may result in management, including pharmacotherapy, in primary care settings.

Etiology

Environmental factors

Environmental factors are presumed to play a role in the genesis of mood disorders, although the identity of these factors and the nature of their effects in the brain remain poorly understood. Family studies of bipolar disorder and MDD indicate that among monozygotic twin pairs in which one twin is affected, the concordance rate for the co-twin is only about 75% and 50%, respectively, suggesting that nonheritable as well as heritable factors are involved in disease expression. Environmental factors are also suggested by the decreasing age at onset for both MDD and bipolar disorder in successive birth cohorts.

Since some aspects of a major depressive episode resemble a severe stress response (e.g., bereavement), it has been presumed that stressful events constitute one type of environmental factor that may play a role in the development of mood disorders. However, such a link has been difficult to establish. Depressed patients may or may not mention life events or situations that they consider important in precipitating their depressive symptoms. Many patients state that they have no reasons to feel depressed since their social, economic, medical or spiritual status has not significantly changed, an observation that may be corroborated by family members. In particular, patients with recurrent depressive episodes learn that their pattern of depressive or euphoric

symptoms is inappropriate to and not explained by life situations. Other patients report stressors that seem trivial and difficult for the physician to take seriously, suggesting that patients attempt to account for depressive symptoms on the basis of a psychological response to a stressor.

One of the best-studied stressors is the relationship between adult-onset depression and traumatic events occurring in childhood. For example, parental loss in childhood has been associated with an increased risk for the development of MDD in adulthood in some, but not all, studies. However, most of these studies failed to control for the possibility that early parental loss occurred as a result of parental affective illness that led to suicide, accidental death or disturbed family relationships. Having parents with mood disorders increases the risk for developing MDD on a genetic basis, confounding attempts to assign etiological significance to bereavement experiences during childhood.

Nevertheless, some patients who meet criteria for MDD do appear to consistently develop depressive symptoms in response to adverse psychosocial events. Depressive episodes in this subgroup have been termed "neurotic-reactive" or "exogenous" by some classification systems to distinguish them from "endogenous" episodes that appear to have no identifiable external precipitant. This distinction may have theoretical utility but its clinical utility remains elusive, since behavioral signs and symptoms that separate "pathophysiologically based" from "psychologically based" depressions or reliably predict response to pharmacological versus psychotherapeutic treatments have not been established.

Life events that are often associated with the development of pathological mood syndromes in women with MDD or bipolar disorder include pregnancy and delivery. The postpartum period in particular constitutes the epoch of greatest risk for the onset of mood disorders and for recurrence of mood episodes. In one series, 37% of female patients with bipolar disorder and 17% of female patients with unipolar depression experienced their first major depressive episode during pregnancy or the postpartum period. The increased susceptibility to mood disorders during these periods suggests an effect of hormonal changes accompanying these events. Such an interaction may also account for the two-fold increase in the incidence of depression in females relative to males and for the exacerbations of depressive symptoms that commonly occur in depressed women in the 1–2 weeks preceding menses.

While the data have not established a simple relationship between psychosocial stressors and the development of mood disorders, a complex interaction between stress and individual biological predisposition may exist. For example, one of the heritable factors for mood disorders may be an increased susceptibility to the effects of stress. This hypothesis is supported by recent twin and recurrence studies.

Post *et al.* have specifically hypothesized that the genetic risk for mood disorders is conferred by an anomalous susceptibility of limbic neurons to the development of long-term sensitization in response to stress. In such a model, episodes of stress induce permanent changes in the strengths of the synaptic connections of limbic neurons in areas such as the amygdala, such that they may subsequently develop the entire stress response spontaneously in the absence of a new stressor. Antidepressant drugs may exert their prophylactic effects against depressive episodes by preventing abnormal limbic neuronal activity from inducing spontaneous recurrence of the major depressive syndrome. Antidepressant drugs have been shown to decrease metabolic activity in the amygdala in depressed patients with MDD, in nondepressed control subjects and in experimental animals. These drugs have also been shown to decrease neuronal firing rates in the amygdala after chronic administration in animals, suggesting that they may exert direct effects in the amygdala.

Genetics, pharmacogenetics, and gene-environment interactions

Heritability of bipolar affective disorder and major depressive disorder

Twin, adoption, and family studies indicate that genetic factors substantially contribute to the liability for developing bipolar disorder and MDD. Moreover, earlier age of onset appears to be associated with increased transmissibility of both bipolar disorder and MDD. Family studies attempting to subdivide bipolar and unipolar illness have established that the first-degree relatives of adult bipolar probands are at increased risk for both bipolar and unipolar disorders when compared with relatives of unipolar probands or with general population rates. Nevertheless, while it is clear that there is some shared genetic liability between bipolar and unipolar disorder, the data also suggest that bipolar and unipolar disorders are transmitted independently to some extent. There is similar family-based evidence suggesting that there is also a partial genetic overlap between bipolar disorder and schizophrenia.

Taken at face value, adult twin and adoption studies indicate that familial transmission of bipolar disorder is largely a result of genetic factors and that genetic factors are more important in the development of bipolar disorders than of MDD. The heritability of bipolar disorder is estimated to be 60–70%. Recent twin studies of adult MDD report a heritability of approximately 40%. These estimates of the heritability of MDD should be considered low since recent examinations of the stability in the reporting of depressive symptoms indicate that approximately 50% of the variability in reporting diagnoses of MDD may represent fluctuation of symptom reports in mild cases. If heritability estimates for MDD are corrected for the assessment error associated with this type

of reporting attenuation, the heritability of MDD may equal that of bipolar disorder.

Putative genetic loci in mood disorders

There is little evidence that familial forms of affective disorders result from simple genetic defects, such as autosomal dominant or recessive mutations. However, just as for other complex medical conditions with prominent genetic components (such as hypertension, diabetes mellitus, or Alzheimer's disease), there is great interest in identifying genetic variations that contribute to the development of mood disorders. Searches for the genes involved in the etiology of the affective disorders have taken one of two general strategies. The first is linkage (which is usually agnostic about what gene is involved). The second involves testing specific candidate genes by association studies.

There have been several claims linking particular genetic loci to affective disorders. Most notable among these have been a number of genetic linkage studies of bipolar disorder reporting conflicting findings regarding the involvement of chromosome 11 and the X chromosome. More recently, there have been claims of linkage to loci on chromosomes 4, 12, 13, 18, 21, and 22, and a new X chromosome locus. Other investigators have used case-control association approaches for testing the involvement of specific genes in the development of bipolar disorders. At present, none of the putative linkage locations or associations is widely accepted and, in general, positive findings have not been replicated. Currently, there are no genetic tests that help with the diagnosis of the depressive or manic disorders.

Pharmacogenetics of mood disorders

Even though specific genes or DNA sequences have not been identified that predispose to risk for mood disorders, a number of recent studies have demonstrated genetic predispositions to treatment response for the selective serotonin reuptake inhibitors (SSRIs) and for lithium prophylaxis. Response to treatment with SSRIs in major depressive disorder and the depressed phase of bipolar disorder has been linked to sequence differences in a regulatory region of the serotonin transporter gene (5-HTT). Reports suggest that patients with a longer form of the gene promoter region are more likely to respond to SSRIs. Interestingly, the same longer variant of the 5-HTT gene promoter has been associated with good antidepressant response to sleep deprivation. Similar to SSRI response, the long form of the 5-HTT gene has been associated with better response to lithium prophylaxis.

Possible gene-environment interactions and the risk for major depressive disorder

Interestingly, the serotonin transporter gene has also been implicated as a possible mediator of gene-environment effects in depression. Individuals who have the long form of the gene appear to be much more sensitive to adverse life effects, resulting in the development of a depressive episode. Though much work remains to be done in this area, these findings suggest that there may be important gene-environment interactions that predict which individuals will become ill and who will respond to treatment.

Pathophysiology

Neurochemical, neuroendocrine, neurophysiological, neuropathological, and neuropsychological abnormalities have all been demonstrated in mood disorders, suggesting that several systems within the brain are affected in these illnesses. Moreover, biological differences appear to exist across subgroups of subjects meeting criteria for MDD, suggesting that this syndrome is associated with multiple pathophysiologic states. This section highlights some of the brain systems implicated in mood disorders that are likely related to their core features.

Anatomical circuits related to mood disorders

Brain imaging technologies have demonstrated a variety of abnormalities in mood disorders in brain regions implicated in emotional processing or modulation by other types of evidence (Chapter 6). These neuroimaging data in both normal emotional states and in primary and induced mood disorders converge with evidence from lesion analyses to implicate circuits involving the ventral and medial prefrontal cortex (PFC) along with limbic structures such as the amygdala, and related parts of the striatum and thalamus. For example, the findings in unipolar depressed subjects with FPDD of abnormally increased cerebral blood flow (CBF) and metabolism in the ventral PFC, the amygdala and the medial thalamus (Fig. 8.1), coupled with indications of reduced flow in the medial caudate, suggest that two interconnected circuits are involved in the pathophysiology of FPDD: a limbic-thalamo-cortical circuit involving the amygdala, the mediodorsal nucleus (MD) of the thalamus (in the medial thalamus), and the ventrolateral and medial PFC; and a limbic-striatal-pallidal-thalamic circuit involving related parts of the striatum and the ventral pallidum in addition to the components of the other circuit (Fig. 8.2).

The first of these circuits can be conceptualized as an excitatory triangular circuit whereby the amygdala and the

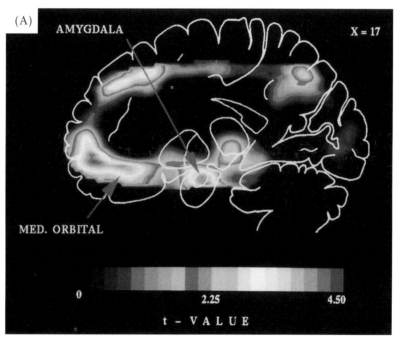

Fig. 8.1 Areas of increased and decreased blood flow in the cortex of unipolar depressed subjects who have FPDD. The sagittal and coronal image slices shown are from an image of t-values, produced by a voxel-by-voxel computation of the t-statistic, and indicate areas where flow is increased (Panel A) or decreased (Panel B) in the depressed group relative to the control group. These t-images were used to generate hypotheses regarding the regions where neurophysiological activity is abnormal in major depression. The presence of abnormal activity in these regions has subsequently been confirmed using both regional blood flow and glucose metabolic image data from independent subject samples.

Panel A. The area of *increased* flow in the left prefrontal cortex extends from the medial orbital cortex to also involve the lateral orbital cortex, the ventrolateral prefrontal cortex, and the pregenual portion of the anterior cingulate gyrus. These "limbic" prefrontal areas interconnect with the amygdala and the medial dorsal nucleus of the thalamus to form the limbic-thalamo-cortical circuit (see text and Fig. 8.2).

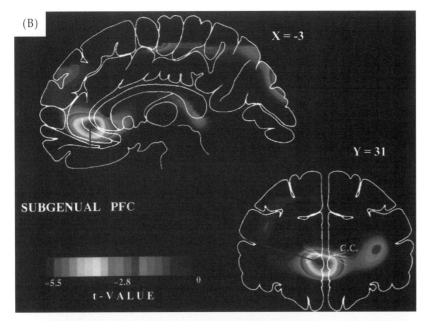

Fig. 8.1 Panel B. The area of *decreased* blood flow in depressed versus control subjects is centered on the left subgenual prefrontal cortex. This is a brain region that has been implicated in the mediation of emotional reactions to social stimuli and in the regulation of monoamine and related neurotransmitter systems, which are the targets of antidepressant drugs. The decreased blood flow to this region is associated with a reduction of cortical gray matter volume. For additional views of these neurophysiological abnormalities, see Fig. 6.6.

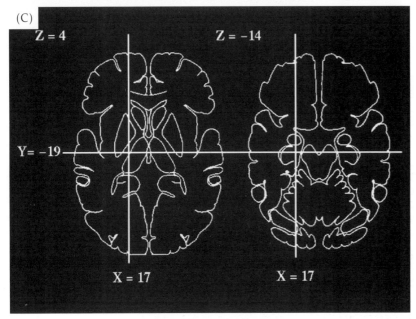

Fig. 8.1 Panel C. The number to the side of each image locates the section in mm from the anterior commissure, with negative Y = posterior, positive X = left hemisphere, and negative Z = ventral to a plane containing both the anterior and the posterior commissures. The orientations of the sagittal and the coronal image slices are indicated on horizontal atlas tracings at the level of the amygdala (Z = −14) and the medial thalamus (Z = 4). The atlas outlines corresponding to each image slice are from Talairach and Tournoux (1988) *Co-Planar Stereotaxic Atlas of the Human Brain*, Stuttgart, Thieme. Left is on the left, and anterior is toward the left for the sagittal section or the page top for the horizontal tracings. Illustration modified from Price, Carmichael, and Drevets, 1996.

prefrontal cortical regions are interconnected by excitatory projections with each other and with the MD. Increased metabolic activity in the amygdala, the medial thalamus and the PFC would presumably reflect increased synaptic activity in these areas, suggesting that synaptic transmission through the limbic-thalamo-cortical circuit is abnormally elevated in FPDD. In ventral frontal lobe tissue removed from depressed patients undergoing neurosurgical treatments, the concentration of the neurotransmitter, aspartic acid, is increased, supporting the hypothesis of increased limbic-thalamo-cortical transmission. Also consistent with this hypothesis, neurosurgical procedures that ameliorate treatment-resistant depression interrupt projections within the limbic-thalamo-cortical or the limbic-striatal-pallidal-thalamic circuits. Other somatic antidepressant treatments may also compensate for the pathophysiology of FPDD by suppressing limbic-thalamo-cortical activity, as antidepressant drug administration is associated with decreased CBF and metabolism in the amygdala, the ventral PFC, and the medial thalamus in depressed patients and with decreased amygdala neuronal firing rates in experimental animals. The areas where abnormal metabolic activity has been identified in unmedicated depressed patients *in vivo* have also been shown to contain histopathological abnormalities post mortem, which include abnormal reductions in cortex volume, glial cell counts and density, and synaptic markers or contacts.

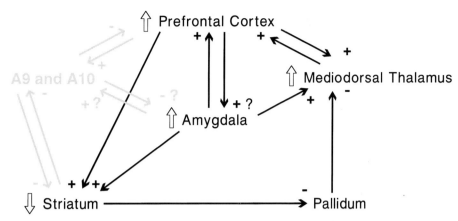

Fig. 8.2 Neuroanatomical circuits hypothesized to participate in the functional anatomy of MDD based on functional neuroimaging and lesion analysis studies. The open arrows adjacent to each region indicate the direction of significant differences in blood flow and glucose metabolism in patients with unipolar depression who have FPDD relative to healthy controls. The regions' monosynaptic connections with each other are illustrated (closed arrows), with + indicating excitatory, – showing inhibitory projections, and ? indicating limited experimental evidence. Portions of the prefrontal cortex (PFC) involve primarily the lateral and medial orbital cortex. The parts of the striatum under consideration are the ventral medial caudate and the nucleus accumbens, which particularly project to the ventral pallidum. In this primary mood disorder, the findings of increased flow and metabolism in the amygdala, the medial thalamus, and the limbic PFC are compatible with other evidence suggesting that synaptic transmission through the limbic-thalamic-cortical circuit is abnormally elevated. In contrast, in major depressive syndromes arising secondary to some neurological disorders, blood flow and metabolic abnormalities have been reported in some of these regions that are opposite in direction with respect to the normative baseline as those shown here. This observation is consistent with evidence from lesion analysis studies that mood disorders may arise by a variety of functional or structural lesions occurring at multiple points within these circuits that affect the synaptic transmission through them in diverse ways.

The major dopaminergic projections from the black substance (A9) and the ventral tegmental area (A10) to these structures are illustrated with the shaded tone. Serotoninergic, noradrenergic, and cholinergic projections into this system exist as well and likely contribute to its overall modulation. Whereas somatic antidepressant therapies influence each of these systems, their therapeutic mechanisms may be associated with enhancing dopaminergic and serotoninergic (especially serotonin$_{1A}$ relative to serotonin$_2$ receptor) function. Both effects would putatively inhibit transmission through the limbic-thalamic-cortical circuit. Other structures and neurotransmitter systems likely play important roles in mood disorders as well, and the circuit shown here is simplified both for clarity and for lack of knowledge. (From Drevets, WC *et al.* (1992) *J Neurosci* 12:3628–3641.)

Subjects with late-onset depression have frontal lobe abnormalities of a different nature (see above). MRI signal hyperintensities appear in the frontal lobe, the caudate and the white matter adjacent to these structures in over 70% of subjects with depression onset after age 60 (Chapter 6). Post-mortem and magnetic resonance spectroscopy data have demonstrated that these signal hyperintensities probably reflect arteriosclerotic/ischemic lesions. As expected in the presence of such lesions, PET images from such elderly depressed patients show diffuse areas of decreased CBF in the PFC, which are presumably accounted for by reduced vascular supply and damaged tissue, rather than by the shifts in local synaptic activity thought to dictate regional metabolic changes in younger depressed patients. When elderly depressed patients are used as their own controls by acquiring scans before and after ECT or antidepressant drug treatment, remission of the depressive syndrome is associated with further CBF decreases in the left PFC. Thus in both young-onset and late-onset depressed patients, left prefrontal activity appears to be elevated in the depressed phase relative to the remitted phase of MDD and, conversely, left prefrontal activity decreases during effective antidepressant treatment.

This circuitry model provides a useful conceptual framework for approaching the depressive syndromes induced by neurological lesions. Induced mood syndromes may also stem from dysfunction within limbic-cortico-striatal-pallidal-thalamic circuits, since lesions involving the prefrontal cortex (i.e., tumors or infarctions) and diseases of the basal ganglia (e.g. Parkinson's or Huntington's disease) are associated with higher rates of depression than other similarly debilitating conditions (Chapter 27). While these disorders all affect limbic-cortical-striatal-pallidal-thalamic circuits, the point of dysfunction is different in each condition, implying that abnormal interaction between elements of this circuit, rather than increased or decreased activity in any single structure, can produce major depressive episodes. The hypothesis that lesions affecting various points within neural circuits that subserve and modulate emotion can give rise to mood disorders is analogous to the case in the motor circuitry (involving the primary and supplemental motor cortices, the dorsal striatum, the dorsal pallidum, and related parts of the thalamus) where dysfunction at multiple sites results in movement disorders.

Distinct abnormalities within limbic-cortical-striatal-pallidal-thalamic circuits could account for clinical differences between depressive subtypes. For example, the sites where lesions can induce bipolar or manic syndromes differ from those where lesions are associated with unipolar depressive syndromes. Cerebrovascular lesions associated with induced manic or bipolar syndromes involve the right ventral PFC, the right striatum, the right thalamus, or the right basotemporal cortex (which may include the amygdala), whereas lesions involving the left PFC and the left caudate are associated with induced unipolar depressive syndromes. Furthermore, degenerative disorders of the basal ganglia associated with unipolar versus bipolar mood syndromes affect synaptic transmission through the limbic-cortical-striatal-pallidal-thalamic circuitry differently. For example, in Parkinson's disease increased striatal-pallidal transmission results from the loss of the inhibitory effects of nigrostriatal dopaminergic neurons, and the course of the induced depression is unipolar and nondelusional (similar to the case in FPDD, where increased striatal-pallidal transmission is hypothesized (Fig. 8.2)). In contrast, in Huntington's disease decreased striatal-pallidal transmission results from the degeneration of striatal neurons, and the course of the secondary mood disorder can be bipolar with or without psychotic features. Finally, the dissimilar regional CBF patterns in bipolar as compared with unipolar depression provides an example of primary depressive subtypes that are associated with distinct abnormalities within the limbic-cortical-striatal-pallidal-thalamic circuitry.

Neuroendocrine abnormalities in major depression

Mood disorders have been associated with neuroendocrine disturbances in the hypothalamic-pituitary-adrenocortical axis, the thyroid axis, and the growth hormone axis. These abnormalities may be related to the neurochemical changes described below and/or involvement of the ventral prefrontal and limbic structures described above. Both the amygdala, where increased metabolism has been found in unipolar depression, and the subgenual PFC and lateral orbital cortex, where abnormal metabolism has been demonstrated in both unipolar and bipolar depression, have extensive connections with the lateral and paraventricular nuclei of the hypothalamus. Disruption of the functional interactions between these structures and the hypothalamus could partly underlie some of the neuroendocrine and autonomic manifestations of mood disorders, as well as the neurovegetative symptoms of the major depressive syndrome (i.e., disturbed sleep, appetite, libido, and energy).

For example, severe depression is associated with hyperactivity of the hypothalamic-pituitary-adrenocortical sys-

tem as indicated by increased CSF levels of corticotrophin releasing factor (CRF), hypersecretion of adrenocorticotrophic hormone (ACTH) and cortisol, and enlargement of the pituitary and adrenal glands. These abnormalities suggest that CRF is hypersecreted in a major depressive episode. Compatible with this hypothesis, the ACTH response to intravenously administered CRF is blunted in depression, and CRF receptor density is decreased in the frontal cortex of suicide victims (presumably reflecting compensatory desensitization or downregulation of CRF receptors due to CRF hypersecretion). In addition, premature escape from the cortisol suppressant effects of dexamethasone is found in 70–85% of patients with bipolar depression and unipolar depressives with FPDD, suggesting that CRF release is disengaged from control by glucocorticoid feedback inhibition. Abnormal dexamethasone suppression is not observed in bereaved subjects with depressive symptoms, so this phenomenon does not simply appear to reflect a correlate of stress.

In some patients with mood disorders, CRF or cortisol levels may conceivably become high enough to contribute to the pathogenesis of some depressive symptoms. For example, the clinical features of Cushing's syndrome include fatigue (100%), anergia (97%), irritability (86%), depressed mood (77%), decreased libido (69%), middle (69%) or terminal (55%) insomnia, anxiety (66%), impaired concentration (66%), crying (63%), appetite disturbance (54%), hopelessness (43%), and guilt (37%). These symptom frequencies are similar to those found in MDD (Table 8.1). Less commonly, elevated glucocorticoid administration (e.g., prednisone treatment) or release (in Cushing's disease) induces manic symptoms. It remains unclear whether increased corticosteroid levels directly induce emotional and neurovegetative symptoms or instead trigger mood syndromes via a separate mechanism.

Neurochemical systems implicated in depression

Neurochemical abnormalities have been consistently identified in the central norepinephrine (NE), serotonin (5-HT), dopamine (DA), acetylcholine (ACh), gamma-aminobutyric acid (GABA), and neuropeptide (i.e., CRF and opiate) systems in the primary mood disorders. Dysfunction within these integrated systems likely contributes to the functional anatomical and neuroendocrine abnormalities described above, as well as to the neuropsychiatric manifestations of mood disorders. However, it remains unclear whether these neurochemical alterations are fundamentally involved in the etiology of mood disorders or instead reflect compensatory changes resulting from pathology in other systems.

Norepinephrine (NE)

The central noradrenergic system has been implicated in major depression by several lines of evidence. Urinary concentrations of the NE metabolite 3-methoxy-4-hydroxyphenylglycol (MHPG) are consistently decreased in patients with bipolar depression and in some patients with unipolar depression. In addition, neuroendocrine (i.e., growth hormone release) and autonomic responses (i.e., heart rate changes) to α-adrenoreceptor agonists (e.g., clonidine) are blunted during both the depressed and re-mitted phases of MDD. Adenylate cyclase responses to β-adrenoreceptor agonists are also diminished in depressed patients, but this abnormality returns to normal with treatment. Finally, β-adrenoreceptor density is abnormally increased in frontal and temporal cortical tissue from suicide victims. Treatment may also reverse this abnormality, as most antidepressant drugs downregulate β-adrenoreceptor density in experimental animals.

Serotonin (5-HT)

Serotonergic function also appears to be altered in depression, as indicated by evidence of deficient 5-HT presynaptic activity and alterations in presynaptic and postsynaptic 5-HT_{1A} receptor density and sensitivity. Some of these changes may not be specific to MDD, as decreased concentrations of the 5-HT metabolite 5-HIAA in the CSF antemortem and in the brainstem postmortem are found in both depressed and nondepressed suicide attempters or victims. These data have led to the hypothesis that lower serotonergic function is associated with suicidal behavior involving planning and resulting in greater medical damage and not specifically with MDD.

Dopamine (DA)

The DA projections from the ventral tegmental area and the substantia nigra into the "limbic" striatum (the medial caudate and the nucleus accumbens) and the medial PFC appear to subserve a "reward-related system" that mediates motivation, hedonia, behavioral reinforcement, and psychomotor activity. Since the emotional experiences and behaviors that appear to be mediated by this mesolimbic DA system are disturbed in mood disorders, it has been implicated as a system where hypofunction could yield the anhedonia, psychomotor retardation and amotivation characterizing a depressive episode and where hyperfunction could account for the euphoria, psychomotor restlessness and hypermotivation observed in mania. The available data support this hypothesis, as reduced DA function in depression is suggested by the consistent findings that antidepressant drugs enhance dopamine receptor sensitivity in limbic structures and that CSF concentrations of the DA metabolite, homovanillic acid, are reduced in nondelusional depressed patients. Moreover, mania has been associated with increased DA function by findings that manic symptoms are reduced by DA receptor antagonists or DA synthesis inhibitors and can be precipitated in euthymic or depressed bipolar patients by DA receptor agonists.

Altered sleep stages in mood disorders

Among the most consistent physiological changes found in MDD or bipolar disorder are abnormalities in the sleep EEG. During a depressive episode, most adults with primary mood disorders demonstrate reduced slow-wave sleep (stages three and four, or "deep sleep"), reduced rapid eye movement (REM) latency (time between sleep onset and REM onset), and increased REM density (time spent in REM sleep). These changes are consistent with depressed patients' subjective impression that their sleep is restless and that they fail to sleep deeply.

The implications these sleep abnormalities hold for the pathophysiology of mood disorders are unclear. Insomnia and sleep EEG abnormalities have been hypothesized to correlate with decreased serotonergic function or with alterations in the ratio of cholinergic-to-aminergic neurotransmission. Sleep EEG changes have also been postulated to corroborate neuroimaging evidence of prefrontal cortical dysfunction in mood disorders, since the PFC has been implicated in the regulation of sleep architecture. Sleep EEG changes are absent in depressed children and early adolescents (who otherwise resemble depressed adults), indicating that they are not fundamental to the development of mood disorders. They may reflect secondary phenomena associated with effects of affective illness or may be associated with an increased risk for the development of depression relatively late in life, given their strong correlation with age.

Some sleep EEG changes encountered in depression may reflect epiphenomena of depressive symptoms, as reduced REM latency has been reported in non-depressed subjects who have been sleep-deprived. Moreover, a contribution of stress or sadness to altered REM density is suggested by studies of *non-depressed*, bereaved elders who, like depressed patients with MDD, show elevated phasic measures of REM sleep although they do not differ from controls on other sleep EEG measures or on subjective evaluation of sleep quality. In contrast, bereaved elders who also meet criteria for a major depressive episode show reduced slow-wave sleep, reduced REM latency and diminished sleep efficiency, similar to depressed patients with MDD. Since depressed-bereaved subjects may experience insomnia, the extent to which nonspecific effects of sleep deprivation account for such sleep EEG changes is unclear.

An intriguing observation regarding sleep disturbances in mood disorders is that a night of total sleep deprivation can transiently alleviate depressive symptoms. Moreover, some bipolar subjects report that sleep deprivation can precipitate hypomanic or manic episodes. As described above, a link between sleep deprivation and antidepressant drug effects (which can both ameliorate depression and precipitate mania) may be the serotonin transporter (5HTT) gene.

Treatment

Management of major depressive disorder

General considerations

The conservative approach to managing mood disorders mandates that patients who meet criteria for a major depressive episode receive antidepressant treatment. The risk of not treating mood disorders is high, and the risk associated with antidepressant treatment is in most cases quite low.

Depression management requires office visits long enough to educate, support, and reassure patients. Frequent follow-up visits are usually needed to ensure that the treatment is tolerated and effective, since patients are often too ill to make decisions or to act on their own behalf. Family members and ancillary healthcare staff may need to be involved in management of the depressed patient because of the impaired insight and judgment that often accompany mood disorders. Follow-up visits should occur at semi-weekly to monthly intervals, depending upon severity, until the patient has at least partially remitted. Once a complete or nearly complete remission has been established, this interval can be increased to two to six months. Follow-up must include monitoring for the development of suicide ideation, psychotic features or mania. (Antidepressant drugs can precipitate mania or hypomania in 0.3% to 1.0% of cases.)

Need for hospitalization and psychiatric referral
A primary reason for hospitalization is suicide prevention. Patients who represent a significant suicide risk ought to be hospitalized until they can be safely managed on an outpatient basis. The assessment of suicidal risk and the management of suicidal behavior are discussed in Chapter 29. Other reasons to hospitalize patients with mood disorders include mania, psychosis, refusal to eat or drink, and inability to manage other medical problems because of depressive symptoms.

As a general rule, depressed patients who require hospitalization also warrant referral to a psychiatrist. Depressed outpatients who develop suicidality, psychosis, or mania or who fail to care for their medical needs also require psychiatric referral. Failure to respond to two six- to eight-week treatment trials, of which at least one involves antidepressant pharmacotherapy, should also prompt referral or consultation with a psychiatrist.

Length of treatment
Once symptom remission has been achieved, maintenance treatment with antidepressant drugs should be continued for a variable length of time. The data from long-term studies of up to five years' duration suggest that antidepressant drugs not only ameliorate the current depressive episode, they can also prevent relapse and recurrence in a majority of cases (Fig. 8.3). Nevertheless, guidelines for the duration of maintenance therapy have not been established. The decision regarding the length of treatment involves consideration of the severity and frequency of previous episodes.

Redevelopment of the depressive syndrome within six months of treatment discontinuation is usually called "relapse" and beyond six months is called "recurrence." The relapse rate increases as the duration of maintenance treatment decreases. Previously, six months was considered an acceptable length of maintenance therapy for most patients. However, the relapse rate for such short treatment duration is unacceptably high. Twelve to eighteen months of maintenance treatment may prove more beneficial for the first one or two episodes of depression.

For the third episode and beyond, longer treatment periods are indicated unless each episode has been separated from the others by several years of remission. Frequent episodes are increasingly being considered a reason for chronic treatment, given the recurrent nature of MDD and its risk of excess mortality and indescribable suffering. The importance of chronic treatment for such cases is highlighted by preliminary indications that up to 30% of patients fail to respond to the antidepressant drug that proved effective in the previous episode if it has been discontinued prior to the current episode. This is an ominous event for clinicians, since identifying another effective agent for such a patient can require trials of several antidepressant drugs.

Selection of treatments
Several safe, effective, and well-tolerated therapeutic options exist for the treatment of major depression. Biological markers or clinical criteria capable of predicting treatment outcome for a specific treatment do not exist. Consequently, the approach to identifying an effective regimen is empirical ("trial-and-error") and in many cases, myriad pharmacologic and nonpharmacological interventions are tried before a successful treatment response is obtained. It is thus imperative that ineffective trials of pharmacotherapy or psychotherapy be amended (e.g., by increasing the dosage) or discontinued to permit initiation of new treatments.

Psychological treatments (psychotherapy)

Management of depression always involves supportive and rehabilitative psychotherapy (see Chapter 21). More specific psychotherapeutic techniques that may prove beneficial in treating MDD include cognitive-behavior therapy (CBT) and interpersonal therapy (IPT). These techniques have shown greater efficacy for treating MDD than other forms of psychotherapy in controlled studies. In contrast to CBT and IPT, insight-directed psychotherapies, which involve examination of subconscious motives, repressed memories, and deep feelings, have not clearly been shown to be effective in depression and may exacerbate depressed patients' feelings of guilt and self-depreciation.

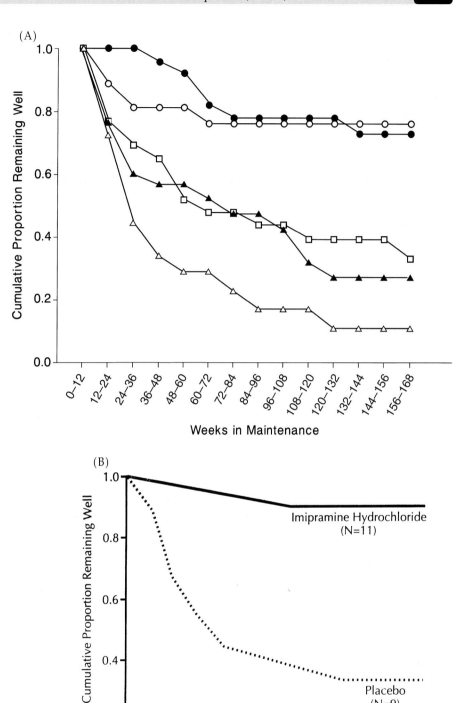

Fig. 8.3 A. Outcome of maintenance therapies in recurrent depression shown as the cumulative proportion of subjects remaining in remission during the three-year treatment period. Open circles represent a group that underwent medication clinic and active imipramine (a tricyclic antidepressant drug); solid circles, a group treated with both interpersonal psychotherapy and active imipramine; squares, a group treated with interpersonal psychotherapy alone; solid triangles, a group treated with interpersonal psychotherapy and placebo; and open triangles, a group that underwent medication clinic and placebo. Reprinted by permission from Frank *et al.* (1990) Arch Gen Psychiatry 47: 1093–1099. **B.** Outcome of maintenance therapies in recurrent depression shown as the cumulative proportion of subjects remaining in remission during years four and five of treatment. At the conclusion of the three-year study summarized in Fig. 8.3A, 20 subjects from the two groups that had received active imipramine were recruited for an additional two-year study in which they were randomized to either continued imipramine treatment or placebo. Although subjects had been in remission for three years prior to being converted to placebo, most relapsed within the one year following imipramine discontinuation. In contrast, 10 of the 11 subjects maintained on imipramine treatment remained free of a recurrence of a depressive episode through year five. Reprinted by permission from Kupfer *et al.* (1992) Arch Gen Psychiatry 49: 769–773.

The theoretical bases for CBT and IPT are distinct. CBT is based upon the hypothesis that depressive emotions arise because patients develop cognitive distortions, in which they view themselves and their circumstances in a consistently negative light. The therapist attempts to help the patient logically challenge such perspectives by training them to recognize such negative thoughts as unrealistic (e.g., changing the thought from "I can't do anything right," to "I do several things well, and no one does everything perfectly"). The patient is thereby guided to develop more positive, realistic and constructive means of assessing their own capabilities and circumstances. The goal of IPT is to enhance the patient's social functioning by improving their ability to effectively deal with stressors and to manage the personal and social consequences of their depressive episode. Within IPT, special techniques have been developed for managing patients who are dealing with grief or loss, interpersonal deficits, or marital problems. The most beneficial psychotherapeutic approach in most cases is likely to be an eclectic one in which elements of all of these techniques are brought to bear on the patient's behalf.

Psychotherapy versus pharmacotherapy as a single treatment
The efficacy of CBT and IPT has been compared to that of pharmacotherapy for the treatment of MDD. Some, if not all, studies showing similar efficacy for psychotherapy and pharmacotherapy appear to suffer from an ascertainment bias, in that most patients referred to such studies have been considered "good candidates" for psychotherapy by the referral source. The general expectation among clinicians is that patients who are relatively mild in severity, are "psychologically-minded" and have retained mood reactivity are more likely to respond to psychotherapy. Mood reactivity implies that a patient is able to feel better when positive life events occur and that their depressive episode may have been precipitated by life events. More severely depressed patients who demonstrate prominent psychomotor disturbances, neurovegetative signs, anhedonia, nonreactive mood, and biological markers for depression are generally not referred for psychotherapy alone.

This distinction has been demonstrated in studies that included a wide variety of patient types in order to assess the psychobiological correlates of psychotherapy response. For example, a recent study included inpatients (n = 32) as well as outpatients (n = 110) and found that a poor outcome with CBT was associated with greater pretreatment symptom severity, unemployment, and sleep-EEG abnormalities. Among the inpatients in particular, poor outcome to CBT was associated with elevated urinary free cortisol levels, male gender, and diagnostic comorbidity. Thus relatively mild, non-chronic depressives who did not demonstrate biological markers for depression were more likely to respond to CBT. An older study divided patients into exogenous and endogenous groups (see above) and found that exogenous patients were at least as likely to respond to CBT as to medications, but that endogenous patients were far more likely to respond to antidepressant drug therapy than to CBT. In a large multicenter trial that compared CBT, IPT, and imipramine, imipramine proved superior to either psychotherapeutic technique for more severely depressed and functionally-impaired patients. In contrast, significant differences between treatments could not be demonstrated for the less severely depressed, less impaired subgroup.

It is likely that the heterogeneity within MDD is responsible for the controversy over whether mood disorders can be treated with psychotherapy alone. At present, no reliable

means of predicting response to psychotherapy as opposed to pharmacotherapy have been established. Reasonable clinical guidelines based upon the extant data are that more severely ill patients or patients with melancholic subtype should receive antidepressant pharmacotherapy, with or without psychotherapy. For mild, non-melancholic cases who are not suicidal and not functionally impaired, a trial of psychotherapy may be a viable option. However, if such patients do not respond to psychotherapy within eight weeks, they should be offered a trial of antidepressant drug treatment.

Psychotherapy as an adjunctive treatment to pharmacotherapy
In addition to the supportive/educational psychotherapy that all patients should receive, adjunctive psychotherapy using more specific approaches such as CBT or IPT can prove invaluable in many cases where patients are receiving antidepressant drugs. Established guidelines for identifying patients likely to benefit from combined therapy are not available. Studies assessing the differential efficacy of using antidepressant drugs in combination with psychotherapy for randomly selected samples have yielded mixed results, with some studies showing a significantly greater response for combined treatment than for drug or talk therapy alone and others showing no benefit for combined therapy over antidepressant drug therapy alone. Thus, it cannot be concluded that all patients require combined therapy.

Patients for whom referral for adjunctive CBT or IPT may be indicated include: (1) depressed patients who have inadequately responded to somatic treatments; (2) those who have improved on antidepressant drugs, but need more intensive rehabilitation for persistent effects of the depressive episode upon self-esteem or interpersonal relationships; (3) patients exhibiting chronic patterns of cognitive distortions (e.g., focusing exclusively on the negative aspects of situations) that have been present irrespective of major depressive episodes; and 4) patients with a history of traumatic life events that have chronically affected self-esteem, emotional stability, or social relationships (e.g., experiences of physical or sexual abuse).

Common errors committed during management of mood disorders include:
1 Failure to detect and diagnose major depressive disorder.
2 Prescription of subtherapeutic doses of antidepressant drugs.
3 Prescription of sedative-hypnotic rather than antidepressant drugs.

PEARLS & PERILS

Pharmacological treatments for depression
General considerations

- Efficacy—management of MDD usually includes treatment with antidepressant drugs because of their relatively high efficacy and relatively mild adverse effect profile. When all patients with MDD are considered together, the efficacy across antidepressant drug classes is similar. Of patients who complete a 6- to 8-week drug treatment trial, about 60% to 70% experience substantial improvement. However, the literature suggests that efficacy may be lower for some subgroups. For example, patients older than age 75 commonly experience only modest therapeutic responses to antidepressant drugs, and patients hospitalized with depression or elderly patients with melancholic subtype may be less responsive to selective serotonin reuptake inhibitors than to tricyclic antidepressants.

- Minimizing adverse effects—since in most cases the efficacy of antidepressant agents appears similar across classes, selection of antidepressant drugs is based largely upon their risk in overdose, side-effect profile, and potential for drug interactions. The importance of considering the latter two categories is magnified for elderly and medically ill patients. For example, cardiovascular effects are of greater concern in the elderly because this population has increased prevalence of concomitant cardiovascular disease and a more limited capacity to adjust to perturbations in cardiovascular function. The tricyclic antidepressant (TCA) agents have Type I antiarrhythmic effects, which, in patients with bundle branch disease, can result in potentially lethal atrial-ventricular conduction block and ventricular arrhythmias. In addition, the most common cardiovascular effect of antidepressant drugs [occurring with the TCAs, the monoamine-oxidase inhibitors (MAOI) and trazodone] is orthostatic hypotension. While in younger patients this side effect is usually inconsequential, in the elderly, orthostatic hypotension increases the risk of falls and hip fractures. Consequently, agents without cardiovascular effects are generally the first choices for treatment in elderly patients.

The anticholinergic effects of the TCAs provide other examples of problems that become exaggerated with old age. Urinary retention or paralytic ileus resulting from TCA use is almost exclusively seen in the elderly. In addition, while younger patients are annoyed by dry mouth and constipation, these side effects can become serious management problems in the elderly where constipation can lead to fecal impaction and dry mouth can preclude the wearing of dentures. Anticholinergic effects can also contribute to acute confusional states or memory impairment in the depressed elderly, although these are rarely seen in younger patients. Patients with late-onset depression, in particular, are at increased risk for developing delirium during treatment with either TCAs or ECT, possibly related to the neuropathologic changes reflected in their MRI scans. Consequently, the newer generation antidepressant drugs that are less likely to produce anticholinergic effects or CNS toxicity are better choices for initial therapy.

- Pharmacokinetic considerations in the elderly and medically ill—several factors associated with normal aging affect the pharmacokinetics of psychotropic drugs. First, the volume-of-distribution (VOD) for most psychoactive drugs, which are highly lipophilic, increases with age as the ratio of fat-to-muscle increases in old age. Second, the clearance of most psychotropic drugs by the liver and the kidney decreases with age. (The polar metabolites of some psychotropic drugs that are generated by hepatic metabolism are excreted by the kidney.) Since the elimination half-life of a drug varies in proportion to its VOD and in inverse proportion to its clearance, both the increasing VOD and the decreasing clearance associated with advancing age work to prolong drug half-life in the elderly. The steady-state concentration of a drug is also inversely proportional to clearance. Thus, as the clearance of most antidepressant drugs decreases in old age, either the magnitude of the dose or the frequency of administration must be reduced to prevent excessive elevations in plasma concentration (see Chapter 26).

An additional factor that may alter pharmacokinetics in the elderly is the increasing prevalence of disease in multiple organ systems with advancing age. This increases the likelihood that hepatic or renal dysfunction may contribute to changes in pharmacokinetics. It also raises the potential for pharmacokinetic and pharmacodynamic drug interactions, since elderly patients are likely to receive treatment with multiple medications.

Classes of antidepressant agents

Seven major classes of antidepressant drugs are now available: the selective serotonin reuptake inhibitors (SSRIs; fluoxetine, sertraline, paroxetine, citalopram, escitalopram, and fluvoxamine), the TCAs (e.g., nortriptyline, desipramine, amitriptyline, imipramine, doxepin), the aminoketones (e.g., bupropion), the triazolopyridines/phenylpiperazines (trazodone and nefazodone), the phenethylamines (e.g., venlafaxine), mirtazapine, and the monoamine oxidase inhibitors (MAOIs; e.g., phenelzine, selegiline, tranylcypromine, and moclobemide). An eighth class, selective norepinephrine reuptake inhibitors, is likely to become available in the near future. While each class contains effective antidepressant agents, substantial differences exist both across and within classes in side-effect profiles, propensity for drug interactions, and extent to which the pharmacokinetics are affected by aging.

Selective serotonin reuptake inhibitors

The SSRIs exert relatively selective inhibition of the reuptake of 5-HT into presynaptic terminals. Following chronic administration this effect results in persistent enhancement of 5-HT neurotransmission putatively through desensitization of the presynaptic 5-HT$_{1A}$ autoreceptor. In contrast, the SSRIs exhibit relatively weak affinities for peripheral or central neurotransmitter receptors. They are consequently free, in most cases, from the troublesome anticholinergic, antihistaminic and antiadrenergic effects of the TCAs. In addition, the SSRIs lack the membrane stabilizing effects of the TCAs, and thus do not affect cardiac conduction. Finally, the SSRIs are not associated with CNS toxicity (i.e., potential for causing seizures) and are unlikely to produce delirium. Therefore, the SSRIs have a wide therapeutic index and are free of many of the adverse effects associated with other classes of antidepressants.

The side effects of the SSRIs are generally limited to the relatively mild adverse effects accompanying excessive blockade of peripheral and central 5-HT reuptake. These most commonly include sexual dysfunction and gastrointestinal effects such as nausea, vomiting, and loose stools. Treatment with the SSRIs can also result in insomnia, anxiety, and restlessness. Sedation is less common during SSRI treatment and occurs more often with paroxetine than with other SSRIs. Fluoxetine-induced nausea and anorexia have been associated with significant weight loss in medically ill depressed patients over age 75.

The incidence of some of the side effects associated with SSRI treatment rises proportionally with drug dose or plasma levels, while the curve relating antidepressant response to dose or plasma levels remains relatively flat. Consequently, bothersome side effects can sometimes be eliminated without sacrificing clinical efficacy by decreasing oral dose. Such adjustments can be accomplished within a few days for most SSRIs, which have elimination half-lives of about one day and require less than one week for new steady-state plasma drug levels to be reached following each dose change. In contrast, achieving a new steady-state for norfluoxetine, the active metabolite of fluoxetine, requires 4–8 weeks.

The SSRIs also differ in their potential for causing pharmacokinetic drug-drug interactions. All of the available SSRIs inhibit the liver enzyme, cytochrome P450 2D6, and thereby slow the metabolism of other drugs cleared by this enzyme system. These drugs include the TCAs (e.g., desipramine), the phenothiazines (e.g., thioridazine), the Type Ic antiarrhythmics (e.g., propafenone, flecainide, and ecainide), and beta-adrenergic antagonists (e.g., metoprolol, propranolol). Paroxetine, fluoxetine, and norfluoxetine are more potent inhibitors of cytochrome P450 2D6 than sertraline, fluvoxamine, citalopram, or escitalopram. Consequently, coadministration of paroxetine or fluoxetine with the TCAs or the Type Ic antiarrhythmics (which have narrow therapeutic indices) requires extreme caution. Fluoxetine and fluvoxamine also inhibit the cytochrome P450 enzyme 3A3/4, and fluvoxamine additionally inhibits the P450 enzyme 1A2 (see Chapter 27). When prescribing an SSRI, physicians should review with patients the drugs that may potentially interact with the SSRI. Of the SSRIs, sertraline, citalopram, and escitalopram appear least likely to produce clinically important drug interactions.

While several studies have now documented the antidepressant efficacy of SSRIs in depressed outpatients, concerns have been raised that the SSRIs may be less effective than the TCAs in depressed inpatients and elderly melancholic patients. The first studies to report a differential efficacy found significantly higher response rates in hospitalized depressed patients treated with the TCA, clomipramine, than in those treated with the SSRIs, citalopram or paroxetine. A more recent study reported that the proportion of elderly depressed patients who remitted during treatment with nortriptyline (82%) was significantly higher than that for matched patients treated with fluoxetine (28%). This difference was magnified in the subset of subjects meeting criteria for melancholic subtype, where 20 of 24 (83%) remitted during nortriptyline treatment compared with only 1 of 10 (10%) during fluoxetine treatment. Such studies comparing the efficacy of TCAs with that of SSRIs have been criticized for their inherent inability to maintain the investigators, blind to the drug administered because of differing side-effect profiles of the TCAs and the SSRIs. Until additional research establishes a differential efficacy for depressive subgroups, a reasonable recommendation may be that severely depressed or melancholic patients who fail to respond to an SSRI or relapse while taking an SSRI ought to receive a therapeutic trial of an agent from another antidepressant drug class.

In summary, the SSRIs generally produce fewer and more benign adverse effects than the TCAs. Of the SSRIs, sertraline, citalopram, and escitalopram possess advantages over fluoxetine or paroxetine for the treatment of elderly and medically ill patients, since their pharmacokinetics are similar in both elderly and younger patients and their inhibitory effects upon the activity of the hepatic isoenzyme P450 2D6 are substantially weaker. Additional research is needed to assess the significance of the aforementioned concerns that the SSRIs are less efficacious in more severely depressed subgroups than agents that block both 5-HT and NE reuptake.

Tricyclic antidepressants

The TCAs are thought to exert their antidepressant effects by inhibiting the reuptake of serotonin (5-HT), norepinephrine (NE) and, to a lesser extent, dopamine (DA) across presynaptic membranes. Their efficacy is well established in patients of all ages. However, the multiple pharmacodynamic actions of the TCAs can result in adverse effects that are particularly problematic in the elderly and medically ill. Their main liability, however, is their lethality in overdose.

The TCAs inhibit Na^+/K^+-dependent ATPase, which accounts for their ability to stabilize excitable membranes. This membrane stabilizing effect slows cardiac conduction and can precipitate arrhythmias or heart block in patients with bundle-branch disease. The risk of cardiac toxicity is highly correlated with plasma levels, accounting in part for the lethality of TCA overdose. Moreover, unintentional TCA overdose may occur at standard oral doses in patients who metabolize TCAs at anomalously slow rates. Thus, the narrow therapeutic index of the TCAs necessitates plasma drug level monitoring in many patients. Plasma level monitoring is particularly important in pediatric and elderly patients, in whom the hepatic metabolism of the TCAs is even more variable.

High TCA levels are also associated with the development of delirium and seizures. Advanced age increases the risk for CNS toxicity, as the plasma level required for the development of TCA-induced delirium decreases as age increases. The incidence of delirium appears particularly high in the presence of cerebrovascular disease (i.e., in post-stroke or late-onset depression).

The TCAs also block muscarinic cholinergic, histaminergic, and α-adrenergic receptors, accounting for a variety of problematic side effects in the elderly. The anticholinergic effects of the TCAs can result in delirium, memory impairment, confusion, sinus tachycardia, urinary hesitancy, constipation, dry mouth, blurred vision, and increased intraocular pressure in the presence of narrow angle glaucoma. The anti-$α_1$-adrenergic effect presumably accounts for the orthostatic hypotension and the consequent two- to three-fold increase in the risk of falls and hip fractures associated with TCA use in the elderly. The antihistaminic effects of the TCAs are thought to confer their potential for producing sedation, which frequently limits the ability to achieve therapeutic doses in elderly patients. Finally, treatment with the TCAs is commonly associated with weight gain.

Besides the cognitive impairment associated with the anticholinergic and sedative properties of the TCAs, impaired mentation or arousal can also result from pharmacodynamic interactions between the TCAs and other drugs that exert sedative (e.g., alcohol, benzodiazepines), anticholinergic or antihistaminic effects. Pharmacokinetic interactions can occur with agents that inhibit the activity of the hepatic isoenzyme P450 2D6 and 3A4 (e.g., the SSRIs), which slow the metabolism of TCAs and may increase plasma concentrations to toxic levels. Conversely, agents that induce the activity of the P450 enzymes (e.g., phenobarbital, carbamazepine) can lower TCA concentrations to subtherapeutic levels.

The sedative and anticholinergic effects associated with the tertiary amine TCAs (e.g., amitriptyline, doxepin, imipramine) are generally greater than those of the secondary amine TCAs (e.g., nortriptyline and desipramine), making the latter agents better choices for most patients. In the elderly, dropout rates commonly exceed 50% in clinical trials in which tertiary amine TCAs are used. In contrast, dropout rates are often less than 10% in trials using the secondary amine, nortriptyline. Nortriptyline may also be less likely to produce orthostatic hypotension than other TCAs.

Bupropion

Bupropion is an aminoketone that weakly inhibits DA reuptake, has multiple and complicated effects upon noradrenergic function, and has been reported to increase firing activity of 5-HT neurons. Because of its novel mechanism, bupropion often proves to be useful in patients who have failed other treatments. Bupropion produces no significant effects upon the cardiovascular system and does not cause sedation or cognitive impairment.

Bupropion is associated with the development of seizures in approximately 0.4% of patients treated at doses up to 450 mg/day. (Patients with seizure disorders or bulimia may be at increased risk for seizures.) However, the incidence of seizures increases seven-fold between doses of 450 and 600 mg/day. While these doses exceed the recommended upper limit of 450 mg/day, this disproportionate increase in seizure risk causes concern in the elderly population, where the pharmacokinetics are not well studied. (Large interindividual variations in metabolism exist even among young subjects.) This is an important concern because the metabolism of bupropion is complex, and higher levels of its three metabolites may contribute to the risk of seizures. Therapeutic drug monitoring has not been adequately established for bupropion as a means to guide dose adjustments in order to avoid the increased risk of metabolite accumulation. The narrow therapeutic index of bupropion with regard to the development of seizures appears to have been widened by the availability of sustained release preparations, which appear to have lowered the seizure incidence at doses of 300 mg per day. Bupropion is a potent inhibitor of the hepatic enzyme cytochrome P450 2D6.

Triazolopyridines/Phenylpiperazines

Trazodone is a triazolopyridine, which is a potent 5-HT2 receptor antagonist. (Its ability to block 5-HT reuptake at clinical doses is negligible.) Trazodone and its metabolite m-chlorophenylpiperazine also block α-adrenoreceptors. Trazodone lacks anticholinergic effects and exerts minimal effects upon cardiac conduction, although it has been associated with arrhythmias in patients with preexisting cardiac disease. Trazodone is unlikely to cause clinically significant pharmacokinetic drug-drug interactions and has a pharmacokinetic profile that is not substantially altered by age or intercurrent disease. Trazodone's use has been limited by its most common side effect, sedation, and by its propensity to cause orthostatic hypotension (presumably due to antagonism of α-adrenoreceptors). These effects can also result in clinically significant pharmacodynamic interactions with other drugs that decrease arousal or impair cognitive performance, or with adrenergic agents that affect blood pressure. In addition, trazodone can rarely produce priapism.

Nefazodone, a phenylpiperazine, is less likely to produce sedation or orthostatic hypotension than trazodone. Like trazodone, nefazodone blocks 5-HT2 receptors, but unlike trazodone, nefazodone (along with its active metabolites) may exert significant reuptake inhibition of 5-HT at clinical doses. Similar to trazodone, nefazodone possesses minimal affinity for muscarinic cholinergic or histaminergic receptors. However, nefazodone has substantially weaker affinity for α-adrenoreceptors than trazodone, which presumably accounts for its decreased risk for producing orthostatic hypotension. Relative to other new generation antidepressant drugs such as the SSRIs and venlafaxine, nefazodone appears less likely to produce sexual dysfunction or sleep disturbances. Nefazodone does not inhibit cytochrome P450 2D6 but can lead to clinically important drug interactions through its inhibition of cytochrome P450 3A4.

Venlafaxine

Venlafaxine is a phenethylamine that inhibits uptake of 5-HT and NE. Venlafaxine is devoid of affinity for brain muscarinic cholinergic, histaminergic, or adrenergic receptors, and appears to lack any propensity to produce arrhythmias or seizures. Its side-effect profile resembles that of the SSRIs, with nausea, dizziness, insomnia, dry mouth, and sexual dysfunction being the most common adverse effects. Less commonly, patients treated with venlafaxine may develop sustained diastolic blood pressure elevation, necessitating regular blood pressure monitoring during treatment. The incidence of this adverse effect is dependent upon dosage. Venlafaxine has a relatively low propensity for altering the metabolism of other drugs at usual clinical doses, but it may have dangerous interactions in combination with monoamine oxidase inhibitors.

Mirtazapine

Mirtazapine is a tetracyclic antidepressant in the piperazino-azepine group of compounds. Its structure is unrelated to the TCA, MAOI, or SSRI classes of antidepressants. Mirtazapine appears to act as a mixed antagonist with blockage of alpha-adrenergic receptors, histamine H2 receptors, and post-synaptic 5HT2 and 5HT3 serotonin receptors. Compared to placebo, the main side effects associated with mirtazapine are somnolence, increased appetite, and weight gain. The usual dose is between 15 mg and 45 mg per day, depending on weight and side effects. Mirtazapine can be used in conjunction with SSRIs or venlafaxine, or a switch can be made directly from an SSRI to mirtazapine without a tapering period. Because there can be serious interactions with MAOIs, it is usually recommended that there be a washout period of 10–14 days before switching between mirtazapine and an MAOI.

Mirtazapine has been shown in a variety of studies to be as effective as SSRIs in the treatment of hospitalized and outpatient depressed individuals, in the elderly, and in several ethnic groups. In several of these same studies, mirtazapine was demonstrated to have an earlier onset of action than SSRIs and to be associated with more weight gain (at least initially in the course of treatment). Several studies have documented efficacy of mirtazapine alone and in combination with an SSRI in treatment-refractory MDD.

Monoamine oxidase inhibitors

MAOIs inhibit the oxidative enzymes located within synaptic terminals that degrade monoamine neurotransmitters, resulting in increased concentrations of NE, 5-HT, and DA within the synaptic cleft. The clinical use of these agents has generally been limited to patients who are refractory to other antidepressant drugs because of their potentially life-threatening pharmacodynamic interactions with sympathomimetic drugs or tyramine-containing foods and beverages. The former include the sympathomimetic amines, phenylpropanolamine and pseudoephedrine. Sympathomimetic amines may be contained in some over-the-counter decongestant preparations. The use of MAOIs in the elderly is also limited by their more common cardiovascular effect, orthostatic hypotension.

The enzyme responsible for the metabolism of tyramine is MAO-A, and blockade of MAO-A is thus responsible for the production of acute hypertensive crisis following tyramine ingestion. The MAOIs previously available in the US were irreversible inhibitors of both MAO-A and MAO-B (i.e., phenelzine, isocarboxazid, tranylcypromine). While it was initially hoped that selegiline, a selective inhibitor of MAO-B, might not have this liability, selegiline loses its specificity for MAO-B in the doses required to achieve antidepressant effects.

More recently, reversible inhibitors of MAO (RIMAs; i.e., moclobemide, brofaromine) have been developed that may have a lower potential for dangerous interactions with tyramine. Moclobemide also appears to have better tolerability than either the irreversible inhibitors of MAO or the tertiary amine TCAs, amitriptyline or clomipramine. Thus the enhanced safety and tolerability of the RIMAs may expand usage of MAOI agents as they become more widely available.

There has been tremendous interest in the use of St John's Wort (which contains an MAOI) for the treatment of depression. Despite much public discussion, there is little data from well-controlled trials to support its use.

Selective norepinephrine reuptake inhibitors

Though no norepinephrine reuptake inhibitors have current approval for use in the treatment of depression in the US, several drugs that selectively block norepinephrine reuptake are in use for other indications, are available for use in other countries, or may receive approval in the US in the near future. Reboxetine is used as an antidepressant in Europe and a close related compound, duloxetine, may become available in the near future in the U.S. Currently, atomoxetine has been approved for use in the U.S. for the treatment of attention-deficit hyperactivity disorder (ADHD), but this drug is also likely to have antidepressant properties. The main side effects noted for atomoxetine in the treatment of ADHD are gastrointestinal distress and a general sense of nervousness. There is little literature to date demonstrating the relative efficacy of this class of drugs versus other antidepressants. However, this is likely to be an area of active research over the next few years.

Other somatic therapies for depression
Electroconvulsive therapy (ECT)
ECT remains the most effective treatment for major depressive episodes. The indications for ECT along with its safety, efficacy, and side effects, are discussed in Chapter 23. This treatment is often life saving for depressed patients who fail to respond to antidepressant drugs or who, because of suicidal intent or refusal to take in food or liquids, cannot safely wait the three weeks typically required for the onset of antidepressant drug efficacy. Following ECT, most patients require maintenance antidepressant pharmacotherapy to prevent relapse.

Phototherapy
Phototherapy is used in cases of MDD where a winter-seasonal pattern of depressive episodes is evident. This therapy involves daily exposure to ultraviolet light at wavelengths similar to sunlight, using phototherapy devices marketed for this indication. Data assessing dosage and long-term adverse effects are still accumulating. Recent findings suggest that oral ingestion of melatonin may have similar efficacy as phototherapy for winter-seasonal depression.

Exercise
A few recent studies suggest that regular exercise may hasten recovery from depression and help prevent relapse. This should be prescribed only as an adjunct to other treatment.

Management of bipolar disorder

General considerations
The recurrent nature of the bipolar disorders and the high morbidity and mortality associated with them make it imperative that patients with bipolar I or bipolar II disorder receive aggressive treatment. The treatment imperative for cyclothymic disorder is less clear. Although the depressive phases of these disorders can often be managed on an outpatient basis, full manic episodes or the presence of psychotic symptoms in manic or depressive phases are indications for hospitalization. With aggressive management approxi-

CONSIDER CONSULTATION FOR DEPRESSION WHEN ...

- Depressed patients develop:
  - serious suicidal ideation, intent or plans
  - delusions or hallucinations
  - mania
  - violent or threatening speech or behavior
  - malnutrition or dehydration resulting from reduced food or fluid intake
  - disability
  - noncompliance with treatments for other medical disorders.
- Depressed patients have failed to respond to two trials of antidepressant treatment, involving pharmacological agents from two distinct antidepressant drug classes, taken at adequate therapeutic doses for sufficient time periods (usually six weeks).
- The physician is uncomfortable with managing the symptoms, signs, or risks associated with the major depressive syndrome or with assessing the response or adverse effects of antidepressant treatment.

mately 85% of patients with bipolar disorder show marked improvement. The main impediments to successful treatment are recognition of the diagnosis by clinicians and compliance with medications by patients.

Mood stabilizing agents, such as lithium salts, valproate, or carbamazepine, constitute the mainstay of medical management for the bipolar disorders, particularly for maintenance treatment. During acute phases of either manic or depressive episodes, antipsychotic medications, minor tranquilizers, antidepressant medications, or electroconvulsive therapy may also be indicated. Initial treatment approaches for acute manic and depressive episodes and for maintenance therapy are outlined below. These have recently been described in detail by the American Psychiatric Association in the form of Practice Guidelines.

As with all serious psychiatric or behavioral disorders, medications should be part of a comprehensive treatment approach involving education, family therapy, and behavioral management. Management of severe manic episodes can pose difficult challenges. As described below, there is ample evidence for the rational choice of pharmacological agents to manage each of the phases of bipolar disorder. In contrast, few formal studies have addressed the application of specific social or psychotherapeutic interventions. Brief family therapy, which includes the goal of acceptance of the illness by the patient and their family, is usually helpful. Though there is no evidence that psychosocial factors cause bipolar disorder, stressful life events may influence the timing and severity of episodes. The identification of potential precipitating stress factors and the exploration of possible future stressors is a major goal of family-based intervention. This involves the family in plans to minimize future stresses and enhances their acceptance of the need for continued treatment following resolution of the acute episode. In the absence of appropriate pharmacological management, there is no evidence for the efficacy of individual or family psychotherapeutic interventions.

Classes of pharmacological agents for bipolar disorder

The main pharmacological intervention for acute manic and acute depressive episodes in bipolar I disorder and for depressive episodes in bipolar II disorder involves the use of the mood-stabilizing agents: lithium, valproate, and carbamazepine. More recently, studies have appeared supporting the use of the anticonvulsant lamotrigine.

Lithium

Lithium has been shown to be effective in the acute treatment of manic and depressive episodes and in the prevention of recurrence. Lithium may also decrease mood instability in general and can be useful in the treatment of cyclothymia and hypomania. It is available as the carbonate or the citrate salt and comes in tablet, capsule, or liquid form.

The correlation between oral dosage and serum lithium levels is variable across patients, but it is relatively stable within individuals. Peak serum levels occur 1–2 hours following ingestion, except for the slow release form, which reaches peak levels in 4–6 hours. Since both the therapeutic and the toxic effects of lithium correlate with serum levels, serum level monitoring is required. Steady-state levels are reached 5–7 days following initiation of therapy or change of dosage. Serum levels should be measured approximately 12 hours after the most recent dose (trough level).

Lithium is excreted principally by the kidneys and has a half-life between 14 and 30 hours. The clearance of lithium decreases with age in association with diminished glomerular function. Lithium levels can change with hydration, and episodes of dehydration may lead to toxic serum levels. Additionally, renal failure or sodium deficiency increases lithium serum levels. Thiazide diuretics increase lithium levels by 30–50%, and nonsteroidal anti-inflammatory agents or angiotensin converting enzyme-inhibiting antihypertensive agents may also increase serum levels.

The majority of patients taking lithium experiences side effects. Most are of little clinical significance or can be reduced by lowering the dosage. Dose-related side effects include polyuria, polydipsia, weight gain, poor concentration, tremor, sedation, and gastrointestinal disturbance. Patients may also experience hair loss, acne, and edema. Nausea, vomiting, and diarrhea can be managed by giving lithium with meals or using lithium citrate rather than carbonate. Polyuria and polydipsia can be moderated by the use of amelioride. A small proportion of patients may develop hypothyroidism following several months of lithium

treatment. Lithium-induced hypothyroidism can usually be reversed by administration of levothyroxine or discontinuation of lithium. Notably, patients who develop lithium-induced hypothyroidism are at increased risk of experiencing a depressive episode and possibly the onset of rapid cycling between manic and depressive episodes. A frequently debated topic is whether long-term lithium use results in irreversible kidney damage. Up to one-fifth of patients treated for more than ten years display morphological changes in the kidney on histological examination. However, these changes have not been related to the development of renal insufficiency or to changes in glomerular filtration rates. It is prudent to measure thyroid hormone and creatinine levels once or twice per year during lithium treatment.

The usual 12-hour post-dose therapeutic serum level of lithium is 0.8 to 1.2 meq per liter. Serum levels of 0.6 to 0.8 meq per liter may be adequate in some elderly patients and reduce the risk of central nervous system side effects in this age group. The daily dose necessary to achieve this trough level is variable across individuals but usually ranges between 900 mg and 1800 mg per day of lithium carbonate. This can be divided in two to three doses to decrease gastrointestinal side effects. However, many individuals are able to tolerate once-a-day dosing, usually administered at bedtime.

Toxic side effects are usually encountered at trough blood levels above 1.5 meq per liter. Early indicators of intoxication include nausea, vomiting, diarrhea, blurred vision, vertigo, confusion, and marked tremor of the extremities. If serum levels rise above 2.0 meq per liter, life-threatening adverse effects are more likely, including seizures, cardiac arrhythmias, or coma. For severe toxicity or overdosage, the only reliable method of rapidly removing excess lithium is dialysis. However, at lower levels of toxicity the patient may be treated with fluids, electrolyte management, and prevention of further gastrointestinal absorption.

The mechanism of action of lithium as a mood stabilizer is unclear. Lithium inhibits several enzymes in the inositol phosphate signaling pathway at therapeutic concentrations as well as decreases phosphorylation of receptor-related proteins. Part of the problem with determining the therapeutic mechanism of lithium is its effects on many cellular processes as well as the lack of meaningful animal models of mania.

Anticonvulsant therapy

Recently, certain anticonvulsants have become established as mood-stabilizing agents. They have proven particularly useful for patients who experience significant adverse effects with lithium or who have been poorly responsive to lithium. The two most widely studied agents are valproate and carbamazepine. Like lithium, the mechanism of action of the anticonvulsants in treating mania is unclear but may involve decreasing neuronal membrane excitability.

Valproate is available in capsule and liquid form, with the most commonly prescribed formulation for bipolar disorder being divalproex sodium. Although not as extensively studied as lithium, the therapeutic range for the treatment of either acute mania or maintenance therapy for mania is the same as or higher than that considered effective for epilepsy (50 to 125 μg/ml, with some patients requiring levels up to 150 μg/ml). Divalproex sodium is usually initiated at 750–1,000 mg daily in two or three divided doses, and the total daily dosage is then increased as tolerated to between 1,000 and 2,500 mg. Valproate is rapidly absorbed and peak serum levels are usually reached within two hours. The plasma half-life is 6–16 hours. Valproate is extensively metabolized by the liver and is highly protein bound in serum. Drug interactions may occur with other medications that are metabolized by the liver or are extensively protein bound. The common side effects of valproate include sedation and gastrointestinal distress, which usually resolve with dose adjustment or continued treatment. Valproate has rarely been associated with hepatotoxicity (which has been fatal in some children under the age of ten) and blood dyscrasias (i.e., thrombocytopenia), so baseline liver function and hematologic screening is indicated prior to initiating treatment, once during the first few weeks of treatment, and every 6–12 months during maintenance treatment.

Carbamazepine is available in a variety of forms. Treatment is generally aimed at achieving serum levels between 4 and 15 μg/ml. Maintenance doses range from 200 mg to 1600 mg per day and average about 1000 mg per day. Carbamazepine is principally metabolized by the liver and induces hepatic microsomal enzymes such that, with continued treatment, its half-life decreases from between 20 and 60 hours to between 5 and 25 hours. The total daily dosage and frequency of administration may thus require adjustments over time to maintain efficacy. Carbamazepine also has important drug interactions with drugs that inhibit microsomal enzyme induction or with drugs that are also metabolized by hepatic cytochrome P450 enzymes (e.g., 3A4). In addition, carbamazepine is highly protein bound and may interact with drugs that are extensively protein bound. Carbamazepine may produce neurological side effects such as ataxia and blurred vision. These are usually dose-limited and transient in nature, except in elderly patients, who are typically more sensitive to these effects. Most patients develop a mild asymptomatic leukopenia. Rarely, serious agranulocytosis, aplastic anemia, or hepatic failure may develop. During the first few months of treatment, frequent monitoring of complete blood counts, platelet counts, and liver function tests is recommended. During maintenance treatment the frequency of these laboratory analyses may be reduced to every 3–4 months.

Several other anticonvulsants have been used to treat bipolar disorder. Recently, lamotrigine has been found to be efficacious in two well-controlled trials. Like valproate and carbamazepine, this drug may work through a decrease in neuronal excitability mediated by prolonging the inactivation of sodium channels. The dosages range from 300 to 500 mg per day for acute bipolar depression. The drug is started at low doses and advanced cautiously over several weeks to potentially therapeutic doses in order to minimize the risk of an uncommon rash that is very rarely fatal. The risk of rash is increased with concomitant valproate administration. Otherwise, there are few reported side effects. Lamotrigine is also effective maintenance treatment, particularly for the depressed phase of the illness. The usefulness of other anticonvulsants in the management of bipolar disorder is uncertain; these anticonvulsants include topiramate, gabapentin, phenytoin, and the 10-keto analog of carbamazepine, oxcarbazepine.

Antipsychotic agents and benzodiazepines

Antipsychotic agents (e.g., haloperidol, thiothixene, trifluoperazine, clozapine, and risperidone) and benzodiazepine agonists (i.e., clonazepam and lorazepam) have been shown to be useful adjunctive treatments for acute mania. Antipsychotic agents are especially helpful when the manic or depressive phases are associated with psychotic features. Recently, the second-generation antipsychotics olanzapine, risperidone, and quetiapine have been shown to be effective in controlled trials; aripiprazole and ziprasidone have also shown promise. In the absence of psychotic symptoms, the benzodiazepines may be effective for reducing motor hyperactivity and agitation. The benzodiazepines offer sedation without the extrapyramidal side effects associated with the antipsychotic drugs (i.e., dystonia, dyskinesia, akathisia, or parkinsonian-like syndromes). However, chronic use of benzodiazepines may result in the development of tolerance and dependence.

Antidepressants

Although antidepressant medications have been well studied in the treatment of MDD, their use in the depressed phase of bipolar disorder is controversial. Antidepressants are more effective than placebo in treating bipolar depression, but there is little evidence that they are more effective than lithium or other mood-stabilizing agents. In addition, virtually all antidepressant agents have been reported to precipitate mania in some patients with bipolar disorder, and some studies have suggested that the use of antidepressants in patients during the depressed phase of bipolar disorder may increase the risk of developing rapid cycling or mixed bipolar states. Nevertheless, some patients with bipolar disorder require the combination of an antidepressant agent and a mood-stabilizing agent to alleviate or prevent depressive episodes. The dosing of antidepressant drugs in depressed patients with bipolar disorder is more complicated than in patients with unipolar depression, as some improve on relatively low dosages but become manic at modestly higher dosages. Generally, the treatment of patients with bipolar disorder with antidepressant drugs requires consultation with a specialist.

Electroconvulsive therapy

ECT is effective for both the depressed and the manic phases of bipolar disorder. ECT may be the treatment of choice for managing acute manic episodes when mood stabilizing agents or antidepressant drugs are contraindicated (e.g., in pregnancy or the presence of serious medical disorders). The usefulness of ECT for maintenance treatment of bipolar disorder has not been established.

ECT may have interactions with other antimanic treatments. The use of ECT in the presence of lithium therapy may result in confusional states. Consequently, lithium is usually discontinued prior to ECT. The use of the anticonvulsant mood stabilizers, valproate and carbamazepine, may decrease the efficacy of ECT by raising seizure threshold.

Treatment of acute mania

The initial treatment of an acute manic episode involves the use of antipsychotic agents, mood-stabilizing agents (e.g., lithium), or ECT. Antidepressant medications should be discontinued because they may worsen mania. It is imperative that an adequate serum level of a mood-stabilizing agent be achieved rapidly. Underlying medical conditions such as hypothyroidism should be identified and treated. Benzodiazepines may be used for severe agitation. If psychotic features are present, antipsychotic agents are usually indicated.

Acute treatment of depressive episodes

If a patient is not taking a mood-stabilizing agent such as lithium, one should be aggressively instituted. For patients who are receiving adequate dosages of mood-stabilizing agents, additional treatment with ECT or antidepressant drugs may be required (with or without specific psychotherapy). If the depressed phase includes psychotic features, adjunctive treatment with antipsychotic drugs is usually necessary.

Treatment of rapid cycling or mixed episodes

Most studies suggest that patients experiencing mixed episodes of manic and depressive symptoms should be treated as if they were manic. Antidepressant drugs should be avoided. Similarly, patients undergoing very rapid changes between depressed and manic states should be treated primarily with mood-stabilizing agents such as lithium, valproate, or ECT, but not with antidepressant drugs. Care should be taken to ensure that thyroid function is adequate and that other general medical disorders are identified and treated.

Prophylaxis or maintenance treatment

Overwhelming data suggest that prophylactic treatment of patients with bipolar disorder decreases the frequency and severity of subsequent manic and depressive episodes. The best-studied mood-stabilizing agent for long-term maintenance therapy is lithium. However, studies from patients being treated for both epilepsy and bipolar disorder suggest that valproate, carbamazepine, and lamotrigine are also effective maintenance treatments. A critical aspect of maintenance therapy is continued patient education and supportive psychotherapy. Education and supervision are also necessary to improve medication compliance. One of the most common reasons for recurrent mood episodes is patient-initiated discontinuation of medication following periods of improved health. Compliance appears particularly important in light of anecdotal evidence suggesting that patients who experience episodes after discontinuing lithium may be less responsive to reinstitution of lithium therapy. When maintenance therapy is terminated, discontinuation should be gradual to minimize the risk of relapse.

CONSIDER CONSULTATION FOR MANIA WHEN . . .

- The current manic episode is the patient's first.
- The patient is under 16 years of age.
- The manic episode occurred while the patient was receiving a therapeutic dose of lithium (e.g., as documented by serum levels).
- The patient develops:
  - suicidal ideation
  - delusions or hallucinations
  - violent or threatening speech or behavior
  - malnutrition or dehydration due to reduced food or fluid intake
  - disability
  - noncompliance with treatments for other medical disorders
  - catatonia
  - agitation inadequately controlled by current intervention.
- The physician is uncomfortable with managing the symptoms, signs, or risks associated with the manic syndrome (which can rapidly escalate) or with assessing the response or adverse effects of antimanic treatment.

Annotated bibliography

American Psychiatric Association (2000) Practice guideline for the treatment of patients with major depressive disorder (revision), *Am J Psychiatry* 157(Apr Suppl).

An overview of current viewpoints regarding the treatment in major depressive disorder.

American Psychiatric Association (2002) Practice guideline for the treatment of patients with bipolar disorder, *Am J Psychiatry* 159(Apr Suppl).

A succinct overview of the state-of-the-art in bipolar disorder treatment.

Davis, K, Charney, DS, Coyle, J, and Nemeroff, CB (eds) (2002) *Psychopharmacology: The Fifth Generation of Progress*, New York, Lippincott, Williams & Wilkins.

This text contains a current and comprehensive compendium of reviews of various aspects of the pharmacological management of mood disorders and the extant data regarding neuroendocrine, neurophysiological, and neurochemical studies in depression and mania.

Goodwin, FK and Jamison, KR (1990) *Manic-depressive Illness*, New York, Oxford University Press.

A comprehensive overview of the clinical presentation, natural history, epidemiology, and treatment of bipolar disorder.

Keck, PE Jr, Nelson, EB, and McElroy SL (2003) Advances in the pharmacologic treatment of bipolar depression, *Biol Psychiatry* 53(8):671–9.

A concise review of new advances in the treatment of the depressed phase of bipolar disorder emphasizing the efficacy of coadministration of antidepressants or atypical antipsychotics with a mood stabilizer.

Preskorn, SH (1999) *Outpatient Management of Depression: A Guide for the Primary-Care Practitioner*, 2nd Edition, Caddo, OK, Professional Communications, Inc.

A pocket-sized text that offers practical guidelines for primary care physicians in the diagnosis and pharmacological management of major depressive disorder. Dr Preskorn includes clinically relevant pharmacokinetic and pharmacodynamic information regarding the newer generation antidepressant agents.

CHAPTER 9

Anxiety Disorders

Laura J. Bierut, MD

Introduction

Anxiety disorders are among the most common psychiatric disturbances and affect up to one-sixth of the general population in a year. Though seldom life threatening, these disorders result in a tremendous amount of impairment and disability, potentially limiting an individual's social and occupational interactions. The sheer number of affected individuals results in an enormous cost to society. Given the frequency of anxiety disorders in the general population, primary care physicians often evaluate, diagnose, and treat patients presenting with these disorders. Direct nonpsychiatric medical treatment may account for over one half of the cost of patient care.

Anxiety, a feeling of fear and apprehension, may be a component of any psychiatric illness or may represent an independent anxiety disorder. Anxiety disorders are chronic illnesses, often remitting and relapsing, and patients are frequently afflicted with multiple different anxiety syndromes. Two factors significantly associated with these illnesses are female gender and lower socioeconomic status.

This chapter describes the diagnosis and management of three common anxiety disorders: panic disorder, phobias, and generalized anxiety disorder.

Panic disorder

Clinical features

The hallmark of panic disorder is panic attacks (see Table 9.1). These episodes of severe acute anxiety develop abruptly and reach their zenith within minutes. Numerous physical symptoms associated with autonomic nervous system arousal accompany these attacks, including a pounding heart, chest pain, shortness of breath, sweating, lightheadedness, and others (see Box 9.1). In addition, patients experience symptoms that can be considered as more psy-

chological such as a fear of losing control. Gradually, these physical and psychological symptoms subside and completely resolve within a short period of time, though some residual anxiousness can last for hours or days.

Many individuals are able to distinctly recall their first episode of panic. Initially, this can be triggered by an event, such as an intimidating social situation, a physically dangerous situation, or a loss of a loved one; subsequent panic attacks then can occur without any precipitant. For instance, many patients report being awakened from their sleep by panic attacks.

DIAGNOSIS

Table 9.1 Panic attacks

Discriminating feature

1 Discrete period of intense fear.

Consistent features

1 Pounding heart.
2 Sweating.
3 Chills or hot flashes.
4 Trembling.
5 Sensation of smothering.
6 Feeling of choking.
7 Chest pain.
8 Numbness.
9 Feeling faint.
10 Feelings of unreality or being detached.
11 Fear of losing control.
12 Fear of dying.
13 Nausea.

Variable features

1 May occur at any age.
2 Initial attacks can be triggered by an event, but subsequent attacks may have no precipitant.

Box 9.1 Panic attacks

DIAGNOSTIC CRITERIA

A discrete period of intense fear or discomfort, in which four (or more) of the following symptoms developed abruptly and reached a peak within ten minutes:

- palpitations, pounding heart, or accelerated heart rate
- sweating
- trembling or shaking
- sensations of shortness of breath or smothering
- feeling of choking
- chest pain or discomfort
- nausea or abdominal distress
- feeling dizzy, unsteady, lightheaded, or faint
- derealization (feelings of unreality) or
- depersonalization (being detached from oneself)
- fear of losing control or going crazy
- fear of dying
- paresthesias (numbness or tingling sensations)
- chills or hot flushes

Adapted from American Psychiatric Association (2000) Diagnostic and Statistical Manual of Mental Disorders, 4th Edition, Text Revision. Washington D.C., American Psychiatric Association.

Box 9.2 Panic disorder with/without agoraphobia

DIAGNOSTIC CRITERIA

A. Both (1) and (2):
1 Recurrent, unexpected panic attacks.
2 At least one of the attacks has been followed by one month (or more) of one (or more) of the following:
   (a) persistent concern about having additional attacks
   (b) worry about the implications of the attack or its consequences (e.g., losing control, having a heart attack, "going crazy")
   (c) a significant change in behavior related to the attacks.

B. The presence/absence of agoraphobia.

C. The panic attacks are not due to the direct physiological effects of a substance (e.g., a drug of abuse, a medication) or a general medical condition (e.g., hyperthyroidism).

D. The panic attacks are not better accounted for by another mental disorder such as social phobia (e.g., occurring on exposure to feared social situations), specific phobia (e.g., on exposure to a specific phobic situation), obsessive-compulsive disorder (e.g., on exposure to dirt in someone with an obsession about contamination), post-traumatic stress disorder (e.g., in response to stimuli associated with a severe stressor), or separation anxiety disorder (e.g., in response to being away from home or close relatives).

Adapted from American Psychiatric Association (2000) Diagnostic and Statistical Manual of Mental Disorders, 4th Edition, Text Revision. Washington, D.C., American Psychiatric Association.

Alone, panic attacks do not automatically lead to the diagnosis of panic disorder. A clustering of recurrent, unexpected panic attacks along with concern of future panic attacks, worry about the results of panic attacks, or a significant change in behavior must occur before the diagnosis of panic disorder is made (see Box 9.2 and Table 9.2).

Case 9.1 highlights the onset of panic disorder years after a first panic attack. Unfortunately, panic disorder can lead to further impairment. Recurrent panic attacks can cause anticipatory anxiety about future attacks, and as a result, an individual limits activities in an attempt to avoid potential attacks. This can lead to the development of agoraphobia, that is, a fear of situations from which escape might be difficult or in which help may not be available. Panic disorder is associated with agoraphobia in 25–50% of cases. Case 9.2 describes panic disorder with the subsequent development of agoraphobia.

Another common complication of panic disorder is depression. Panic disorder and major depression co-occur more often than expected by chance alone. Major depression occurs in 50–65% of individuals with a history of panic disorder. It is often difficult to determine whether the clinical presentation represents two individual disorders or one disorder causing the other. Nonetheless, when symptoms of major depression and panic occur, both illnesses should be diagnosed and treated appropriately.

Panic disorder and substance dependence also co-occur more often than expected. About one-third of individuals with panic disorder will suffer from substance abuse or substance dependence in their lifetime. Both disorders must be recognized and treated for successful results.

Table 9.2 Panic disorder

DIAGNOSIS

Discriminating feature

1 Recurrent, unexpected panic attacks.

Consistent features

1 Persistent concern about additional attacks.
2 Worry about the consequences of attacks.
3 Significant change in behaviour.

Variable features

1 Onset usually in late adolescence through mid-30s.
2 Waxing and waning lifelong course.
3 Often associated with major depression, substance misuse, and agoraphobia.
4 May cluster in families.

Ms A first had a panic attack in high school. Subsequently, she had an attack about once a year, but she had no associated worries and continued all her usual activities. While in her mid 20s, Ms A had another panic attack at a workplace meeting where she had to participate in a group discussion. Following this attack, she had several panic attacks per week with no precipitant. She grew anxious about having further attacks and began avoiding meetings at work. Fearful that she had heart problems, she visited her physician, and at that time she was diagnosed with panic disorder.

A 37-year-old single woman presented for treatment because "I've had panic attacks off and on for ten years . . . worse the past six months." The first panic attack occurred when she was driving. Her symptoms were initially evaluated in an emergency room and the diagnosis of panic attack was made. At that time, the patient responded to reassurance. For a year or so after the initial attack, the attacks occurred rarely while driving but unprovoked attacks began to happen more often at home and other places. The attacks appeared suddenly and peaked within 2–3 minutes with symptoms that included shortness of breath, feelings of choking, perspiring, dizziness, racing heart, "trembling," hot flashes, nausea, derealization, and fear of going crazy. Each attack lasted 15–30 minutes. The patient was also awakened at night by panic attacks—she thought the symptoms were indicative of early menopause. The attacks occurred three or more times a week.

The fear of having another attack was associated with disability—the patient restricted driving, only driving to work or to provide transportation for her son to school or other activities. Nevertheless, she had experienced panic attacks when another person drove. She avoided being in places from which escape was difficult—she was afraid of airplanes, tunnels, boats, and elevators. She went to the grocery store or to the mall only when she believed there would be few people around.

She denied any exacerbation of anxiety in social situations. She did not associate panic attacks with a specific phobia. Her mood was good, and she described an interest in activities that was frustrated by her fear of having a panic attack. She denied thoughts of death or suicide. She denied repetitive thoughts and repetitive behaviors to alleviate anxiety.

In DSM-IV-TR, there are two diagnoses for panic disorder: panic disorder without agoraphobia and panic disorder with agoraphobia. The patient described here was diagnosed with panic disorder with agoraphobia.

Suicide attempts have been identified as a complication of panic disorder independent from comorbid major depression and alcohol dependence. In a general community survey, 20% of subjects with panic disorder had made a suicide attempt. Other work suggests that males with panic disorder, but not females, are at increased risk of sudden cardiovascular death. Thus, panic disorder may have a lethal outcome.

Panic disorder has a variable long-term course. In follow-up studies of individuals treated for panic disorder, 30% were well, 40–50% were improved, and 20–30% were the same or had worsening of symptoms. Overall, panic disorder remains a lifelong illness with a waxing and waning course.

Differential diagnosis

Panic attacks are a common feature of many psychiatric disturbances including major depression, substance intoxication (e.g., stimulants), substance withdrawal (e.g., alcohol), psychosis, and other anxiety disorders. In the initial evaluation of panic attacks, the physician should look for the presence of other psychiatric illnesses and, if found, determine whether the disorder is causative of the panic attacks or, alternatively, comorbid with panic disorder.

Medical causes for panic attacks including hyperthyroidism and pregnancy must be ruled out. In medically ill patients, an evaluation of panic attacks and panic disorders can be difficult since many disorders may contribute to anxiety symptoms. In these patients, a review of anxiety symptoms focusing on the first time symptoms occurred is helpful. Since panic disorder is a lifelong illness with an onset generally before the age of 40 years, a history of previous panic attacks starting at a young age is crucial in making a diagnosis of panic disorder.

Case 9.3 highlights the evaluation of panic disorder in a medically ill man.

The key feature in the diagnosis of panic disorder is unexpected, untriggered panic attacks with subsequent development of anxiety. Panic attacks are differentiated from phobias by the absence of a triggering factor for panic attacks. Panic disorder differs from generalized anxiety disorders by the discrete episodes of panic.

Family history

There is a striking clustering of panic disorder within families. Family members of an individual with panic disorder are at 3–8 times greater risk of developing panic disorder compared with the general population. Twin studies also support a genetic component to panic disorder with monozygotic twins more often afflicted than dizygotic twins given a co-twin with panic disorder.

Mr J is a 56-year-old man with a history of hypertension, diabetes, and coronary artery disease who presents with chest pain and tachycardia. Over the past four months, Mr J has had four emergency room visits for similar complaints. Other than a mildly elevated blood pressure, his physical exam is unremarkable. Blood glucose is adequately controlled and electrocardiogram shows no significant changes. Since these episodes have recurred over a short period of time, further history of these episodes is obtained.

Mr J reports that these episodes come out of the blue. On further probing, it becomes clear that Mr J had similar episodes beginning in his 20s and occurring a few times a year, but he sought no medical treatment at that time. Be-

cause he now has medical problems, he assumes he is having a heart attack when he has these symptoms. Given this history, panic disorder is strongly suspected.

Since it is impossible to accurately apportion the cause of these symptoms to each illness, a multi-pronged approach is taken to optimize the management of each illness. Mr J's blood pressure is closely monitored for several weeks and pharmacological control is optimized. Similarly, glucose is monitored to avoid hypoglycemic episodes. At the same time, treatment for panic disorder is initiated. Over the next several months, Mr J stabilizes and has only rare episodes of tachycardia and chest pain.

Epidemiology

Panic disorder is a relatively common disorder with a 2.2% one-year prevalence and 3.4% lifetime prevalence in the general population. Women are 2–3 times more likely to be affected than men. The onset of panic disorder typically occurs in the age range from adolescence till the mid 30s.

Treatment

There are three major treatment approaches to panic disorder: pharmacological management, cognitive behavioral therapy, and a combination of both. The responses to pharmacotherapy and cognitive behavioral therapy are similar, and combination therapy has a somewhat superior response. Patient choice and availability of therapy direct treatment.

Long-term pharmacological management focuses on treatment with antidepressant medications: selective serotonin reuptake inhibitors (SSRIs), tricyclic antidepressants, monoamine oxidase inhibitors (MAO inhibitors), and unique antidepressant classes. Antidepressant medications have

been shown to be effective in reducing the occurrence of panic attacks. Treatment requires several weeks to become effective at a full antidepressant dose and is recommended to continue for at least 12 months. Many patients will require long-term treatment and indefinite maintenance on antidepressant medications is recommended. High potency benzodiazepines are also effective in the treatment of panic disorder. Relief is more immediate, however, long-term use with benzodiazepines can lead to tolerance and dependence. Recent trials of anticonvulsants involving medications such as gabapentin and related drugs may have demonstrated a role for these compounds in the management of panic disorder.

Brief cognitive behavioral therapy is useful in the treatment of panic disorder, and referral to a therapist trained in cognitive behavioral therapy can be effective. The cognitive aspect includes the re-framing of thoughts, so that the patient no longer immediately assumes that he or she will die when autonomic nervous system symptoms begin. Behavioral treatment includes relaxation techniques. Case 9.4 describes the co-occurrence of panic disorder and major depression.

Ms S is a 35-year-old woman who presents to her family physician complaining of headaches and stress. She reports that she has been stressed over the past four months but is unable to give any specific precipitants to this stress. She sometimes develops an abrupt fear that she will die. She also has sweating, hot flashes, palpitations, and light-headedness. These episodes last approximately 20 minutes and then completely resolve. She is now worried that something terrible is wrong with her, so she is limiting her activities.

Ms S denies any alcohol or substance use; however, she endorses low mood over the last several years. She describes crying spells, decreased energy, poor concentration, and feelings of guilt. She has trouble falling asleep. There has been no

weight change, no psychotic symptoms, and no thoughts of hurting herself.

Ms S has both panic disorder and major depression. In an attempt to treat both groups of symptoms, her physician prescribes an antidepressant medication, fluoxetine, 20 mg daily. When the patient experiences a worsening of her anxiety with the first dose, the medication is restarted at a lower dose (10 mg every other day) and then gradually increased to 20 mg a day. Over several weeks, the patient experiences a gradual reduction in both depressive symptoms and panic attacks. She remains symptom free for several months, and she and her physician decide to continue long-term treatment.

Panic disorder

Onset: usually late adolescence till mid 30s.

Course: waxing and waning lifelong illness.

Lifetime prevalence: 3.4% (2–3 times more women than men affected).

Familial disease: risk in first-degree relatives 3–8 times greater than general population.

Comorbidity: often associated with major depression, substance misuse, and agoraphobia.

Treatment

Pharmacologic: selective serotonin reuptake inhibitors, tricyclic antidepressants, monoamine oxidase inhibitors, and benzodiazepines. Newer agents, such as gabapentin and related compounds, may also be efficacious.

Psychotherapy: cognitive behavioral therapy.

Phobias

Clinical features

A phobia is an excessive fear surrounding a specific event or object (see Table 9.3). This event or object almost invariably provokes an immediate anxiety response even though the individual recognizes that the fear is unreasonable. As a result of this excessive fear, affected individuals avoid situations and limit activities. Phobic disorders have been divided into three major categories: specific phobia, social phobia, and agoraphobia.

Table 9.3 Phobias

Discriminating feature

1 Marked, unreasonable fear cued by a specific object or situation.

Consistent features

1 Exposure to the stimulus almost invariably provokes anxiety.
2 The phobic situation or object is either avoided or endured with intense anxiety.
3 There is impairment in occupational or social functioning.

Variable features

1 Onset usually in childhood through early adulthood.
2 Childhood fears may be transient.
3 Adolescent and adulthood fears persist lifelong.
4 Commonly associated with major depression and substance misuse.
5 May cluster in families.

Specific phobias

Specific phobias are fears targeted at a specific object or situation, for instance a fear of heights or a fear of specific animals (see Box 9.3). Specific phobias occurring in childhood are often transitory and not clinically significant. However, phobias that persist into adulthood seldom remit. An isolated fear may not significantly affect an individual's lifestyle, but a specific phobia can cause significant impairment in job performance or social relationships depending on the phobic stimulus and a person's daily responsibilities.

Box 9.3 Specific phobia

A. Marked and persistent fear that is excessive or unreasonable, cued by the presence or anticipation of a specific object or situation (e.g., flying, heights, animals, receiving an injection, seeing blood).
B. Exposure to the phobic stimulus almost invariably provokes an immediate anxiety response, which may take the form of a situationally bound or situationally predisposed panic attack. Note: in children, the anxiety may be expressed by crying, tantrums, freezing, or clinging.
C. The person recognizes that the fear is excessive or unreasonable. Note: in children, this feature may be absent.
D. The phobic situation(s) is avoided or else is endured with intense anxiety or distress.
E. The avoidance, anxious anticipation, or distress in the feared situation(s) interferes significantly with the person's normal routine, occupational (or academic) functioning, or social activities or relationships, or there is marked distress about having the phobia.
F. In individuals under age 18 years, the duration is at least six months.
G. The anxiety, panic attacks, or phobic avoidance associated with the specific object or situation are not better accounted for by another mental disorder, such as obsessive-compulsive disorder (e.g., fear of dirt in someone with an obsession about contamination), post-traumatic stress disorder (e.g., avoidance of stimuli associated with a severe stressor), separation anxiety disorder (e.g., avoidance of school), social phobia (e.g., avoidance of social situations because of fear of embarrassment), panic disorder with agoraphobia, or agoraphobia without history of panic disorder.

Adapted from American Psychiatric Association (2000) Diagnostic and Statistical Manual of Mental Disorders, 4th Edition, Text Revision. Washington, D.C., American Psychiatric Association.

Social phobia

Social phobia is a fear caused by social situations (see Box 9.4). These fears include a fear of eating in public, speaking in public, or embarrassing oneself in some way. Social phobia is the most common type of phobia and can be extremely impairing because it impinges upon relationships and social interactions. Unfortunately, social phobias often are unrecognized by physicians and go untreated. Case 9.5 illustrates

---

Box 9.4 Social phobia

A. A marked and persistent fear of one or more social or performance situations in which the person is exposed to unfamiliar people or to possible scrutiny by others. The individual fears that he or she will act in a way (or show anxiety symptoms) that will be humiliating or embarrassing. Note: in children, there must be evidence of the capacity for age-appropriate social relationships with familiar people and the anxiety must occur in peer settings, not just in interactions with adults.

B. Exposure to the feared social situation almost invariably provokes anxiety, which may take the form of a situationally bound or situationally predisposed panic attack. Note: in children, the anxiety may be expressed by crying, tantrums, freezing, or shrinking from social situations with unfamiliar people.

C. The person recognizes that the fear is excessive or unreasonable. Note: in children, this feature may be absent.

D. The feared social or performance situations are avoided or else are endured with intense anxiety or distress.

E. The avoidance, anxious anticipation, or distress in the feared social or performance situation(s) interferes significantly with the person's normal routine, occupational (academic) functioning, or social activities or relationships, or there is marked distress about having the phobia.

F. In individuals under age 18 years, the duration is at least six months.

G. The fear or avoidance is not due to the direct physiological effects of a substance (e.g., a drug of abuse, a medication) or a general medical condition and is not better accounted for by another mental disorder (e.g., panic disorder with or without agoraphobia, separation anxiety disorder, body dysmorphic disorder, a pervasive developmental disorder, or schizoid personality disorder).

H. If a general medical condition or another mental disorder is present, the fear in Criterion A is unrelated to it, e.g., the fear is not of stuttering, trembling in Parkinson's disease, or exhibiting abnormal eating behavior in anorexia nervosa or bulimia nervosa.

From American Psychiatric Association (2000) Diagnostic and Statistical Manual of Mental Disorders, 4th Edition, Text Revision. Washington, D.C., American Psychiatric Association.

---

a case of social phobia with a significant restriction of social activities.

Agoraphobia

Agoraphobia is the fear of being in a situation from which escape might be difficult or in which help might not be available. Although agoraphobia has been linked historically with panic disorder and has generally been considered a complication of panic disorder, epidemiological surveys demonstrate the existence of agoraphobia without panic disorder. Agoraphobia causes impairment since individuals do not attempt activities or require a companion for activities. Agoraphobia often develops after the onset of social phobia and further limits an individual's social functioning.

Phobias are often associated with comorbid psychiatric illness, primarily major depression, substance dependence, and other anxiety disorders. The lifetime prevalence of major depression is about 20% in individuals with phobias. Substance abuse or dependence complicates about a quarter of phobic disorder cases. Phobias are also often associated with panic attacks and generalized anxiety disorder.

Differential diagnosis

Patients are often able to clearly describe phobias when asked. The symptoms of the phobia can be consistent with a panic attack, but the episodes are always triggered by the phobic stimulus as opposed to the untriggered panic attacks experienced in panic disorder. Since comorbid illnesses are often associated with phobias, disorders such as major depression and substance abuse should be evaluated.

Family history

The rates of phobic disorders in families are less well studied than for many other psychiatric disorders. Family studies demonstrate a familial aggregation with up to a three-fold risk to relatives. Twin studies have shown evidence of a genetic predisposition to phobias.

Epidemiology

Phobic disorders are common in the general population. A recent epidemiological survey estimated the following one-year and lifetime prevalences, respectively: specific phobia—5.5% and 11.3%; social phobia—4.5% and 13.3%; and agoraphobia—2.3% and 6.7%. Women are affected 1.5–2 times more often than men. The onset of phobias occurs in childhood to early adulthood, and the natural history for phobias that persist into adulthood is a chronic and lifelong course.

Treatment

Treatment for phobias includes both pharmacological and

Mr M had the onset of social phobia in high school. He became anxious whenever he had to speak with someone new. Although he had excellent grades, he chose not to attend college; instead he began working at a loading dock. He was able to function adequately in this job since he had little contact with new people. At the age of 40, he still lived at home and had few friends. The friends he did have dated back to childhood.

Ms D is a 40-year-old executive with a severe phobia about flying. She avoids flying whenever possible. When a family reunion was planned several thousand miles from her home, she was confronted with either flying or not attending. She discussed this situation with her physician who prescribed alprazolam 1 mg to be taken before each flight. Though she did experience some anxiety, she was able to tolerate the flight and enjoy her family reunion.

psychotherapeutic interventions, alone or in combination, and the approach is often based upon the chronicity and intensity of the phobia. For instance, an isolated phobia that does not impinge on an individual's everyday life may require only episodic treatment with no long-term management necessary. On the other hand, if the phobic disorder is causing frequent distress, a long-term treatment approach should be considered. Case 9.6 describes treatment of a fear of flying associated with mild impairment.

The pharmacologic management of phobias, in particular social phobia, focuses on treatment with selective serotonin reuptake inhibitors. Treatment is recommended to continue for several months in order to obtain full response and maximize remission. In general, long-term treatment is indicated for 12 months or more to sustain remission. Lifelong treatment should be considered in cases with a long history of significant impairment. Though selective serotonin reuptake inhibitors are considered the first-line choice in the pharmacologic treatment of social phobias, additional agents, such as gabapentin and related compounds, are under study and may be efficacious. Psychotherapeutic approaches rely primarily on behavioral therapy as a long-term treatment approach. A patient is exposed to the feared stimulus, either through imagery or actual exposure, until the associated anxiety diminishes.

Generalized anxiety disorder

Clinical features

Generalized anxiety disorder (GAD) is another common disorder in the family of anxiety disorders. As opposed to panic disorder and phobias that are characterized by discrete episodes of anxiety, GAD is associated with chronic, continuous, low-grade anxiety (see Table 9.4). Symptoms of GAD are out of proportion to the situation and cause clinical distress (see Box 9.5). GAD co-occurs with several other psychiatric illnesses, including major depression, substance abuse or dependence, and other anxiety disorders. Case 9.7 describes GAD complicated by asthma.

Phobia

- Onset: childhood till early adulthood.
- Course: chronic.
- Lifetime prevalence: specific phobia 11.3%; social phobia 13.3%; and agoraphobia without panic disorder 6.7%.
- Familial disease: some familial clustering.
- Comorbidity: often associated with major depression, substance misuse.

Treatment

- Pharmacologic: selective serotonin reuptake inhibitors. (Monamine oxidase inhibitors, benzodiazepines, and beta-blockers may be considered in some cases.) Newer agents, such as gabapentin and related compounds, may also be efficacious.
- Psychotherapy: behavioral therapy.

Table 9.4 Generalized anxiety disorder

Discriminating feature

1 Excessive anxiety and worry.

Consistent features

1 Feeling keyed up.
2 Feeling easily fatigued.
3 Difficulty concentrating.
4 Irritability.
5 Muscle tension.
6 Sleep disturbance.
7 Impaired occupational or social functioning.

Variable features

1 Onset often in childhood or adolescence.
2 Often a chronic lifelong course.
3 Often associated with major depression and substance misuse.
4 May cluster in families.

Box 9.5 Generalized anxiety disorder

A. Excessive anxiety and worry (apprehensive expectation), occurring more days than not for at least six months, about a number of events or activities (such as work or school performance).
B. The person finds it difficult to control the worry.
C. The anxiety and worry are associated with three (or more) of the following six symptoms (with at least some symptoms present for more days than not for the past six months. **Note**: only one item is required for children).
   1 restlessness or feeling keyed up or on edge
   2 being easily fatigued
   3 difficulty concentrating or mind going blank
   4 irritability
   5 muscle tension
   6 sleep disturbance (difficulty falling or staying asleep, or restless unsatisfying sleep).
D. The focus of the anxiety and worry is not confined to features of an Axis I disorder; e.g., the anxiety or worry is not about having a panic attack (as in panic disorder), being embarrassed in public (as in social phobia), being contaminated (as in obsessive-compulsive disorder), being away from home or close relatives (as in separation anxiety disorder), gaining weight (as in anorexia nervosa), having multiple physical complaints (as in somatization disorder), or having a serious illness (as in hypochondriasis), and the anxiety and worry do not occur exclusively during post-traumatic stress disorder.
E. The anxiety, worry, or physical symptoms cause clinically significant distress or impairment on social, occupational, or other important areas of functioning.
F. The disturbance is not due to the direct physiological effects of a substance (e.g., a drug of abuse, a medication) or a general medical condition (e.g., hyperthyroidism) and does not occur exclusively during a mood disorder, a psychotic disorder, or a pervasive developmental disorder.

From American Psychiatric Association (2000) Diagnostic and Statistical Manual of Mental Disorders, 4th Edition, Text Revision. Washington, D.C., American Psychiatric Association.

Differential diagnosis

Symptoms of GAD are very general and may fit into other disorders, such as major depression. GAD often has an insidious onset and an indolent course. After screening for the presence of medical disorders, major depression, substance dependence, or other anxiety disorders as a cause of the symptoms, the diagnosis of GAD is made. Case 9.8 describes GAD.

Family history

Family and twin studies support familial transmission in the development of GAD with evidence of a partial genetic predisposition.

Epidemiology

The one-year and lifetime prevalences of GAD are 3.1% and 5.1%, respectively. Women are affected almost twice as often as men. The onset of GAD occurs at a young age, and many patients describe being anxious their whole lives. The course of illness is continuous and chronic.

Treatment

As in other anxiety disorders, standard treatment for GAD includes antidepressant medications (selective serotonin reuptake inhibitors and others) and benzodiazepines. In addition, buspirone, a unique anxiolytic agent, is effective in GAD. Again, long-term treatment must be considered given the chronicity of GAD and the high rate of relapse. Since GAD is a chronic illness, psychotherapy is often recommended.

Pathophysiology of anxiety disorders

An understanding of the biologic basis of anxiety is unfolding with pharmacological, animal, and imaging studies. Panic attacks can be reproduced pharmacologically. Infusions of sodium lactate or respiration of 5% carbon dioxide

---

CASE 9.7

Ms C is a 50-year-old obese woman with asthma requiring treatment with theophylline and inhalers. She presents with anxiety, which she describes as impinging on her relationships. Ms C describes herself as a lifelong "worrier." She is on edge all the time, easily fatigued, and irritable. She denies symptoms of major depression, and there is no evidence of substance abuse.

Her anxiety symptoms are attributed initially to her obesity, asthma, and medications. An attempt to manage her asthma without theophylline is unsuccessful. Although theophylline appears to be contributing to her anxiety, Ms C has a history of anxiety independent from the medication. Thus, it is decided to treat the anxiety symptoms as part of a GAD complex complicated by medical problems and medications.

Ms C is treated with diazepam 5 mg three times daily with some symptomatic relief. The symptoms of worrying and irritability are diminished, but the fatigue continues. Ms C considers this a significant improvement.

A 34-year-old married woman presents with a chief complaint of "Worry . . . past 17 to 18 years." The worry is present most days and the patient recognizes that her worry is excessive. She worries about finances, her marriage, her job, and her future. She tries to control the worry with constant activity, largely involving her job as a health care provider. The patient relates her excessive worry to an inability to make career decisions: "my life is on hold."

She endorses feeling restless and tense with increased irritability and difficulty sleeping. The tension is associated with shoulder and upper back pain for which the patient has sought medical consultation and finds over-the-counter analgesics ineffective. Other anxiety symptoms include excessive perspiration, queasiness, intermittent constipation, and a dry mouth. She denies ever experiencing panic attacks, and social situations do not elicit a worsening of worry or anxiety.

The clinician is not able to elicit a disabling specific phobia. The patient reports good mood and a loss of interest in activities like going to movies, but she indicates that she enjoys her work and sexual relations and relates the decreased interest to excessive worry. She denies fatigue, feelings of worthlessness or guilt, and problems with concentration. She denies thoughts of death, thoughts of suicide, and thoughts of homicide. Although her work exposes her to unfortunate events, including the death of patients that she cares for and the counseling of grieving families, she takes pride in her ability to provide appropriate care and denies ever having been exposed to extreme trauma or feeling threatened by death. She denies drinking alcohol or taking any illicit drugs. By her description, she has been happily married for 12 years. Her children are doing well in school, although she worries about them.

Physical exam is unremarkable. Mental status examination reveals a patient carefully dressed in attire typical of her profession who has a furrowed brow and either sits on the edge of the chair or, at times, moves around restlessly in the chair. Speech and flow of thought are unremarkable, although she becomes irritable as the examination progresses. She is not psychotic. The patient is oriented with a superior fund of knowledge. Insight into illness is adequate—she understands that her worry is excessive—and she has the judgment to seek treatment.

Laboratory studies, including a urine drug screen, do not reveal any new findings. She is given a diagnosis of generalized anxiety disorder.

Generalized anxiety disorder

Onset: over half of cases begin in childhood or adolescence.

Course: chronic.

Lifetime prevalence: 5.1% (twice as many women as men are affected).

Familial disease: some familial clustering.

Comorbidity: often associated with major depression or substance misuse.

Treatment

Selective serotonin reuptake inhibitors, tricyclic antidepressants, benzodiazepines, and buspirone.

---

mixtures cause panic attacks in individuals with panic disorder, whereas control subjects without panic disorder are unaffected. This susceptibility to pharmacologically induced panic attacks has led to a "false suffocation alarm" theory of panic disorder that proposes a brainstem hypersensitivity to carbon dioxide. Similarly, benzodiazepine receptors, which are linked to gamma-aminobutyric acid (GABA) and are extensively distributed throughout the brain, are hypothesized to be key in the etiology of anxiety. Since benzodiazepines can block anxiety, these receptors may be fundamentally involved in the genesis of anxiety.

Animal studies have implicated other areas of the brain that may cause anxiety. The locus ceruleus, which contains more than 50% of all noradrenergic neurons, has extensive projections throughout the brain. Stimulation of this center in animals produces a fear and anxiety response, whereas ablation of this center reduces anxiety responses.

Finally, imaging studies may provide a functional understanding of anxiety disorders. Imaging techniques, such as positron emission tomography (PET), can demonstrate areas of activation in anxiety states. In combination with pharmacological and animal studies, an integrated understanding of the physiology of anxiety in humans is developing.

Special issues

Anxiety disorders in primary care

Treatment begins with diagnosis (see *Key clinical questions and what they unlock*). Because one-sixth of the population suffers from anxiety disorders, primary care physicians care for the majority of these cases. Patients can present to their primary care physician or to emergency rooms with anxiety masquerading as various physical complaints, such as chest pain or gastrointestinal distress. An awareness of the high prevalence of anxiety disorders aids in its recognition.

Anxiety disorders are diagnosed by clinical history. Thus, the signs and symptoms of anxiety disorders should be elicited from patients with a focus on the onset of the symptoms and the triggering events. At the same time, screening for other medical and psychiatric disorders is necessary. Specifically, the presence of major depression and substance misuse should be evaluated.

KEY CLINICAL QUESTIONS AND WHAT THEY UNLOCK

- *Are there discrete episodes of anxiety or is the patient troubled by chronic worry in the absence of anxiety attacks?*
  Panic attacks and chronic worry are associated with many types of psychiatric disorders, but chronic worry in the absence of panic attacks suggests consideration of generalized anxiety disorder (GAD).

- *Do the panic attacks occur in response to a specific trigger or do they appear unexpectedly?*
  Panic disorder is associated with the absence of an environmental cue, even if initial attacks are sometimes associated with a specific circumstance or circumstances. Specific phobias can elicit an anxiety attack when exposure to the phobia occurs even when the "exposure" is subtle—a person with a phobia of flying can, for example, have a panic attack when asked about purchasing airline tickets. The anxiety attacks associated with social phobia are disabling in a social context such as public speaking or eating a meal in a restaurant.

- *Are the anxiety attacks associated with a sufficient number of symptoms to meet criteria for major depression?*
  Identification of a depressive syndrome increases the risk of an adverse outcome such as suicide and biases treatment towards antidepressant medications (SSRIs, tricyclic antidepressants, MAOIs) that have antipanic effects and away from benzodiazepines.

- *Does excessive use of alcohol or use of illicit drugs complicate the clinical picture?*
  Self-medication with alcohol complicates the administration of benzodiazepines due to overlapping side effects (e.g., memory problems). In addition, alcohol withdrawal and stimulant (e.g., cocaine, amphetamines) intoxication are associated with anxiety symptoms, including panic attacks.

- *What is disabling about the symptoms of anxiety?*
  Defining the types of dysfunction—problems performing work, for example—helps justify treatment beyond patient education and reassurance, enhances the evaluation of interventions, and facilitates decisions about referral.

The diagnosis of anxiety disorder and comorbid conditions lead treatment decisions. Antidepressants can be used to treat anxiety disorders and concomitant major depression. Comorbid substance dependence also points to treatment with antidepressants, because there is abuse potential with benzodiazepine treatment. Psychotherapy is an effective option that will appeal to some patients. The two major tools in the pharmacotherapeutic arsenal readily employed by primary care physicians to treat anxiety are antidepressants and benzodiazepines. Antidepressants are effective anxiolytics; they have evidence of long-term efficacy with no abuse potential. However, it often takes several weeks before there is clinical evidence of a response, and side effects are often troublesome. Benzodiazepines are effective quickly, but they do not adequately treat an accompanying depression and they have the potential for abuse.

Selective serotonin reuptake inhibitors (SSRIs) (citalopram, fluoxetine, fluvoxamine, sertraline, and paroxetine) have been shown to be effective in the treatment of some anxiety disorders. Though some SSRIs have received approval from the Federal Drug Administration (FDA) for the treatment of specific anxiety disorders, it is likely that all SSRIs have similar effectiveness. The effective dosage appears to be in the standard antidepressant range. The advantage of SSRIs is that the side-effect profile is generally mild and well tolerated by patients. Also, it is difficult to successfully suicide by overdose. Disadvantages of SSRIs include an increase in anxiety in the initial phase of treatment. Starting at the lowest possible dosage and gradually increasing can minimize this. Long-term treatment is often well tolerated.

Tricyclic antidepressants (imipramine, amitriptyline, desipramine, nortriptyline, and others) have been extensively studied. Although imipramine is the most commonly studied of this group, all tricyclics are likely to be equally effective. These antidepressants should be prescribed at the same doses used to treat major depression, for example, imipramine 150 mg per day or nortriptyline 75 mg per day. The advantage of the tricyclic antidepressants is that they have been most extensively studied and have been consistently effective. A common side effect is sedation, which may be beneficial for an anxious patient. The major disadvantage of this class of medication is the side-effect profile. They have strong anticholinergic side effects, such as dry mouth, blurred vision, and constipation, along with orthostatic hypotension. These side effects can be minimized by choosing a secondary amine tricyclic (desipramine or nortriptyline), but these side effects can still limit the effective dose. Also, the tricyclic antidepressants are potentially lethal in overdose. As a result, tricyclic antidepressants are not a first-line treatment choice.

Monoamine oxidase inhibitors (isocarboxazid, phenelzine, and tranylcypromine) are a second classic treatment for many anxiety disorders. Optimal doses again are in the therapeutic range for an antidepressant effect. The advantage of this group is its consistent efficacy in numerous clinical trials. A major disadvantage is that the patient must adhere to a strict tyramine-free diet (elimination of cheeses, aged meats, wines, and other foods) because hypertensive crises can occur with ingestion of tyramine or an over-the-counter sympathomimetic such as pseudoephedrine. Because the MAO inhibitors are irreversible inhibitors, several weeks must pass before this enzyme system returns to functioning. Potential for lethal overdose is present. Given these disadvantages, MAO inhibitors are used only in refractory cases.

High potency benzodiazepines (alprazolam and clonazepam), along with many of the other benzodiazepines, are

PEARLS & PERILS

A clinical approach to anxiety in primary care

Prevalence:
- one-sixth of the population suffers from an anxiety disorder.

Diagnosis:
- diagnosis is made by clinical history. An awareness of the high prevalence of these disorders aids in recognition. An assessment for the presence of comorbid major depression and substance misuse is necessary.

Treatment:
- Pharmacologic: antidepressants and benzodiazepines are the two major classes of medications used for the treatment of anxiety.

Antidepressants:
- Advantages: antidepressants can treat comorbid depression and there is no abuse potential.
- Disadvantages: several weeks of treatment with antidepressants are required before there is an anxiolytic effect. Some antidepressants are lethal in overdose. There are often more side effects with antidepressants than with benzodiazepines.

Benzodiazepines:
- Advantages: benzodiazepines provide immediate relief from anxiety.
- Disadvantages: benzodiazepines do not adequately treat comorbid major depression. Benzodiazepines may be misused.

CONSIDER CONSULTATION WHEN...

- Anxiety disorder is complicated by comorbid substance misuse, major depression, or other psychiatric disorders.
- Anxiety disorder is associated with a concurrent medical illness, particularly if the medical illness has overlapping symptoms (for example, asthma, diabetes, atrial fibrillation).
- The diagnosis is uncertain because the patient does not appear to meet criteria for a specific disorder.
- A trial of psychotherapy is desired.
- The patient has not responded to treatment.

1 Reassess diagnosis: with increased information from follow-up care, a reassessment of the initial diagnosis of an anxiety disorder is necessary. A medical or other psychiatric disorder may have become evident and better explain the clinical picture. The presence of an untreated comorbid condition such as substance dependence, major depression, or medical illness leads to treatment-resistant anxiety.

2 Reassess treatment: treatment failures are often the result of patient non-compliance, insufficient dose, and time-limited drug trials. Medications are not effective if not taken. Patients with anxiety disorders are often sensitive to side effects of medications and so discontinue the drug. Starting at the lowest possible dosage and gradually increasing the dose may minimize this. A common mistake with the treatment of anxiety is prescribing inadequate dosages of medications, particularly antidepressant medications. The anxiolytic dose for antidepressant medications is in the same range as for the antidepressant effect, and treatment must continue at this level for at least six weeks before considering it a treatment failure.

3 Consider referral: if a patient is not responding and a reassessment of diagnosis and treatment does not lead to a reason for treatment resistance, consider referral to a therapist for psychotherapy or a psychiatrist for further evaluation and treatment.

effective in the treatment of anxiety syndromes. The response to treatment is rapid, and patients feel almost immediate relief. However, these medications have abuse potential, which is a significant concern in patients with comorbid substance dependence. Depression, which is a frequent comorbid condition, is not adequately treated with benzodiazepines alone.

Other medications used to treat specific anxiety syndromes include buspirone and beta-blockers. Buspirone is a specific anxiolytic agent that does not have abuse potential. Similar to the antidepressants, buspirone requires several weeks at a therapeutic dosage before a response is seen. Unfortunately, many patients are unable to tolerate this delay and do not remain compliant with treatment. Beta-blockers may suppress some autonomic symptoms of anxiety, but they are not considered a first-line choice of treatment (see *Pearls & Perils*).

Treatment-resistant anxiety

Anxiety disorders are highly treatable, but when a patient does not respond, the following steps may be taken to evaluate the case.

Conclusions

Anxiety disorders are among the most common psychiatric disorders and result in significant impairment in social and occupational functioning. Fortunately, these disorders are responsive to both pharmacological and psychotherapeutic treatment. Recognition and treatment of these disorders will improve the quality of life for many.

Annotated bibliography

Andreasen, NC and Black, DW (2001) *Introductory Textbook of Psychiatry*, 3rd Edition, Washington, D.C., American Psychiatric Publishing, Inc.

This is a simple, clear, and factual textbook written primarily for medical students and residents in psychiatry. However, it is an excellent book for any physician who treats psychiatric patients.

Barlow, DH (2002) *Anxiety and Its Disorders: the nature and treatment of anxiety and panic*, 2nd Edition, New York, The Guilford Press. *This is an excellent resource on anxiety disorders. It is comprehensive and includes theoretical aspects of anxiety.*

Goodwin, DW and Guze, SB (1996) *Psychiatric Diagnosis*, 5th Edition, New York, Oxford University Press. *This book provides a concise, well-written summary of many psychiatric diagnoses including panic disorder and phobic disorders. There is a richness to this book that is rare in standard medical texts.*

Sadock, BJ and Sadock, VA (eds) (2000) *Kaplan and Sadock's Comprehensive Textbook of Psychiatry*, 7th Edition, Baltimore, MD, Lippincott, Williams & Wilkins. *This is a comprehensive two-volume textbook of psychiatry. It covers many areas in an indepth manner.*

American Psychiatric Association (2000) *Diagnostic and Statistical Manual of Mental Disorders*, 4th Edition, Text Revision, Washington, D.C., American Psychiatric Association. *This book provides the official nomenclature for psychiatric diagnosis, which is a consensus of current formulations in psychiatry. It briefly describes diagnostic features, subtypes, associated features, prevalence, course, and differential diagnosis for each psychiatric diagnosis.*

CHAPTER 10

Anxiety Disorders: Obsessive-Compulsive Disorder

Elliot C. Nelson, MD

Introduction

The ability to voluntarily control one's own thoughts is, understandably, something that almost everyone takes for granted. In individuals with obsessive-compulsive disorder (OCD) this ability is unfortunately no longer intact (see Case 10.1).

Definitions

The DSM-IV criteria for a diagnosis of OCD are listed in Box 10.1. The most common description of an obsessive thought is "it just popped into my head." Compulsions are behaviors (including mental acts) either performed in response to an obsession or according to stereotyped rules. While most

One day at the age of 22, Mrs L was at home caring for her three-year-old daughter when ". . . I just saw her and saw the knife. I had this thought and became terribly afraid that I would kill her." Mrs L reported that she became almost immobile. "All I did was cry. I didn't know what was the matter with me." She loved her daughter and so could not understand why these thoughts were present. They terrified her and she began to fear that she might act on them.

Because of these fears, she immediately went to see her gynecologist who referred her to an outpatient mental health clinic. The two-week wait for her first appointment seemed endless especially since she began to have thoughts that she might poison someone. When she saw the therapist, he told her that the stress from her problematic marriage caused the thoughts to be directed at her daughter, the object of that marriage, and recommended that she stay busy. Mrs L found the advice to be somewhat helpful and, over an eight-month period, the thoughts gradually dissipated.

During the ensuing two decades, Mrs L had a variety of other obsessions including fears that she would steal things, that she had cancer and other diseases, and that if something was not in its assigned place, harm would somehow come to her loved ones. She was much less bothered by these obsessions and, because she did not realize that they were symptoms of an illness, she never sought treatment for them. The diagnosis of OCD was not made until it was suggested by a friend, to whom Mrs L confided when the homicidal obsessions returned 27 years later.

At that time, Mrs L was mailing a condolence card to a friend when she suddenly had a thought that she had killed someone. After mailing the card, she began to worry that she had written a confession on the card and to wonder when the police would arrive. She soon had similar thoughts regarding a bank deposit slip. She stopped serving coffee to her clients at work because she feared that she might poison them. During trips to the grocery store she was plagued by thoughts that she might have placed poison into someone's milk carton. Thoughts that she had hit someone caused her to go back and check to see that she had not done so, making otherwise short car trips take hours.

After her brother called to say that he planned to visit her and intended to bring his grandson along, Mrs L began to worry that she would kill the child. She concluded that she was obligated to kill herself to protect the child, but would wait to do so until her brother actually arrived so as to save him an extra trip for her funeral. Fortunately, at this time she instead sought help.

Box 10.1 Obsessive-compulsive disorder

A. Either obsessions or compulsions:

Obsessions as defined by 1, 2, 3, and 4:

1 recurrent and persistent thoughts, impulses, or images that are experienced, at some time during the disturbance, as intrusive and inappropriate and that cause marked anxiety or distress

2 the thoughts, impulses, or images are not simply excessive worries about real-life problems

3 the person attempts to ignore or suppress such thoughts, impulses, or images, or to neutralize them with some other thought or action

4 the person recognizes that the obsessional thoughts, impulses, or images are a product of his or her own mind (not imposed from without as in thought insertion).

Compulsions as defined by 1 or 2:

1 repetitive behaviors (e.g., hand washing, ordering, checking) or mental acts (e.g., praying, counting, repeating words silently) that the person feels driven to perform in response to an obsession, or according to rules that must be applied rigidly

2 the behaviors or mental acts are aimed at preventing or reducing distress or preventing some dreaded event or situation; however, these behaviors or mental acts either are not connected in a realistic way with what they are designed to neutralize or prevent or are clearly excessive.

B. At some point during the course of the disorder, the person has recognized that the obsessions or compulsions are excessive or unreasonable. **Note**: this does not apply to children.

C. The obsessions or compulsions cause marked distress, are time consuming (take more than one hour a day), or significantly interfere with the person's normal routine, occupational (or academic) functioning, or usual social activities or relationships.

D. If another Axis 1 disorder is present, the content of the obsessions or compulsions is not restricted to it (e.g., preoccupation with food in the presence of an eating disorder; hair pulling in the presence of trichotillomania; concern with appearance in the presence of body dysmorphic disorder; preoccupation with drugs in the presence of a substance use disorder; preoccupation with having a serious illness in the presence of hypochondriasis; preoccupation with sexual urges or fantasies in the presence of a paraphilia; or guilty ruminations in the presence of major depressive disorder).

E. The disturbance is not due to the direct physiological effects of a substance (e.g., a drug of abuse, a medication) or a general medical condition.

Specify if:

With poor insight: if, for most of the time during the current episode, the person does not recognize that the obsessions and compulsions are excessive or unreasonable.

From American Psychiatric Association (2000) Diagnostic and Statistical Manual of Mental Disorders, 4th Edition, Text Revision, Washington, D.C., American Psychiatric Association.

---

individuals with OCD generally consider their symptoms to be excessive or unrealistic, good insight is not always present. For this reason, an ability to specify "with poor insight" was added to DSM-IV.

The most common obsessions involve fears of contamination or of harming oneself or others (see Table 10.1 for a more extensive list). The most common compulsions involve checking or washing (Table 10.2). Consistent with strong underlying biological determinants, OCD symptoms have been observed to be very similar across extremely diverse cultures. The severity of any one particular OCD symptom may vary markedly over time or across subjects.

Brief historical background

OCD has been well described for many centuries. The medical literature of the 19th century, particularly that of Germany and France, includes clear depictions of OCD symptoms. One topic vigorously debated in the literature of that period was whether insight should be a criterion for the diagnosis of OCD. Freud's description of OCD displayed a

TABLE 10.1

Content of primary obsessions from DSM-IV field trials

Content of obsession	Percentage of subjects reporting symptom as primary obsession across five sites
Contamination	37.8
Fear of harming oneself or others	23.6
Symmetry	10.0
Somatic	7.2
Religious	5.9
Sexual	5.5
Hoarding	4.8
Unacceptable urges	4.3
Miscellaneous	1.0

From Foa *et al.* (1995) *Am J Psychiatry* 152:90–96. Reprinted with permission.

TABLE 10.2	Type of primary compulsions from DSM-IV field trials	
	Type of compulsion	Percentage of subjects reporting symptom as primary compulsion across five sites
	Checking	28.2
	Cleaning/washing	26.6
	Miscellaneous	11.8
	Repeating	11.1
	Mental rituals	10.9
	Ordering	5.7
	Hoarding/collecting	3.5
	Counting	2.1

From Foa *et al.* (1995) *Am J Psychiatry* 152:90–96. Reprinted with permission.

precise understanding of the intrusive nature of obsessive thoughts.

Epidemiology

Until the 1980s, OCD was believed to be a rare psychiatric illness with a lifetime prevalence rate of 0.05% most often quoted. The goal of the Epidemiology Catchment Area (ECA) study, a five-center investigation published in the 1980s, was to estimate the prevalence rates of a variety of psychiatric disorders in the United States. Trained lay interviewers administered a structured interview to assess the presence or absence of psychiatric illness(es). One of the most surprising findings of the ECA study was that the lifetime prevalence rate of OCD ranged from 1.9% to 3.3% across sites. Since the publication of these results, similar rates have been reported from numerous countries. Studies in clinical populations have led to estimates of the rate of OCD in psychiatric outpatients varying from 0.6% to 10%. Estimates derived from similar work examining psychiatric inpatients range from 0.1% to 4.0%.

The gender ratio of OCD sufferers obtained from community samples has typically suggested a mild predominance among women. The gender ratio obtained from adult clinical samples has been near unity while that from children and adolescents has tended to show a small male predominance. The most common age of OCD onset has been reported to be in the late teens or early 20s with a somewhat earlier onset seen in males. It is not unusual for symptoms to begin during the first decade of life; onset after 35 years of age is fairly rare.

Comorbidity

The most common comorbid illness seen among individuals presenting for treatment of OCD is major depressive disorder (MDD); approximately 30% meet criteria for the disorder and up to 83% report individual depressive symptoms (e.g., low mood). The lifetime prevalence rate for comorbid MDD in those with OCD has been reported to be nearly 70%. It has become apparent that a higher than expected rate of bipolar disorder is also observed among those with OCD. The degree to which this excess comorbidity can be attributed to induction of mania during treatment with antidepressants is unclear.

Higher than population rates of comorbid social anxiety disorder (social phobia), panic disorder with and without agoraphobia, and simple phobia have also been reported among those with OCD. As seen with other anxiety disorders, increased rates of alcohol and other substance abuse and dependence have been noted. These individuals often describe their substance use as self-medicating in an attempt to control their anxiety and other OCD symptoms. Individuals with OCD also demonstrate an increased rate of disorders whose symptoms largely involve preoccupation with their bodies. These illnesses include anorexia nervosa, body dysmorphic disorder and hypochondriasis.

Tourette syndrome and chronic motor tic occur at varying rates among OCD patients. Because Tourette syndrome is a considerably rarer illness, the overall rate seen among those with OCD tends to be fairly low. The rate of OCD reported among individuals with Tourette syndrome is as high as 89% or as low as 2% depending upon the criteria used to delineate a complex motor tic from a compulsion.

Rates of personality disorders, illnesses involving a pervasive pattern of impaired interpersonal interactions with onset in adolescence or early adult life, also have been found to be substantially elevated among those with OCD. Reports suggest that avoidant and dependent personality disorders are actually more common among individuals with OCD than obsessive-compulsive personality disorder. Interestingly, pharmacologic treatment of OCD results in a significant decrease in the rate of these illnesses, which are generally considered medication nonresponsive and are thought to potentially require long-term psychotherapy.

Differential diagnosis

Individuals with MDD often manifest repetitive negative thoughts, termed ruminations, that differ from obsessions in that they occur only in the context of low mood and, as such, rarely seem intrusive. Ruminations often take the form of brooding over past events; obsessions are more often concerns about the present or future.

Individuals with OCD commonly experience panic attacks when faced with stimuli or situations related to their fears (see Table 10.3). In panic disorder, unlike OCD, the panic attacks at least initially occur without provocation. In social anxiety disorder, intrusive thoughts (when present) are limited to feared social situations. In generalized anxiety

Table 10.3 Obsessive-compulsive disorder

Discriminating feature

1 Obsessions or compulsions that cause marked distress, interfere with functioning, or are present for more than one hour daily.

Consistent features

1 Insight preserved
    • thoughts perceived as unwanted
    • behaviors felt to be excessive.
2 Both obsessions and compulsions present.
3 Not entirely related to another illness.
4 Not caused by substance use or general medical condition.

Variable features

1 Panic attacks in response to symptom-provoking stimuli.
2 Comorbid affective disorders.
3 Substance abuse.
4 Other anxiety disorders.
5 Tics or Tourette's syndrome.
6 Eating disorders.
7 Association of symptom exacerbations with streptococcal infections.
8 Family members affected.
9 Insight into current symptoms.
10 Willingness to challenge symptoms in behavior therapy.

disorder, excessive worry about life circumstances is present, but it is not experienced as intrusive and generally involves typical life issues (e.g., fear of losing a job).

In body dysmorphic disorder, the individual becomes preoccupied with a real or imagined defect in appearance. If the defect is real, the concerns are felt to be grossly excessive. The thoughts driving the individual's absorption are usually described as intrusive and may often be accompanied by frequent checking behaviors. Although these thoughts and behaviors are phenomonologically indistinguishable from those of OCD, the presence of other obsessions and compulsions meeting criteria is required for an additional diagnosis of OCD. Similarly, the preoccupation with body habitus seen in anorexia nervosa commonly involves intrusive thoughts that may lead to frequent checking of weight and appearance, but comorbid OCD is not diagnosed unless other symptoms meeting criteria are present.

Tics are sudden, rapid, stereotyped movements. They do not occur in response to obsessive thoughts and generally involve only bodily movements rather than goal-directed behaviors. Individuals with Tourette syndrome also have verbal tics that may involve grunting, groaning, or profane utterances. This differs from individuals with OCD who may have fears that they will begin to curse at work, school, or in a place of worship, but who do not actually do so.

Individuals who have difficulty controlling various impulsive behaviors often describe themselves as compulsive, but the behaviors in which they engage (i.e. gambling, sexual activity, substance abuse, shoplifting, etc.) are initially experienced as pleasure-generating. True compulsions are not enjoyable behaviors, although the relief that may result from performing them may be described as a positive or pleasurable experience. Individuals with obsessive-compulsive personality disorder tend to be miserly, rigid, cold, perfectionistic, and preoccupied with rules and details. They may hoard worthless or worn-out objects, but not to the degree where the objects are a fire hazard or make travel through the house treacherous. They differ from individuals with OCD in that neither obsessions nor compulsions comprise a major part of their clinical presentation.

Natural history

Early studies examining the natural history of OCD suggested that patients tend to separate into three groups: those with chronic, unremitting illness; those whose illness partially remits to the point where social functioning is relatively spared; and those with an episodic course that includes periods of complete remission. It is believed that only about 10% of those with OCD demonstrate the chronic, unremitting course.

PANDAS

The acronym PANDAS—pediatric autoimmune neuropsychiatric disorders associated with streptococcal infections— has been coined to refer to a subgroup of OCD patients with early-onset illness whose symptoms display acute exacerbations following Group A streptococcal infections. The symptoms displayed by these individuals commonly include tics, emotional lability, separation anxiety, and attentional problems. Recognition of this subgroup has led to exciting new areas of research (described below) that include the use of novel treatment modalities.

Twin, family, and molecular genetic studies

Two twin studies have examined the genetic epidemiology of OCD symptoms. In a large sample of adult female twins, factors roughly corresponding to obsessions and compulsions derived from a self-administered questionnaire were found to have heritabilities of 33% and 26%, respectively. The other study reported data from two large samples of twin children (from Missouri and the Netherlands) whose parents completed questionnaires from which OCD symptom scores were obtained. The heritability of these OCD symptom scores was found to vary between 51% and 58%.

Early family studies of OCD were limited by a variety of methodological difficulties but typically noted a higher than expected rate of OCD among first-degree relatives. Several groups have personally interviewed first-degree relatives of OCD probands. The parents of children with OCD have consistently been found to display greater than population rates of both clinical and subclinical OCD. Interestingly, the primary symptom of probands and their ill parents was reported in one study to overlap only 13.3% of the time, a pattern more suggestive of genetic effects than an environment or learning model. As has been observed with other psychiatric disorders, greater risk of illness in first-degree relatives has been reported for probands with early onset OCD. Two studies included direct interviews of the first-degree relatives of both adults with OCD and normal controls. One found a significantly higher rate of subclinical, but not clinical OCD in patients' relatives. The other reported a significantly higher rate of OCD in the relatives of cases versus controls, but observed that this finding was entirely the result of OCD diagnosed in the relatives of probands with early-onset illness. This latter study also noted significantly higher rates of other anxiety disorders and affective disorders in the relatives of cases versus those of controls.

Several groups have reported evidence for a genetic relationship between Tourette syndrome (TS), chronic motor tic disorder (CMT), and OCD. One study compared the rates of OCD, TS, and CMT among adoptive and biologic relatives of TS probands, with and without OCD. None of the adoptive relatives met criteria for these disorders. Among the biologic relatives, the rates of none of these illnesses differed between the relatives of TS probands with and without OCD, and those of both groups were increased compared with population rates.

One report examined the rates of OCD and tics in the first-degree relatives of children admitted for the treatment of PANDAS. The rates of OCD and tics in these individuals were observed to be higher than those reported in the general population.

Candidate gene studies of OCD have not yet produced any positive findings that have been adequately replicated. A genome-wide linkage study of early-onset OCD has been performed but did not yield positive findings; no LOD score greater than two was reported for any region. The present characterization of OCD will likely prove to be a syndrome that occurs via a variety of pathophysiologic routes, some of which are genetically-mediated or involve gene-environment interactions.

Treatment

Freud provided a cogent description of OCD symptoms that accompanied his hypotheses regarding the underlying conflicts and his recommended course of treatment. Unfortunately, attempts to apply Freud's views and methods to the treatment of OCD proved fruitless, leading psychiatrists to view OCD as a treatment-resistant illness for many years. OCD also has been observed to display relatively low rates of placebo response across treatment studies. In a two-week, single-blinded trial of placebo in 30 individuals with OCD assessed with several different scales designed to rate OCD symptoms, no significant difference across any scale or subscale with placebo treatment was found.

Pharmacotherapy

The cornerstone of OCD pharmacotherapy is the class of antidepressants known as the serotonin reuptake inhibitors (SRIs). In a series of sequential trials that began in the mid to late 1980s with clomipramine, SRIs have been shown to have superior efficacy to either placebo or other types of antidepressants. There are some important differences that must be kept in mind when prescribing SRIs for the treatment of OCD versus their use for depression. First, the time course required to treat OCD with these drugs is substantially more prolonged (with improvement occurring over 10–12 weeks or longer) than that typically required to treat depression (commonly 3–6 weeks), and so it is important to allow a greater length of time to pass before making dosage increases. Second, the rate of response in OCD treatment is not as high as that observed in the treatment of depression. Third, a higher medication dose may be required for successful treatment of OCD, and responders often need to remain on medication for a substantially longer time period. When clomipramine was stopped abruptly in 21 responders in one study, 19 had a relapse of OCD symptoms and another became depressed. Gradual reductions in medication dosage over a period of months, after an adequate response has occurred, may allow patients to maintain a response at a lower overall dose. Successful discontinuation of medication with maintenance of response is possible for some responders; this goal is much more likely to be achieved in those whose treatment included the concomitant use of behavior therapy.

Clomipramine, a potent SRI, was the first to receive approval as an OCD treatment in the U.S. It is a tricyclic (TCA) antidepressant that has anticholinergic, antihistaminergic, and anti-alpha$_1$ adrenergic effects as well as an active metabolite that is a potent norepinephrine (NE) uptake inhibitor. In a large multi-center double-blind comparison with placebo in non-depressed individuals with OCD, the mean reduction in OCD symptoms after ten weeks of clomipramine treatment (mean dose 218.8 mg) was 44% as compared with 5% with placebo treatment. The rate of response, defined as at least a 35% reduction in OCD symptoms, was 60% with clomipramine versus 7% with placebo. The typical dose range in treating OCD is 100 to 250 mg. Common side effects of clomipramine include dry mouth, dizziness, tremor, somnolence, constipation, and fatigue. As with other tricyclics, overdose with clomipramine carries a substantial risk of death and, for this reason, care must be taken with its prescription to potentially suicidal patients. It is important to remember that elderly patients may metabolize clomipramine more slowly and that they have a substantial risk of dangerous falls with orthostatic hypotension. Although clomipramine has well-established antiobsessional efficacy, its use has been somewhat limited by the wide range of adverse effects that are a natural consequence of the drug's diverse actions. Because of this limitation and the not inconsequential rate of OCD non-response seen with every drug thus far studied, a series of subsequent investigations have examined the use of other SRIs for OCD treatment.

The other SRIs for which antiobsessional efficacy has been established all lack substantial cholinergic, histaminergic, or alpha$_1$ adrenergic activity. Because of their specificity, these drugs are referred to as selective SRIs (SSRIs). One study compared various doses of fluoxetine (20, 40, and 60 mg) with placebo and found significantly better response rates, defined as a 35% reduction in OCD symptoms, with active drug at each of the three dosages. However, the response rate of 35.1% at 60 mg fluoxetine versus 8.5% with placebo was lower than the prior study with clomipramine, heralding a trend that would be observed across this set of studies with rates of active drug response gradually declining and rates of placebo response increasing. In clinical practice, the use of fluoxetine at doses of 80 mg or more in the treatment of OCD is not unusual. Common side effects of fluoxetine include nausea, diarrhea, decreased appetite, dry mouth, insomnia, somnolence, and anxiety with some tendency for these side effects to be seen at a greater frequency with higher medication dosage. Fluoxetine's half-life, the longest of the SSRIs, is further prolonged in elderly patients.

Fluvoxamine has also been proven to possess substantial efficacy in the treatment of OCD with well established superiority to placebo and other antidepressants. In a large 10-week trial, 53% of fluvoxamine-treated patients responded, defined as having a 25% reduction in OCD symptoms, versus 18% of those treated with placebo. It is interesting to note that 20% of OCD patients who have had an unsatisfactory response to either clomipramine or fluoxetine were observed to respond to fluvoxamine, although the primary mechanism of action of these drugs is believed to be identical. The range of fluvoxamine doses used to treat OCD is commonly 150 to 300 mg. The side effect profile of fluvoxamine overlaps with that of fluoxetine although nausea and sedation are seen more commonly with the former and restlessness and insomnia more often with the latter.

Similarly, sertraline (at doses ranging from 50 to 200 mg), paroxetine (at doses ranging from 20 to 60 mg), and most recently citalopram (at doses ranging from 20 to 60 mg) have been demonstrated to be superior to placebo in treating OCD. The reduction in OCD symptoms seen with these drugs versus placebo was also less than that of the initial studies with clomipramine. These drugs have fairly similar side-effect profiles to the other SSRIs. Paroxetine has some mild anticholinergic activity and a shorter half-life that may result in greater risk of SSRI discontinuation symptoms.

Several groups have performed meta-analyses that suggest that clomipramine may have antiobsessional efficacy superior to the SSRIs. The major issue is whether the greater reduction in OCD symptoms observed with clomipramine is a true reflection of superior efficacy or a result of a temporal selection bias as the more responsive patients, perhaps with less comorbid illness, are removed from the pool available for pharmacotherapeutic trials. Several direct comparisons of clomipramine and an SSRI have been performed and have generally found no significant difference in efficacy between medications.

Because for most OCD patients a response to a SRI is limited to a significant reduction, but not a complete remission, in symptoms with improvement in quality of life, a number of agents have been used in an attempt to augment this response. The only agents with documented superiority to placebo in augmenting the effect of a SRI for OCD are antipsychotics. Initially, augmentation therapy with the older agents haloperidol and pimozide was reported to result in a significant decrease in OCD symptoms that was limited to patients with either comorbid TS or CMT. These findings led to trials of atypical antipsychotic augmentation. Risperidone has demonstrated efficacy, not limited to patients with comorbid tic disorders, in a placebo-controlled, double-blind study. Olanzapine and quetiapine have shown similar efficacy in open trials. Another augmentation strategy used with less definitive success involves combining clomipramine with an SSRI. However, given the ability of some SSRIs (i.e., fluoxetine, fluvoxamine, and paroxetine) to strongly inhibit the liver enzyme cytochrome P450 2D6, care must be taken to avoid dangerously high clomipramine levels with such combinations (i.e., making slow dose increases and frequently monitoring clomipramine blood levels). Another option that has been used successfully in research trials involves the intravenous administration of clomipramine, and more recently citalopram, to individuals who had not responded to, or poorly tolerated, oral agents.

The treatment of OCD symptoms in children with PANDAS has generally included the use of SRIs, as described above, in combination with other therapy directed at the autoimmune aspect of the illness. In one placebo-controlled, three-armed trial in which pre-entry psychotropic medications were continued, intravenous immunoglobulin and plasma exchange were each observed to demonstrate efficacy superior to placebo. A placebo-controlled crossover trial of penicillin prophylaxis failed to demonstrate any benefits in terms of recurrent OCD symptoms in children with a history of PANDAS. A small, open label trial of antibiotic treatment of sentinel PANDAS episodes reported that initial OCD symptoms responded well as did recurrences that accompanied subsequent infections.

Behavior therapy

Behavior therapy begins with the therapist obtaining a detailed history not only of the types of obsessions and compulsions that are being experienced but also of the specific situations that increase symptoms and the rituals or avoidance behaviors that subsequently occur. For each specific type of behavior (e.g., checking doorknobs), the therapist constructs a hierarchy that orders symptoms from those with the lowest (e.g., checking the closet door) to those with the highest levels of associated anxiety (e.g., checking the home's outer doors when leaving for an extended vacation). The patient is trained in various means of anxiety reduction. The therapist then accompanies the patient in an exposure to a situation that the patient would have previously handled by either avoidance behavior or the performance of rituals. The patient is instructed not to perform compulsive behaviors and to remain in the situation until a reduction in anxiety occurs. The patient may benefit from seeing the therapist perform the exposure at the same time without subsequent ritualizing (participant modeling).

The stimuli for the initial exposures are chosen to cause a tolerable, but not extreme, degree of anxiety. Situations that the patient perceives to be intolerably anxiety-provoking may be first approached via an imaginal exposure, in which the patient mentally visualizes the activity rather then directly confronting it. Although the obsessive thoughts typically linger for a period of weeks after the individual stops performing the compulsive behaviors, with successful completion of exposures, the patient eventually habituates to the involved stimuli with no resulting occurrence of symptoms. Optimally, generalization occurs such that the patient also habituates to situations similar, but not identical, to the exposure. The therapy then proceeds up the patient's hierarchy to more anxiety-producing exposures. Flooding, which involves starting near the top of the sufferer's hierarchy, has not been found to be more effective; it also may be associated with a higher rate of treatment discontinuation. Cognitive restructuring techniques are often employed in therapy to assist OCD sufferers with redefining how they view themselves, their priorities, and their capabilities apart from their illness. Alternative approaches that also have been reported to be beneficial include group behavioral therapy and a program of self assessment and self-administered behavior therapy called BT STEPS. Case 10.2 describes one woman's experience of behavior therapy.

CASE 10.2

Mrs T reported, "I've always been a perfectionist." While growing up she tended to be somewhat territorial around the home, "I didn't want anyone messing with my stuff." In her late teens she began to worry excessively about hairs accumulating on clothing and other household surfaces. The thoughts were intrusive and led to rituals involving repeatedly shaking out the laundry and wiping the surfaces to remove the hair. Other compulsions were soon added involving ordering and arranging household items.

These symptoms continued at a level that the patient found annoying, but tolerable, until her marriage at 32 years of age necessitated her having to incorporate her husband's presence into her routine. She experienced an increase in her obsessions and compulsions that led her to request that her husband restrict their social activities, including time outside the home and having guests visit their house (to limit exposures and allow more time for rituals).

The amount of time involved in performing the compulsive behaviors gradually increased such that, for example, it eventually would take Mrs T an hour to wipe down the kitchen after a meal. This behavior would continue "until it feels right." Although her husband was very supportive, Mrs T's symptoms began to substantially restrict their activities. At his urging, she first presented for treatment at age 37. She was seen by a psychiatrist who recommended that she be hospitalized for treatment of depression. She did not have symptoms meeting criteria for depression at that time and so sought care elsewhere. She was next evaluated over several sessions by a behavior therapist who forewarned both Mrs T and her husband that therapy would be very effortful. She became concerned by his warnings and chose not to proceed at that time.

Mrs T next presented for evaluation at 39 years of age. Her symptoms had worsened somewhat, and she was now spending more than three hours per day engaged in rituals. She was given information on therapeutic alternatives including medication and behavior therapy; she chose to be treated with a combination of both modalities. She was begun on fluoxetine 20 mg daily and the process of acquiring the detailed history required for behavior therapy was begun. After one week she increased her fluoxetine dose to 40 mg, as instructed. On this dose she began to feel less energetic, more depressed, and somewhat jittery. For this reason, fluoxetine was discontinued and she was begun on clomipramine 50 mg daily, which was later increased to 100 mg per day. On the higher dose, she had complaints of dry mouth, sedation, and orthostatic hypotension, but they were deemed tolerable.

Before formally beginning behavior therapy, Mrs T noted a reduction in her anxiety and reported that it was considerably easier for her to delay completing her rituals. She related this improvement to the medication. Mrs T's behavior therapist established several hierarchies including one involving the shaking of clothes and others focusing on her wiping surfaces only once and leaving objects out of place. Mrs T's husband was involved with her in the therapy and remained extremely supportive. Mrs T began working through each hierarchy with most exposures actually done in her home. She made continuous progress with her behavioral assignments and was able to complete all three hierarchies over an eight-month period. A clomipramine taper was begun at this time with the reduction in dose proceeding gradually at 25 mg every two months. The clomipramine was eventually discontinued with Mrs T continuing to do very well without any OCD symptoms whatsoever.

Most studies using behavior therapy to treat OCD have reported success rates at least comparable to pharmacotherapeutic trials. A meta-analysis reported that the rates of much and moderate improvement across studies were 51% and 39%, respectively, and that after a follow-up period of months to years, more than 70% had maintained this level of improvement. It is important to recognize that the direct applicability of the behavior therapy literature to clinical practice is highly dependent on the quality of the therapists who are readily available. Also, a not insignificant number of patients will either refuse behavior therapy or not adequately engage in it. Several studies examined whether greater benefit was seen with combined behavior therapy and medication treatment versus either modality alone and reported either equivocal or negative results. One study found that children with OCD who had previously not responded to behavior therapy displayed a significant response to fluvoxamine and a significantly greater response when it was combined with additional behavior therapy. In another investigation of adults who had failed to respond to fluoxetine, a trial of cognitive-behavior therapy led to a significant reduction in OCD symptoms. In clinical practice, the concomitant use of appropriate pharmacotherapeutic agents often will allow patients to proceed with behavioral treatment. The current standard of care involves, at the very least, making all patients aware of both medication and behavioral treatment options.

Psychosurgery

A variety of psychosurgical procedures have been performed on patients with OCD including cingulotomy, orbital undercutting, anterior capsulotomy, bifrontal tractotomy, and bimedial leucotomy. Although generally good success rates have been reported, in most studies surgical candidates were not limited to individuals with treatment-resistant illness. Because of the reported success of these procedures that share the feature of interrupting connections between frontal lobe and basal ganglia structures, a model implicating involvement of these areas in the pathophysiology of OCD has gained considerable acceptance.

Swedish researchers evaluated ten patients with incapacitating, treatment-resistant OCD before and one year after capsulotomy and noted significant reductions in anxiety and OCD symptoms. Although cingulotomy has been reported to be less effective than other procedures, it has been the primary procedure performed in the United States. A reevaluation of 33 patients who had undergone at least one cingulotomy over a 25-year period at the Massachusetts General Hospital found that only 9% had been treated preoperatively with behavior therapy. In the 14 patients for whom adequate assessment of postoperative symptoms could be made, six reported no improvement and eight moderate to marked improvement. In a prospective study by the same group, cingulotomy was performed only on individu-

KEY CLINICAL QUESTIONS AND WHAT THEY UNLOCK

- *Did OCD symptoms present abruptly in a preadolescent?* Children who present with an acute onset of OCD, tics, emotional lability, separation anxiety, or attention problems may have pediatric autoimmune neuropsychiatric disorders associated with streptococcal infections (PANDAS). Although treatment with SRIs is typical, other interventions (described in the text) not usually prescribed for OCD should also be considered.
- *Is the patient with OCD symptoms currently depressed?* Treatment of symptoms with an SRI may be preferable to initiating behavioral therapy.
- *Has the OCD sufferer experienced episodes of mania in the past?* Treatment with a medication that is thought to stabilize mood (e.g., lithium) is advisable before starting an SRI.
- *Does the patient have OCD and tics?* Inadequate response to an SRI leads to consideration of the addition of an antipsychotic, particularly newer medications (e.g., risperidone, olanzapine, and quetiapine).
- *Does the patient with OCD suffer from other anxiety-related disorders such as post-traumatic stress disorder (PTSD), social anxiety disorder or panic disorder?* Interventions, particularly behavior therapy, need to be prioritized to the most severe symptoms/disorder.
- *If a patient with schizophrenia presents with OCD, are the symptoms new?* Treatment with newer antipsychotic agents ("atypical antipsychotics") may induce OCD symptoms and decreasing the antipsychotic dose, switching to another antipsychotic, or adding an SRI are reasonable options.
- *What are the options if SRI treatment of OCD is inadequate?* Partial SRI effectiveness suggests the implementation of augmentation strategies such as behavior therapy (even if this has failed as monotherapy). Absence of benefit from one SRI suggests a trial of another SRI.

als with an established history of non-response to multiple medication trials and behavior therapy. When participants were evaluated two years postoperatively, 5 of 18 patients were conservatively classified as responders and another three individuals as partial responders. An alternative approach involving the stereotactic implantation of electrodes bilaterally into the internal capsule in order to enable long-term electrical stimulation (deep brain stimulation) in individuals with intractable OCD has reportedly led to improvement in symptoms that waned when the stimulation was temporarily discontinued. Neurosurgical referral should be reserved for individuals with chronic, debilitating OCD who have not had an adequate response to repeated, well-documented trials of conventional therapies (including both pharmacotherapy and behavior therapy) and preference should be given to national or, at the very least, regional centers with clinical expertise in this area.

Pathophysiology

Association with neurologic illness

As our understanding of the functional neuroanatomy underlying the symptoms of OCD has gradually evolved, a relatively clear picture has begun to emerge. The relative success of neurosurgical treatments that tended to interrupt cortical connections to basal ganglia structures caused researchers to focus attention on these areas. The presence of OCD symptoms has been reported to be associated with diseases in which the pathophysiology is known to involve the basal ganglia (e.g. post-encephalitic parkinsonism, Huntington's disease, blepharospasm). Similarly, the realization that higher than expected rates of OCD are found in individuals with Sydenham's chorea, an illness involving the post-streptococcal infection formation of autoantibodies to the caudate nucleus, eventually resulted in the first description of PANDAS. Basal ganglia involvement has been implicated in TS, an illness that is also a component of PANDAS and with which comorbid OCD is quite common. Case reports have also associated OCD with infarct or injury to the caudate nucleus or globus pallidus.

Neuroimaging

The most consistent findings from early positron emission tomography (PET) studies of OCD were either unilateral or bilateral increases in glucose or oxygen metabolism in the orbital frontal cortex. After pharmacologic treatment, significantly decreased orbital frontal glucose metabolism was observed bilaterally with the right-sided difference correlating significantly with the decrease in OCD symptoms. Similarly, a decrease in midfrontal, right anterior frontal, and left caudate glucose metabolism has been reported with medication treatment. In another important study involving PET scans before and after ten weeks of treatment with either medication or behavior therapy, responders to each treatment modality were found to have decreased glucose metabolism in the head of the right caudate nucleus. This was the first example in which the successful treatment of a mental illness with two very different types of treatment was shown to produce similar effects on brain metabolism. A later PET study of individuals with OCD before and after paroxetine treatment found that non-depressed individuals with OCD who responded to paroxetine displayed decreased metabolism in the right caudate, right ventrolateral prefrontal cortex, bilateral orbital frontal cortex, and thalamus. Also, improvement in OCD symptoms was found to be correlated with pretreatment glucose metabolism in the right caudate nucleus. An MRI study of treatment-naïve children with OCD observed that the children had bilaterally increased thalamic volumes that declined after paroxetine treatment,

with volumetric changes correlated with OCD symptom response. Other studies have reported that lower pretreatment orbital frontal blood flow was associated with response to fluvoxamine and higher posterior cingulate cortex pretreatment blood flow was associated with response to either fluvoxamine or cingulotomy.

Activation studies, in which symptoms are provoked during the scan, have provided another useful means of visualizing the functional neuroanatomy of OCD. One PET study used a subtraction method in which a control scan was subtracted from the activation scan in order to create a difference image to examine medication-free OCD subjects. For example, subjects were presented with a neutral stimulus (e.g., a sterile glove) in the first scan and then a stimulus chosen to provoke OCD symptoms (e.g., a contaminated glove) in the second scan. Significantly increased blood flow in the left anterior orbital frontal cortex that was positively correlated with the subjects' assessment of the change in the degree of their OCD symptoms was found. Other regions that demonstrated significant increased blood flow with symptom provocation included the right caudate nucleus and the midline anterior cingulate cortex, but changes in these regions were not correlated with increased OCD symptoms. Another group studied four subjects with OCD across a variety of stimuli designed to provoke OCD symptoms to varying degrees and examined correlations between the degree of symptoms reported and blood flow in various regions. Changes in blood flow were found to be positively correlated with OCD symptom intensity in a variety of structures, including the right inferior frontal cortex, right caudate nucleus, right globus pallidus, and right thalamus.

In children with PANDAS, the size of the caudate, putamen, and globus pallidus has been reported to be increased. Case reports comparing children with PANDAS, before and after successful treatment, have observed that the size of these structures decreased after treatment.

These PET and MRI studies of OCD have generated a great deal of excitement that may be better understood with an appreciation of the underlying neuroanatomical interconnections. A loop has been described that connects the orbital frontal cortex, caudate nucleus, globus pallidus, and thalamus (from which there is a feedback connection to the orbital frontal cortex). Researchers have hypothesized that the excitatory and inhibitory interconnections within this loop may result in increased risk of self-sustained firing. Components of this loop have been implicated in the pathophysiology of OCD by several converging lines of investigation: (1) PET and MRI studies demonstrating increased activity in resting subjects with further increases noted in activation studies involving symptom provocation; (2) the occurrence of OCD symptoms associated with neurological illnesses (including PANDAS) whose pathology involves these regions; and (3) the observation that an improvement in OCD symptoms may result from the psychosurgical interruption of these connections. Although a comprehensive model accounting for basal ganglia and orbital frontal cortex involvement and adequately explaining the specificity of SRIs has yet to be cogently presented, it is hoped that continued improvement in our understanding over the next decade may lead to the development of improved OCD treatments.

OCD in a family practice setting

For physicians working in a primary care setting, illnesses like OCD may seem far removed from typical medical practice. Many psychiatrists also report that they encounter a very limited number of OCD sufferers. These patients, as epidemiological research confirms, are actually present to a greater extent than is generally appreciated. When one does not ask an OCD patient directly about the specific symptoms from which the individual suffers, the information may not be transmitted to the physician.

If one has reason to suspect the presence of OCD, it is important to screen for OCD symptoms. The Yale-Brown Obsessive Compulsive Scale (Y-BOCS) is a very useful instrument for this purpose. The Y-BOCS contains fairly comprehensive lists of obsessions and compulsions that may be presented to appropriate patients to assist in making the diagnosis of OCD. The value of this approach is derived from the fact that most patients with OCD have insight into their symptoms and often consider them to be embarrassing idiosyncracies. These patients often fail to recognize their own pathology when vague screening questions are posed to them in an attempt to determine if they have ever had intrusive thoughts or engaged in repetitive behaviors. Some common scenarios in which the possibility of OCD should be entertained are suggested in Box 10.2.

BOX 10.2

When to think about OCD and related illnesses

- A patient without substantial risk factors requests an HIV test and then seems dissatisfied with the negative result and asks to be retested.
- A patient presents across time with fears of cancer involving multiple sites of origin.
- A patient has chapped or shiny, erythematous hands without a clear explanation.
- A patient requests that a plastic surgeon correct a defect visible only to the patient.
- A patient repeatedly states, "You don't understand."
- A parent repeatedly brings a well child in for unnecessary examinations.
- A patient discontinues several medications after 2–3 days for vague reasons.
- A patient is constantly asking repetitive questions about a variety of illnesses.
- A patient continually arrives late for appointments without any clear explanation.

CASE 10.3

Mr V first presented for psychiatric evaluation at age 32 during a period of high situational stress. He reported a three-week history of frequent crying spells, increased anxiety with palpitations, sleep disturbance with terminal insomnia, decreased appetite that had resulted in a 15 lb weight loss over a one-month period, poor concentration, fatigue, lack of enjoyment of activities, and feelings of hopelessness, helplessness, and worthlessness. He was diagnosed with depression and initially treated with imipramine and alprazolam. Because of concerns regarding right bundle branch block on EKG, the imipramine was quickly discontinued and trazodone therapy begun. Mr V responded well to this combination and his depressive symptoms completely remitted. The alprazolam was gradually tapered and Mr V continued to do well.

Several months later, Mr V began to complain of throat irritation, and he was seen eventually by an otolaryngologist who recommended a tonsillectomy and adenoidectomy. The surgery was performed without incident, but post-operatively, Mr V continued to complain of throat irritation. Mr V was seen in consultation by another otolaryngologist who also could find no clear organic etiology for Mr V's complaints. Buspirone was added because of anxiety Mr V was experiencing including fears that he would lose his job and be unable to support his wife and their new child as a result of his throat irritation. Mr V's symptoms improved but did not entirely remit. Alprazolam was restarted and further improvement occurred, enabling Mr V to return to work.

At this time, Mr V reported that he had been examining his throat often in an attempt to find an explanation of his symptoms. He also reported intrusive thoughts about swallowing, clearing his throat, and blinking his eyes. He spontaneously voiced additional symptoms dating to childhood including touching compulsions, obsessive thoughts about staring at the sun, and compulsions to repeat certain words. Mr V continued to have infrequent symptoms that worsened with situational stressors. He remained on trazodone and buspirone. A trial of fluoxetine was attempted, but could not be completed because of sedation. He later developed symptoms that included checking rituals involving doors, appliances, and his son and a resurgence of touching compulsions necessitating his having to touch certain objects up to four times.

Mr V has remained somewhat symptomatic, but he has not wanted to proceed with a trial of behavior therapy or consider a change in medication. He has, however, continued to function fairly well at work and home.

With cost containment and other economic issues continuing to drive changes in medical practice in the United States, it is likely that the role of primary care physicians will continue to expand. Increasingly, these practitioners will have an additional burden of acting as effective gatekeepers who must make appropriate referrals to a variety of specialty care physicians and other caregivers. Although many primary care physicians routinely refer their patients with OCD to psychiatrists, these practitioners are increasingly being asked to handle the pharmacologic aspects of treatment in conjunction with a behavior therapist or other health care provider. These physicians must therefore possess a good understanding of the clinical management of OCD and set a reasonable standard for the level of comfort beyond which a referral to a psychiatrist should be made. Some helpful reminders of the basic tenets of OCD treatment are presented in the *Pearls & Perils* box.

CONSIDER CONSULTATION WHEN...

- The patient presents with atypical symptoms (e.g., a pervasive lack of insight).
- The patient quickly terminates multiple medication trials secondary to perceived side effects.
- Prominent symptoms persist after a trial of an SRI of typically adequate dose and duration.
- Symptoms worsen after the start of a medication trial.
- The patient's symptoms include avoidance behavior or rituals, and the treating physician is unfamiliar with behavior therapy.
- The patient has a comorbid psychiatric disorder with which the treating physician lacks expertise.
- The patient's symptom exacerbations appear to be associated with recent streptococcal infections.
- The patient presents with suicidal ideation or plan or has made a recent suicide attempt.
- The patient has a history of bipolar disorder or develops manic symptoms in response to an SRI.

Treatment of obsessive-compulsive disorder

PEARLS & PERILS

- Make patients aware of the relative efficacy and side effects of available therapies.
- Higher medication dosages may be needed than those typically used to treat depression.
- Time to respond is longer than in depression, so increase medication dose slowly.
- Risk of relapse may be increased with abrupt discontinuation of medication.
- Lower doses may achieve comparable effects with fewer side effects later in treatment.
- Behavior therapy is beneficial for most OCD sufferers, but remains underutilized.
- Use the Y-BOCS to screen for additional OCD symptoms even when the diagnosis is not in doubt. The patient almost always has other symptoms not appreciated as OCD-related.
- Use the Y-BOCS to monitor treatment response. OCD patients often forget early gains.
- Educate family members regarding alternatives to offering the sufferer reassurance.
- Self-help groups (i.e., Obsessive Compulsive Foundation (OCF)) allow the patient and family to meet others with similar difficulties and hear how these individuals have coped and progressed.

OCD is a fascinating illness in which each sufferer may have diverse symptoms requiring individualized treatment. Research aimed at improving our understanding of the pathophysiology underlying OCD is ongoing; it also may lead to a better understanding of normal brain functioning. Although the treatment of patients with OCD may be time-consuming, it is extremely satisfying to assist these individuals in their attempts to regain the freedoms that we so readily take for granted.

Annotated bibliography

Foa, EB and Wilson, R (1991) *Stop Obsessing! How to overcome your obsessions and compulsions*, Bantam Doubleday Dell, New York.
This breakthrough book, written by internationally renowned authorities on treating anxiety disorders, has already helped thousands of people enjoy a life free from excessive fears and rituals. This newly revised edition incorporates even more effective exercises.

Jenike, MA, Baer, L, and Minichiello, WE (eds) (1998) *Obsessive-compulsive Disorders: Practical management*, 3rd Edition, Mosby, Chicago, IL.
A text for medical and other professionals that provides an excellent review of the clinical presentation, assessment, treatment, and underlying pathophysiology of OCD.

March, JS and Mulle, K (1998) *OCD in Children and Adolescents: A cognitive-behavioral treatment manual*, The Guilford Press, New York.
This manual describes a cognitive-behavioral treatment for OCD symptoms in children that incorporates insights from the authors' extensive clinical experience. Rating scales, patient handouts, and resources for parents are also included.

Penzel, F (2000) *Obsessive-compulsive Disorders: A complete guide to getting well and staying well*, New York, Oxford University Press.
This book was written to help sufferers, their families, and those who would help them and discusses the entire spectrum of these disorders, from the classic form characterized by intrusive, repetitive, and often unpleasant thoughts to body dysmorphic disorder, trichotillomania, compulsive skin picking, and compulsive nail biting.

Schwartz, JM and Beyette, B (1997) *Brain lock: Free yourself from obsessive-compulsive behavior*, HarperCollins, New York.
Dr Schwartz's revolutionary Four-Step method helps patients defeat their irrational impulses by a process of Relabeling, Reattributing, Refocusing, and Revaluing.

CHAPTER 11

Cognitive Disorders: Delirium and Amnestic Disorder

Keith E. Isenberg, MD

Introduction

Cognitive disorders involve impairments of memory and information processing that represent a loss of previous capacity. Diagnostic criteria for delirium, dementia, and amnestic disorder facilitate the recognition of these syndromes. Current nosology (DSM-IV-TR) etiologically relates the specific syndromes to nonpsychiatric disorders ("due to a general medical condition") or specific substances causing either intoxication or implicated in withdrawal ("substance-induced"). The term *organic mental disorder* was deleted from DSM-IV because the word *organic* was felt to imply that other psychiatric disorders (or "nonorganic" syndromes) were not associated with biological findings. Dementias (chronic brain syndromes associated with memory impairment and other cognitive deficits) are discussed in this chapter primarily as they pertain to the differential diagnosis of delirium and amnestic disorder; further description of dementia can be found in Chapter 12.

This chapter focuses on delirium, a disorder characterized by the acute onset of altered consciousness and change in cognition or perception, and amnestic disorder, memory impairment in the absence of other significant cognitive deficits. Classification of delirium and amnestic disorder as caused by drugs or general medical disorders recognizes the importance of extrinsic factors in the causation of both syndromes. In a specific patient, delirium and amnestic disorder may both occur as a result of the same etiological factor, such as alcohol use. The amnestic disorder associated with alcoholism, Korsakoff's syndrome, is often preceded by a delirium, Wernicke's encephalopathy. Delirium and amnestic disorder are considered separately because delirium, like dementia, is a manifestation of global cognitive dysfunction, whereas amnestic disorder is a relatively specific impairment of memory. The purpose of this chapter is to provide a systematic approach to these disorders that enhances the prevention, recognition, and treatment of the disorders.

Delirium

Diagnosis

Delirium is characterized by the rapid onset of impaired consciousness and perceptual changes or altered cognition; the syndrome typically has a fluctuating course. Regardless of the cause of delirium, evidence should exist to support the presence of DSM-IV-TR Criteria A, B, and C (Box 11.1).

Etiological specification directs interventions aimed at alleviating delirium. The assignment of Not Otherwise Specified (NOS) should be rare. Physicians have long associated these clinical findings with numerous medical conditions, attaching various names to delirium. The historical lack of uniform terminology and the often subtle onset of delirium probably contribute to underdiagnosis of the syndrome. Timely recognition and treatment of delirium improve the quality of patient care and may reduce the use of services. Consistent features of the syndrome are described in Table 11.1, and suggestions for eliciting common symptoms can be found in Box 11.2, which outlines an examination to establish the presence of signs of delirium.

Although much of the information can be gleaned from direct examination, interview and evaluation of collateral sources may be critical, particularly for a patient who is stuporous or obtunded. Case 11.1 provides an example of the complexities that may be involved in evaluating acute mental status changes. The symptoms associated with delirium are readily apparent in this case, and appropriate management is described. This case illustrates most of the important conditions associated with delirium: drug intoxication, sedative-hypnotic (including alcohol) withdrawal, and

Box 11.1 Delirium

DIAGNOSTIC CRITERIA

A. Disturbance of consciousness (i.e., reduced clarity of awareness of the environment) with reduced ability to focus, sustain, or shift attention.

B. A change in cognition (such as memory deficit, disorientation, language disturbance) or the development of a perceptual disturbance that is not better accounted for by a preexisting, established, or evolving dementia.

C. The disturbance develops over a short period of time (usually hours to days) and tends to fluctuate during the course of the day.

Delirium due to a general medical condition
   There is evidence from the history, physical examination, or laboratory findings that the disturbance is caused by the direct physiological consequences of a general medical condition.

Substance intoxication delirium
   There is evidence from the history, physical examination, or laboratory findings of either 1 or 2:

   1 the symptoms in criteria A and B developed during substance intoxication
   2 medication use is etiologically related to the disturbance.

Substance withdrawal delirium
   There is evidence from the history, physical examination, or laboratory findings that the symptoms in criteria A and B developed during, or shortly after, a withdrawal syndrome.

Delirium due to multiple etiologies
   There is evidence from the history, physical examination, or laboratory findings that the delirium has more than one etiology (e.g., more than one etiological general medical condition, a general medical condition plus substance intoxication or medication side effect).

Delirium not otherwise specified
   This category should be used to diagnose a delirium that does not meet criteria for any of the specific types of delirium described above.

Modified from American Psychiatric Association (2000) Diagnostic and Statistical Manual of Mental Disorders, 4th Edition, Text Revision, Washington, D.C., American Psychiatric Association.

Table 11.1 Delirium

DIAGNOSIS

Discriminating features

1 Waxing and waning awareness.
2 Acute onset of cognitive dysfunction.

Consistent features

1 Disorientation, usually to time.
2 Memory impairment, particularly recent memory.
3 Hallucinations, typically visual, and misperceptions.
4 Language dysfunction, such as an impaired ability to name objects.
5 Definable cause.

Variable features

1 Hyperactivity and/or hypoactivity.
2 Mood disturbance.
3 Alteration in sleep-wake cycle.
4 Delusions.
5 Impaired judgment.
6 Dreamlike experience for patient.

environment. Although the disturbance of consciousness may be manifested as "clouding" or somnolence, delirium is more generally associated with reduced responsiveness to the surroundings. During examination, the patient may respond to questions by perseverating with the answer to a previously asked question. It may be necessary to repeat questions because the patient is distracted by irrelevant stimuli. The reduced awareness may be so severe that it is impossible to interview the patient. Interviews of collateral sources (such as family or hospital staff) may be necessary to establish onset of reduced awareness. The patient described in Case 11.1 was usually inattentive and often lethargic.

Disturbances of cognition, a critical aspect of delirium, can affect orientation, memory, and language. Individuals without delirium can respond to name (oriented to name), provide an appropriate name for the current location (oriented to place), and know the day, month, season, and year with accuracy for the date within one or two days (oriented to date). Disorientation may be the first sign of mild delirium. Confusion regarding the date is common, disorientation to place is probably less common, and disorientation to name is rare in delirium. Although disorientation may be observed in other disorders, such as dementia and mental retardation, a recent change in a previously oriented person suggests delirium. The patient in Case 11.1 was, at times, oriented only to name.

Memory impairment usually involves recent events and affects the quality of the history elicited from the patient. Recall, which is also involved, can be assessed by asking the patient to remember several unrelated items or a simple sentence, making certain that the information was processed

metabolic encephalopathy. Each condition probably played a role in this case, which is indicative of multifactorial etiology. Finally, hospital course was prolonged and the postdischarge outcome, placement in a nursing home, was poor; these are unfortunately common results of delirium.

Clinical features

Patients with delirium have an impaired awareness of the

Evaluation of delirium

Disturbance of consciousness

- Patient may be difficult to arouse. For instance, patient may have evidence of excessive sleepiness during the examination, in the chart, or from collateral sources.
- Patient may not attend to a question or task because of a lack of focus.
- Patient may not complete an answer to a question or complete a task because he or she is distractible, showing a failure to sustain attention.
- Patient may not be able to shift attention as indicated by perseveration in speech or task.
- Patient may have difficulty repeating numbers (digit span) or reverse spelling (e.g., of a common word such as "world") because of inattention.

Change in cognition

- Patient may be disoriented to person, place, and/or time.
- Patient may have problems involving memory and ability to recall.
  - Short-term memory may be examined by having the patient repeat three unrelated words (also a test of attention) and then recall those words five minutes later, prompting with categories if unprompted effort is unsuccessful.
  - Examine the patient's recall of recent events (social, personal).
  - Examine the patient's recall of remote events (historical, personal).
- Evaluate language. For example: see whether the patient can name objects such as a watch, pencil, or key. Document inappropriate word use or word substitution.
- Patient may have altered perception. For example: illusions, hallucinations.

Acute onset and fluctuating course

- This information may be obtained both by observation of the patient and from collateral sources such as the patient's family, facility staff, or chart.

by requesting that the patient repeat the provided information. (Failure to attend to the task is indicative of impaired attention.) After involving the patient in other tasks for several minutes (for example, by gathering more history or performing other aspects of the mental status examination), an inquiry is made about the remembered material. Remote memory is relatively spared. Like orientation, the patient's memory in Case 11.1 was impaired. At worst, the patient was unable to give accurate information about his family (compatible with loss of remote memory); even when he was mildly affected, the patient had difficulty with recall.

Language dysfunction can be manifested as an impaired ability to name objects. Speech may be rambling, perhaps re-lated to an inability to attend to tasks, or incoherent, because of unpredictable switching from topic to topic. The patient described in Case 11.1 was difficult to interview because of rambling speech.

Perceptual disturbances associated with delirium include illusions and hallucinations. Illusions represent the improper labeling of stimuli. Body parts may be perceived as distorted, shadows as real objects, and loud sounds as threatening. Hallucinations represent perceptual experiences in the absence of relevant stimuli. Hallucinations may be simple, such as the visualization of stars or lights, or they may be complex with a patient conversing with nonexistent visitors. When present, illusions and hallucinations can be associated with delusions, or false beliefs that are not shared with others (such as the patient's family). For example, the misinterpretation of a loud sound as a gunshot may be elaborated into an execution, and a patient may become afraid of being the next to be executed. Hallucinated visitors may be described as stealing things or as messengers from God. In delirium, illusions and hallucinations tend to be fragmentary, transitory, and visual.

The perceptual disturbances of delirium have been compared with those reported in dreams. Clearly, the experience of illusions and hallucinations has a bizarre aspect that is shared with many dreams. Interestingly, patients afflicted with multiple episodes of delirium may have similar perceptual disturbances during each episode. At times, particularly in the evening, the patient described in Case 11.1 attended to nonexistent visual stimuli. When disoriented to place, he substituted locations other than the hospital and acted as if the substitutions were valid, a form of confabulation that is delusional. Management of the patient was complicated by assaultive behavior towards staff that occurred as the result of perceptual symptoms.

Symptoms of delirium develop rapidly on a time scale measured in hours to days. The patient in Case 11.1 had an acute onset in the immediate postoperative period. Presentation of mild delirium can be subtle because of the fluctuating course. Careful review of the patient's chart may reveal a notation by hospital staff of "confusion" at night 1–2 days before more obvious manifestations of delirium. The sleep-wake cycle may be disturbed, with somnolence during the day and agitated insomnia at night. Case 11.1 describes a patient who was alert and knowledgeable at times, only to decompensate at other times, particularly in the evening. Variation in awareness may further tax a patient's comprehension of events; sleep and dreaming fade into the hallucinations and somnolence of delirium. Numerous medical personnel documented an acute onset and a fluctuating course for the patient described in Case 11.1. The individual arriving in the office or emergency room with delirium and no collateral source may be a diagnostic problem because the patient may not be able to provide a reliable history.

Mr S was admitted to outpatient surgery for transurethral resection of what proved to be a bladder carcinoma. The patient was premedicated with 100 μg of fentanyl (a narcotic), 1.5 mg of midazolam (a benzodiazepine), and 15 mg of ephedrine (a sympathomimetic, used as a pressor during spinal anesthesia), all given intravenously. The operation was performed without complication while the patient was under spinal anesthesia, which was chosen because of a history of heavy alcohol consumption. After the procedure, 1 g of vancomycin (an antibiotic) was given intravenously.

During recovery the patient complained of bladder pain, which was managed with 10 mg of oxybutynin (an anticholinergic) given orally. When this did not alleviate the complaints, repeated doses of intravenous meperidine (a narcotic) to a total dose of 190 mg were also given. The patient was agitated, confused, and unable to follow commands, necessitating a prolonged stay in the recovery room and repeated doses of midazolam to a total dose of 8 mg. Vital signs, including oxygen saturation per pulse oximetry, were unremarkable, but as the patient's mental status deteriorated, blood pressure increased to 190/95 and was managed with 5 mg of labetalol (a selective α_1 and nonselective β adrenergic antagonist) given intravenously.

The patient was transferred from the recovery room to the urology ward, where agitation, diaphoresis, combativeness, orientation only to person and place, and inability to follow commands were noted. These symptoms were worse at night. At times the patient was observed to be lethargic, particularly during the day. The physical examination was not revealing. The patient was afebrile; his electrolytes and complete blood count (CBC) were unremarkable. The internist noted a history of heavy drinking and suggested postoperative delirium caused by alcohol withdrawal. Symptoms were managed with haloperidol (a neuroleptic) and various benzodiazepines.

The patient was transferred from the urology ward to the medicine ward three days postoperatively because his mental status had improved only slightly. The patient was initially noted to be tremulous, uncooperative, and oriented to person, month, and year, but he did not know the place. Electrolytes were within normal limits; magnesium was normal. Elevated creatine kinase (peaked at 946 IU/ml 3 days postoperatively), not associated with a cardiac source, was judged to be from agitation. The creatine kinase returned to normal over the next several days. Serum glutamic oxaloacetic transaminase (SGOT; aspartate aminotransferase [AST]) and lactate dehydrogenase (LDH) were elevated slightly (twice normal) but decreased to normal; serum glutamate pyruvate transferase (SGPT; alanine aminotransferase (ALT)) and bilirubin were normal. Total protein and albumin were slightly decreased. Orientation and cooperation continued to vary remarkably over the course of a day.

A neurology consultant agreed that the patient was suffering from delirium tremens and thought the patient had peripheral neuropathy and chronic cognitive dysfunction secondary to alcohol abuse. He recommended oral and intramuscular vitamin supplementation, including thia-

mine, as well as continued use of chlordiazepoxide. An ammonia level, recommended by the neurologist, was within normal limits four days postoperatively.

Six days postoperatively, a psychiatrist was consulted. He noted a chief complaint of, "Do you have a match?" The patient was oriented to person but not to place; however, he was able to give the day, month, and year, missing the date by three days. His fund of knowledge was good; for example, he gave the full names of the president, the vice-president, and the president's wife. Simple contrasts and comparisons were performed without difficulty. The patient recalled three of three items immediately and two of three items at five minutes despite prompting. The family noted concerns about preexisting chronic cognitive impairment, suggestive of alcoholic dementia in addition to delirium. The psychiatrist confirmed the diagnosis of alcohol dependence, concurred with the diagnosis of delirium tremens, and agreed that further evaluation, particularly for central nervous system (CNS) lesions (such as metastatic tumor to the brain) was wise. Computed tomography (CT) of the head with contrast was obtained 1 week postoperatively and showed two small, ill-defined foci of low attenuation consistent with prior ischemic disease but otherwise normal for age. The patient was switched from chlordiazepoxide and diazepam (long half-life benzodiazepines) to lorazepam (a short half-life benzodiazepine), facilitating the intermittent administration of an intramuscular benzodiazepine for severe agitation and minimizing the risk of drug accumulation.

Persistent confusion ten days after the operation led to a search for causes of delirium other than alcohol withdrawal. The CBC, electrolytes, and other blood chemistries were repeated and were within normal limits or much improved relative to initial evaluations. The patient was afebrile and cultures of blood and urine were negative. Thyroid studies were unremarkable, as were B_{12} and folate levels. An electroencephalogram (EEG) obtained 11 days postoperatively showed background slowing indicative of a mild diffuse encephalopathy. The patient had an elevated ammonia level of 44.5 μmol/L (expected range 9 to 33 μmol/L) 12 days postoperatively; the elevated ammonia persisted throughout the remainder of the hospitalization. Consultation among the specialists involved suggested that no further workup was indicated, a recommendation accepted by the patient's family. Benzodiazepines were discontinued; efforts to manage a sleep-wake disturbance and psychosis with haloperidol failed, but the patient slept through the night on 25 mg of thioridazine (a neuroleptic) taken at bedtime every night. The patient was felt to have chronic hepatic encephalopathy and was transferred to a nursing home facility on a 30-g protein diet.

Mr S's cognitive function and ammonia levels were followed in the nursing home during a two-month recuperation. Thioridazine was tapered and discontinued. Memory and cognition improved gradually but substantially; ammonia levels slowly returned to normal. At the time of discharge from the nursing home facility, the patient was without clinically obvious signs of delirium or dementia.

Other symptoms of delirium show greater variability (see Box 11. 3) and are discussed before etiology is systematically considered. Many symptoms variably present in delirium were previously regarded as critical components of the syndrome; however, the simplified criteria codified in DSM-IV-TR should facilitate diagnosis by avoiding the requirement of these more variable features of delirium.

Delirium is usually associated with a disturbance of motor activity. Patients may be described as hyperactive compared with their usual selves; hypoactive compared with their usual selves; or suffering from a mixture, with hypoactivity on some occasions and hyperactivity at others. Hyperactivity is manifest as a purposeless restlessness that may make management particularly difficult. It has been suggested that management difficulties (e.g., the patient removing various medical devices, wandering the halls, and entering other patients' rooms) bring the hyperactive variant of delirium to medical attention more often than the hypoactive variant. The patient in Case 11.1 was hyperactive at times, particularly at night. Delirium tremens represents a classical hyperactive delirium. Individuals with delirium who are hypoactive tend to show little spontaneous movement and are more likely to make little effort to assist in self-care even if they are apparently awake. This hypoactivity can merge into the inactivity of stupor. The patient described in Case 11.1 notes daytime lethargy. Solvent exposure can be associated with a quiet delirium that may proceed to respiratory or cardiac arrest and death. Fluctuation in course, a critical component of delirium, may be observed as a variation in motor activity, with the patient being inactive at times (perhaps during the day) and hyperactive at other times (perhaps during the evening), as exemplified by Case 11.1.

Mood disturbance is an important aspect of delirium that, like motor activity, does not lend itself to simple description and classification. Aberrant mood is apparently fueled to some extent by the perceptual experiences of the patient who is delirious. The patient who experiences hallucinations with an amusing content may be jocular and euphoric. More commonly the patient suffers from depressed mood and morbid perceptual disturbances, which may place the patient at risk of suicide. A fearful mood is probably most common, and even familiar surroundings can be perceived as threatening. For example, the patient who is delirious may find vivid hallucinations of snakes and insects unbearable. The individual in Case 11.1 was usually irritable.

Current diagnostic criteria recognize the importance of psychotic symptoms in delirium by specifying the presence of perceptual disturbances or memory impairment. The implication of this approach is that psychotic symptoms such as visual hallucinations need not be invariably present. Language disturbance can be of psychotic proportion, with the disjointed speech suggestive of a formal thought disorder. Although it seems plausible that the presence of psychotic symptoms in delirium would have treatment implications,

this has not been demonstrated. Indeed, delirium tremens, a typically psychotic disorder, is better treated with benzodiazepines than antipsychotics.

Disturbances of perception and memory leave the individual who is delirious vulnerable to the consequences of impaired judgment. The agitated patient may be particularly difficult to manage because he or she is less readily redirectable by verbal approaches. An inability to distinguish reality from hallucinations and delusions facilitates behavior that puts the patient at risk of harm to self or others. Impaired judgment, occurring in many psychiatric disorders, is not specific to delirium.

Neurological signs are commonly seen in delirium. Some types of delirium have been classically associated with specific signs, such as asterixis in hepatic encephalopathy or ataxia and ophthalmoplegia in Wernicke's encephalopathy. The suggestion that these signs are part of specific syndromes of delirium has led some scholars to suggest that classification of delirium ought to be type-specific. However, neurological signs are not invariably present in any etiologically specific syndrome, nor is any sign syndrome-specific. Specifying subsyndromes of delirium based on the presence of particular neurological signs appears untenable. A general, simplified approach to diagnosing acute cognitive impairment, exemplified by DSM-IV-TR, enhances recognition of delirium.

Classification of delirium as a reversible disorder, as specified by older nosologies, ignores the mortality associated with the condition. Delirium is a common feature of the final stages of disorders such as various cancers and congestive heart failure. Treatment of delirium when death is expected minimizes the distressing impact of psychotic symptoms. The designation of delirium as *reversible* appears to have been intended to facilitate distinguishing delirium from the relatively irreversible dementias. Delirium in patients who are chronically cognitively impaired appears to be associated with persistent residual symptoms, perhaps accelerating the course of dementia but more importantly suggesting irreversible changes induced by delirium. Criteria that emphasize reversibility are likely to exacerbate the failure to recognize delirium in patients who are demented or dying.

Psychometric evaluation of patients who are delirious is not very useful clinically. Instruments are available that allow screening for cognitive impairment, such as the Mini-Mental State Examination (MMSE), or help physicians rate the symptoms of delirium, such as the Delirium Rating Scale. The interpretation of instruments that screen for cognitive impairment is confounded by intelligence, educational attainment, and socioeconomic status, which are interrelated variables. The use of screening and rating instruments typically requires that the patient participate systematically in the evaluation. Consciousness is particularly difficult to rate reliably. Furthermore, fluctuating course may permit a mild delirium to go undetected if the patient does not have

TABLE 11.2

Causes of delirium

	Percentage			
	Purdie, Honigman, and Rosen, 1981 (n = 100)	Newton and Janati, 1986 (n = 100)	Sirois, 1988 (n = 100)	Francis, Martin and Kapoor, 1990 (n = 50)
Drug intoxication	22	17	9	14
Withdrawal	6	—	13	—
Metabolic	6	43	19	4
Intracranial	15	10	15	2
Infection	8	12	6	8
Fluid and electrolyte imbalance	3	12	4	8
Functional	16	—	—	—
Postsurgical	—	6	—	—
Multiple	24	—	34	64

Categories correspond roughly to those employed in a prospective study of delirium in the elderly (Francis, Martin, and Kapoor, 1990). Adjustments were made to reflect conditions that were found in the other series and relevance to the general practitioner. Categories such as drug intoxication or infection apply to patients who appear to have delirium as the result of processes related to this category only. One series (Newton and Janati, 1986) does not appear to have considered multiple causes as a category. The relative contribution of each category to the etiology of delirium in each case series is likely to reflect the diagnostic criteria employed for the diagnosis of delirium, the criteria for etiological assignment, and most relevant to the primary care physician, referral bias. For example, one retrospective series of patients seen by psychiatric consultants (Newton and Janati, 1986) notes referral for evaluation of delirium after anesthesia in six instances, a cause of delirium that is likely to be rare in samples generated from hospital admissions (Purdie, Honigman, and Rosen, 1981; Francis, Martin, and Kapoor, 1990). A study of elderly patients excluded nursing home admissions and patients with dementia (Francis, Martin, and Kapoor) although poor predelirium functioning is likely to increase the risk of delirium and alter etiological classification (Purdie, Honigman, and Rosen). The elderly, perhaps because of multiple medical problems, may be particularly likely to suffer from a multifactorial disorder.

significant impairment at the time of examination. Lethargy and uncooperativeness, problems noted in Case 11.1, limit the use of screening instruments. Prospective studies of delirium are complicated by the significant number of cases that were probably undetected because patients could not participate in the systematic evaluation required for reliable research. Screening instruments and rating scales are not as specific to delirium as would be desired; the difficulty of employing screening and rating instruments in systematic studies suggests caution in the clinical implementation of such approaches. The physician is advised to incorporate questions about orientation and memory into every examination and make the diagnosis of delirium based on history, physical evaluation, and laboratory tests, minimizing the use of psychometric techniques.

Ascertaining the cause of delirium often leads directly to intervention, appropriate treatment of the cause and ideally to resolution of the delirium. Case 11.1 is illustrative of the process of determining specific causes of delirium. Additionally, Table 11.1 lists causes of delirium as reported in four case series.

DSM-IV-TR describes the following four broad etiological diagnostic categories for delirium: (1) substance-induced delirium, either during intoxication or withdrawal; (2) delirium caused by a general medical condition; (3) delirium resulting from multiple etiologies; and (4) delirium NOS.

Etiology is considered within the framework proposed in DSM-IV-TR and uses the categories outlined in Table 11.2. An exhaustive list of diagnostic possibilities is beyond the scope of this presentation; the physician is encouraged to review other sources for a more complete presentation of etiological possibilities (see Annotated bibliography).

Drug intoxication is arguably the most important etiological category because in some cases delirium is preventable. Drug-intoxication delirium specifically refers to the direct effect of drugs on the brain rather than an indirect effect mediated by systemic toxicity. Intoxication may arise during the administration of drugs at usually effective doses and is thus a side effect of treatment. Intoxication may also arise when doses of a medication larger than those usually recommended are used therapeutically as part of the treatment plan, when larger than usual doses are taken in an intentional or accidental overdose, or when drugs are taken illegally for recreational purposes. Delirium can occur as the result of accidental or intentional exposure to an inducing substance in a work setting. Finally, delirium *may* occur as the result of intentional poisoning. Recreational drug use, occupational exposure, and intentional poisoning often involve compounds with which most physicians are unlikely to be familiar (such as organic solvents or heavy metals). Consideration of these drugs as etiological agents may benefit from consultation with more knowledgeable specialists (physicians familiar

TABLE 11.3

Therapeutic agents associated with drug-intoxication delirium

Analgesics:
  Narcotics (meperidine)
  Nonsteroidal anti-inflammatory drugs
  Acetaminophen
Anesthetics
Antiasthmatics (theophylline)
Anticholinergics:
  Procedure premedicants (atropine)
  Tricyclic antidepressants and related compounds
    (amitriptyline, maprotiline)
  Antiemetics (meclizine)
  *Antipsychotics (chlorpromazine)
  CNS-active antihistamines (diphenhydramine)
  Antiparkinsonians (benztropine)
  Cycloplegics and mydriatics (atropine)
  Proprietary medications (atropine, scopolamine)
Anticonvulsants (any)
Antihypertensives (beta-blockers such as propranolol or
  methyldopa)
Antimicrobials (antibiotics, antifungal antiprotozoans,
  antivirals, etc)
Antineoplastics (methotrexate, procarbazine)
Bismuth compounds

Cardiac compounds (digitalis, lidocaine)
Cholinesterase inhibitors
Corticosteroids
Gastrointestinal drugs:
  H_2 antagonists (cimetidine)
  Proton pump inhibitors
Herbal medications (jimsonweed, pennyroyal, ma huang,
    eucalyptus; all herbal remedies can also be implicated in drug-drug
    interactions and symptomatology due to adulteration)

Immunosuppressants
Intravenous immunoglobulins
Lithium
Monoclonal antibodies
Muscle relaxants
Antiparkinsonian agents (levodopa [L-dopa])
Antidepressants (any)
Sedative-hypnotics (any)
  Barbiturates
  Ethanol
  Benzodiazepines
Vaccines

These drugs are associated with delirium because of their direct effects on the CNS. General classes of compounds are listed, followed by notation in parentheses of appropriate specific important examples. In some cases, multiple compounds appear to present a similar risk (such as antibiotics and anticonvulsants). In others, a specific drug (cimetidine, for example) appears to pose an increased risk relative to other compounds from that class.

* Also may be associated with a nonanticholinergic delirium (e.g., neuroleptic malignant syndrome).

with the effects of drugs of abuse, such as emergency room physicians, psychiatrists, occupational medicine physicians, toxicologists, and forensic specialists). The elderly and the medically ill, particularly those with CNS disease, are likely to be at greater risk of delirium from drug intoxication than the young and healthy.

Any prescribed drug is a possible cause of delirium, particularly in patients who are at risk for delirium (Table 11.3). After establishing the presence of clinical signs indicative of delirium, a thorough medication history should be obtained. A list of recently prescribed and current medications should be reviewed to note dose, particularly in relation to usually efficacious doses and duration of treatment relative to the onset of symptoms. The initiation of treatment with a medication in the hours or days before the onset of delirium should heighten suspicion that this drug plays a role in the disorder. Consideration should be given to obtaining drug levels; levels are helpful for compounds like lithium and the anticonvulsants. The decision to obtain a drug level should be partly dependent on an estimate of the need for continuing therapy with each specific drug. Drug levels can only

serve as a guide because toxicity has been documented in some cases (involving lithium or anticonvulsants, for example) at therapeutic levels. Toxicological screens of blood and urine, as well as screens for drugs of abuse, that employ standard testing batteries may be helpful, particularly for patients without collateral sources. Consultation regarding testing for nonprescribed substances may be helpful if recreational drugs, occupational exposure, or poisoning are suspected.

The task of medication evaluation is more straightforward for the primary care physician than the consultant, given greater patient familiarity. In some cases, drugs are discontinued but, because of the recurrence of symptoms for which the drug is indicated, need to be added back. The physician with knowledge of the patient's longitudinal course is in the best position to assess benefits, risks, and alternatives in this circumstance. The assessment of pharmacological risks and benefits is a recurring task as long as the patient remains delirious, since drugs administered to manage the patient who is delirious can exacerbate or cause delirium (see Case 11.1 and the following paragraphs). A useful rule of thumb is that CNS-active drugs are more likely culprits in causing delirium than compounds with little or no known CNS effect.

Anesthetics may be associated with delirium (Table 11.3). Some classes of anesthetics (barbiturates, benzodiazepines, and opioids) are associated with delirium when used for other purposes (see below). A difficulty in attributing delirium to a specific anesthetic utilization is that anesthetics are associated with procedures. Each patient brings a specific risk profile to a procedure, hopefully well defined in advance but never a complete certainty, and, even for elective procedures, some deficit in well-being is the basis for subjecting the patient to the intervention. This profile has some effect on the risk of any and all complications but may particularly have an impact on the risk of delirium. In turn, procedures may have relatively specific risks (e.g., chemical peritonitis and cholecystectomy) as well as more general complications (pneumonia) that contribute to the appearance of delirium. Most procedures involve exposure to more than one anesthetic agent. Disentangling an association between an anesthetic or a type of anesthetic and delirium is thus complicated by host and procedure risks. Even when a particular drug is implicated as a risk factor for delirium (e.g., meperidine—see below), the risk is small and other options (e.g., morphine, fentanyl) are not risk-free. Case 11.1 illustrates the complexities of disentangling the effects of anesthesia from other factors. Concerns about the risk of general anesthesia influenced the treatment team to chose spinal anesthesia rather than expose a patient with alcoholism to general anesthesia. Many small, randomized clinical trials suggest that regional anesthesia carries the same risk for delirium as general anesthesia. Despite the efforts of the treatment team to minimize the risk of general anesthesia, the patient developed delirium.

Drugs with anticholinergic properties are an especially important cause of delirium (see Table 11.3). The observation that belladonna alkaloids, mixtures of atropine and scopolamine, cause delirium dates to antiquity. Atropine and scopolamine intoxication are associated with dilated pupils, blurred vision, flushed face, dry skin and mucous membranes, tachycardia, diminished or absent bowel sounds, urinary retention, increased blood pressure, and fever. Unfortunately, these signs are usually absent in the case of delirium associated with other potent antimuscarinic drugs, such as tricyclic antidepressants (TCAs), which have many other effects (antihistaminic, for example). The weight of current evidence favors anticholinergic effects as the most likely cause of delirium for the classes of drugs listed under the anticholinergic headings in Table 11.3. Physostigmine, an inhibitor of acetylcholinesterase, can be given intravenously to reverse anticholinergic delirium and should be used in severe poisoning. However, the increase in cholinergic tone may be associated with side effects that can be severe (such as bradycardia). Physostigmine also has a short half-life, so it

should be used judiciously. Anticholinergic drugs have been used to induce delirium in experimental settings, and the apparent importance of cholinergic mechanisms in cognition suggests a more general role for this system in the etiology of delirium. Just before the onset of delirium, the patient described in Case 11.1 received a relatively typical dose of the anticholinergic drug oxybutynin to facilitate bladder emptying. Although this drug is a potent antimuscarinic agent with occasional CNS side effects, delirium appears to be a relatively uncommon problem. Despite the appearance of delirium shortly after the administration of oxybutynin, the drug probably had little to do with the disorder in this case.

Drugs with sedative-hypnotic properties are associated with delirium. Medications in this class, including alcohol, are associated with intoxication, which has symptoms that overlap with delirium. Severe intoxication that is persistent and associated with the need for extensive evaluation and treatment is indicative of delirium. Historically, bromide compounds were associated with severe and prolonged delirium; these compounds are rarely used at present. Barbiturates are associated with delirium, but indications for the use of drugs from this class have narrowed considerably over the years. Barbiturate-induced delirium may be as likely from illicit use as from therapeutic administration. Benzodiazepines have replaced barbiturates for many indications and are probably less likely to be the sole agent inducing delirium. The sedative and amnestic effects of benzodiazepines may contribute to delirium in patients with multiple causes of delirium. For example, benzodiazepines have been implicated as a risk factor for postoperative delirium. Other sedative hypnotics (for example, chloral hydrate) are associated with intoxication delirium. These compounds, like barbiturates, are probably more likely to cause delirium than benzodiazepines. The most commonly used drug with sedative properties is ethanol; alcohol intoxication is associated with delirium.

The patient described in Case 11.1 required large doses of a short-acting benzodiazepine in the immediate postoperative period, which, although indicated, may have contributed to the patient's delirium. As the patient's illness persisted, he was switched from benzodiazepines with a long half-life and active metabolites (diazepam and chlordiazepoxide) to benzodiazepines with a shorter half-life and essentially no active metabolites (lorazepam) to minimize the risk of exacerbating his condition. Finally, the benzodiazepines were discontinued when a diagnosis of hepatic encephalopathy was suspected, terminating the contribution to delirium by these compounds. It is probable that withdrawal from sedative-hypnotic drugs is a more important cause of delirium than sedative-hypnotic intoxication.

Opioids administered in the recovery room may have exacerbated delirium in the patient in Case 11.1. Meperidine is the opioid most commonly associated with delirium. Perhaps the anticholinergic properties of the meperidine metabolite, normeperidine, contribute to the potential for delirium. Because other opioids may cause delirium, it is prudent to consider any opioid administered to a patient as a possible cause of a delirium. The suspicion that meperidine played a role in the induction of delirium in Case 11.1 is heightened by the observation that the doses employed are at least twofold to threefold greater than usually effective doses. Premedication with fentanyl is unlikely to have played a role in the induction of delirium in Case 11.1 because the drug was used once at a typical dose. Supplementation of opioid analgesia with other approaches (such as acetaminophen or nonsteroidal analgesics) may reduce the risk of opioid delirium.

Multiple other classes of drugs have been implicated in the etiology of delirium (Tables 11.3–11.5). The association of delirium with many therapeutic drugs is often based on a single case, several case reports, or small case series. Information about symptomatology in these reports tends to be poor, and in some cases systemic drug effects (for example, hyponatremia) may account for delirium rather than direct intoxication. Polypharmacy may be a risk factor for delirium, although the risk may be confounded by concurrent medical illnesses that initiated the polypharmacy. A physician suspecting that a drug is involved as the cause of delirium should consider an estimate of the likelihood that a drug has CNS effects. CNS-active drugs (for example, antidepressants) are probably more likely culprits in the cause of delirium than compounds with little or no known CNS effects (most antibiotics, for example). Nevertheless, it is prudent to consider every drug administered to a patient who is delirious as a possible cause. The patient in Case 11.1 received vancomycin, an antibiotic, and ephedrine, a sympathomimetic. Both compounds, particularly the antibiotic, are somewhat unusual causes of delirium, and although the route of administration would favor effects on the brain, they were used at usual doses on a single occasion. It is unlikely that either vancomycin or ephedrine played a role in the observed delirium.

Illicitly used drugs can cause delirium (see Table 11.4); many of these compounds also have therapeutic applications. Knowledge that the individual under consideration has a history of illicit drug or alcohol use should suggest strong consideration of illicit drugs as causative of delirium. Given that young people are more likely to use illicit drugs than the elderly, appearance of delirium in individuals aged 15–30 should prompt consideration of illicit drugs. Finally, some compounds that cause delirium are poisons (see Table 11.5). Detecting delirium from these compounds may require specialized evaluation.

Delirium tremens represents the classic drug withdrawal delirium. Similar withdrawal deliria have been described for withdrawal from various sedative-hypnotics. Although benzodiazepines are less likely to be associated with severe withdrawal than other compounds, withdrawal delirium

TABLE 11.4

Illegally used substances associated with drug intoxication delirium

Amphetamines and related drugs
Cocaine
Hallucinogens (such as lysergic acid diethylamide or LSD)
Inhalants
Marijuana and related drugs
Opioids
Phencyclidine and related drugs
Sedative-hypnotics (including ethanol)

Compounds are listed by class. Some compounds (such as marijuana) may rarely be associated with delirium, whereas others (for example, inhalants) are probably often associated with delirium.

TABLE 11.5

Poisons associated with drug intoxication delirium

Organic solvents	Hydrogen sulfide
Aliphatic hydrocarbons (propane)	Refrigerants (Freon)
Aromatic hydrocarbons (benzene)	Metals (arsenic, mercury, acid lead)
Halogenated hydrocarbons (carbon tetrachloride)	Organophosphate insecticides
Alcohols (ethylene glycol, methanol)	Biological poisons
	Animals (snake or spider venom)
Gasoline and kerosene	Plants (jimsonweed, morning glory)
Carbon monoxide	Mushrooms (Amanita species)
Carbon disulfide	

Classes of toxin are listed and followed by representative examples, when appropriate. Exposure may be accidental (snake or spider venom), occupational (carbon tetrachloride) or the result of intentional poisoning (arsenic). In some cases (organic solvents, refrigerants), exposure may be accidental or part of a pattern of abuse.

has been reported. Although extremely rare, withdrawal delirium has been described for drugs from other classes of therapeutic compounds. The patient in Case 11.1 was known to be a heavy drinker, and when he was carefully interviewed it was shown that he fulfilled criteria for alcohol dependence. No alcohol had been consumed by this person in the 24 hours before the onset of delirium, which is somewhat different from the more usual appearance of delirium tremens 72 to 96 hours after the last drink. The rapid onset of delirium in this patient is suggestive of the involvement of other factors in its onset, although alcohol withdrawal was

TABLE 11.6	**Laboratory evaluation**	
Electrolytes	Calcium
CBC, particularly white blood cell count	Head scan (CT/MRI, with/without contrast)
Glucose	Arterial blood gases
Blood urea nitrogen (BUN)/ creatinine	Venereal disease research laboratory (VDRL)/rapid plasma reagin (RPR)
Electrocardiogram (EKG)	
Urinalysis (urine culture)	Human immunodeficiency virus (HIV)
Chest x-ray (sputum culture)	
Drug toxicology Screen/drug levels	Blood cultures
SGOT/SGPT/LDH, bilirubin, total protein/albumin, ammonia level	Thyroid tests
	B_{12}/folate
	EEG
	Lumbar puncture

probably the most important aspect of the first phase of the delirium.

Patients who develop delirium tremens often have other complicating conditions (for example, malnutrition or infection) and need to be thoroughly evaluated for other causes of delirium. Delirium tremens rarely lasts more than ten days, and when the patient's symptoms of delirium persisted beyond this period, further diagnostic evaluation was performed. The patient in Case 11.1 developed hepatic encephalopathy, probably during the course of delirium tremens.

So many medical conditions are associated with delirium that it is beyond the scope of this chapter to detail most of them. Types of disorder are mentioned in Table 11.2. Sometimes, particularly in the elderly, medical disorders coexist with delirium, with little information from the history or physical examination to provide guidance regarding the cause. Laboratory evaluation may be crucial, and even if a particular cause is clear, it may suggest unsuspected difficulties (such as electrolyte imbalance or drug use). Laboratory tests and procedures to evaluate delirium are listed in Table 11.6 in an order that roughly reflects the complexity, invasiveness, and usefulness of the test. The history and physical examination should suggest a more specific approach, although some patients (most notably the elderly) present problems in a fashion that may merit consideration of evaluative procedures such as EEG.

Metabolic encephalopathies such as hepatic encephalopathy are the most important single type of general medical disorder associated with delirium. Unfortunately, the term *encephalopathy* has been used in various ways, although many neurologists appear to apply the term in a fashion that is similar to the use of *delirium*. The term *metabolic encephalopathy* is used here to describe delirium resulting from the disruption of the internal milieu caused by the failure of usual compensatory mechanisms. Encephalopathy encompasses organ failure, such as occurs in hepatic encephalopathy as well as vitamin deficiencies, such as the lack of thiamine that is thought to underlie Wernicke's encephalopathy. For largely historical reasons, infection and disturbances of fluids and electrolytes are usually not considered metabolic encephalopathies. Intracranial processes, infection, and possibly fluid and electrolyte disturbances are sufficiently common and require a sufficiently distinct diagnostic process that these classes of etiological factors warrant separate consideration.

Metabolic encephalopathies are systemic disorders. Failure of vital organs such as the liver, heart, kidney, and lung is associated with delirium; acute failure may rapidly progress to coma and death. Disorders of endocrine organs such as the pancreas and the thyroid are also associated with delirium. The thyroid and pancreas are interesting because too much activity produces symptoms (such as hyperthyroidism or hypoglycemia from an insulinoma) as well as too little activity (for example, hypothyroidism or diabetes mellitus). Cancer of various kinds can cause delirium through multiple systemic effects, although hypercalcemia is one common mechanism. The systemic effects of cancer, which are potentially correctable, should be distinguished from metastasis to the brain and the toxic effects of treatment (antineoplastics, perhaps interacting with radiotherapy of the brain). In many instances (including hypercapnia and hypercalcemia), it appears that the rapidity with which changes occur is a factor in the development of delirium. The patient who is chronically hypercapnic may tolerate higher levels of CO_2 than the person who develops acute changes.

It is particularly important to distinguish the failure of homeostatic mechanisms, such as those that occur in hepatic encephalopathy, from the toxicity of drugs used to treat problems caused by the failing organ. For example, efforts were made to minimize drug toxicity in Case 11.1, attempting to separate the effects of benzodiazepines and neuroleptics from symptoms caused by alcohol withdrawal and hepatic encephalopathy. The clinical decision to employ neuroleptics (such as haloperidol) rather than benzodiazepines was made on the presumption that neuroleptics would be less toxic to the CNS than benzodiazepines. The longitudinal course of the patient's illness suggested the possibility of hepatic encephalopathy in addition to delirium tremens; the best available laboratory test for hepatic encephalopathy, a measurement of ammonia levels, supported the diagnosis. Although no signs of Wernicke's encephalopathy were observed in this patient, thiamine supplementation (initially parenteral) was provided to treat this disorder and minimize the risk of Korsakoff's syndrome (see the section on amnestic disorders).

Disturbances of fluid (such as dehydration and water intoxication) and electrolytes (for example, increases or decreases in serum sodium or potassium) have been treated separately from the metabolic encephalopathies in many descriptions of delirium. The ability of patients who are medically ill or elderly to regulate water and electrolyte balance is often impaired. Several prospective studies have identified elevations in BUN, largely reflecting dehydration, to be a predictor of delirium. In many cases, problems with fluids and electrolytes arise from or are exacerbated by medication administration, particularly diuretics. Disturbances of fluid and electrolytes are to some extent iatrogenic complications of drug administration. For example, a physician's awareness that medications such as diuretics can cause delirium via hyponatremia should lead to systematic evaluation of fluid and electrolyte status in patients who are at risk. Drugs such as lithium, the TCAs and cisplatin, which are associated with delirium via direct CNS effects, can cause systemic fluid and electrolyte disorders. Disturbances of fluids and electrolytes may be more commonly associated with delirium from multiple causes than with being the sole causes of delirium.

Infection is often associated with delirium, particularly in the elderly. Fever and delirium have been historically associated. Delirium may be a sign of an infection and precede the onset of fever, or delirium may appear at the height of the fever. In some instances, delirium may appear after the fever has resolved. The observation that many elderly people have an infectious delirium without fever suggests that an infection can produce delirium in the absence of fever. Further consideration was given to infectious disease without a fever as a cause for delirium in Case 11.1 when the delirium did not resolve as expected. Some evidence suggests that host susceptibility plays a role in the likelihood that delirium will develop after an infection.

Infections associated with delirium involve numerous organs and various microorganisms. The brain is considered separately because it seems reasonable that the systemic effects of infection, such as those that produce fever, are distinct from the effects of direct involvement of the brain (see below). The numerous types of infectious disease that can cause delirium cannot be adequately considered here, but some general guidance based on available literature can be provided. Given the increased risk of delirium from afebrile infection in the elderly, infection of commonly affected organs (such as the lungs or bladder) should be given priority consideration at presentation. Clear signs of systemic toxicity from a bacteremia should be addressed with cultures, treatment, and consideration of the source.

Infections of the nervous system cause delirium. Viruses such as herpes simplex and influenza cause encephalitis that is associated with delirium; distinguishing the systemic effects of influenza from the direct effects of the virus on the brain may be difficult. Acquired immunodeficiency syndrome (AIDS) causes a dementia that may be preceded by delirium; equally important, the immunocompromised status of these patients predisposes them to other intracranial infectious processes such as cytomegalovirus encephalitis, cryptococcosis, and *Toxoplasma gondii* infection. Delirium is probably a sufficiently unusual symptom of AIDS dementia that consideration of other intracranial processes, such as the noted infections, is wise. Delirium has been associated with various types of meningitis, most notably the pneumococcal and tuberculous types. Asceptic meningitis mimics bacterial meningitis and can be caused by antibiotics, nonsteroidal anti-inflammatory drugs and exposure to intravenous immunoglobulins and monoclonal antibodies.

Bacteria can cause an abscess that presents with delirium, probably as the result of processes similar to other intracranial masses. The presence of infection outside the CNS, particularly in areas of the head near the brain (such as the sinuses or the ear), suggests the diagnosis of abscess. Neurosyphilis can have the symptom-complex of delirium. Various fungal and parasitic conditions may feature delirium as an important aspect of the course. Finally, some individuals develop a postinfectious encephalomyelitis after an infectious illness (usually viral) or after immunization. Delirium is an important part of the course of this illness and is thought to be the result of cell-mediated immunity.

Other intracranial processes are associated with delirium. These heterogeneous disorders represent direct insults to the brain, with acute global impairment as one possible result. Mass lesions, either benign (subdural hematoma) or cancerous (glioblastoma), may have delirium as a presenting complication. Although bladder cancer usually spreads locally, the unusual presentation and course in the patient in Case 11.1 suggested consideration of metastases to the head; an imaging study was obtained despite the minimal evidence of other neurological signs.

Head trauma is commonly associated with delirium. The typical case of head trauma involves a young adult who has been drinking ethanol and is subsequently involved in an accident, suggesting a multifactorial cause for many cases of delirium from head trauma. Loss of consciousness is often followed by delirium. Finally, head trauma can be associated with multiple other injuries, some of which have systemic effects that can cause delirium. The immobility necessary to manage many orthopedic injuries aggravates the course and management of the delirium associated with head trauma.

Epilepsy is associated with delirium, either as an ictal phenomenon, a postictal phenomenon, or an interictal phenomenon. Ictal deliria are associated with generalized absence (petit mal) status and complex partial status, situations that constitute medical emergencies. Postictal and interictal deliria must be distinguished from the toxicity of anticonvulsants.

Several pathological processes involving the vasculature of the CNS are associated with delirium. Infarction, embolism, and hemorrhage can cause delirium. Hypertensive encephalopathy and, less commonly, migraine are associated with delirium. Inflammation and necrosis of CNS vasculature occurs in several vasculitides, most notably systemic lupus erythematosus, and can produce a delirium. All these disorders appear to cause delirium as a direct consequence of CNS involvement.

Inspection of Table 11.1 suggests that the most important cause of delirium is multifactorial. This observation should not be surprising because serious medical illness predisposes a patient to delirium. Furthermore, the patient series with the largest portion of delirium caused by multiple factors is composed of elderly patients who were admitted to a general medical ward, suggesting that age is also a risk factor for delirium from multiple factors. Dementia and other types of preexisting CNS pathologic conditions are thought to predispose a patient to delirium. It seems reasonable to suspect polypharmacy as a risk factor for multifactorial delirium, although underlying medical illnesses may explain much of the increased risk. Regardless of risk factors, many deliria are the result of more than one etiological factor.

One type of typically multifactorial delirium, which occurs after surgery, is particularly interesting since delirium may be the first manifestation of complications. As noted above, delirium has been associated with virtually every type of medical procedure. Cardiovascular surgery, particularly following cardiotomy, is a risk factor for the development of delirium. Independent of surgical repair, fractures seem to be a risk factor for delirium, particularly in the elderly. Similarly, burns may predispose a patient to a multifactorial type of delirium. The onset of agitated postoperative delirium in the recovery room, as occurred with Case 11.1, is thought to develop in about 2% of surgical cases. Other patients become delirious in the days after the procedure, and the rate of delirium in the 30 days after an operation is about 40%. Risk factors associated with delirium after elective surgery include poor preoperative cognitive status, poor preoperative function, and abnormal preoperative serum sodium, potassium, or glucose. The risk associated with abnormal preoperative laboratory test results is particularly important since corrective action before surgery may diminish the risk of delirium. Preoperative evaluation of electrolytes should be part of the preparation for invasive procedures. Drugs associated with an increased risk of postsurgical delirium include ethanol, benzodiazepines, and meperidine; other narcotics are not so clearly associated with increased risk of delirium. Consideration should be given to a period of abstinence or perhaps even specific treatment when elective surgery is planned for a patient suffering from drug or alcohol problems. The patient in Case 11.1 apparently represents an example of a delirium caused by multiple factors, with onset in the immediate postoperative period.

Not all cases of delirium have an identifiable cause. Although the rate at which delirium occurs is unknown, it should not be surprising, given the enormous number of possible causes, that it is not always possible to identify the etiological agent or agents with certainty during a brief episode of delirium. The diagnosis of delirium NOS is appropriate in these rare circumstances. This designation may be appropriate for deliria thought to arise from sensory deprivation. Although sensory deprivation may predispose an individual to delirium, attributing delirium to sensory deprivation as the sole etiological agent is controversial. If phenomena such as sensory deprivation, immobilization, and sleep deprivation cause delirium, they probably do so in patients who are already at risk, such as the elderly, patients with dementia, and patients who have suffered an insult to the CNS.

Natural history

The natural history of delirium is poorly understood, in part because the syndrome has received many different labels in the past and in part because the disorder is underrecognized. Delirium may be the presenting manifestation of numerous disorders, as exemplified by the onset of hepatic encephalopathy in Case 11.1. Although its onset is acute by definition and according to current literature, initial symptoms of mild delirium can be subtle. An insidious onset appears possible when symptoms are present most prominently at night. Furthermore, the fluctuating course of delirium may allow a patient to appear relatively normal during a single interview. Careful review of charting by other physicians and hospital staff is a necessary component of the evaluation for delirium.

Some types of delirium are limited in duration. For example, delirium tremens has a relatively typical onset and duration. Postoperative delirium that occurs outside of the recovery suite is said to be often preceded by a lucid interval of one or two days. In both cases the duration of delirium is typically 4–7 days, with more complicated and severe cases lasting slightly longer.

Death can be a result of delirium. Studies of delirium have demonstrated that death occurs more often in patients who are delirious than in matched controls, although the portion of cases with this outcome varies remarkably from series to series. Presumably the risk of death is largely attributable to the risk associated with the severity of the causative illness (or illnesses). Similarly, dementia is said to be an outcome of delirium. The process that converts delirium into dementia is unknown. Chronic exposure to organic solvents appears to produce an irreversible syndrome of cognitive impairment, suggesting that sustained exposure to a noxious agent is one pathway from delirium to dementia. Dementia is usually associated with neuronal loss; perhaps prolonged delirium produces dementia through cell death. Additional cell death would explain the irreversible deficits that are thought to occur when delirium is superimposed on dementia. Finally, the process by which Wernicke's encephalopahy (a form of delirium) merges into Korsakoff's syndrome (a type of amnestic disorder) is unknown. What is unequivocal is the observation that patients who are delirious have more complicated courses, longer hospital stays, and poorer outcomes than matched patients without delirium.

Differential diagnosis

The key issue in the diagnosis of delirium is recognition. Distinguishing the disorder from other psychiatric disorders is relatively straightforward once consideration is given to delirium. Physicians who care for hospital inpatients who are acutely ill should recognize that at least one of ten patients (higher in the elderly) is delirious at some point during hospitalization. Questions about memory and orientation should be incorporated into the examination of all patients (see Box 11.2). The clinician reviewing the patient chart should consider the possibility of delirium by looking for signs of a fluctuating course and altered consciousness. Finally, appearance of complications such as infection should immediately alert the physician to the possibility of delirium and stimulate an examination that considers signs of delirium and a search for additional causes of delirium. The payoff for the patient and the doctor is a less complicated course of illness and possibly a reduced length of stay. Appropriate recognition and treatment of delirium is good medical practice, even in terminally ill patients, if the management of symptoms results in an amelioration of symptoms (for example, hallucinations).

Delirium can be readily distinguished from dementia, although they may occur concurrently (Table 11.7). The most important distinction is the acuteness of onset. Rapid deterioration (hours to days) in the mental functioning of any patient, regardless of prior cognitive status, should suggest delirium. Fluctuation in the course of dementia is possible, but it is rarely as dramatic as is typical of delirium. Patients who are demented generally have a clear consciousness. Patients who are delirious are more likely to have disorganized thought whereas patients with dementia have impoverished thought. Current diagnostic criteria for dementia emphasize neurological signs such as apraxias and agnosias; these are

presumably rare signs during delirium in the absence of another CNS process associated with these findings.

Depression and mania rarely present with a picture typical of delirium. Nevertheless, one series notes a substantial number of patients with a psychiatric disorder who had signs and symptoms suggestive of delirium (see Box 11.1). The distinction between delirium and mood disorder is made by ascertaining the presence of sufficient symptoms of depression or mania to meet criteria for an affective episode. A prior history of affective illness supports the diagnosis of mood disorder. Distinguishing delirium from schizophrenia and schizophrenia-like illnesses is performed similarly. Catatonia is associated with affective disorders, schizophrenia, or delirium; a careful history, physical examination, and laboratory evaluation should suggest the underlying disorder. As is the case with dementia, delirium can be superimposed on any other psychiatric condition. Acute onset and a rapidly fluctuating course of cognitive impairment strongly suggest the presence of delirium.

Genetics and family history

Delirium is the psychiatric disorder most clearly caused by extrinsic influences, and for this reason it has been little studied from a family-history perspective. Studying the effects of experimental infection on the performance of healthy volunteers suggests that individual variation in cognitive impairment is large, even in the face of clinically similar infections. This observation suggests a limited role for intrinsic, possibly genetic, factors in the risk of developing delirium. Other risk factors, such as severe medical illness, presence of known brain disease, age, and possibly polypharmacy, seem more important than any genetic contribution.

Epidemiology

Delirium is a common psychiatric disorder among patients who are medically ill. Accurate estimates are difficult to obtain and are sensitive to patient referral sources in addition to the variable presence in any clinical sample of the risk factors

	Clinical features that distinguish delirium from dementia		
Feature	**Delirium**		**Dementia**
Onset	Acute: hours to days		Insidious: months to a year or more
Course	Fluctuating, generally lasts days to weeks		Chronic with stable or, in the case of presumptive dementia of the Alzheimer's type, gradually worsening function
Consciousness	Decreased awareness and alertness, sometimes with stupor		Usually clear
Perception	Hallucinations, typically visual, are often part of the syndrome		Hallucinations, typically visual, and delusions are often a feature of midphase dementia of the Alzheimer's type
Thought	Disorganized		Impoverished

TABLE 11.7

mentioned above. A reasonable estimate is that about 10–15% of medically ill inpatients suffer from delirium; this estimate increases to 15–20% if the patient population is over age 65. Postoperative delirium occurs in about one-third of surgical cases; the incidence of delirium is higher in patients who undergo open-heart surgery. Only about one in ten patients suffering from delirium is likely to receive the diagnosis.

Pathophysiology

The final common pathway that produces the cognitive impairment characteristic of delirium is unknown. Signs and symptoms of delirium are sufficiently characteristic that a common pathway presumably exists. The disturbance of consciousness that has been so difficult to define, at least historically, is relatively uncommon in many other neuropsychiatric disorders. Any pathophysiological mechanism should be sufficiently general to apply to most cases of delirium, regardless of cause. A theory of delirium must also accommodate the vulnerability conferred by age, dementia, other types of structural brain disease, systemic illness, and polypharmacy. An adequate pathophysiological understanding of delirium is likely to illuminate the understanding of mental mechanisms relevant to phenomena such as consciousness and hallucinations. A review of current hypotheses about pathophysiological mechanisms of delirium provides a helpful framework for considering the disorder. Theories can be described as fitting into the following four general and not mutually exclusive categories: (1) disturbance of cortical metabolism, (2) disturbances of electrical excitability, (3) dysfunction in a neurotransmitter system or systems, and (4) neurohumoral hypotheses.

One of the oldest hypotheses is that delirium represents cerebral insufficiency caused by a generalized lack of a critical CNS metabolic need. This notion is derived from the observation that delirium is associated with a decrease in brain electrical activity, reflected in the appearance of slow waves (delta and theta) in the EEG. Furthermore, deficits in the availability of critical cerebral metabolites—O_2 in hypoxia and glucose in hypoglycemia—are known to be associated with delirium. Oxygen and glucose are critical to the function of all neurons, an attractive aspect to a theory that would explain the global dysfunction of delirium. Functional imaging studies, such as positron emission tomography (PET) and single photon emission computed tomography (SPECT), of patients suffering from chronic exposure to organic solvents suggest global decreases in cerebral metabolism that are particularly striking in the frontal and temporal lobes. These findings were generally not associated with structural lesions as detected by typical structural imaging methods (CT and magnetic resonance imaging [MRI]). Decreased cerebral perfusion has been reported for the early stages of delirium tremens, neuropsychiatric manifestations

of systemic lupus erythematosus and hepatic encephalopathy. Unfortunately, patients with CNS lupus and liver failure may also show atrophy, confounding the interpretation of scanning. Furthermore, magnetic resonance spectroscopy findings may be different in hepatic encephalopathy and neuropsychiatric systemic lupus erythematosus. Presumably, marginalization of neuronal function by different initial processes produces perfusion deficits associated with cortical insufficiency and "global" symptomatology (the disturbance in consciousness). "Specific" aspects of delirium (disorientation and visual hallucinations, for example) would reflect the relatively greater sensitivity of neurons (perhaps those in the frontal or temporal lobes) associated with these cognitive impairments to deprivation of critical metabolic needs than other nerve cells.

The function of the nervous system is dependent on the ability of nerve cells to generate and efficiently transmit electrical signals. Neurons have the capacity to rapidly move ions in and out of the cell, generating action potentials, a process that is sensitive to the ionic milieu. Alterations in fluid and electrolyte status disrupt this process and are clearly causes of delirium, whether because of a decrease (for example, hyponatremia or hypoosmolality) or an increase (such as in hypernatremia or hyperosmolality). Disturbances of critical metabolic needs, such as those that occur in decreased cerebral blood flow, hypoxia, or hypoglycemia, would affect ionic transmission indirectly by impairing the ability of nerve cells to appropriately pump ions. It is estimated that as much as one-half of brain metabolic work is devoted to Na^+/K^+ ATPase function, suggesting that mild perturbations of metabolic function (e.g., as might occur as the result of fever) would impair ion regulation and neurotransmission. As with the previous hypothesis that delirium is caused by a decrement in critical metabolic components, certain populations of nerve cells would presumably be more sensitive to ionic disturbance than others.

The hypothesis that dysfunction of a specific population of neurons causes the symptoms of delirium is attractive when considering the role of a particular neurotransmitter system in delirium. Involvement of the CNS cholinergic system in delirium is an especially robust concept. Drugs with antimuscarinic properties are known common causes of delirium. Furthermore, overcoming cholinergic blockage by treating patients with the acetylcholinesterase inhibitor physostigmine reverses the symptoms of delirium, at least temporarily. Donepezil, rivastigmine, and galantamine, cholinesterase inhibitors with much longer duration of effect than physostigmine, may reduce the risk of delirium and have also been used to treat delirium. Numerous lines of evidence implicate the cholinergic system in memory impairment, a key aspect of delirium.

However, the specificity of the cholinergic hypothesis of delirium is open to question. Serotonin syndrome, seemingly the result of excessive serotonergic neurotransmission, and neuroleptic malignant syndrome, apparently reflecting inhibited dopaminergic neurotransmission, may reflect delirium initiated via other neurotransmitter systems. The associated clinical characteristics of these syndromes (e.g., facial flushing with serotonin syndrome, rigidity with neuroleptic malignant syndrome) seem different from the associated features of anticholinergic syndromes (e.g., prominent dry mouth). Physostigmine may reverse delirium in situations that are not the result of obvious anticholinergic effects. Donepezil has been associated with delirium in at least one instance, however. Furthermore, organophosphate insecticides (see Table 11.5) cause delirium, presumably via inhibiting cholinesterase and increasing cholinergic tone. Anticholinesterase drugs are indicated in the treatment of dementia, particularly dementia of the Alzheimer's type (DAT), and are thought to work by reversing cholinergic deficits associated with dementia. Although cholinergic deficits may explain the somewhat similar defects in memory noted for delirium and dementia, it is unclear how cholinergic mechanisms can cause the acute change of consciousness typical of delirium yet not cause similar symptoms in dementia.

Various other neurotransmitter systems have been implicated in delirium. As noted above, serotonin syndrome and neuroleptic malignant syndrome involve serotonin and dopamine, respectively. More generally, the signs of autonomic instability characteristic of delirium tremens and some other deliria suggest the involvement of central catecholaminergic neurons in delirium. Excess dopaminergic neurotransmission has been associated with psychosis regardless of the type of psychiatric illness and may account for the psychotic symptoms often observed in delirium. Sedative-hypnotics, such as benzodiazepines and barbiturates, appear to exert CNS effects largely through γ-aminobutyric acid (GABA$_A$) receptors; some evidence in animals suggests dysregulation of receptor expression during withdrawal. Hypotheses to explain the CNS dysfunction seen in hepatic encephalopathy invoke dysregulation of GABAergic and glutamatergic systems. These systems are widely distributed yet appear to have regional specificity by virtue of subtype-specific receptor expression. It may be possible to study the role of the various neurotransmitter systems in delirium by employing system-specific ligands in functional imaging studies.

Neurohumoral hypotheses of delirium have been advanced. The notion that stress facilitates the appearance of delirium suggests involvement of stress hormones, such as corticosteroids. Whereas stress from sleep deprivation, immobility, and extreme alteration of the sensory environment (either overload or deprivation) may predispose to delirium, it appears unlikely that these factors are sole etiological agents. Equally important, treatment with corticosteroids is not always associated with a psychiatric disorder. Corticosteroids are probably as likely to cause mania or depression

as delirium. A corticosteroid hypothesis is interesting because of the capacity of this and other hormones (and perhaps vitamins such as thiamine) to exert an effect on most neurons, resulting in global dysfunction. The relatively greater impact of a hormone on specific populations of neurons would account for specific symptoms (for example, hallucinations).

These hypotheses are not mutually exclusive. For example, it is possible that cholinergic neurons are more sensitive to metabolic deprivation, ionic disturbance, and neurohumoral factors than (for the sake of argument) adrenergic neurons. Furthermore, acute disruption of the function of cholinergic neurons could disturb consciousness through an effect mediated by the reticular system, producing dysfunction of many other nerve cells because cholinergic cells have a wide distribution in the brain. The point to this line of reasoning is merely to illustrate the concept that the hypotheses outlined previously do not necessarily exclude each other. However, an approach to the pathophysiology of delirium such as outlined here produces hypotheses that are testable at the systems, cellular, and molecular levels.

Prevention, management, and treatment

Prevention of delirium holds promise for moderating the frequency of this complication of severe illness. Risk factors such as impairments of vision and hearing can often be mitigated by relatively simple interventions such as assuring that assistive devices (e.g., hearing aids) are available. Depression is a treatable illness that has been identified as a risk factor for delirium. Identification of patients with dementia can result in labor-intensive environmental interventions such as frequent orientation. Ascertaining that a patient uses alcohol to excess or is very malnourished should prompt administration of thiamine to reduce the risk of Wernicke's encephalopathy. Signs of alcohol withdrawal such as unexpected sinus tachycardia/hypertension should prompt consideration of early administration of benzodiazepines. Finally, fluid and electrolyte abnormalities may be predisposing factors in addition to causes of delirium, and aggressive correction may blunt the risk of delirium.

Clinical trials provide a mixed picture of the effectiveness of prevention. In part, this situation reflects heterogeneity among the various trials; it also reflects design features such as small size, nonrandom design, and within-trial patient sample heterogeneity. Potentially effective interventions include reorientation, environmental cueing, and patient mobilization. These low-technology efforts can be considered good nursing care with the caveat that the current hospital environment places a premium on staff mastery of high technology skills (e.g., electronic medical record management). Reduction in rates of delirium should improve the quality of care and shorten average length of hospital stay with a positive impact on the cost of health care. However, cost savings have not been adequately demonstrated and the labor-

KEY CLINICAL QUESTIONS AND WHAT THEY UNLOCK

Delirium

- *When and how rapidly did the change in thinking occur?*
  Delirium is associated with acute onset of cognitive dysfunction, typically over hours. Dementia has a more chronic course. Since these two disorders can co-occur and dementia may be a risk factor for delirium, the task may be obtaining a history of an acute change superimposed on chronic cognitive dysfunction. Depression and mania can have a relatively acute onset, but affective symptoms are usually much more prominent than cognitive symptoms and are usually present longer than would be expected with delirium. Schizophrenia is a chronic condition associated with mild cognitive dysfunction. Catatonia, an uncommon syndrome of disturbance in movement and communication, is associated with affective disorders, schizophrenia, and delirium and illustrates the importance of a longitudinal history in disentangling delirium from other psychiatric disorders.

- *Is a cause identifiable? What additional information needs to be gathered to address possible causes?*
  The search for a cause is critical yet many patients have multiple causes, complicating treatment. Rapidly working through plausible causes is key and may involve consultation with other physicians. Failure of delirium to resolve will result in further investigations.

- *How necessary is each current medication and are alternatives available that may pose less risk of inducing delirium?*
  Upon suspecting delirium, a thorough review of current medications often results in the discontinuation of some that are no longer necessary. In cases where pharmacotherapy is necessary, substitution of alternatives

that are associated with less risk of delirium should be attempted.

- *Are behavioral interventions in place to manage troublesome behavior? Should medications be used to treat symptoms of delirium?*
  Provision of frequent reorientation, correction of sensory deficits, and reassurance in the presence of a consistent routine are important management techniques that may maximize patient comfort and minimize disruptive behavior. Unmanageable agitation that puts the patient or others at risk is a common reason to initiate pharmacotherapy with agents such as haloperidol. Antipsychotic treatment should be considered if the patient has prominent hallucinations and delusions. Delirium associated with alcohol or sedative/hypnotic withdrawal usually benefits from treatment with a benzodiazepine.

- *Has the diagnosis, treatment, and prognosis been discussed with the patient? Family? Others involved in the care and treatment of the patient?*
  A simple description of the situation to the patient is warranted when the patient is aware enough to respond, but retention of the information is likely to be poor and repetition is prudent. During an episode of delirium, it is more useful to communicate the diagnosis, treatment, and prognosis to the patient's family and friends since delirium is not present in all patients with a given medical problem, the disorder prolongs recovery and, in some instances (dementia, terminal illness), recovery may be poor or not expected. A description provided to medical providers can facilitate interventions and anticipate problems. A follow-up visit with the patient after recovery is probably the best way to address patient concerns effectively.

---

intensive nature of preventive interventions may actually result in minimal savings. Finally, sustaining quality programs such as a delirium prevention effort can be difficult due to a loss of focus on this objective in the face of ever-changing and competing problems. A multi-site delirium prevention trial targetted to a somewhat homogeneous population (e.g., patients undergoing hip replacement) with incorporation of a cost-benefit analysis seems warranted.

Establishing the cause of delirium is the most critical aspect of treatment because treatment of the causative disorders usually reverses most symptoms of delirium. The treatment of the numerous disorders listed previously and in Table 11.1 constitutes much of the practice of medicine and involves topics beyond the scope of this chapter. As Case 11.1 exemplifies, the existence of delirium may involve multiple possible causes.

General observations about the process of evaluation provide guidance for treatment (see *Key clinical questions and what they unlock*). The history and physical examination are

the starting points for most diagnoses and are thus critical to the etiology of delirium. A systematic approach to laboratory tests guided by the history and physical examination is appropriate (see Table 11.6). Laboratory tests may be critical for the patient who is incoherent or obtunded and has no readily available collateral source. Consultants may be helpful in sorting out etiology, particularly for the individual with multiple possible causes. Patients who abuse alcohol or drugs and patients suffering from malnutrition should receive parenteral vitamins, particularly thiamine, to prevent delirium caused by vitamin deficiency, such as Wernicke's encephalopathy.

An approach to considering the role of possible drug intoxication in cases of delirium is suggested in Fig. 11.1. Drugs should be discontinued if the indication is uncertain or the repercussions of discontinuation are minimal. Doses, in conjunction with appropriate drug levels, should be carefully considered for pharmacological agents deemed necessary and should be lowered if at all possible. Another agent with a

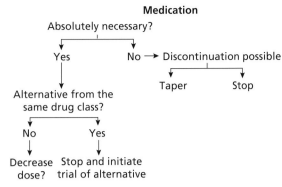

Medication

Absolutely necessary?

Yes

No → Discontinuation possible

Taper   Stop

Alternative from the same drug class?

No   Yes

Decrease dose?   Stop and initiate trial of alternative

Fig. 11.1 Managing possible drug intoxication delirium. Evaluation of many critical drugs (for example, digoxin) can be difficult because the condition for which the compound is indicated (such as congestive heart failure) may also be associated with delirium. Determining drug levels may be helpful under these circumstances. Measuring drug concentrations can also be useful if elevated drug levels are clearly associated with delirium (for example, carbamazepine, TCAs). In some cases, indications for 'absolutely necessary' drugs may be unclear, and diagnostic evaluation may suggest that a drug can be discontinued. Initiation of trials with alternative medications should give some consideration to the half-lives of both compounds, since the alternative also poses some risk of inducing delirium and concurrent administration of both drugs would presumably increase the risk. Discontinuation by tapering may be useful for drugs associated with withdrawal symptoms (such as sedative-hypnotics) and permit the selection of a lower, presumably more appropriate, dose at which delirium is not a problem. Application of the algorithm in cases of polypharmacy (probably the typical situation) is best accomplished if drugs are considered from most important to least important.

lower risk of inducing delirium or a nonpharmacological treatment may be substituted. If a single agent is deemed to be the probable cause of delirium, cessation of administration is likely to be followed by relatively rapid improvement, although exceptions are known (for example, lithium and bromide compounds). Observation of improvement supports the hypothesis that the particular drug was the cause. Given that serious medical illness is a risk factor for delirium, the more typical approach to consideration of drug intoxication is to make multiple changes in a regimen that involves many compounds.

An important aspect of delirium management is manipulation of the patient's environment to enhance cognitive status. Many interventions date to antiquity and are similar to the preventive efforts described previously. Sensory stimulation is modulated to match the patient's apparent state of awareness and, if possible, expressed wishes. Lethargic patients are provided with modest amounts of sensory stimulus, and hyperactive patients are placed in environments that minimize stimulation. The hospital routine is modified to emphasize daytime activity and nighttime sleep. Explanations of events as they unfold are provided (typically repeatedly) in a direct and simple fashion. Family members

are involved in reassuring the patient and making the environment more like home. Finally, the use of restraints is minimized and targeted to the situation. Nevertheless, the need to protect the integrity of life-sustaining medical devices (such as endotracheal tubes and central lines) may necessitate the use of restraints, as do life-threatening behaviors directed toward others (assaultive behavior towards staff) and self (for example, a suicide attempt or wandering away). Although good nursing management is critical to the care of delirious patients, effects on course are modest at best.

Antipsychotic medication plays a role in the management of delirium. Many patients suffer from hallucinations, and some have delusions that impair their understanding. Because the experiences are real to the patient, they can lead to dangerous behavior. Antipsychotic drugs also have sedative properties that are likely to contribute to effectiveness. Haloperidol is the drug of choice because it has minimal anticholinergic (and thereby presumably deliriogenic) and cardiovascular effects. A prospective randomized trial indicated that haloperidol was better tolerated and more effective treatment of delirium in patients with AIDS than lorazepam. The medication can be given intravenously (a common method, although it is not a route of administration that has been approved by the Food and Drug Administration [FDA]), intramuscularly, or orally. Therapy may be initiated parenterally with modest doses (0.5–5 mg, lower doses in the elderly), and as the patient is stabilized administration may be switched to the oral route. As the patient's mental status improves, the drug is tapered and discontinued. Much larger doses can be employed if the clinical situation poses sufficient risk to the patient. Haloperidol is associated with various neuromuscular syndromes, the most important during short-term use being an acute dystonia or dystonias. Droperidol is an alternative with a shorter half-life and perhaps a more rapid onset of action. Newer antipsychotics such as risperidone, olanzapine, and quetiapine have been used to manage delirium because these drugs are less likely to be associated with the extrapyramidal side effects seen with haloperidol and droperidol. Effectiveness is unclear, however, and these drugs may have other risks.

Benzodiazepines are the drug of choice for sedative-hypnotic withdrawal delirium, including delirium tremens. Members of this class may also be useful adjuncts to pharmacological treatment of other types of delirium with haloperidol, presumably by potentiating the sedative properties of haloperidol. Neuroleptics are not appropriate as sole agents for the management of alcohol withdrawal delirium, however, because they are associated with higher mortality, more complications, and longer duration of delirium than sedative-hypnotic agents in controlled trials. Neuroleptics should be avoided as sole agents for the management in other types of sedative-hypnotic withdrawal as well. The role of second-generation antipsychotics in sedative-hypnotic delirium is ambiguous at present, but they probably should also not be used as sole management agents, given the wealth of data regarding the effectiveness of sedative-hypnotic drugs in the management of sedative-hypnotic delirium. The differential utility of sedative-hypnotics and antipsychotics in the management of different types of delirium underscores the importance of diagnosis.

Lorazepam is the preferred benzodiazepine because it is effective when administered via various routes (intravenously, intramuscularly, and orally), thus facilitating emergency management and permitting the switch to an oral formulation for subsequent treatment. The drug does not have active metabolites and has a modest half-life, which minimizes accumulation of active drug yet provides coverage for a number of hours. Other commonly used short-acting benzodiazepines include midazolam and oxazepam. Drawbacks of the benzodiazepines include amnestic effects, which probably contribute to the propensity of these compounds to cause delirium. Benzodiazepines also cause ataxia and can be oversedating. Acute benzodiazepine toxicity is reversible with flumazenil. However, since this short-acting drug can induce withdrawal and cause seizures (at higher doses), its use should be reserved for emergent toxicity. Chlordiazepoxide, a long-acting compound, is used in sedative-hypnotic withdrawal because its long half-life facilitates management by titration to the desired effect and discontinuation. Cessation of administration is followed by a gradual fall in drug levels, ameliorating the subsequent withdrawal symptoms. This and other long-acting sedative-hypnotics (such as clonazepam and phenobarbital) may be useful in some cases of sedative-hypnotic delirium. However, these compounds are not necessarily more effective; they may have a narrower therapeutic index (barbiturates); and because of drug accumulation, they may be more deliriogenic.

Special topics

The importance of delirium as a clinical entity has sometimes been discounted. The argument is that delirium is really a proxy for an underlying cause or causes. Addressing the etiological condition (or conditions) presumably makes the presence or absence of delirium a moot point. Unfortunately, this argument ignores the fact that delirium can be the presentation for virtually any condition, particularly in patients who are at risk of delirium. Controlled observation has repeatedly demonstrated that patients who are delirious suffer greater morbidity and probably greater mortality than matched patients without delirium. Physicians should be particularly concerned about the iatrogenic aspects of delirium. Downplaying the importance of delirium reduces the quality of patient care.

Similar arguments about quality of life underlie the suggestion that delirium should be recognized and addressed in the terminally ill. For instance, most patients dying of cancer develop a delirium during their last days. The cause is likely to be multifactorial, since multiple organs fail. The goal of recognition is to provide treatment that is palliative and ameliorates the disturbing hallucinations and delusions, as well as providing more restful sleep.

Psychiatrists are commonly consulted to establish the diagnosis of delirium and advise about management. Other specialists (for example, neurologists, internists, and physicians with various subspecialties) are perhaps more likely to be consulted to evaluate and treat causative disorders. Case 11.1, which involves an obviously complicated patient, exemplifies a coordinated approach to evaluation and treatment. It is reasonable to expect the consulting psychiatrist to examine any hospital-based referral with the diagnosis of delirium in mind. Probably the most common diagnostic issue (after failure to consider delirium) is the inability of the referring physician to distinguish delirium from other psychiatric disorders. Patients with preexisting psychiatric disorders can be particularly difficult to evaluate. The widespread use of medications such as haloperidol and lorazepam makes physicians in acute care settings aware that psychotropics can be used to manage delirium. Psychiatrists can be helpful when considering alternative choices and evaluating patients for side effects. They can also suggest a reasonable approach to tapering medications.

Psychiatric consultation may be particularly useful when drugs are thought to play an etiological role. Psychotropic drugs are often implicated in cases of delirium. Probably the best-studied example is the risk of delirium from TCAs. About 5% of patients hospitalized for psychiatric reasons develop delirium when treated with TCAs. TCA-induced delirium is correlated with drug level, age, and female gender. A psychiatrist is the appropriate consultant to evaluate patients who are delirious and receiving any psychotropic drug, not only to consider the etiological role of the drugs but also to advise regarding alternative management. Patients who experience delirium as the result of illicit drug use should be advised to cease using illicit substances. They are likely to need treatment of drug dependence beyond resolution of the delirium (see Chapter 14).

CONSIDER CONSULTATION WHEN...

- The diagnosis of delirium is uncertain, particularly if the history and symptoms suggest another or an additional psychiatric disorder (such as depression or dementia).
- Management with usually effective approaches (for example, haloperidol or restraints) is not sufficient to allow treatment of concurrent medical conditions, particularly when behavior is a danger to self or others.
- Symptoms of delirium fail to resolve despite apparent resolution of causative/contributive medical conditions.

In summary, delirium is a common complication of drug treatment (particularly when CNS-active compounds are used) and many medical conditions. Useful criteria exist for establishing the diagnosis. Patients can be systematically evaluated, the diagnosis can be established, and treatment can be initiated in a straightforward fashion (see *Pearls & Perils*). Treatment is largely directed at the underlying cause; neuroleptics (such as haloperidol) and benzodiazepines (such as lorazepam) may be an important part of patient management. Prevention and early recognition are likely to diminish morbidity and mortality.

Delirium

- Delirium afflicts at least one in ten hospitalized patients.
- Most cases of delirium are not recognized.
- Delirium is associated with death, longer hospital stay, and disability.
- Age, dementia, other types of coarse brain disease, severe systemic illness, and dehydration put patients at risk for developing delirium.
- Acute onset and fluctuating course of a disturbance of consciousness strongly suggest the diagnosis of delirium.
- Abnormalities of orientation, memory, language ability, and perception (for example, visual hallucinations) establish the diagnosis.
- Review of current drug therapy and medical conditions is important in the diagnostic evaluation to find causes.
- Many patients have multiple possible causes of delirium.
- Treatment of delirium is directed at the cause or causes.
- Patient safety and comfort should be sustained by judicious use of neuroleptics (for example, haloperidol) and benzodiazepines (for example, lorazepam).
- Nursing interventions enhance the quality of patient care.
- Restraints may be required in life-threatening circumstances.
- Individuals with dementia who develop delirium may not return to predelirium cognitive functioning after resolution of delirium.
- Delirium is a common aspect of terminal illnesses.
- Most patients with delirium who are not terminally ill recover.

Amnestic disorders

Amnestic disorders represent cognitive disorders that are largely, if not solely, a disturbance of memory (Box 11.3). As is the case with the more global cognitive disorders of delirium and dementia, amnestic disorders are classified on an etiological basis as either resulting from a general medical condition or induced by a specific substance. DSM-IV diagnostic criteria A, B, and C must be met for every case of suspected amnestic disorder. Etiological specification should focus on general medical conditions, since amnestic disorder caused by drugs and toxins independent of malnutrition and apart from intoxication or withdrawal is rare. The clinical description of patients with amnesia over the past 40 years has contributed significantly to the understanding of the mechanisms responsible for memory, providing knowledge useful to clinicians and basic scientists (Table 11.8).

Amnestic disorders are important to the primary care physician because the recognition of individuals at risk for

Box 11.3 Amnestic disorder

A. The development of memory impairment as manifested by impairment in the ability to learn new information or the inability to recall previously learned information.
B. The memory disturbance causes significant impairment in social or occupational functioning and represents a significant decline from a previous level of functioning.
C. The memory disturbance does not occur exclusively during the course of a delirium or a dementia and persists beyond the usual duration of substance intoxication or withdrawal.

Amnestic disorder due to a general medical condition
There is evidence from the history, physical examination, or laboratory findings that the disturbance is the direct physiological consequence of a general medical condition (including physical trauma).

Specify if:
- transient: if memory impairment lasts for one month or less
- chronic: if memory impairment lasts for more than one month

Substance-induced persisting amnestic disorder
There is evidence from the history, physical examination, or laboratory findings that the memory disturbance is etiologically related to the persisting effects of substance use (e.g., a drug of abuse, a medication).

Amnestic disorder not otherwise specified
This category should be used to diagnose an amnestic disorder that does not meet criteria for any of the specific types described in this section.
Modified from American Psychiatric Association (2000) Diagnostic and Statistical Manual of Mental Disorders, 4th Edition, Text Revision, Washington, D.C., American Psychiatric Association.

Table 11.8 Amnestic disorder

DIAGNOSIS

Discriminating features

1 Difficulty remembering the past, particularly recent events.
2 Impaired ability to learn new information.
3 Absence of other clinically significant cognitive dysfunction, particularly that seen in delirium and dementia.
4 Substantial change from previous function.

Consistent features

1 Social or occupational dysfunction of variable severity.
2 Clear consciousness.
3 Definable cause.

Variable features

1 Confabulation.
2 Poor insight.
3 Bad judgment.
4 Inability to perform activities of daily living outside of an institution.
5 Disorientation.
6 Indifference to memory problems.

amnestic disorders should diminish the probability that patients will experience the devastating and often irreversible effects of chronic amnestic disorder. A case report of Korsakoff's syndrome is provided (Case 11.2).

Diagnosis

Amnestic disorders are characterized by memory failure (Box 11.3). Patients afflicted with these disorders suffer from an impaired ability to learn new material (anterograde amnesia), as well as a significant deficit in the recall of previously learned information (retrograde amnesia). The ability to remember the distant past, material learned long before the onset of the amnestic disorder, is conserved. The ability to immediately repeat information (such as digit span) is also preserved. A profound amnesia can produce disorientation to time and place with sustained orientation to person, although this is not an essential feature. The patient in Case 11.2 had impaired recall and an inability to learn new material, although his immediate repetition ability and remote memory were good.

The memory disturbance results in substantial impairment of social and occupational functioning and represents a significant decline from previous status. Severe amnesia can impair the affected individual to the extent that custodial care is required to sustain activities of daily life.

Chronic amnesia is often complicated by an indifference to the memory deficits, although this is a variable feature of the disorder. The potentially profound effects of amnesia on the ability of an affected individual to lead a normal life are the impetus for prevention and recognition. The patient in Case 11.2 required assistance with all activities of daily living because amnesia made it impossible for him to run a household; he lived with his son, who managed his affairs. The patient was unable to return to his job as a laborer; he was indifferent to this turn of events.

Other features of amnestic disorders are not invariant (see Table 11.8) but occur at a sufficient rate that they are important. Many patients with memory problems respond to questions with incorrect answers as a result of confusing remembered events that occurred at different times, of using completely fabricated material, or a mixture of both. It may be difficult to discern that this is occurring without reliable collateral sources. In the extreme case, fantastic information is offered voluntarily; this form of confabulation tends to occur early in the course of chronic amnestic disorders. Fantastic confabulation appears to be similar to a delusion, although the patient is unlikely to sustain the content because of memory problems.

Severe amnestic disorder is commonly associated with a lack of insight into the condition, which further complicates the course of chronic profound amnesia. Patients may become agitated when poor memory leads to disagreements with others. The associated features of amnestic disorder obviously contribute to the disability seen from the disorder.

Current criteria emphasize the exclusion of delirium and dementia as part of the diagnosis of amnestic disorder. Examination of patients along the lines suggested in Boxes 11.1 and 11.3 facilitates the distinction between amnestic disorder and dementia or delirium, which are disorders involving more global cognitive impairment. The distinction of amnestic disorders from dementia hinges on the absence of other signs of clinically significant cognitive impairment in amnestic disorders. Delirium and dementia typically involve impaired perception with disturbances such as visual hallucinations, which are rare, unrelated occurrences in amnestic disorder. Delirium characteristically involves a disturbance of consciousness that is not part of amnestic disorder. The patient described in Case 11.2 was significantly impaired by poor memory without clear signs and symptoms of either delirium or dementia.

Amnestic disorders are classified on the basis of an underlying general medical condition (Box 11.4) or as substance induced (Box 11.5). Transient forms of amnestic disorder are seen in transient global amnesia, as a manifestation of a seizure, and after head injury.

Recovery from an amnestic disorder after head injury can take considerably longer than recovery from other disorders associated with transient amnestic disorder. Next to head injury, transient global amnesia is the second most common

Mr W is a 55-year-old man who was referred for evaluation and treatment of memory problems. He had long been described as acting strange but was brought to the emergency room when he was found wandering about at work with no idea as to what he was supposed to be doing. He had been sent home from work two days before but returned to work with the same problem.

He had a long history of alcohol dependence complicated by withdrawal, seizures, and a right frontal hematoma. He was not intoxicated when he arrived at the hospital, nor did he show any signs of withdrawal during the hospitalization. No evidence was obtained from collateral sources to suggest recent head trauma or recent seizures. A brother carried the diagnosis of mental retardation. Mr W had only an eighth-grade education, which complicated the evaluation of his intellect, although he had worked as a laborer for the same employer for several years.

The patient did not have any focal or lateralizing neurological signs. At the time of initial evaluation he was alert and oriented in all three spheres. No psychotic symptoms were elicited, although the patient did not feel he had a problem. He recalled three of three items at one minute but only one of three items at five minutes. Simple arithmetic was not a problem (subtraction from 20 by threes), and he could perform simple comparisons (apple and orange). He could not perform more difficult arithmetic or make more complicated comparisons, difficulties that were attributed to his lack of education. The patient could repeat six digits forward and four in reverse, although he had a great deal of difficulty learning the task of reversing the digits.

An emergent CT scan of the head showed mild cerebellar vermian atrophy and a tiny low-density lesion of uncertain origin lateral to the left frontal horn. He was advised to stop drinking and was given thiamine. He was without impairment of consciousness throughout the hospitalization. Mr W left the hospital against medical advice but returned for an EEG two weeks later; his EEG was normal.

When evaluated by a psychiatrist in an office visit one week after his hospitalization, his recall and other tests of cognitive function were unchanged. His chief complaint concerned physical symptoms such as swollen feet and shortness of breath, which were not obvious on examination. The patient had no memory of the hospitalization.

Consideration was given to neuropsychological testing, particularly a comparison of intelligence quotient (IQ) as measured by a standardized test such as the Wechsler Adult Intelligence Scale (WAIS) with memory as measured by a standardized test such as the Wechsler Memory Scale-Revised (WMS-R). Poor compliance and an inability to accurately determine baseline intellectual function (the patient's rural school district was no longer in existence because of consolidation) suggested that testing would not be useful. This decision was discussed with the patient's son and the primary care physician; they agreed.

Mr W had symptoms of depression that included low mood, poor energy, poor sleep, a history of poor appetite, and thoughts of death. He was treated with an antidepressant. He was also treated with thiamine throughout the follow-up period. Mr W's symptoms of depression improved, but he showed consistent difficulty with recall over the next nine months. He was oriented and eventually he was able to learn the name of the current president. The patient read the paper, but his reporting of current events was inaccurate; he mixed events from the remote past with current events. He lived with his son, who provided for his needs and monitored his environment. The patient was felt to be disabled by his memory problems. The patient was repeatedly advised to avoid alcohol use but was known to be drinking intermittently when he was lost to follow-up evaluation.

---

type of transient amnestic disorder. A disorder of acute onset and short duration (24 hours or less), transient global amnesia is not associated with focal neurological signs or symptoms. Amnestic disorder as a manifestation of epilepsy can be distinguished from transient global amnesia by the brief duration (less than one hour) and recurrent nature of epileptic amnesia.

Partial complex seizures are a relatively rare cause of a brief amnestic disorder; most patients with epilepsy have other obvious signs and symptoms of nervous system involvement as part of the seizure. An amnestic disorder resulting from electroconvulsive therapy (ECT) is uncommon; rarely patients relate remote memory loss, a problem unlike amnestic disorder. Most patients who receive ECT have some memory loss that is partly attributable to the induced seizure, but the memory loss is also probably related both to the electricity used to induce the seizure and the anesthetic agents that are part of the procedure (see Chapter 23). Cerebrovascular disease can cause a short period of amnesia, but these episodes of transient ischemic amnesia are usually associated with focal neurological signs.

The most common medical condition associated with chronic amnestic disorder is thiamine deficiency as the result of malnutrition. In Western societies the preceding delirium (Wernicke's encephalopathy) and resulting memory problems (Korsakoff's syndrome) almost always occur in people who are addicted to alcohol. Amnestic disorder as the result of a cerebral infection reverses slowly or not at all. Anoxia can produce irreversible amnestic disorder. Bilateral surgical removal of temporal lobe structures, usually performed to control intractable seizures, produces an amnestic disorder. Neoplasm and cerebral vascular disease can cause an amnestic disorder but are unlikely to be the sole cause; usually other signs and symptoms of CNS involvement are present.

The use of ethanol, the most important substance associated with amnestic disorder, appears to produce a persisting amnestic disorder in an indirect manner involving thiamine

Medical conditions associated with amnestic disorder

- Transient global amnesia
- Head injury
- Seizures
  - Epilepsy/partial complex seizures
  - ECT
- Malnutrition
- Thiamine deficiency (Wernicke-Korsakoff syndrome)
- Cerebral infection (e.g., herpes encephalitis)
- Anoxia
- Surgical intervention
  - Removal of all or a significant portion of the temporal lobe
- Neoplasm
- Cerebral vascular disease
  - Posterior cerebral artery

Some of the listed conditions (such as seizures or cerebral vascular disease) do not usually cause amnesia without other clinically significant neurological signs or symptoms and are thus unusual causes of amnestic disorder.

Substances associated with substance-induced persisting amnestic disorder

- Sedative-hypnotics
  - Alcohol
  - Barbiturates
- Anticonvulsants
- Methotrexate (intrathecal)
- Heavy metals
  - Lead
  - Mercury
- Organophosphate insecticides
- Carbon monoxide
- Industrial solvents

Caution should be used in attributing amnestic disorder to any of these substances. For example, thiamine deficiency is a far more common cause of chronic amnestic disorder.

deficiency. Other sedative-hypnotic compounds also may cause a persistent amnestic disorder, although these drugs are more commonly associated with amnesia during intoxication or withdrawal, conditions distinct from amnestic disorder. The compounds listed in Box 11.5 are rare causes of amnestic disorder.

Neuropsychological testing is an important adjunct to the evaluation and diagnosis of chronic amnestic disorder. The brevity of transient global amnesia and amnestic disorder associated with epilepsy severely limits the usefulness of testing in brief episodes of amnesia. The most widely used memory instrument is the Wechsler Memory Scale (WMS-R). Psychological instruments are useful for documenting the absence of more generalized cognitive impairment and providing an estimate of the rate of recovery in generally reversible amnestic disorders (for example, after head injury). Unfortunately, testing may reveal abnormalities of doubtful or unknown clinical relevance.

Natural history

The natural history of amnestic disorders reflects the specific course. The duration of amnestic disorder should be specified as either transient or chronic. By definition, transient amnestic disorders last no more than one month. The following discussion of the natural history of amnestic disorder is based on a distinction between transient and chronic disorders.

Transient global amnesia is a benign transient amnestic disorder. Patients, typically in late middle age, experience a relatively sudden onset of memory failure. Many cases are preceded by some type of emotional or physical stress (such as running and swimming, sexual relations, or medical procedures). Men and women are probably equally affected. Patients are alert and have at most only minor neurological signs; laboratory studies are generally uninformative, although recent functional imaging studies suggest the presence of a bilateral decrease in temporal lobe perfusion. Symptoms resolve gradually over hours to a day or perhaps a bit longer; as noted previously, epileptic amnestic disorder generally is of even briefer duration. The affected individual is left with amnesia for the period of the disturbance (anterograde amnesia) and for about an hour before the onset of amnesia (retrograde amnesia). No greater impediment than the amnesia is observed in patients who experience a single episode of transient global amnesia; only about 10% of patients experience repeated episodes. Transient amnestic disorder as the result of seizures is associated with a greater risk of recurrence; consideration of partial complex seizures should be given to patients with apparently recurrent transient global amnesia.

Head trauma is associated with amnesia of variable duration. Even in the absence of loss of consciousness or other neurological findings, mild head injury can produce amnesia that lasts an hour or so. The more severe the injury, the more prolonged the amnesia. Interestingly, the duration of amnesia predicts a significant portion of the disability resulting from head trauma. The longer the amnesia, the greater is the resulting disability. Amnestic disorder from head trauma is usually associated with neuropsychological findings, although the presence of other clinically significant cognitive difficulties should suggest either delirium or dementia. Delirium often occurs after head injury and a significant minority of patients develops dementia rather than amnestic disorder. Head trauma and presumably the associated amnestic disorder are usually seen in young patients, particularly those who use alcohol or drugs. Older age is probably associated with a worse prognosis.

Bilateral lesions involving temporal lobe structures (such as surgical removal or anoxia) typically produce irreversible chronic amnestic disorder. The most famous patient with amnestic disorder suffered anterograde and retrograde memory loss after bilateral removal of the medial temporal lobe in 1953 to alleviate intractable epilepsy. This individual is of above average intelligence but because of profound memory impairment is unable to live independently.

Patients with Korsakoff's syndrome tend to be men 50–60 years old with alcohol addiction; females may have an earlier onset of the disorder. Most have additional complications of alcoholism, as did the patient in Case 11.2. Although many patients with Korsakoff's syndrome have Wernicke's encephalopathy, some have a more insidious onset of Korsakoff's syndrome without a clear preceding delirium. Some individuals show modest recovery with the passage of time, particularly if they abstain from alcohol. Abstinence and proper diet may lead to a better outcome. Nevertheless, these older malnourished individuals are likely to require custodial care for the remainder of their lives; death is commonly the result of the medical complications of alcoholism.

Differential diagnosis

The separation of amnestic disorder from the more generalized cognitive dysfunction characteristic of delirium and dementia (see *Key clinical questions and what they unlock—amnestic disorder*) is sufficiently important that the criteria for amnestic disorder insist that delirium and dementia be excluded (Box 11.3). Many of the medical conditions associated with amnestic disorder are also associated with delirium and dementia (see Boxes 11.4 and 11.5). Dementia is characterized by the presence of memory dysfunction and clear evidence of at least two kinds of additional cognitive impairment, including aphasia (disturbance of language), agnosia (failure to identify objects despite intact sensory function), apraxia (inability to perform motor tasks despite intact motor function), or disturbance of executive function (skills involved in planning, sequencing, organizing, and abstracting). Amnestic disorder is largely a disorder of memory without clinically significant impairment of other cognitive function. Although patients with amnestic disorder may provide imaginary events to fill in missing memory, they do not suffer from the visual hallucinations and persecutory delusions so commonly seen in many patients with dementia of the Alzheimer's type (DAT). Finally, the course of amnestic disorder is variable, depending on its cause, whereas dementias tend to be static or, in the case of DAT, progressive.

KEY CLINICAL QUESTIONS AND WHAT THEY UNLOCK

Amnestic disorder

- *Is the pathology restricted to memory or do the deficits involve other elements of psychopathology?*
  Memory problems, particularly an inability to learn new information, are the *sine qua non* of amnestic disorder. Delirium and dementia are more global disorders of cognitive function, which have significant and frequently prominent memory dysfunction; demonstrating deficits in other areas of psychopathology—for example, executive dysfunction in the case of dementia or deficits in attention in the case of delirium—suggests these disorders. Sometimes an episode of delirium precedes the onset of amnestic disorder—Wernicke's preceding Korsakoff's, for example. Acute intoxication with drugs having sedative-hypnotic properties—for example, alcohol, benzodiazepines and related drugs, barbiturates—can be associated with prominent memory deficits (blackouts). Memory deficits associated with intoxication are state dependent (associated with the state of intoxication) and are limited, the period of deficit resolving with elimination of the drug. Depression and mania can be associated with "memory" deficits although affective symptoms should substantiate an affective diagnosis. Similarly, schizophrenia is associated with psychosis or a relatively bizarre defect state that can be distinguished from amnestic disorder. Patients with some causes of amnestic syndrome (e.g., Korsakoff's syndrome) have deficits readily detectable by relatively sophisticated neuropsychological testing that are not clinically relevant—demonstration of deficits beyond memory problems on clinical examination should suggest a dementia diagnosis.
- *Is the memory deficit transient or chronic?*
  Transient global amnesia is the classic transient amnestic disorder and Korsakoff's syndrome is the classic chronic amnestic syndrome. Transient syndromes are likely to resolve without long-term sequelae. Chronic amnestic disorder is likely to require sustained high intensity care for patient safety (e.g., nursing home). During the initial phase of amnestic disorder—the first month—there may be ambiguity about the eventual outcome and, if ambiguity exists regarding the eventual outcome, patients should be given a diagnosis of provisional transient global amnesia.

Delirium is a disorder of impaired consciousness, a cognitive function that is preserved in amnestic disorder. Patients who are amnestic should do well on tasks that reflect attention, such as digit span, whereas patients who are delirious typically do not. Patients with delirium, like many patients afflicted with dementia, tend to have perceptual disturbances such as illusions or visual and auditory hallucinations. Language dysfunction, such as an inability to name objects or rambling incoherent speech, is common in delirium. The course of delirium fluctuates on a time span that is measured in hours, which is unusual in amnestic disorder.

Drugs with sedative-hypnotic properties, most notably alcohol, can cause transitory memory disturbances during intoxication or withdrawal. Interestingly, alcoholic blackout is commonly associated with an inability to retrieve learned material in the absence of alcohol; reexposure may bring back memories of material learned during previous blackouts. This characteristic, a form of state-dependent learning, distinguishes the blackout from the inability of the person who is amnestic to learn new material. Amnestic symptoms that develop during intoxication or withdrawal are classified as part of a particular type of substance-induced intoxication or withdrawal.

Epilepsy and cerebrovascular disease cause amnesia but rarely cause amnestic disorder. Patients experiencing amnestic disorder attributed either to seizures or cerebrovascular disease should be carefully evaluated to elicit clinically significant neurological signs and symptoms. Individuals suffering from seizures are likely to benefit from anticonvulsant therapy, whereas no treatment is indicated for transient global amnesia. Furthermore, patients who suffer from transient amnestic episodes caused by ictal phenomena without initial evidence of epilepsy will probably develop clear seizures. Cerebrovascular disease is associated with a relatively poor outcome because of an increased risk of myocardial infarction and stroke.

Amnestic disorders must be distinguished from the poorly understood dissociative states (see Chapter 18). Primary care physicians also need to be aware that apparent memory problems can be the result of malingering or factitious (self-induced) disorder. A key to the distinction between malingering, factitious disorder, and the dissociative states on the one hand and amnestic disorder on the other lies in the ability to ascertain a cause for the amnestic disorders. Etiological conditions should be temporally related to the onset of amnestic disorder. A great deal of information is available about etiological factors associated with amnestic disorder, many of which are common disorders (for example, alcoholism and head trauma) that may occur in patients with dissociative states. Historically, the so-called psychogenic amnesias have been separated from amnestic disorder on the basis of lost personal memories in the face of adequate function on formal memory testing observed in psychogenic amnesia. Several case reports suggest that autobiographical memories may be lost as a result of CNS lesions and advise caution in the application of this distinction. Primary care providers would probably be wise to refer any cases of suspected dissociative state, malingering, or factitious disorder to specialists with an interest in these controversial and probably rare disorders.

Most other psychiatric disorders are readily distinguished from amnestic disorder. Patients with other psychiatric disorders (such as depression, anxiety disorders, or mania) may complain of poor memory and in some cases exhibit poor performance on formal testing. However, most patients with amnestic disorder are unaware of the extent of their memory problems. The presence of symptoms suggestive of a psychiatric disorder (for example, suicidal ideation and poor appetite suggest depression) other than amnestic disorder in a patient who complains of poor memory should lead to a thorough evaluation to estimate the possibility that he or she meets criteria for a disorder other than amnestic disorder. The individual in Case 11.2 exhibited a significant number of depressive symptoms and appears to have benefited from treatment. Perhaps some of the apparent reversal of memory difficulties in this person is attributable to appropriate antidepressant treatment.

Genetics and family history

Like delirium, amnestic disorder is likely to be almost entirely the product of environmental insults on the brain, with little familiality or evidence for genetic effects. Transient global amnesia has been rarely noted to be familial. Interestingly, the disorder most closely associated with transient global amnesia, migraine, shows significant family loading. Further study of transient global amnesia will help researchers estimate the extent of familiality and perhaps relate it to migraine in some instances.

Korsakoff's syndrome was postulated to be the result of a genetic defect in an enzyme called transketolase that requires thiamine pyrophosphate as a cofactor. At present, no variation in the transketolase gene of patients with Wernicke-Korsakoff syndrome has been described. Patients who develop thiamine deficiency as the result of malnutrition from other causes have been described; amnestic disorder in these cases is virtually indistinguishable from that seen in people with alcoholism. The enduring puzzle is that only a fraction of people with alcoholism develop amnestic disorder. Whereas a significant underestimate of clinical cases is probable (see the following section), the familiality (if any) of Korsakoff's syndrome in people with alcoholism needs to be separated from the familiality of alcoholism and related medical conditions.

Epidemiology

The epidemiology of amnestic disorder is closely related to the epidemiology of the causative disorders. The occurrences of transient global amnesia, a brief benign disorder, and Wernicke-Korsakoff syndrome, typically a chronic state, are relatively well understood. At least four population-based studies provide an estimate of the annual incidence of transient global amnesia, with numbers ranging from 3–10 cases per 100,000 people. Patients who suffer from transient global amnesia are at little risk of suffering from epilepsy and cerebrovascular disease, although there seems to be increased risk of migraine.

Korsakoff's syndrome is much more common than transient global amnesia. Estimates of prevalence based on postmortem series suggest a prevalence of 0.8% to 2.8%. The higher estimates are derived from Australia, where an epidemic of Korsakoff's syndrome appeared to occur in the 1970s and early 1980s. A community-based study from The Netherlands suggests a prevalence of about five cases per 10,000 people, an order of magnitude lower than the postmortem estimates. These findings suggest that although prevalences based on postmortem series may overestimate the occurrence of Wernicke-Korsakoff syndrome, a substantial number of cases are not recognized in living patients. Furthermore, the Australian experience suggests that rates are tied to environmental factors such as per capita alcohol consumption and dietary thiamine supplementation. Primary preventive measures, such as thiamine supplementation and education about the consequences of excessive alcohol intake, may have the desirable effect of reducing the prevalence of Korsakoff's syndrome.

Pathophysiology

To understand what is known about the pathophysiology of amnestic disorder, it is necessary to develop some general principles about learning and memory. First and foremost, memory is an integral aspect of thinking and is thus involved in most cognitive processes. Clinically, this observation is substantiated most obviously by noting that memory is impaired in other global disorders of cognitive functioning, such as dementia and delirium. Memory consists of multiple processes, many of which are difficult to define and poorly understood. In amnestic disorder, patients can repeat digits or words immediately after presentation but are unable to retain the information much beyond this brief period; patients who are delirious have difficulty performing both tasks.

Patients with amnestic disorder also have variable problems retrieving information learned before the onset of the causative disorder (for example, after head trauma or surgery). These observations, supported by much additional data reviewed in the annotated bibliography, suggest that the process of learning involves acquisition (indicated by the ability to repeat information immediately after presentation), retention (storing the data), and retrieval (repetition of some or all of the information when desired). The processes are bounded by an element of time in the sense that the process of learning takes some time to occur (minutes to hours). Time, as marked by the pathological event responsible for the impaired memory of amnestic disorder, delineates the difficulties in learning new items (anterograde amnesia) and retrieving older memories (retrograde amnesia) from

memories of the distant past (remote memory), which are more likely to be spared.

The study of patients with amnesia has shown that these individuals do not lack the capability of learning new material. In particular, they can learn and retain complex procedural skills (such as reading words as they appear in a mirror) despite an inability to remember the content or nature of the task. Observations such as this suggest that amnestic disorder typically involves a type of memory that requires some conscious effort, unlike more automatic memory that is associated with many motor tasks, for example. The memory impaired in amnestic disorder is heavily but not solely related to verbal output. A more general observation is that memory is distributed in specific neural networks serving different functions; some of these functions, such as those involved in execution of the mirror-reading task, are spared in amnestic disorder. Finally, the observation that patients develop amnestic disorder as the result of lesions in different parts of the brain suggests that the memory systems involved in amnestic disorder are distributed and interconnected.

The exploration of clinical cases provides a great deal of information about the anatomical basis of amnestic disorder. The surprising memory deficits of the most famous patient with amnestic disorder were initially interpreted as the failure of all memory, because no learning could be demonstrated despite the preservation of intellect. Subsequent research has demonstrated the ability of this patient and other similarly affected individuals to learn and preserve the ability to execute various tasks (such as the mirror-reading test) even though they were unaware of having previously practiced such tasks. Since the site of surgical intervention was known, it was surmised that the hippocampus and associated structures performed critical learning and memory functions. Unilateral lesions are generally not associated with amnestic disorder. Mapping pathologically affected regions of the brain with scanning techniques (CT and MRI) in this individual and others with chronic amnestic disorder confirmed the original hypothesis. Chronic amnestic disorder associated with anoxia and carbon monoxide poisoning is presumably the result of hippocampal neuronal loss, which can be seen at autopsy. Functional scanning data (from PET and SPECT images) support the belief that temporal lobe structures such as the hippocampus and associated subcortical regions are involved in the pathophysiology of amnesia that is associated with disorders without clear pathology, such as transient global amnesia and epilepsy.

The neuroanatomical basis of Korsakoff's syndrome has been a more controversial subject. Acute pathological changes associated with Wernicke-Korsakoff syndrome have been described in the mammillary bodies and associated structures. Microscopic hemorrhages, hyperplasia of blood vessel walls with proliferation of capillaries, and glial proliferation with initial sparing of neurons but later

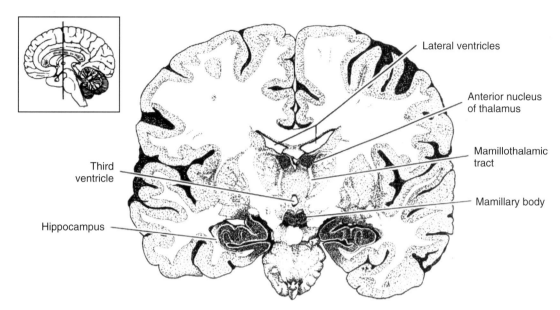

Fig. 11.2 Neuroanatomical structures implicated in amnestic disorder.

Two separate but interconnected systems have been implicated in amnestic disorder and are readily visualized in this line drawing of a brain slice taken at the level indicated in the inset. Externally, this slice would be in front of the ear. The ventricles are indicated; clear areas otherwise correspond to white matter, lightly stippled areas to gray matter, and dark areas to sulci. Neuroanatomical regions thought to be involved in amnestic disorder are heavily stippled. The hippocampus and related structures implicated in amnestic disorder are indicated on the left; the mammillary body, mammillothalamic tract, and thalamic regions involved in Korsakoff's syndrome are on the right.

This slice shows neuroanatomical structures in two dimensions; all structures extend in anterior and posterior directions, with the hippocampus and related structures occupying an extensive portion of the temporal lobe. Bilateral lesions of either region are usually required for amnestic disorder. The dorsal medial thalamic nucleus is not shown, and the involvement of this structure in amnestic disorder is controversial.

development of neuronal chromatolysis are observed in Wernicke's encephalopathy; the affected regions in Korsakoff's syndrome show atrophy as a result of neuronal loss and discoloration. Involvement of thalamic nuclei has been unequivocal, although disagreement exists as to which regions of the thalamus are included. The best available information suggests that the anterior thalamus and possibly the medial dorsal nucleus of the thalamus, in addition to the mammillary bodies, are affected in Korsakoff's syndrome. Korsakoff's syndrome is also likely to involve the interconnection between the mammillary bodies and the thalamus, i.e., the mammillothalamic tract. The thalamic nuclei, the mammillary bodies and this connection have been referred to as diencephalic memory structures.

Brain MRI studies of patients with Korsakoff's syndrome have confirmed reductions in mammillary body and thalamic volume but have also demonstrated correlation between hippocampal volume reductions and anterograde memory deficits. The hippocampus and associated cortex projects to the mammillary bodies and the anterior thalamus largely through the fornix. Older work suggests that lesions of the fornix are not associated with amnesia although more recent work in monkeys and rats questions the solidity of this ob-

servation. An alternative to considering the hippocampus and the diencephalic systems separately is the proposal that an "extended" hippocampal memory system involves the hippocampus and associated regions, the diencephalic structures and connections between hippocampal and diencephalic regions, largely but not entirely through the fornix.

Additional controversy regarding the pathophysiology of Korsakoff's syndrome surrounds the role of the frontal lobes in the resulting disability. Cortical atrophy, particularly in the frontal lobes, is observed in many autopsies and neuroimaging studies. The distinction between Korsakoff's syndrome and a dementia related to chronic ethanol consumption would be difficult if patients with Korsakoff's syndrome show additional chronic cognitive impairment, perhaps because of frontal lobe pathological changes. It is unclear why some regions of the brain are selectively affected by thiamine deficiency when it appears that all brain cells require a continuous supply of thiamine.

A related issue is the importance of ethanol in causing the pathological condition. Ethanol has direct neuronal toxicity, at least in culture systems and in developing animals. It has been difficult to show pathological effects of ethanol on the brain of mature animals. In humans who are alcoholic, direct neuronal toxicity has been hard to demonstrate because the interpretation of postmortem lesions is confounded at least to some extent by the complex premortem pathologic state associated with death in people with alcoholism. Patients at risk for Wernicke-Korsakoff syndrome probably develop thiamine deficiency as the result of reduced dietary intake, decreased intestinal absorption, and depletion of thiamine stores. Although the mechanism by which thiamine deficiency causes Korsakoff's syndrome is unknown, thiamine is critically involved in glucose metabolism; perhaps deficiency of thiamine produces a relative deficiency in the function of a neurotransmitter system such as acetylcholine involved in memory.

Management and treatment

The treatment of amnestic disorder involves the treatment of the associated conditions. Enhancing memory by teaching patients mnemonic devices is of no proven benefit. Addressing the various conditions requires distinguishing one condition from the other, including the separation of transient conditions from chronic amnestic disorder. Transient global amnesia does not need to be treated except to keep the patient safe. Epileptic amnestic disorder should be addressed by treating the underlying partial complex seizures with an appropriate anticonvulsant. Transient ischemic amnesia and amnestic stroke should be distinguished from amnestic disorders largely for prognostic reasons at present.

Treatment of head injury is a complex issue commonly complicated by other injuries. Recovery from even minor head injury can be prolonged by the presence of symptoms described under the rubric of "postconcussive syndrome," although the boundaries of this entity are poorly defined. Hopefully, further study of patients who have suffered varying degrees of brain trauma will further define the relationship between amnestic disorder, other trauma, and the postconcussive syndrome.

As noted previously, supplementation of dietary sources with thiamine may decrease the prevalence of Wernicke-Korsakoff syndrome. Public education about the consequences of excessive alcohol consumption may also reduce the prevalence of Korsakoff's syndrome. Patients who come to a physician with malnutrition, especially patients who are alcoholic or suspected of being alcoholic, should receive additional vitamin supplementation, particularly thiamine. The management of delirium ought to include the administration of parenteral thiamine, hopefully preventing Korsakoff's syndrome. The continued administration of thiamine to patients with Korsakoff's syndrome is of unknown benefit but of little harm; it probably makes good sense, since these individuals are likely to have other pathologic disorders as well as continue to drink. Most vitamin preparations are adequate. Patients with chronic amnestic disorder, regardless of the cause, probably require custodial care, usually in an institution such as a nursing home. These individuals can survive a long time, with prognosis likely to reflect the associated medical conditions.

Amnestic disorder is cognitive impairment limited to the most obvious type of memory in humans (see *Pearls & Perils*). The disorder should be classified according to the signs and symptoms indicative of an etiological condition and further characterized on the basis of amnesia duration. The presence of clinically significant cognitive impairment suggests other disorders, particularly delirium and dementia, even if amnesia is present. Chronic amnestic disorder often results in profound disability requiring custodial care.

PEARLS & PERILS

Amnestic disorder

- Amnestic disorder is restricted to memory dysfunction.
- Other disorders associated with amnesia (dementia and delirium) need to be considered and excluded.
- Amnestic disorder may be brief in duration (for example, transient global amnesia) or chronic (such as Korsakoff's syndrome).
- Prognosis reflects underlying condition and duration.
- Chronic amnestic disorder may require custodial care to sustain life.
- Korsakoff's syndrome (thiamine deficiency), usually seen in people who are alcoholic, is a common but preventable disorder.

CONSIDER CONSULTATION WHEN...

- The diagnosis of amnestic disorder is unclear, particularly if the patient has features of dementia, delirium, dissociative states, or malingering.
- The likely etiological condition is treatable by a specialist (for example, alcohol dependence or epilepsy) or may benefit from rehabilitation (such as a head injury).

Annotated bibliography

American Psychiatric Association (2000) *Diagnostic and Statistical Manual of Mental Disorders*, 4th Edition, Text Revision (DSM-IV-TR). Washington, DC, American Psychiatric Association.
This book supports diagnostic criteria for delirium and amnestic disorder with a presentation of essential information that allows the busy practitioner to rapidly develop a diagnosis.
American Psychiatric Association (1999) Practice guideline for the treatment of patients with delirium, *Am J Psychiatr* 156:1–20.
Expert consensus document providing information on evaluation as well as treatment.

Cook, IA (2004) *Guideline Watch: Practice guideline for the treatment of patients with delirium*, Arlington, VA: American Psychiatric Association.
Available online at http://www.psych.org/psych_pract/treatg/pg/prac_guide.cfm.
Updates the practice guideline, providing an online resource for current practice.
Kopelman, MD (1995) The Korsakoff syndrome, *Br J Psychiatry* 166: 151.

This article provides an excellent review of this form of amnestic disorder; it also presents related memory concepts in a succinct and thorough fashion.
Lipowski, ZJ (1990) *Delirium: acute confusional states*, New York, Oxford University Press.
An extensive review of delirium that remains useful because of completeness although somewhat dated.

CHAPTER 12

Cognitive Disorders: Dementias

Eugene H. Rubin, MD, PhD

Introduction

Dementia is a syndrome characterized by deterioration in memory and other cognitive functions that interferes with a person's ability to manage everyday activities. Functions involving higher level cortical integration are often involved, including general intellect; abilities to plan, organize, and reason; orientation; speech; mathematical skills; visuospatial abilities; and motor planning. Changes in personality are common. Psychotic symptoms, including delusions and hallucinations, often appear as the illness progresses. Most dementias are progressive disorders that rob a person of what it is to be human. Over a period of years, a highly successful and productive person may be reduced to an individual who no longer recognizes her spouse or children and requires full-time nursing care.

Although there are many illnesses leading to the syndrome of dementia, dementia of the Alzheimer type (DAT) is by far the most common cause in North America, accounting for 60–70% of progressive dementias. Only a small percentage of dementias are a result of processes that can be interrupted, stabilized, or reversed. Memory changes or other evidence of compromised brain function that interferes with daily activities are not normal and should not be dismissed with "what do you expect for an 80-year-old." When such changes occur, it is imperative to evaluate and diagnose the illness responsible for the breakdown of brain function. As effective treatments become available, early diagnosis will become even more important. Diagnosis is also the first step in long-term planning for both patients and families.

DAT is common, occurring in 5–10% of people age 65 and older. Its prevalence increases dramatically with advancing age; over one-third of people age 85 and older suffer from DAT. Major progress in elucidating the pathophysiologic mechanisms responsible for this disorder is occurring. Current pharmacologic treatments can stabilize symptoms for

about a year. Treatments based on the pathophysiologic mechanisms underlying this disorder are being developed and have the potential to interfere with disease progression. In fact, it is conceivable that such treatments could be initiated prior to the observation of clinical symptoms and prevent the clinical manifestation of illness. This would require the ability to diagnose the illness prior to symptom onset, which may become feasible with advances in imaging amyloid accumulation.

This chapter will focus on DAT. Lewy body dementia, frontotemporal dementia, and vascular dementia will also be briefly discussed. These four types of dementias account for the large majority of progressive dementias.

Dementia of the Alzheimer type (DAT)

Diagnosis

DAT is a slowly progressive dementia that eventually involves many cortical brain functions (Box 12.1 and Table 12.1). It is important to emphasize that symptoms represent change from a person's baseline, are gradually progressive, and interfere with general ability to function.

If an individual always has had a tendency to misplace glasses or keys, then such a complaint is not a symptom of a progressive dementia. A substantial increase in the frequency of losing such objects may be more concerning, however. Objective memory testing is useful in documenting changes over time. Some age-related cognitive changes occur normally but not to the extent that they interfere with the ability to keep up with key activities. Name recall may become slightly more difficult. Performance on tasks requiring both speed and memory may decrease somewhat with age. Complex tasks requiring attention to many events simultaneously become more difficult. These changes, however, are subtle and rarely interfere with everyday social or occupa-

A 68-year-old corporate president, Mr A, has been the patient of a primary care physician for 25 years and has enjoyed excellent health except for periodic upper respiratory infections and mild arthritis. During an annual checkup, Mrs A pulls the physician aside and relates that Mr A has become more absentminded over the last year. He is still working full time, apparently without difficulties, but she has become aware that he misplaces keys and forgets where he parks the car when he goes shopping. These behaviors are new. She states that he still remembers everyday messages and would remember the details of dinner at a restaurant the previous night. He would remember a wedding from several weeks ago, but he might not be as accurate with details of that event as he would have been ten years ago. It has become harder for him to organize documents for tax preparation. Occasionally he forgets an appointment, which he never did before. He has become a little more socially withdrawn.

When the physician evaluates Mr A, he states that he feels fine and that he is doing well in terms of his memory and thinking skills. Routine blood tests, including tests for thyroid hormone and vitamin B$_{12}$, are all normal. A neurologic exam reveals no abnormalities. On several brief cognitive batteries, such as the Short Blessed Test (described by Katzman and colleagues) and the Mini-Mental Status Exam (described by Folstein and colleagues), Mr A scores perfectly. The physician reviews with Mr and Mrs A that Mr A's laboratory work and exam are normal and that the reported changes in his memory and function are subtle and of unknown significance. The physician emphasizes the need for careful follow-up in order to see if symptoms progress over time.

There is little change over the next year. The following year, however, Mrs A reports that there has been definite, slowly progressive slippage. Mr A still works full time, but their son who works with him reports that his father is starting to forget earlier business decisions and to mix up accounts. This has not occurred frequently, but it is often enough that other company executives are concerned. Mrs A reports that Mr A seemed more confused during a vacation to Europe. In past years, he enjoyed planning such trips, but this year he asked her to take over. She has noticed that he not only has difficulties remembering names but he also repeats stories without realizing it. He forgets to tell her that someone has called and forgets appointments more often. She also has noticed that he is less able to recall certain words and that she has been completing sentences for him. At Mr A's request, Mrs A had assumed responsibility for paying bills and keeping track of investments. He had always been accurate in leaving an 18–20% tip at restaurants, but lately he leaves from 10–30% without apparent intent.

When the physician interviews Mr A, he states that everything is fine other than forgetting a name occasionally. Everything is okay at work, and he is beginning to think about retirement. His performance on cognitive testing is still within normal limits, but he does not fully remember a name and address that is part of a brief cognitive test. The physician orders a head magnetic resonance imaging study, which shows mild global atrophy. The physician talks with the couple and indicates that these subtle cognitive changes may represent the very mild stages of DAT. He reviews information about this disorder and suggests that they learn more by contacting the Alzheimer's Association. He encourages Mr A to maintain enjoyable activities and exercise. After reviewing the risks and benefits of pharmacotherapy, all agree that Mr A will start on a cholinesterase inhibitor. Subsequently, the physician sees Mr A every three or four months, and he remains cognitively stable for the next 15 months.

After this 15-month respite, the illness progresses again and over the next two years, Mr A has increasing difficulty with memory, orientation, judgment, visuospatial skills, speech, and behavior. The clinical diagnosis of DAT is confirmed by the nature and progression of his symptoms. He has trouble remembering the details of an event from several days ago. If he does not write down a phone message, it is likely forgotten. He still drives but has lost his car at malls on several occasions. He forgot his wife's birthday for the first time. He thought that a visit from a son two weeks ago occurred several months ago. He is no longer able to program his VCR. He reads much less and has noticeable trouble finding words when speaking. He can no longer manipulate figures mentally. In an attempt to draw a clock indicating 2:45, he sketches three hands—one pointing to each number. On brief cognitive testing, his short-term memory is obviously compromised.

During the following year, Mr A becomes irritable and at times physically threatening. He is more secluded and spends much of his time sitting and watching TV. He is certain that his family is stealing from him. On occasion, he believes that the people on TV are actually in his house. He imagines people in his yard and hears their conversations. Eventually, agitation coupled with increasing incontinence necessitates nursing home admission.

This vignette demonstrates a typical history of a person with DAT. As treatments are discovered that delay the biochemical and neuropathologic changes, it will be important to initiate such treatment early in the course of the illness.

tional function. If changes begin to have an impact on function, the clinician should become increasingly concerned that such changes could be the initial manifestation of DAT.

As noted, the case history described previously is typical of DAT. The earliest clinical symptoms typically involve subtle memory changes. Other early, common symptoms are increasing passivity and withdrawal. The first to observe such changes is often a collateral source, such as a spouse, child, or close friend. Collateral source observations of these early symptoms are usually more accurate than reports from the patient. It is not rare for patients to deny symptoms even when cognitive failure is evident to all who are close to them. It is important to integrate the history from both the collateral source and the patient.

Box 12.1 Dementia of the Alzheimer's type

DIAGNOSTIC CRITERIA

A. The development of multiple cognitive deficits manifested by both

1 memory impairment (impaired ability to learn new information or to recall previously learned information)

2 one (or more) of the following cognitive disturbances:
- aphasia (language disturbance)
- apraxia (impaired ability to carry out motor activities despite intact motor function)
- agnosia (failure to recognize or identify objects despite intact sensory function)
- disturbance in executive functioning (i.e., planning, organizing, sequencing, abstracting).

B. The cognitive deficits in criteria A1 and A2 each cause significant impairment in social or occupational functioning and represent a significant decline from a previous level of functioning.

C. The course is characterized by gradual onset and continuing cognitive decline.

D. The cognitive deficits in criteria A1 and A2 are not due to any of the following:
- other central nervous system conditions that cause progressive deficits in memory and cognition (e.g., cerebrovascular disease, Parkinson's disease, Huntington's disease, subdural hematoma, normal-pressure hydrocephalus, brain tumor)
- systemic conditions that are known to cause dementia (e.g., hypothyroidism, vitamin B_{12} or folic acid deficiency, niacin deficiency, hypercalcemia, neurosyphilis, HIV infection)
- substance-induced conditions.

E. The deficits do not occur exclusively during the course of a delirium.

F. The disturbance is not better accounted for by another Axis I disorder (e.g., major depressive disorder, schizophrenia).

Adapted from American Psychiatric Association (2000) Diagnostic and Statistical Manual of Mental Disorders, 4th Edition, Text Revision. Washington, D.C., American Psychiatric Association.

Table 12.1 Dementia of the Alzheimer's type

DIAGNOSIS

Discriminating features

1 Gradual, progressive deterioration involving multiple cognitive functions, including memory, that eventually interferes with ability to function. Speech, learning, reasoning, mathematical skills, visuospatial abilities, and complex motor skills may be involved.

Consistent features

1 Personality changes (for example, more passive and less interested) are common early in the illness.
2 Agitation, delusions, and hallucinations may occur with illness progression.
3 Complete inability to perform basic activities of daily living eventually occurs.

Variable features

1 Depression.
2 Progressive aphasia preceding or accompanying cognitive deterioration.
3 Social inappropriateness preceding or accompanying cognitive deterioration.
4 Mild Parkinsonian features accompanying cognitive deterioration.

Note that variable features 2, 3, and 4 could also suggest non-DAT dementias.

Natural history

DAT is a progressive disorder that leads to deterioration in most brain functions over several years. The illness usually presents with subtle changes in memory and personality, however, more focal presentations can occur (see below). Illness progression can be monitored by asking a series of questions pertaining to cognitive and behavioral changes at each visit. These questions coupled with neurologic and mental status examinations can be sufficient. Some clinicians administer brief cognitive batteries, such as the Short Blessed Test or Mini-Mental Status Exam, every 6–12 months. More

detailed global staging instruments are also available and are helpful for clinical research. The group from the Alzheimer's Disease Research Center at Washington University has developed and refined the Clinical Dementia Rating Scale (CDR). This scale has been shown to be reliable and useful for staging illness as very mild, mild, moderate, or severe based on six individually rated domains: memory, orientation, judgment and problem solving, home and hobbies, community affairs, and personal care. By using such scales in longitudinal studies, an accurate description of the rate and nature of progression has been elucidated.

DAT in its earliest clinical stages can be difficult to diagnose because the symptoms can remain subtle for several years. Eventually, perhaps over a period of several years, symptoms become consistent and progressive enough to support a diagnosis of very mild or mild DAT. Memory changes start to interfere with everyday function. If the patient is still working, performance most likely deteriorates to a level where co-workers become aware that something is wrong. If the person is retired, the collateral source may acknowledge that their loved one's memory and thinking have deteriorated to a point that would prohibit a pre-retirement level of function. Stories are repeated; messages are forgotten. It is common that affected people who are involved in volunteer organizations are encouraged to give up positions of leadership because of poor performance. Money management abilities deteriorate. At this very mild or mild stage of illness, patients still can be active with family and friends. They may not be able to organize vacations, but they may still enjoy traveling with family members. Hobbies are still maintained although they are performed less well. Bowling or golf partners may report that their friend has trouble calculating the score or becomes mixed up with the number of strokes already played. Activities around the home are usually maintained, although perhaps at a less intense level; selfcare in terms of grooming, toileting, and eating is not yet influenced. Once a mild stage of illness is reached, over half of patients progress to a moderate or severe stage of disease over the next 15 months. Within three years, 80% of people with mild DAT progress beyond the mild stage, and more than half are either severely demented or dead.

The moderate stage of dementia is characterized by substantial memory loss. Patients retain little from events or conversations. They may forget that their caregivers are their spouses; they may not recognize their children. It becomes difficult to take them to gatherings or restaurants because their social judgment is compromised. They are unable to help with chores. They require help with dressing, bathing, and eating. Wandering and agitation occur frequently. Such people may become increasingly withdrawn. They may sit in front of the television all day with little evidence of attentiveness. In mild stages of DAT, some patients may believe that people are stealing from them. These suspicions can increase in intensity and frequency during moderate stages. Hallucinations and delusions are common during this moderate stage of illness. Behavioral disturbances, including wandering, agitation, and psychotic symptoms, are difficult for the family to manage without help. Education, knowledge about community resources, and support groups for caregivers are essential and are provided by the Alzheimer's Association and its local chapters.

During the severe stage of illness, memory abilities are almost totally destroyed. Patients may not recognize themselves or their loved ones. Incontinence is typical, and nursing home admission is commonly necessary. People with severe DAT may be either mobile or bedridden. When mobile, they do not participate in activities even though they may be brought into the room where such activities are occurring.

The progression from the very mildest stage of the illness to the mild stage may be very gradual, that is, it may take many years. Once the mild stage is reached, progression to the severe stage usually occurs over one to five years. Death may not occur for many years after the illness has reached the severe stage. In otherwise healthy people with mild DAT, about half are still alive after eight years; however, almost all are in the severely demented stage of illness. Therefore, once this illness clearly declares itself and reaches a mild stage of severity, it will rob a person of most important brain functions over the next few years, leaving a severely incapacitated, totally dependent individual for many more years until death ends the ordeal.

Less common presentations

On occasion, DAT can begin with symptoms suggestive of more focal brain pathology. Most cortical and subcortical regions are involved in advanced DAT; however, early illness may involve discrete brain regions before the pathological changes become more generalized. Diagnosing DAT is difficult when the illness begins with predominantly focal symptoms. For instance, DAT may disproportionately attack frontotemporal regions of the brain early in the disease process, and the first symptoms may be coarse and grossly inappropriate behaviors with only minimal cognitive changes. Such symptoms are also seen in a less common group of dementias known as frontotemporal dementias (FTD, see below). Treatments that help stabilize patients with DAT such as cholinesterase inhibitors may not be beneficial in people suffering from non-DAT, frontotemporal dementias. Furthermore, as treatments become more based on underlying mechanisms, it will become increasingly important for diagnostic tools to be developed that allow the clinician to differentiate among the various causes of this clinical presentation.

Some patients with DAT may have symptoms of mild parkinsonism. Psychotic symptoms may also be present. Although such symptoms may occur in DAT, their presence may increase the chances that the dementia is not DAT, but dementia with Lewy bodies (DLB, see below). Similarly, some patients with DAT may present with a marked aphasia; however, such presentations can also occur in a group of rare dementias pathologically distinct from DAT.

Currently, clinicians need to be aware that, although DAT may have unusual presentations, the more atypical the symptoms, the more likely that other, less common types of dementia may be responsible.

Differential diagnosis

Many illnesses can cause the syndrome of dementia; however, DAT, either alone or with other dementing disorders, is the most common cause of dementia among the elderly in North America. Accurate diagnosis will become increasingly important as treatments become more specific. Drugs that interfere with amyloid deposition may prove effective in slowing the progression of DAT, but they would be unlikely to influence the natural history of vascular dementia.

Examples of non-DAT dementias are listed in Box 12.2.

A major goal in evaluating patients with dementia is to determine whether diseases other than DAT are causing or contributing to the dementia. If so, treating the primary disorder may halt the progression of the dementia or possibly reverse it. Unfortunately, very few patients have truly reversible dementias. Two of the more common causes of reversible dementia are medications and major depression.

Examples of dementias other than DAT

Non-Alzheimer primary CNS degenerative disorders
- Parkinson's disease with dementia
- Dementia with Lewy bodies
- Progressive supranuclear palsy
- Huntington's disease
- Non-Alzheimer frontotemporal dementias (including Pick's disease)

Other CNS Disorders
- Vascular dementias
- Major depression
- Brain injury
- CNS infections
- Neoplasms involving CNS
- Hydrocephalus
- Subdural hematoma

Disorders related to exogenous substances
- Medication induced
- Substance abuse induced

Systemic disorders
- Endocrine disorders—thyroid, parathyroid
- Cardiovascular disorders
- Immune system disorders
- Hepatic disorders
- Renal disorders
- Nutritional deficits—vitamin B_{12} deficiency

KEY CLINICAL QUESTIONS AND WHAT THEY UNLOCK

- *Has there been a change in memory over the last year or two that is now interfering with the patient's everyday function?*
- *Has there been a change in the patient's ability to remember important information regarding recent events, that is, events that have occurred over the last several days? If so, are these changes interfering with the patient's activities and function?*
- *Could the patient master new information of particular personal interest to the same level as she could have several years ago? For instance, if the patient likes to play card games, could she become as skillful at a new card game as she could have several years ago? (It might take somewhat longer to master. The important question to establish is whether the same level of skill could be attained.)*
- *Is the patient having more difficulty performing tasks that require organizational skills such as keeping up with bills, maintaining the checkbook, or organizing papers for tax preparation? If the patient has never performed these tasks, would it be much more difficult for him to learn how to do them now in comparison to several years earlier? (Many of us were never good at these tasks; the important information is whether there is a change in such abilities.)*
- *Could the patient handle a previous job or role in a volunteer organization with the memory and thinking skills that she currently has?*
- *Did cognitive changes start in a subtle manner and gradually progress over time?*
  Answers to these questions that indicate increasing difficulty with cognitive function over time are very consistent with a dementia, especially DAT.
- *When memory changes are very mild, are any of the following occurring often?*
    Visual hallucinations: that is, seeing things that are not there, especially well-formed scenes such as a group of children playing.
    Symptoms suggestive of mild Parkinson's disease.
    Repeated periods of marked cognitive fluctuation.
  When this group of symptoms occurs in a person with very mild memory changes, Lewy body dementia should be seriously considered.
- *When cognitive changes are very mild, does the patient often exhibit obviously crude and embarrassing behaviors in public settings? For example, a previously quiet and socially proper individual routinely may tell loud and inappropriate jokes to perfect strangers.*
  A positive answer to this question suggests the possibility of frontotemporal dementia.

The evaluation of a patient with dementia starts with a careful history from knowledgeable collateral sources and the patient, which may require multiple visits and examinations over time. A physical examination, including neurologic and mental status examinations, is important. Brief or more formal cognitive testing is often valuable to establish a baseline for comparison as the illness progresses. In evaluating a patient with dementia, many clinicians routinely measure thyroid hormone and vitamin B_{12} levels. Other tests may be useful including tests of liver and renal function. Measuring plasma levels of currently used medications can be helpful. Computerized tomography or magnetic resonance imaging of the brain is usually indicated to rule out structural lesions that could be responsible for symptoms. Dementias with unusual symptoms like motor neuron disease should be referred to a specialist for further evaluation.

Parkinson's disease with dementia

Patients with Parkinson's disease (PD) are at high risk for both depression and dementia. Approximately 50% of people with Parkinson's disease have had or will subsequently develop major depression. Approximately 30% of patients with Parkinson's disease develop a dementia. The relationship between dementia and PD is complex. People with DAT are at increased risk for developing extrapyramidal symptoms such as bradykinesia, tremor, gait disturbance, and rigidity, and they may have anatomical changes in the substantia nigra consistent with PD. Patients who develop PD without initial symptoms of cognitive impairment have an increased risk of developing a dementia; however, the pathological changes related to dementia are varied. In addition to evidence of PD involving the substantia nigra, typical pathologic findings of Alzheimer's disease with widely distributed senile plaques and neurofibrillary tangles may be present. Other patients may have evidence of PD together with cortical Lewy bodies (see below) but be without evidence of Alzheimer's disease. The overlap between DAT, Parkinson's disease, and Lewy body dementia (see below) both in terms of clinical symptoms as well as pathological changes is a rapidly evolving clinical and research area.

Dementia with Lewy bodies

A syndrome referred to as dementia with Lewy bodies (DLB) may be one of the more common dementias, perhaps accounting for 15–20% of dementias. The brains of people with this illness contain intraneuronal cortical Lewy bodies, with or without the presence of amyloid plaques. Neurofibrillary tangles are frequently absent. The neuropathology of Alzheimer's disease is defined by the presence of amyloid plaques and cortical neurofibrillary tangles. However, in some patients, Lewy bodies also may be present in the cortex and yet the patients have classic symptoms of DAT. DLB may be related to abnormalities in a synaptic protein called synuclein. Although clinical and pathological overlap may exist between DLB and Alzheimer's disease, the core pathological abnormality involving synuclein suggests that DLB has a different pathophysiology than Alzheimer's disease.

Several clinical features increase the likelihood of DLB, although clinical differentiation between DAT and DLB is not always clear. These clinical features include recurrent, marked fluctuation in cognitive abilities, visual hallucinations at an early stage of illness when cognitive abilities are relatively intact, parkinsonian features, and frequent falls. Psychiatrists may see these patients because the visual hallucinations, sometimes accompanied with auditory hallucinations, can be dramatic. DLB progresses gradually and eventually cognitive deterioration becomes dominant. At the moderate stages of this illness, patients' symptoms may resemble those seen in DAT. Patients suffering from DLB are extremely sensitive to the motor side effects of antipsychotic medications, and a careful risk/benefit assessment is necessary when deciding whether to use such agents. As is true in patients with DAT, cholinesterase inhibitors may be beneficial in people with DLB. As more is learned about the pathophysiology of this disorder, more specific treatments will be developed.

Frontotemporal dementias

Frontotemporal dementias (FTD) also have clinical symptoms that help differentiate these dementias from DAT. FTD may occur in people in their 40s, 50s, and 60s, that is, the age of onset may be younger than in the majority of patients with DAT. The clinical presentation of FTD is dominated by gradual but substantial changes involving social behavior. At a time when cognitive changes are subtle, crude and disinhibited behaviors occur. Loved ones are frequently surprised and embarrassed by inappropriate public displays, which may involve crude language, inappropriate jokes, and lack of social sensitivity. Patients often lack insight. Changes in language may be evident, including repeating phrases and echoing words. Eventually a poverty of speech may occur, and mutism is not uncommon. There are likely to be clinical subtypes of FTD depending on the relative involvement of certain regions of the frontal cortex and the anterior temporal lobe.

The illness gradually progresses and eventually patients with FTD may be indistinguishable from people with DAT. The pathology associated with FTD varies, but it usually involves neuronal cell loss. Some patients have some of the changes associated with Pick's disease, that is, cell loss, Pick's cells, and Pick's bodies. Therefore, Pick's disease is a subtype of FTD. FTD may involve abnormalities of the tau protein. As the pathophysiology becomes clearer, specific treatments should become available. As for now, treatment is supportive and non-specific.

Vascular dementia

Vascular dementia is thought to result from the consequences of cerebrovascular disease. Risk factors are the same as those that predispose patients to cerebrovascular disease including hypertension, heart disease, and disorders leading to cerebral emboli. The precise relationship of cerebral infarcts to dementia requires further research. The number, location, and size of infarcts necessary for symptoms of dementia are not well characterized. Most agree that multiple strokes involving large areas of the brain compromise cognitive function. However, the role of single discrete lesions or multiple clinically silent lesions detected by brain imaging studies is uncertain. Evidence of strokes from clinical history, clinical examination, and imaging coupled with cognitive changes time-linked to the cerebrovascular event suggests the diagnosis of vascular dementia.

The course of symptoms will vary substantially depending on the nature of the infarct. Cerebrovascular disease is common, and people who die without clinical evidence of dementia can have significant numbers of small infarcts. Patients dying with Alzheimer's disease but with no clinical evidence of cerebrovascular disease similarly can have multiple, small, scattered infarcts. Patients with DAT can also have clinically evident infarcts. Infarcts can worsen the symptoms of DAT. Pure vascular dementia in the absence of Alzheimer's disease occurs, but separating such cases from patients with mixed vascular dementia and DAT is difficult. Vascular dementias have a fluctuating course but can progress rapidly. Minimizing the risk of future cerebrovascular events may slow the progression of pure vascular dementia if the reason for progression is recurrent infarcts.

Vascular events in the brain may either cause or exacerbate many psychiatric disorders including depression, mania, and DAT. "Silent infarcts" may not be silent but may manifest as behavioral changes. Our understanding of the exact relationship of infarcts and dementia is still evolving. Certainly, minimizing risk factors for a cerebrovascular event is sound advice. Exercise, a healthy diet with attention to cholesterol and triglyceride levels, blood pressure regulation, and avoiding cigarettes can help minimize the contribution of cerebrovascular events to the presentation or progression of dementia.

PEARLS & PERILS

- Although DAT often presents with subtle changes in memory and personality, presentations suggesting initial focal pathology can occur.
- Contrary to earlier beliefs, truly reversible dementias in the elderly are not common. Medication-induced dementia and dementia of depression are two types of potentially reversible dementias.
- Patients with DAT can also have symptomatic or silent cerebral infarcts.
- Pure vascular dementia in the absence of Alzheimer's disease may be difficult to differentiate from a mixed dementia caused by Alzheimer's disease and cerebral infarcts.

Epidemiology

The incidence and prevalence of DAT increases dramatically with age. The illness is rare in people younger than age 50. Approximately 1% of people age 60 to 64 have symptoms of DAT. In older people, the prevalence of the illness doubles every five years, and more than one-third of seniors age 85 and older suffer from DAT. In the year 2000, there were about 35 million people in the U.S. 65 years of age and older. Between 2000 and 2030, there will be a doubling of that number of people to 70 million. Between the years 2000 and 2050, the number of people in the U.S. age 85 and older will increase from about 4 million to about 19 million. If we are unable to prevent or delay the onset of DAT, the number of people with this disorder will quadruple by 2050.

Although DAT is common in both women and men, it occurs more often in women. Women outlive men, and 70% of people age 85 and older are women. Therefore, the absolute number of women with this disease will greatly exceed the number of men. Genetic factors, environmental factors, and the interaction of genetic with environmental factors all play roles in causing DAT. There are a small number of families with autosomal dominant forms of DAT. Although these families probably account for less than 1% of all cases, the elucidation of the specific genetic abnormalities in these families has helped clarify the pathophysiology underlying the more common forms of the illness. The genetic mutations in these rare families all influence the accumulation or elimination of beta-amyloid, a polypeptide formed from the metabolism of a cellular protein, amyloid precursor protein. Mouse models of AD have been developed based on the discoveries of these genetic mutations.

A more common genetic risk factor for developing DAT involves apolipoprotein E subtypes (ApoE). These apolipoproteins are involved in cholesterol and fatty acid transport and perhaps the clearance of various other brain constituents. There are three ApoE subtypes, ApoE2, 3, and 4; each person has two copies of the ApoE allele. Each subtype differs from the others by one or two amino acids. People with one copy of the ApoE4 allele are at an increased risk for developing DAT, and those with two copies of ApoE4 are at a substantially increased risk. The reason for this relationship is not fully understood, but it may involve differential influence of the various forms of ApoE on the clearance of amyloid. The degree of increased risk varies in different populations. For instance, the risk of developing DAT associated with ApoE4 is substantially higher in Caucasians than in African Americans. Although the risk is increased in people with two copies of ApoE4, there are a number of people with two copies of ApoE4 who never develop the illness, and there are many people who have no copies of ApoE4 who do develop DAT. Currently, the determination of an individual's ApoE subtype is generally not recommended. This may change once ApoE4-specific treatments are developed or if preventive treatments become available.

Although less clearly understood, there is increasing evidence of relationships between brain cholesterol homeostasis, risk factors for stroke, and the development or worsening of DAT. Whether there is a direct relationship between cholesterol and the mechanisms underlying DAT or an indirect relationship with "silent" infarcts interacting with AD pathology in a synergistic manner or both will be clarified over time.

Repeated head trauma may also increase the risk of developing DAT. People with ApoE4 may have an increased susceptibility to CNS damage from repeated head trauma. Such a relationship would demonstrate an interesting interaction between environment and genetics.

Another environmental influence may be level of education. Several studies have demonstrated an inverse relationship between educational level and the risk of developing dementia. The reason for such a relationship is unclear. Some believe that formal education may be correlated with increased synaptic connections, forming a reserve that may help delay the clinical manifestations of DAT.

It is probable that many more genetic and environmental factors related to the development of DAT will be discovered. Such discoveries may lead to a variety of treatment options. Some of these treatments may only be effective in people with specific genetic risk factors.

Pathophysiology

Alzheimer's disease is defined by clinical course coupled with characteristic pathologic findings in the brain. At the level of the whole brain, atrophy can be evident; however, there is great variability in its degree and location. Usually primary motor and sensory areas are affected less than association regions. In some cases, disproportionate focal atrophy is evident with brain imaging studies and can be substantial.

At the microscopic level, neuronal loss can be dramatic. Senile plaques, consisting of beta-amyloid together with many other substances, occur in large numbers throughout many cortical regions. Some plaques are diffuse in appearance; others have dense central cores. Some plaques have components of deteriorating intracellular neuronal material referred to as neuritic changes, some do not. There is great heterogeneity in plaque type, burden, and location in the brains of people who died during similar stages of illness. Although neocortical plaques can occur in small clumps in a few areas of the cortex in people without dementia, the presence of multiple plaques in several regions of the cortex is highly suggestive of Alzheimer's disease.

Intraneuronal neurofibrillary tangles are another neuropathologic feature of most patients with Alzheimer's disease. An abnormally phosphorylated cytoskeletal protein called tau is a major component of tangles. The number and location of tangles is also quite variable in people with DAT. With age, tangles increasingly accumulate in areas in and near the hippocampus in the absence of Alzheimer's disease. With DAT, tangles increase in and near the hippocampus as well as many neocortical regions. The presence of neocortical tangles is usually indicative of a pathological condition.

DAT is usually associated with both amyloid plaques and neurofibrillary tangles. The relationship between plaque formation and the development of neurofibrillary tangles is unclear. Some evidence suggests that an increase in cortical plaques triggers events that lead to an increased rate of accumulation of neocortical tangles.

Other neuropathologic abnormalities can be seen in the brains of people affected by Alzheimer's disease, including Hirano bodies, granulovacuolar degeneration, and, on occasion, Lewy bodies. The presence of Lewy bodies makes the neuropathologic differentiation of DAT and DLB difficult at times. Little is known about the relationship of these changes to neuronal loss, plaques, and tangles.

Substantial progress has been made in understanding the molecular biology and genetics of Alzheimer's disease. As mentioned earlier, there are rare, familial forms of Alzheimer's disease that are inherited in an autosomal dominant pattern. The mutations responsible for these familial forms and the proteins involved in several of these mutations have been identified. This genetic information has led to the development of animal models of the disease, and data from several avenues of research have converged on the hypothesis that Alzheimer's disease is caused by excessive accumulation of beta-amyloid, a polypeptide derived from amyloid precursor protein. Factors that increase the formation of beta-amyloid fibrils and amyloid-containing plaques or inhibit the removal of beta-amyloid enhance the risk of Alzheimer's disease (see Fig. 12.1). According to this hypothesis, excessive amyloid can lead directly to changes that cause the dysfunction and destruction of neurons. For instance, destruction may be caused by immune reactions, activation of proteins that cause cell death, or the production or release of free radicals or other toxic substances. The balance between accumulation and clearance of amyloid may be influenced by genetic factors, such as apoliprotein E subtype, or environmental factors. Although substantial evidence supports this "amyloid cascade" hypothesis, it is still a work in progress. It is possible that amyloid is not directly responsible; amyloid accumulation may correlate with a yet to be discovered process that is etiologically responsible. There are many complex relationships involving the relationship of amyloid with other pathological changes such as tangle formation (related to accumulation of abnormal tau protein) and Lewy body formation (related to synuclein accumulation) that are not yet fully understood.

Even if the accumulation of amyloid is causally related to Alzheimer's disease, accumulation alone is not sufficient to cause symptoms. Significant minorities of cognitively healthy, elderly people have amyloid plaques at autopsy. In some of these cognitively healthy people, plaques are few and found in patches, that is, large regions of brain are without plaques. In others, however, plaques are plentiful, and brains resemble those of people with Alzheimer's disease. If these people lived another few years, it is likely that they would have developed symptoms of DAT; therefore, this group might be considered as having "presymptomatic" DAT. Once methods are available to measure amyloid *in vivo*, "presymptomatic" Alzheimer's disease can be studied. Such methods are in development.

Even once beta-amyloid fibrils and plaques have accumulated, it is likely that genetic and environmental factors exist that can delay subsequent events leading to neural dysfunction and destruction. The illness progresses over a period of several years once the destructive cascade is triggered. This fact suggests that the damage is caused by a continuing process and that different interventions may be helpful depending on the stage of the pathology. When *in vivo* beta-amyloid imaging techniques become a reality, people at high risk, that is, accumulating excessive amounts of amyloid, will be identifiable. If the amyloid cascade could be blocked in these high-risk people, the progression of the illness could be prevented prior to the appearance of clinical symptoms. Agents are now under development that can interfere with the accumulation of beta-amyloid, disrupt its aggregation

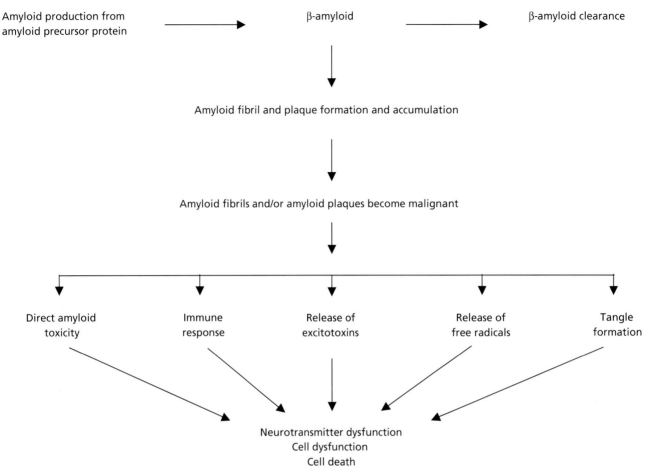

Fig. 12.1 Possible role of amyloid in Alzheimer's disease.

into fibrils, and enhance its clearance. This is obviously an exciting and important area of research.

Treatment

DAT is an illness that affects patients together with their families and loved ones. Current treatment strategies include biopsychosocial approaches. Biologic treatment includes pharmacotherapy for cognitive and other psychiatric symptoms of the illness. Psychosocial intervention involves educational programs, resource referrals, and psychologic support systems for patients and caregivers. The Alzheimer's Association provides expertise in resource referrals.

An early phase of treatment involves teaching the patient and the family about Alzheimer's disease. Emphasizing to the caregiver that changes in behavior are not the patient's fault but are a result of gradual CNS deterioration helps minimize blame and stress. The abilities of patients and their families to accept and understand the implications of a diagnosis of DAT vary greatly, and it is important to individualize the manner in which this information is conveyed.

Discussions may require several visits. Appropriate referrals to reading material, the Alzheimer's Association, and social services should be done in a timely but sensitive manner. Many elderly are appropriately fearful of the diagnosis of DAT, and words need to be chosen carefully. If the diagnosis is likely but uncertain, it is important to indicate that there is uncertainty and explain that time will be necessary to clarify the diagnosis. It will become clear from careful follow-up whether the cognitive changes represent the early stages of DAT. Patients and their families need to know so that planning can begin. If a patient and his family have not yet formalized an advanced directive regarding health care, this should be addressed. The course of the illness is gradual but progressive, and medical, financial, and legal plans should be made with patients' full input. People's reactions to learning about the illness vary from fear to relief. Insight may be compromised even early in the illness. This phase of treatment, that is, disclosure of the diagnosis and education, can be the most difficult for the physician. Patients and families are usually appreciative of a direct but caring approach.

General principles of pharmacologic management in the elderly are reviewed in Chapter 26. Patients with DAT are frequently sensitive to cognitive-impairing side effects of medications and, therefore, simplifying pharmacologic regimens and minimizing doses of necessary medications can help improve cognitive function.

Cognitive symptoms

As CNS destruction occurs, various neurotransmitter systems are compromised. The central acetylcholinergic system is involved in memory and learning. It had been thought that the cholinergic system is selectively involved in DAT, and initial pharmacologic strategies involving acetylcholine analogous to dopaminergic strategies in treating Parkinson's disease were proposed. Although it has become apparent that multiple other CNS transmitter systems are involved in DAT, cholinergic replacement strategies have been investigated. Increasing acetylcholinergic function by inhibiting metabolism via acetylcholinesterase has been successful in producing agents that are more effective than placebo in delaying progression of the illness. Since 1993 several cholinesterase inhibitors have become available. Tacrine is historically important because it was the first such agent shown to delay the progression of DAT. Liver enzymes needed to be monitored in people taking tacrine, and a large number of people could not tolerate the dose necessary to slow disease progression. Subsequently, donepezil, rivastigmine, and galantamine have been approved in the U.S. for treatment of DAT. Although there are some differences among these three drugs, all are cholinesterase inhibitors, and they have overlapping side-effect profiles and similar efficacy. It is likely that some patients may tolerate one agent better than another.

It is important to explain to patients and families what to expect from treatment with cholinesterase inhibitors. Although some patients may demonstrate mild improvement, the major benefit from these agents is a delay in symptom progression by about 6–12 months. On average (and with substantial variation among patients), people with DAT who are treated with these agents maintain cognitive performance for six months or more and subsequently stay six months or more ahead of where they would have been had they taken a placebo. Although deterioration eventually returns, this 6–12 month benefit can be maintained for a significant period of time. If the medication is stopped, deterioration to the level expected had the patient not taken the medication is common. Although the magnitude of benefit from these drugs may not be dramatic, maintaining abilities for an extra six months or more can be clinically important. If families expect dramatic improvement instead of short-term stabilization, they may be disappointed when they do not see improvement. If they understand what to expect, compliance is likely to be better.

Cholinesterase inhibitors can also help with non-cognitive symptoms of DAT. Personality changes, affective symptoms, psychotic symptoms, wandering, and agitation can be part of the natural history of DAT. Several of these non-cognitive symptoms may stabilize or improve with cholinesterase inhibitor treatment. The stabilization that can occur with this class of drugs may help lessen caregiver burden and delay nursing home admission.

Cholinesterase inhibitors can help patients with mild to moderate DAT. Studies are ongoing to see if such treatment is helpful in the earlier stages of illness. These medications are costly and have side effects. Delaying treatment may not be in a patient's best interest, but neither is treating subtle changes for which an etiology has not yet been clarified. The clinician should be careful not to commit someone to long-term treatment unless the spectrum of symptoms is consistent with DAT or other dementias shown to be responsive to cholinesterase inhibitors.

In addition to cholinesterase inhibitors, vitamin E may slow functional impairment in people who are in the moderate stage of severity of DAT. Large doses (1,000 IU twice a day) were used in the major study demonstrating this effect. It is not known if smaller doses are helpful or if vitamin E can be beneficial in earlier stages of illness. One should be cautious using vitamin E in people with a diathesis for bleeding or in people taking blood thinning agents. Also, there is a recent report that high doses of vitamin E may be related to a slight increase in mortality (Miller *et al.*, 2005).

Cholinesterase inhibitors may also be helpful in delaying the cognitive deterioration associated with DLB. Some of the non-cognitive symptoms of DLB may also respond to cholinesterase inhibitors. This class of agent does not appear to be beneficial in the treatment of frontotemporal dementias.

In late 2003, memantine was approved for the treatment of moderate to severe DAT. This agent is an antagonist of a glutamate receptor known as the N-methyl-D-aspartate (NMDA) receptor. This agent may help protect cells from damage caused by excessive stimulation from glutamate. Memantine can slow the rate of functional deterioration in people with moderate to severe dementia. At the current time, its efficacy in mild dementia has not been established. More research is needed to evaluate possible additive benefits of memantine with cholinesterase inhibitors at different stages of DAT.

There have been epidemiologic studies suggesting that people treated with anti-inflammatory drugs have lower risks for developing DAT. Such correlations from epidemiologic studies do not mean, however, that anti-inflammatory agents actually cause decreased risk. In fact, studies examining the use of both older and newer non-steroidal anti-inflammatory drugs have not, for the most part, supported their efficacy in treating patients with DAT. Similarly, there have been epidemiologic studies suggesting that estrogen use may correlate with decreased risk of developing DAT. More recent studies, however, do not support the use of hormone replacement therapy for preventing cognitive decline. Furthermore, a large multicenter federally sponsored study examining the use of estrogens to treat DAT concluded that such treatment was ineffective.

Recent research suggests that cholesterol may increase amyloid accumulation. Some studies suggest that decreases in cholesterol levels may correlate with a decreased risk of DAT. Trials of statins for the treatment of DAT are currently ongoing. From prior experience with both anti-inflammatory drugs and estrogens, it is prudent to wait for results from large, well-designed studies before considering the use of statins for the treatment of DAT.

Depressive symptoms

Depressive symptoms are common in DAT, as discussed in Chapter 26. It may be difficult to determine whether such symptoms represent a concurrent major depressive disorder since depressive symptoms in people with DAT may fluctuate more than in people without DAT. If depressive symptoms such as dysphoria, markedly diminished interest, substantial fatigue, guilt, and low self-esteem are present and interfere with function, they should be addressed. Suicidal thoughts should always be carefully evaluated. Treatment will depend on the frequency of symptoms and the degree of discomfort and disability they create. Patients who become severely dysphoric and apathetic may stop eating and become very withdrawn. Their sleep may become disrupted, and they may develop delusions of sin or guilt as well as hallucinations. Untreated, such patients can die from suicide, self-neglect, or exacerbation of other medical disorders, including heart disease and diabetes. Symptoms of dementia may be confounded by additional cognitive decline resulting from depression.

Although there is not a great deal of research on the responsivity of depressive symptoms to treatment in patients with DAT, clinically significant depressive symptoms generally respond to treatment. Treatment options include pharmacotherapies, psychotherapies, and electroconvulsive therapy (ECT), depending on the severity of symptoms, the nature of family support, and the patient's cognitive ability. Severely depressed patients, even with concurrent DAT, may have a gratifying response to ECT. During treatment they may become confused; however, shortly after the course of ECT the confusion usually improves, and their mood, appetite, activities, and self-care return to levels present before the depression began. Once such depressive symptoms are successfully treated, maintaining remission may require either maintenance ECT (see Chapter 23) or maintenance pharmacotherapy.

If a patient in the very mild stages of dementia has depressive symptoms that are not life threatening (that is, suicidal ideations or plans are absent and adequate selfcare is maintained), psychotherapeutic approaches and/or pharma-cotherapies can be helpful. Patients and their families benefit from supportive therapy. Behavioral approaches may help with mild symptoms. The initiation of a cholinesterase inhibitor may also help with some of the behavioral symptoms of DAT, as well as provide short-term stabilization of cognitive symptoms. Frequent contact between the treatment team and patient where mood is assessed and practical information is exchanged can lead to symptomatic improvement. Specific psychotherapies may be helpful depending on the patient's ability to understand and actively participate in such approaches. Antidepressant medications can be effective especially when coupled with support and advice. Tricyclic antidepressants, especially those with high anticholinergic properties such as amitriptyline, are not good choices for the cognitively impaired elderly patient. In addition to interfering with cognition and having peripheral anticholinergic side effects, these agents can cause orthostatic hypotension and sedation. Selective serotonin reuptake inhibitors (SSRIs), such as fluoxetine, paroxetine, sertraline, citalopram, or other new generation antidepressants, such as venlafaxine or mirtazapine, are often prescribed. Many of these drugs are inhibitors of various P450 enzymes in the liver, and, therefore, the physician needs to be aware of the potential for pharmacokinetic interactions. Starting with low doses, building gradually to therapeutic levels, and being aware of the potential for drug interactions and long half-lives are important principles.

Each of these agents has specific advantages and disadvantages, and the clinician should become familiar with several agents, including a few SSRIs and a few of the other new agents. Monoamine oxidase inhibitors have been reported to be excellent antidepressants in the elderly; however, concerns exist about dietary complications, potentially severe drug interactions, and compliance. Especially during early stages of treatment, patients should be closely monitored. Side effects should be assessed frequently in order to determine whether benefits of treatment outweigh risks. Once depressive symptoms resolve, treatment should be maintained for about six months before considering a gradual withdrawal of the antidepressant. When tapering patients off medications, frequent visits are important to evaluate whether symptoms are returning. If symptoms reappear, increasing the dose of medication can minimize morbidity. The natural history of depressive symptoms in dementia is unknown, and, therefore, attention to re-occurrence over the years is necessary.

Psychotic symptoms

Psychotic symptoms often occur during the course of DAT. Although hallucinations and delusions may respond to judicious use of low doses of antipsychotic medication, these agents have potentially severe side effects in elderly patients with dementia, including Parkinsonian symptoms, orthostasis, falls, sedation, confusion, tardive dyskinesia, and weight gain. Before initiating treatment, it is important to evaluate how disruptive and uncomfortable the symptoms are to the patient and caregivers. If the symptoms do not seem overly distressing, explaining that such symptoms are common and teaching simple behavioral approaches may adequately alleviate the discomfort. If symptoms become overwhelming or interfere with function, a course of antipsychotic medication can be helpful.

In some patients, agitation and irritability may be triggered by psychotic symptoms, and substantial improvement in these behaviors is possible with antipsychotic medication. The new generation antipsychotic medications may be better tolerated than the old generation medications, and side effects, especially those related to movement disorders, may occur less often. The risk of movement disorders increases with length of treatment and can occur within months in elderly patients with compromised brain function. Weight gain and the possibility of increasing cardiovascular risk factors should also be considered in terms of risks versus benefits with various antipsychotic agents. Frequent, even if brief, visits are recommended in order to monitor efficacy and side effects. After psychotic symptoms have remitted for a few weeks, dose reduction should be attempted. Medications can sometimes be gradually stopped, and psychotic symptoms remain in remission. However, should symptoms reappear, another decision based on risk versus benefit should be made regarding resuming pharmacotherapy.

Patients with Lewy body dementia are extremely sensitive to movement-disorder side effects of antipsychotic medications. Although hallucinations commonly occur even in early stages of this disorder, extreme caution is advised in the use of antipsychotic medications. A careful assessment of risk versus benefit is imperative. If symptoms are painful or severely disabling and a decision is made for a trial of an antipsychotic medication, initial doses should be very low, and any increases should be gradual with careful follow-up to monitor for the development of parkinsonian side effects or other features of extrapyramidal movement disorders. New generation antipsychotic drugs may have less movement disorder side effects than old generation antipsychotics, however extreme caution in using these drugs is still warranted.

Agitation

Patients in the moderate or late stages of dementia can develop severe irritability and agitation. These behaviors are difficult for a caregiver either at home or in a nursing home. A careful history and observation may reveal precipitating factors in the environment, and behavioral interventions can be initiated. Concomitant medical illnesses, pain, or delirium can also precipitate agitation. If a delirium is caused by a uri-

nary tract infection, an antibiotic might be the treatment of choice for the accompanying agitation. If agitation is primarily related to DAT, and if behavioral approaches have been ineffective, pharmacotherapy together with behavioral management may be required.

Cholinesterase inhibitors may help with some of these behavioral symptoms. Antipsychotic medications can be effective at alleviating agitation, however, the concerns regarding side effects that have been already discussed apply. Agitation can be time limited, and if an antipsychotic is required, the need to continue treatment should be re-evaluated often. Increased attention to behavioral and supportive approaches can be successful in maintaining remission of the agitation once the antipsychotic drug has been discontinued. Some patients require long-term pharmacotherapy, but this should be determined empirically by frequent attempts at dose reduction of these agents. New-generation antipsychotic agents are likely to be better tolerated than old-generation agents (see Chapter 22); however, it is important to monitor side effects including movement disorders, weight gain, and influence on cardiovascular risk factors.

Since antipsychotic medications have substantial side effects, other agents have been studied for efficacy in treating agitation or aggressiveness. Agents as diverse as trazodone, beta-blockers, valproic acid, lithium, and buspirone have been tested. Well-designed, clinical studies are necessary to help define which agents may be helpful in treating these problem behaviors. A variety of other behaviors can be disabling and disruptive. Some patients have hypomanic behaviors. Little is known about the efficacy of antimanic agents such as lithium or valproic acid in treating these behaviors. Some patients with moderate to severe illness exhibit loud and repetitive screaming behavior. These patients may respond to behavioral or low-dose pharmacologic interventions, but some do not improve and are difficult management challenges.

The treatments discussed in this section can be helpful but usually do not lead to significant improvement of cognitive functioning. As advances in understanding the pathophysiology of Alzheimer's disease are made, substantial progress can be expected in early diagnosis and effective treatments (see *Consider consultation when . . .*).

CONSIDER CONSULTATION WHEN...

- There is diagnostic confusion.
- The patient's behavior becomes dangerous to himself or others.
- Psychiatric symptoms are not responding to behavioral intervention or standard use of psychotropic medications.
- Psychotropic management becomes complicated as a result of side effects or interactions with other medications.

PEARLS & PERILS

- Pharmacologic treatments for DAT are under active investigation, and it is likely that a variety of agents that work via different mechanisms will become available over the next several years.
- Education of caregivers as well as patients about DAT is crucial.
- Depressive symptoms are common in DAT and should be carefully evaluated and treated.
- Psychotic symptoms should be evaluated in light of how disruptive and uncomfortable they are for patient and caregivers. Antipsychotic medication may be beneficial. Side effects should be monitored carefully. Frequent attempts should be made to decrease the dose and discontinue these medications while evaluating the presence and severity of target symptoms.
- Agitation can be precipitated by medical illness, pain, or delirium in patients with DAT. Therefore, these conditions should be addressed in the agitated patient.

Summary and special considerations

In the past, when an elderly person became extremely forgetful, it was labeled "senility" and considered a part of the aging process. Few physicians were interested in treating these frail, elderly people. Over the last 25 years, increased attention has been devoted to diagnosis, staging, and elucidation of the natural history of dementia. The majority of people who live into their mid-80s can enjoy cognitive health. Severe cognitive deterioration is not inevitable.

Advances in molecular genetics and neurobiology coupled with careful diagnostic and descriptive clinical research have led to major advances in the understanding of dementing disorders. Therapeutic nihilism has been replaced by excitement about future therapeutic possibilities. This chapter has attempted to review some of these advances and reflect the excitement that exists in the field of dementia research. The primary care practitioner is the front-line physician in treating dementia. Although geriatricians, geriatric psychia-trists, and geriatric neurologists can provide consultation, there are too few specialists to provide primary care for the millions of patients affected. The more the primary care practitioner becomes interested in evaluating mental status, including cognition, mood, and psychosis, the better equipped he or she will be to help these patients and their families. Helpful treatments, both somatic and psychosocial, are currently available. New and exciting diagnostic approaches and treatments will become available over the next decade. Staying current with this rapidly advancing field will be an exciting challenge for all of us.

Acknowledgment

I would like to acknowledge the support of the Washington University Alzheimer's Disease Research Center (National Institutes of Health grants P50 AG05681) and the editorial assistance of Dorothy Kinscherf.

Annotated bibliography

Coffey, CE and Cummings, JL (eds) (2000) *The American Psychiatric Press Textbook of Geriatric Neuropsychiatry*, 2nd Edition, Washington, D.C., American Psychiatric Press.
  This is a superb book, containing excellent chapters which address geriatric psychiatric disorders as well as reviews of CNS structure and function.

Cummings, JL (ed.) (2003) *The Neuropsychiatry of Alzheimer's Disease and Related Dementias*, London, Martin Dunitz.
  This is a useful and beautifully illustrated book that succinctly reviews the common forms of dementia with good attention to neuropsychiatric aspects.

Cummings, JL and Cole, G (2002) Alzheimer disease, *JAMA* 287:2335–2338.
  This is a useful and well-written review.

Jacobson, SA, Pies, RW, and Greenblatt, DJ (2002) *Handbook of Geriatric Psychopharmacology*, Washington, DC, American Psychiatric Publishing, Inc.
  This is a very useful geriatric psychopharmacology text.

Morris, JC, Galvin, J, and Holtzman, D (eds) (in press) *Handbook of Dementing Illnesses*, 2nd Edition, New York, Marcel Dekker, Inc.
  This book contains excellent reviews of Alzheimer's disease and other dementias.

CHAPTER 13

Schizophrenia and Related Disorders

John W. Newcomer, MD, Peter Fahnestock, MD, and Dan Haupt, MD

Introduction

This chapter provides an overview of schizophrenia and related psychotic disorders, including schizophreniform disorder, brief psychotic disorder, schizoaffective disorder, and delusional disorder. A common term for this group of disorders is the "nonaffective psychoses." Though other psychiatric illnesses outside this category—most notably the mood disorders—may present with psychotic symptoms, the disorders discussed in this chapter are set apart by the primacy of the psychotic disturbance. The particular case of schizoaffective disorder, a controversial disorder because of its admixture of psychotic and mood symptoms that is being diagnosed with increasing frequency, is discussed toward the end of this chapter.

Schizophrenia and related disorders are very common. According to national surveys supported by the National Institutes of Mental Health (NIMH), over 1 million individuals in the United States are likely to suffer currently from schizophrenia. Medical comorbidity occurs often in schizophrenia. In addition, antipsychotic medications are associated with obesity and related impairments in glucose and lipid metabolism. Psychiatrists benefit from collaborative relationships with primary care physicians in treating comorbidities and medication side effects experienced by their patients. Primary care physicians are thus essential members of the team providing health care to patients with schizophrenia. In some cases, primary care providers are responsible for psychiatric management.

As a group, schizophrenia and related psychotic disorders present an array of some of the most striking and disabling behavioral disturbances found in clinical practice. Psychotic symptoms are a source of enormous subjective distress and disturb various aspects of physical, psychological, occupa-

tional, and social functioning. An elevated mortality rate (estimated at eight times the base rate for the general population) results from comorbid medical conditions and successful suicide (10% of patients with schizophrenia die by suicide). The adverse effect of the illness on general adherence to medical treatment contributes to the problems that clinicians face in treating these patients. These disorders are devastating to families as well, creating chronic stress and psychological burden that fall especially hard on the principal caregiver and a financial burden that can have long-lasting effects. The central primary care issue involves minimizing morbidity, mortality, and the adverse effects of these disorders.

Schizophrenia is among the most common of the "severe mental illnesses," as reported by the National Advisory Mental Health Council (NAMHC) (Table 13.1). Its report underscored that, despite persistent myth, severe mental illnesses like schizophrenia and delusional disorder are readily definable and treatable. Recent research advances in diagnosis and treatment permit many people with severe mental illnesses to be treated as outpatients and have allowed millions of individuals to return to productive lives. Numerous well-controlled clinical trials have established the efficacy of specific treatments and the scientific basis for making clinical decisions, putting the management of severe mental illnesses on a par with other medical or surgical conditions (Fig. 13.1).

Unfortunately, schizophrenia and related disorders are typical of severe mental illnesses with respect to chronicity and cost to society, closely matching the overall costs of medical conditions such as respiratory and cardiovascular disease (CVD) (Table 13.2). The NAMHC report also included a detailed cost comparison of diabetes and schizophrenia (Table 13.3), demonstrating comparable direct treatment costs but a greater potential for reducing morbidity and mortality costs through the adequate treatment of schizophrenia.

The purpose of this chapter is to provide the primary care clinician as well as the psychiatrist with information regarding the evaluation, diagnosis, and management of patients with schizophrenia and related disorders. The latest information on the epidemiology, course, symptom definitions, differential diagnoses, etiology, pathophysiology, and treatment for schizophrenia and related disorders is summarized. Most of this chapter deals specifically with schizophrenia because of its higher prevalence, cost to society and the correspondingly larger amount of research and clinical experience available relative to other nonaffective psychoses. The information presented for schizophrenia is largely applicable to related disorders. Important differences are discussed in the separate sections dedicated to each of these disorders.

Epidemiology, risk factors, and age of onset

The most commonly cited lifetime prevalence of schizophrenia is 1.0%. The National Comorbidity Survey (NCS), which showed that 0.7% of the general population has a "nonaffective psychosis" at some point in their lives, was based on a stratified multistage area probability sample of individuals aged 15–54 years in the non-institutionalized civilian population of the 48 contiguous states in the United States. The NCS represents the state-of-the-art for epidemiologic surveys of psychiatric disorder prevalence.

The ECA survey, comprising samples of over 3,000 subjects at each of several sites in the U.S., found a slightly greater lifetime prevalence of 1.0 to 1.5% of the general population. This survey controlled for differences in age, sex, and ethnicity across the different sites and found no consistent confounding relationship between any demographic variable and the prevalence of schizophrenia. The ECA sampled

TABLE 13.1	Percentages of US adults with severe mental disorders	
Diagnosis		**Percentage of adults (ages 18 years and above)**
Schizophrenia		1.5
Manic-depressive illness (bipolar disorder)		1.0
Major depression		1.1
Panic disorder		0.4
Obsessive-compulsive disorder		0.6
Any of these diagnoses		2.8[a]

[a] A person may have more than one diagnosis at the same time. The percentages for each individual diagnosis cannot be added together to obtain the total percentage of the study population with any disorder.
From National Advisory Mental Health Council (1993) Health care reform for Americans with severe mental illnesses: report of the National Advisory Mental Health Council, *Am J Psychiatry* 150: 1447–1465. Copyright 1993, the American Psychiatric Association; http://AJP.psychiatryonline.org. Reprinted by permission.

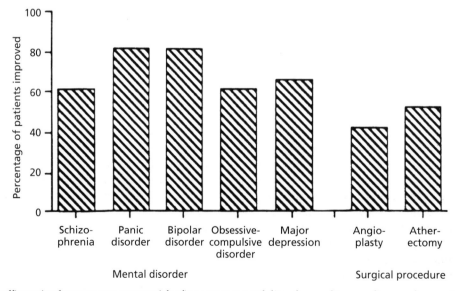

Fig. 13.1 Treatment efficacy (early treatment outcome) for five severe mental disorders and two cardiovascular surgical procedures. From *Am J Psychiatry* (1993) 150:1447–1465. Copyright 1993, the American Psychiatric Association; http://AJP.psychiatryonline.org. Reprinted by permission.

TABLE 13.2

Costs of respiratory disease, cardiovascular disease, and mental illness in 1990

Type of cost	Amount (billions of dollars)		
	Respiratory disease[a]	Cardiovascular disease[a]	Mental illness[b]
Direct	57	85	67
Indirect	42	75	75
Other, related	0	0	6
Total	99	160	148

[a] Unpublished data from the National Heart, Lung, and Blood Institute.

[b] See also Rice, DP and Miller, LS (1998) Health economics and cost implications of anxiety and other mental disorders in the United States, *Br J Psychiatry* 173 (suppl 34):4–9.

Adapted from National Advisory Mental Health Council (1993) Health care reform for Americans with severe mental illnesses: report of the National Advisory Mental Health Council, *Am J Psychiatry* 150:1447–1465. Copyright 1993, the American Psychiatric Association; http://AJP.psychiatryonline.org. Reprinted by permission.

psychiatric institutions more heavily than did the NCS, which may explain the greater prevalence found, as schizophrenic patients are more likely to be institutionalized than patients with most other psychiatric disorders. Overall, a remarkably consistent 1% prevalence rate for schizophrenia has been confirmed across large numbers of studies covering most of the globe. Notably, the prevalence of all nonaffective psychoses in the first-degree relatives of patients with schizophrenia is five-fold higher than the prevalence in relatives of unscreened controls.

The lifetime prevalence of other "nonaffective psychoses" is harder to estimate because of changing diagnostic criteria for these entities over the past several decades, which is a particular problem for schizoaffective disorder, and the smaller number of studies addressing the prevalence of these disorders. Kendler and colleagues estimated the prevalence of delusional disorder to be 0.024–0.030% and the prevalence of "other nonaffective psychoses" (inclusive of delusional disorder, schizophreniform disorder and atypical psychosis) to be 0.7–0.8%.

Risk factors (e.g., genetic factors, substance abuse, perinatal injury) for the development of schizophrenia have historically been difficult to identify and, when found, to replicate. This inconsistency is in part a result of study-related methodologic problems and in part the consequence of studying a heterogeneous disorder with different risk factors across different individuals. Recent evidence suggests that early life (e.g., prenatal) injury may increase the risk of developing schizophrenia. For example, several studies have reported that patients with schizophrenia have a higher chance of being born to mothers exposed to influenza in the second trimester, suggesting that maternal-infant second trimester viral infection may contribute to the risk for the development of the disorder. However, this association has not always been replicated. In addition, there is strong evidence that schizophrenia and related psychoses have a genetic component. Several lines of converging evidence suggest that schizophrenia may be best conceptualized as a neurodevelopmental disorder related to genetic susceptibility and early brain insults that subsequently lead to progressive endogenous excitotoxic injury in critical brain regions. The role of genetic factors, environmental insults, and excitotoxic injury in the development of schizophrenia is discussed below in the section on Etiology and Pathophysiology.

While the lifetime risk of developing schizophrenia is not different for males and females, males have an earlier age of illness onset (Table 13.4). In addition, males may have a more chronic course, although this is less clear. When studies control for numerous potentially confounding factors, there is no convincing evidence for differences in relative rates of schizophrenia across different racial or ethnic groups, or in urban versus rural settings. Lower socioeconomic status, certainly as a consequence of the disorders and perhaps as a purely non-specific contributing risk or stressor, is associated with having a nonaffective psychotic disorder. Similarly, substance abuse and adverse life events have been described as either causally related to the onset time for schizophrenia or, alternatively, a psychosocial consequence of illness onset with its disruptions of multiple aspects of normal functioning. Sorting out issues of cause versus consequence require careful, often prospective (i.e., expensive), studies with large sample sizes. Despite the importance of risk factors to primary prevention, issues related to separating cause and consequence remain unsettled for schizophrenia and schizoaffective disorder and relatively unstudied for delusional disorder.

TABLE 13.3 Comparative costs of schizophrenia and diabetes

Type of cost	Amount (billions of dollars)
Cost of schizophrenia (1990 estimates)[a]	
Direct	18
Patient care	17
Related	1
Indirect	15
Morbidity	11
Mortality	1
Other	3
Total	33
Cost of diabetes in 1990[b]	
Direct	17
Hospitalization	4
Nursing home	3
Related medical conditions	7
Other	3
Indirect	10
Disability	3
Mortality	7
Total	27

[a] See also Rice, DP (1999) The economic impact of schizophrenia, *J Clin Psychiatry* 60 (Suppl 1):4–6; discussion 28–30.

[b] Data from Huse, DM *et al.* (1989) The economic costs of non-insulin-dependent diabetes mellitus, *JAMA* 262:2708–2713. Copyright © 1989, American Medical Association. All rights reserved. Reprinted by permission.

Adapted from National Advisory Mental Health Council (1993) Health care reform for Americans with severe mental illnesses: report of the National Advisory Mental Health Council, *Am J Psychiatry* 150:1447–1465. Copyright 1993, the American Psychiatric Association; http://AJP.psychiatryonline.org. Reprinted by permission.

TABLE 13.4 Age-distributed risk of first hospitalization for schizophrenia by sex in the British population

By age	Cumulative % of total risk	
	Male	Female
15	1	1
20	11	11
25	31	25
30	51	44
35	70	60
40	81	72
45	91	83
50	96	92
55	100	100

Modified from *Schizophrenia Genesis: the origins of madness* by Irving I. Gottesman. © 1991 by Irving I. Gottesman. Used with permission of Worth Publishers.

Development of the diagnosis of schizophrenia

Schizophrenia has historically been the subject of extensive study. Beginning in the late 19th century, German psychiatrists sought to reproduce the success of Koch, who had identified the infectious etiology of tuberculosis. Like clinician-investigators in many fields of medicine at the time, they sought to identify specific clinical presentations in large series of patients that would correspond to specific underlying organic disease etiologies. Increasingly restrictive criteria are required to move from the description of a clinical syndrome to that of a discrete clinical disorder and from there to a pathophysiologic (i.e., disease) entity (Table 13.5). The development of formal diagnostic criteria for schizophrenia and delusional disorder continues to this day, with the latest iteration of criteria reviewed below.

In 1898, Emil Kraepelin incorporated earlier symptom descriptions into a unified description of symptoms, course and outcome that he labeled "dementia praecox," which is closely related to what is called schizophrenia today. He recognized the typical early onset and asserted that the disorder had a characteristic progressive deteriorating or dementing course. Kraepelin considered dementia praecox to be an "organic" brain disorder. He further described three different "paranoid" or delusional disorders: (1) "paranoia," a rare chronic illness with an insidious onset of fixed delusions (not restricted to "paranoid," or persecutory, delusions) and the absence of hallucinations and the progressive deterioration or dementia; (2) "paraphrenia," a mild form of dementia praecox, with delusions and hallucinations but no progressive deterioration; and (3) "dementia paranoids," a form of dementia praecox that was similar to "paranoia" but

Recent investigations have addressed the special features of those schizophrenia patients presenting with an uncharacteristic age of onset. While early investigators recognized presentations with a late age of onset, some diagnostic systems initially excluded patients with an age of onset over either 40 or 45. The principal diagnostic system in use today (see below) now permits a diagnosis of schizophrenia independent of the age of the individual although early (before age 15) and late (after 45) onset cases are uncommon (see Table 13.4). Studies suggest that late-onset patients are more often of the paranoid subtype and have better premorbid social and occupational functioning in adolescence and early adulthood. In contrast, childhood or juvenile onset cases of schizophrenia have been reported to show greater pre-psychotic impairments in social, developmental, and cognitive functioning.

Levels in the validation of a disease

Levels of disease concept	Criteria for validation
Clinical syndrome	1 Characteristics are distinguishable from other syndromes
	2 Intercorrelated group of symptoms
	3 Consistent clinical picture (stable and homogenous correlational structure of symptoms)
Discrete clinical disorder	4 Explicit inclusion and exclusion rules
	5 Predictable progression of interrelated syndromes as a unit
	6 Rarity of intermediate or combined cases (discrete boundaries from other disorders)
Pathophysiologic entity	7 Identification of biosocial risk factors
	8 Pathophysiologic explanation of symptoms, syndromes, and course
	9 Specific pathway from risk factors to disturbed pathophysiology

had an earlier onset and progressive deterioration. (It is worth noting that the terms "paranoid" and "delusional" are classically synonymous; over time the lay public has come to use the term "paranoid" to refer solely to delusions of persecution.) Kraepelin's writings were based on careful prospective, longitudinal studies of patient outcomes and included excellent descriptions of delusions, hallucinations, certain negative symptoms ("negative" referring to the absence of normal functions; see below), and interesting abnormal stereotyped movements. The latter, occurring in never-medicated patients, have become important as confounders to the interpretation of neuroleptic-induced abnormal movements (e.g., tardive dyskinesia).

First coining the term "schizophrenia" in 1911 in reference to a splitting of mental functions, Eugen Bleuler also described hallucinations, delusions, and other psychotic symptoms. However, he de-emphasized course and outcome and described four symptoms as central to the schizophrenic condition (the 4 As): a disturbance or loosening of *associations*, *autistic* behavior and thought, a disturbance of *affect*, and *ambivalence*. Despite his belief that schizophrenia had an organic basis, he maintained a more psychodynamic view of the disorder, using Freudian theory to explain some psychotic symptoms.

In 1939, Kurt Schneider described a set of "first rank symptoms," which he viewed to be pathognomonic for the diagnosis of schizophrenia: (1) audible thoughts, or the experience of auditory hallucinations of voices speaking one's thoughts aloud; (2) voices arguing, referring to hallucinatory voices usually discussing the patient in the third person; (3) voices commenting on one's actions or activities as they occur; (4) influence playing on the body, where the patient describes being a passive or reluctant recipient of sensations imposed on him by an external agent; (5) thought withdrawal, or the experience of having one's thoughts taken away by some external force; (6) thought insertion, or the experience of having thoughts that are not one's own; (7) diffusion or broadcasting of thoughts, where the patient experiences his thoughts leaving his mind in a manner in which they might be perceived by others; (8) made feelings, where the patient experiences feelings that do not seem to be his own; (9) made impulses, where the patient experiences an impulse to do something that is imposed by some external agent but acting on the impulse (if carried out) is not imposed (10) made volitional acts, where the patient experiences his actions as being under the control of some external force; (11) delusional perception, a two-stage phenomenon where the patient first experiences what they acknowledge to be an ordinary perception (e.g., someone dropping a pencil) that almost immediately takes on delusional importance (e.g., meaning that the patient has been selected for a special mission by the CIA). Although first rank symptoms have inadequate sensitivity and specificity to serve as diagnostic criteria for schizophrenia, they have been reported to occur in up to 80% of patients otherwise diagnosed with schizophrenia.

Following this early period, a proliferation of descriptions and diagnostic criteria were developed for "schizophrenia" and "paranoia" (an early variant of what was to become delusional disorder) that offered explicit inclusion and exclusion rules, the first elements of defining a clinical disorder. However, as recently as three to four decades ago, psychiatric diagnosis was generally an object of derision, and clinicians and researchers were typically unable to achieve even a reasonable level of agreement in diagnosing disorders. The diagnosis of schizophrenia was especially problematic, and it was studied intensively in the U.S.-U.K. Cross National Project. A direct comparison of diagnoses made by staff members of several British and American hospitals showed that diagnoses made in the United States were considerably broader, with significantly more patients diagnosed with schizophrenia whose consensus project diagnosis was affective disorder. This suggested that either clinicians were using inconsistent criteria for making diagnoses or the more worrisome possibility that clinicians were unable to apply the same criteria in a consistent manner, which would obscure any ability to detect real differences in the prevalence of schizophrenia from one location to another.

Concerns about the reliability and validity of existing definitions of schizophrenia led to the World Health Organization (WHO) International Pilot Study of Schizophrenia (IPSS). This international project sought to identify a standardized and reliable means of diagnosing schizophrenia, utilizing the Present State Exam (PSE), a standardized interview, as the principal source of diagnostic data for the study. The development and application of explicit diagnostic criteria over the last 20 years, finally resulting in the *Diagnostic and Statistical Manual of Mental Disorders* (DSM), has led to a dramatic improvement in the reliability of classification of schizophrenia and related disorders.

DSM-IV serves as the official diagnostic guidelines used by the American Psychiatric Association, continuing a focus on objectively verified data concerning the presence or absence of particular symptoms, duration of illness, use of specific exclusions for biological confounds, and the requirement for evidence of functional impairment or clinical deterioration secondary to the disorder. The precursors of the DSM in the United States arose out of the need to classify mental disorders for statistical purposes, which was first attempted in the 1840 census with the single category of "idiocy/insanity." Further development of a nomenclature for severe psychiatric disorders involved collaboration between the American Medico-Psychological Association (eventually the American Psychiatric Association [APA]) and the National Commission on Mental Hygiene to produce terminology for use by the Bureau of the Census in 1917. Later the APA and the New York Academy of Medicine worked together to produce criteria for use in the first edition of the American Medical Association's Standard Classified Nomenclature of Disease. The U.S. Army and the Veterans Administration expanded the scope of this psychiatric nomenclature to accommodate presentations of World War II servicemen and veterans. The World Health Organization, influenced by the efforts of the Army and the Veterans Administration, included 10 categories of psychosis in a new section on mental disorders for the Sixth Edition of the *International Classification of Diseases* (ICD). Beginning with DSM-I in 1952, the APA has published an evolving series of more descriptively explicit classification schemes for use by clinicians and researchers rather than census workers. The current nosology, DSM-IV TR, is intended to be an atheoretical descriptive approach, requiring that any changes made to criteria be substantiated by empirical data, field trials of new criteria, and a "consensus of the field."

The distinctive advantage of standardized operational diagnostic criteria is high levels of agreement, which are essential if studies of pathophysiologic and etiologic mechanisms are to be replicated. The incorporation (or removal) of specific symptoms from psychiatric diagnostic criteria like the DSM continues to revolve around concerns for both reliability and validity. For the past several decades, investigators have also focussed on the study of reliable and validated groups of symptoms within the confusing array of overall schizophrenic psychopathology. The two principal senses of reliability are (1) inter-rater reliability, or the ability of independent clinicians to agree on the presence and severity of a symptom (i.e., symptoms like "orientation" are very easy to get agreement on while others like "emotional withdrawal" are more difficult), and (2) test-retest reliability, or the ability of a single clinician to confirm the presence and same severity of a given symptom at two different points in time.

The two principal senses of validity are (1) construct validity, or the confirmation that specific groups of symptoms correspond to specific underlying pathophysiologies or neural mechanisms (e.g., confirmation that the group of tuberculosis symptoms really should be thought of as a group because they are all caused by *Mycobacterium tuberculosis*), and (2) predictive validity, or the confirmation that the presence or severity of a group of symptoms predicts the course or outcome of the illness. The use of standardized operational diagnostic criteria has produced some predictive validity for schizophrenia, and less for delusional disorder. Construct validity, or the objective verification that the diagnostic groupings are related to distinct underlying pathophysiologic or disease processes, remains to be established.

Clinical presentation and diagnosis

Over time, clinician investigators have assembled a long list of symptoms that have been observed in patients with schizophrenia and related disorders. The symptoms of these disorders are remarkably diverse and reflect disturbances in a broad range of mind/brain function, including behavioral, emotional, perceptual, physical, and cognitive domains. The symptoms that may accompany schizophrenia are outlined below. Although individual symptoms are categorized into different domains, this is to some extent arbitrary as many of these symptoms are complex and multidimensional phenomena.

Symptom descriptions

The behavioral symptoms associated with schizophrenia include bizarre or stereotyped behaviors (e.g., strange hand signals while speaking or repetitive odd speech), motor hyper- or hypo-activity including catatonia, reductions in facial or bodily (e.g., hand) expressiveness and gesturing, poor hygiene, unusual dress, reductions in impulse control (e.g., suicidality), and reduced occupational and social performance. DSM-IV defines and uses as a diagnostic criteria "grossly disorganized behavior" which "may manifest itself in a variety of ways, ranging from childlike silliness to unpredictable agitation . . . [and] may be noted in any form of goal-directed behavior, leading to difficulties in performing activities of daily living such as organizing meals or maintaining hygiene."

Catatonic motor behaviors as defined by DSM-IV can "include a marked decrease in reactivity to the environment, sometimes reaching an extreme degree of complete unawareness (catatonic stupor), maintaining a rigid posture and resisting efforts to be moved (catatonic rigidity), active resistance to instructions or attempts to be moved (catatonic negativism), the assumption of inappropriate or bizarre postures (catatonic posturing), or purposeless and unstimulated excessive motor activity (catatonic excitement) . . . [but these] are nonspecific and may occur in other mental conditions [e.g., mood disorders], in general medical conditions [e.g., hypercalcemia], and Medication-Induced Movement Disorders [e.g., neuroleptic-induced parkinsonism]." DSM-IV identifies three key "negative" symptoms that are manifested behaviorally: (1) affective flattening, "characterized by the person's face appearing immobile and unresponsive, with poor eye contact and reduced body language," (2) alogia or poverty of speech, "manifested by brief, laconic, empty replies . . . [in which the] individual . . . appears to have a diminution of thoughts that is reflected in decreased fluency and productivity of speech," and (3) avolition, one of the characteristic symptoms identified by Kraepelin, described as "an inability to initiate and persist in goal-directed activities."

A variety of emotional disturbances can occur in patients with schizophrenia. They can experience a reduction in emotional tone, feeling, or responsiveness, which may be manifested behaviorally as described previously in a blunting or flattening of affect. The internal, subjective emotional state of patients may become impoverished with a loss of ability to experience pleasure, i.e., anhedonia, and loss of drive or will, i.e., avolition. Patients with schizophrenia can also experience inappropriate emotions (e.g., glee or sadness without evident environmental cues). Although not generally considered to be part of schizophrenia per se, depressed mood and symptoms of depression often occur in patients with schizophrenia. As noted before, it has been estimated that up to 60% of patients with schizophrenia experience an episode of depression at some time over the course of their illness. Taken together with evidence that depression also clusters in the families of patients with schizophrenia, it is reasonable for primary care clinicians to remain alert for the manifestations of depression in the overall management of patients. Notably, this tendency to develop depression often leads to confusion in differentiating schizophrenia from schizoaffective disorder.

The perceptual symptoms associated with schizophrenia consist of illusions and hallucinations. An illusion is defined as a misperception of real sensory data, whereas a hallucination is the experience of perceived sensations that are entirely false (e.g. "hearing" a sound when no sound exists). Hallucinations figure prominently in most diagnostic sys-

tems. They can occur in any sensory domain, but are most commonly auditory and/or visual. Auditory hallucinations can consist of "voices," single or multiple, intelligible or not, subjectively perceived as coming from inside the patient's head or from outside. These voices can speak to each other or to the patient and can range (within and between subjects) from being the patient's helpful allies to being the patient's harshest critic and dreaded enemy. Auditory hallucinations can also include command hallucinations that may instruct the patient to act in various ways, including self-injury. The capacity to resist these commands varies. Because of the personification of such voices, patients may feel that they are locked alone in a struggle with a powerful adversary. It is always important to inquire in detail about hallucinations and any related commands, both because of the obvious risks and because many patients welcome the offer of an alliance that may (with treatment) reduce the strength and authority of their "adversary."

A variety of physical changes are associated with schizophrenia. While soft neurologic signs (e.g., abnormal right-left discrimination, astereognosis, and abnormal finger-thumb opposition) occur in some patients with schizophrenia, their clinical significance is unclear. These patients may be more sensitive to adverse effects of neuroleptic treatment. Patients with schizophrenia can have enlargement of the brain ventricular system and reductions in the volume of specific brain structures detectable by neuroimaging. A disturbance in normal eye tracking function and the central regulation of this tracking defect has been described in patients with schizophrenia and their relatives, offering a promising familial marker. Some findings may have relevance to specific symptoms (e.g., memory deficits, hallucinations) and to generalized hypotheses concerning the pathophysiology of the disorder. Unfortunately, many findings show considerable intersubject variability, and none is diagnostic for the disorder.

The cognitive symptoms of schizophrenia comprise a broad group of disturbances. To be precise, there are two senses of the term "cognitive" used here, one a psychiatric reference to "disorders of thought" and the other a more formal neuropsychological reference to specific mental abilities like memory and attention. The psychiatric meaning can be further divided into so-called disorders of form versus disorders of content. Disorders of content include delusional thinking (discussed below), lack of insight, and the impoverishment of thought content. Disorders of form, or "formal" thought disorders, include disruptions in the associations between ideas ("derailment" or "loosening of associations") and thought blocking (i.e., the sudden interruption of a patient's train of thought). Derailment can range from mild circumstantiality—deviating from the usual line of association but eventually returning to the point—to a loss of the normal associations between words within even a single sentence, resulting in incoherence ("word salad").

In the neuropsychologic domain, schizophrenia is characterized by a variety of specific cognitive deficits. Memory and learning deficits are relatively large compared with deficits in other differentiated elements of cognitive performance. Studies suggest that the memory and learning deficits in schizophrenia are related to ineffective organization and encoding of information. An association between various attentional dysfunctions and schizophrenia has also been reported. Investigators have reported attentional deficits in patients with acute, chronic, and residual schizophrenia and in the clinically unaffected children of parents with schizophrenia. Deficits in selective attention and processing speed have also been reported in patients with schizophrenia and their relatives.

All psychotic disorders can present with delusions. In schizophrenia these can be either bizarre or non-bizarre in nature. (In delusional disorder, by contrast, delusions must by definition be non-bizarre.) DSM-IV defines delusions as "erroneous beliefs that usually involve a misinterpretation of perceptions or experiences . . . [and whose] content may include a variety of themes (e.g., persecutory, referential, somatic, religious, or grandiose) . . . [which] are deemed bizarre if they are clearly implausible and not understandable and do not derive from ordinary life experiences." DSM-IV defines hallucinations as phenomena that "may occur in any sensory modality (e.g., auditory, visual, olfactory, gustatory, and tactile), [with] auditory hallucinations . . . by far the most common" and which "must occur in the context of a clear sensorium." DSM-IV defines the core schizophrenic symptom of disorganized thinking (i.e., "formal thought disorder" or "loosening of associations") in terms of disorganized speech, recognizing that "because mildly disorganized speech is common and nonspecific, the symptom must be severe enough to substantially impair effective communication . . . [with] less severe disorganized thinking or speech . . . occur[ing] during the prodromal and residual periods of schizophrenia."

In addition to the importance of individual symptoms, specific groups of symptoms have been defined with attention to both reliability and validity. A "negative" versus "positive" construct of psychotic symptoms was first articulated by 19th-century neurologists, and it has been refined and extended to define positive, disorganized, and negative symptom groupings in schizophrenia. Positive symptoms are exemplified by hallucinations and delusions. Disorganized symptoms are exemplified by disturbances in the associations between ideas. Negative symptoms are exemplified by blunted affect, emotional withdrawal, and social and occupational deficits. These groups of symptoms tend to cluster together statistically in large patient samples, where all of the symptoms within such a group can be more prominent or less prominent, but tend to occur together as a group. This may sometimes occur as well within individual patients who might, for example, have predominantly negative symptoms at a particular point in time. However, patients typically present with a mixture of different symptom groups. This mixed and varying clinical presentation has confounded efforts to subtype schizophrenia into different disorders with distinct etiologies. Some investigators have hypothesized that different underlying pathophysiologic mechanisms may operate simultaneously in the same patient to produce this varied symptom presentation.

Current diagnostic criteria

The DSM-IV definition for schizophrenia is listed in Box 13.1 with associated features listed in Table 13.6. A recent change in the diagnostic criteria involves the age of onset for the disorder. DSM-III did not permit the diagnosis of schizophrenia when the onset of the disorder was at or after the age of 45 years. This restriction was removed with DSM-III-R and continues to be absent from the DSM-IV.

Box 13.1 Schizophrenia

A. *Characteristic symptoms*: two (or more) of the following, each present for a significant portion of time during a one-month period (or less if successfully treated):
1 delusions
2 hallucinations
3 disorganized speech (e.g., frequent derailment or incoherence)
4 grossly disorganized or catatonic behavior
5 negative symptoms, i.e., affective flattening, alogia, or avolition.
Note: only one criterion A symptom is required if delusions are bizarre or hallucinations consist of a voice keeping up a running commentary on the person's behavior or thoughts, or two or more voices conversing with each other.

B. *Social/occupational dysfunction*: for a significant portion of the time since the onset of the disturbance, one or more major areas of functioning such as work, interpersonal relations, or self-care are markedly below the level achieved prior to the onset (or when the onset is in childhood or adolescence, failure to achieve expected level of interpersonal, academic, or occupational achievement).

C. *Duration*: continuous signs of the disturbance persist for at least six months. This six-month period must include at least one month of symptoms (or less if successfully treated) that meet criterion A (i.e., active-phase symptoms) and may include periods of prodromal or residual symptoms. During these prodromal or residual periods, the signs of the disturbance may be manifested by only negative symptoms or two or more symptoms listed in criterion A present in an attenuated form (e.g., odd beliefs, unusual perceptual experiences).

DIAGNOSTIC CRITERIA

DIAGNOSTIC CRITERIA (continued)

D. *Schizoaffective and mood disorder exclusion*: schizoaffective disorder and mood disorder with psychotic features have been ruled out because either (1) no major depressive, manic, or mixed episodes have occurred concurrently with the active-phase symptoms; or (2) if mood episodes have occurred during active-phase symptoms, their total duration has been brief relative to the duration of the active and residual periods.

E. *Substance/general medical condition exclusion*: the disturbance is not due to the direct physiological effects of a substance (e.g., a drug of abuse, a medication) or a general medical condition.

F. *Relationship to a pervasive developmental disorder*: if there is a history of autistic disorder or another pervasive developmental disorder, the additional diagnosis of schizophrenia is made only if prominent delusions or hallucinations are also present for at least a month (or less if successfully treated).

Classification of longitudinal course (can be applied only after at least one year has elapsed since the initial onset of active-phase symptoms):
- episodic with interepisode residual symptoms (episodes are defined by the reemergence of prominent psychotic symptoms); *also specify if*: with prominent negative symptoms
- episodic with no interepisode residual symptoms
- continuous (prominent psychotic symptoms are present throughout the period of observation); *also specify if*: with prominent negative symptoms
- single episode in partial remission; *also specify if*: with prominent negative symptoms
- single episode in full remission
- other or unspecified pattern.

From American Psychiatric Association (2000) Diagnostic and Statistical Manual of Mental Disorders, 4th Edition, Text Revision, Washington, D.C., American Psychiatric Association.

Table 13.6 Schizophrenia

Discriminating features

1. Two (or more) of the following, each present for a significant portion of time during a one-month period (or less if successfully treated):
   - delusions
   - hallucinations
   - disorganized speech (e.g., frequent derailment or incoherence)
   - grossly disorganized or catatonic behavior
   - negative symptoms, i.e., affective flattening, alogia, or avolition.
2. One or more major areas of functioning are markedly below the level achieved prior to the onset.
3. Continuous signs of the disturbance persist for at least six months.

Consistent features

1. Not due to the effects of substance use or general medical conditions.
2. If there is a history of autistic disorder or another pervasive developmental disorder, the diagnosis of schizophrenia is made only if prominent delusions or hallucinations are also present.
3. Not accounted for by major affective disorder.

Variable features

1. Inappropriate affect.
2. Anhedonia.
3. Dysphoric mood.
4. Disturbances in sleep pattern.
5. Abnormalities of psychomotor activity.
6. Difficulty concentrating.
7. Cognitive dysfunction.
8. Confused or disoriented.
9. Lack of insight.
10. Depersonalization, derealization, and somatic concerns.

The inclusion of late-onset patients in the diagnosis of schizophrenia is based on studies that find more similarities than differences between patients with young adult onset versus later onsets, when both are compared with healthy controls. Specifically, younger and later onset patients have similar levels of positive and negative symptom psychopathology, neuropsychological impairment, and impaired childhood adjustment, as well as similar family histories of schizophrenia. Late-onset patients are better functioning in adolescence and young adulthood (when younger onset patients are typically beginning to develop illness), more often the paranoid subtype, and perhaps more often women. Patients with late-onset schizophrenia should be thoroughly evaluated because presenting symptoms may reflect a medical or neurological condition prevalent in this older population. Childhood-onset schizophrenia (onset of

psychosis by age 12) is a particularly severe form of the disorder. Long controversial, recent data from the NIMH childhood-onset schizophrenia project indicate that diagnostic criteria used in adults can be applied to children and that the childhood diagnosis exists on a continuum with previously identified early-onset schizophrenia. Such very early onset cases are often associated with more severe neurodevelopmental abnormalities and a poor overall prognosis.

Differential diagnosis

Schizophrenia and related disorders can be considered diagnoses of exclusion. The serious prognostic and treatment implications of these disorders further suggest the importance of a validated and reliable diagnostic process. While

KEY CLINICAL QUESTIONS AND WHAT THEY UNLOCK

- *Is the patient experiencing hallucinations (false sensory experiences) and/or delusions (fixed, false beliefs not consistent with cultural norms)?*
- *Has the patient's speech become disorganized, with (for example) frequent derailment or incoherence?*
- *Does the patient demonstrate affective flattening (i.e., diminished expression of emotional states), avolition, alogia, or grossly disorganized/bizarre behavior?*
- *Have the effects of a substance or a general medical condition been ruled out as the cause of the above symptoms?*
- *Do these symptoms occur independently of the symptoms of a major affective disorder, i.e. unipolar depression or bipolar disorder?*

  Affirmative answers to the above questions are strongly suggestive of schizophrenia or a related disorder.

- *Have continuous signs of the condition been present for at least six months?*
- *If the patient is experiencing mood symptoms, are they only present for a minor portion of the duration of the illness, or do they fall short of the criteria for a major affective disorder?*
- *If delusions are present, are they bizarre (i.e., impossible to realistically believe) in nature?*

  Affirmative answers to these additional questions indicate a specific diagnosis of schizophrenia. Note that bizarre delusions are not a requirement, but if present they preclude a diagnosis of delusional disorder.

- *Has the patient's body weight increased substantially since initiation of pharmacotherapy?*

  (An increase in abdominal adiposity is of most concern.)

- *Does the patient have an elevated fasting plasma glucose level?*
- *Does a fasting lipid panel show abnormalities such as elevated total cholesterol, elevated triglycerides, elevated LDL level, or a decreased HDL level?*

  These questions are important indicators of the possible metabolic consequences of antipsychotic treatment. Affirmative answers to any of them—particularly the second and third questions—indicate a need for medical intervention.

---

complete medical and neurological evaluation of any patient presenting with schizophrenia-like symptoms. An abbreviated list of differential diagnostic entities is provided in Box 13.2. This list of possible explanations for psychotic symptoms is difficult to review in the abstract, as factors such as an acute versus insidious onset, relationship to other symptoms, and the presence or absence of physical and/or laboratory findings can sharply narrow the list. A more detailed discussion of the psychiatric presentations of medical and neurological conditions is provided in Chapter 27.

BOX 13.2

Differential diagnosis of schizophrenia-like symptoms

Medical or neurological*
- *Drug-induced intoxications*: especially phencyclidine (PCP), ketamine; also amphetamines, cocaine, hallucinogens, L-dopa, alcohol (e.g., hallucinosis); less commonly agents such as anticholinergic medications, belladonna alkaloids, cimetidine, digitalis, disulfiram
- *Drug-related withdrawal syndromes*: such as alcohol, benzodiazepines, barbiturates, other sedative-hypnotic agents
- *CNS infections*: such as HIV, herpes encephalitis, Creutzfeldt-Jakob disease, neurosyphilis
- *Epilepsy*: especially temporal lobe foci
- *Mass lesions*: including frontal or temporal tumors, subdural/epidural hematoma, normal-pressure hydrocephalus
- *Metabolic abnormalities*: such as acute intermittent porphyria, carbon monoxide poisoning, metachromatic leukodystrophy, heavy metal poisoning (arsenic, manganese, mercury, thallium), homocystinuria, Wilson's disease, Hallervorden-Spatz disease
- *Endocrinopathies*: especially adrenal and thyroid
- *Progressive neurological disorders*: such as Alzheimer's disease, Huntington's disease, Pick's disease
- *Autoimmune disorders*: such as systemic lupus erythematosus, CNS vasculitides
- *Nutritional*: such as B_{12} deficiency, pellagra
- *Psychiatric*: including schizophreniform disorder, brief reactive disorder, schizoaffective disorder, atypical psychosis, delusional disorder, major depressive disorder with psychotic features, bipolar affective disorder with psychotic features, personality disorders (especially schizotypal, schizoid, borderline, paranoid types), autism, mental retardation, malingering, factitious disorder with psychological symptoms.

*Categories are defined for convenience of review and organization. Some entities could be assigned to multiple categories (such as Wilson's disease—metabolic, progressive neurological—and psychiatric disorders).

---

some clinicians may focus on the negative consequences of making the diagnosis of schizophrenia, failing to make this diagnosis when it is appropriate can undermine proper treatment decisions.

The symptoms of schizophrenia reflect a profound disruption of normal functioning in behavioral, emotional, perceptual, physical, and cognitive domains. The range of symptoms found in schizophrenia implicate a broad array of brain functions that can, in turn, be altered by a variety of abnormal processes within the CNS and the periphery. Many of the pathologic processes producing secondary symptoms resembling schizophrenia reflect treatable medical or neurologic conditions. It is critical to perform a

- Schizophrenia and related disorders remain essentially diagnoses of exclusion.
- The serious prognostic and treatment implications of assigning patients diagnoses such as schizophrenia give added importance to the need for careful differential diagnosis in these disorders.
- While many students in psychiatry, psychology, and related fields focus on the negative consequences of making the diagnosis of schizophrenia, one cannot overlook how failing to make this diagnosis when it is appropriate can undermine proper treatment decisions.
- The symptoms of schizophrenia and related disorders reflect a profound disruption of normal functioning in behavioral, emotional, perceptual, physical, and cognitive domains.
- The range of symptoms found in schizophrenia implicate a broad array of brain functions that can, in turn, be altered by a variety of abnormal processes within the CNS and the periphery.
- Many of the pathologic processes that can produce secondary symptoms resembling schizophrenia and delusional disorder are also treatable medical or neurologic conditions.
- It is critical to perform a complete medical and neurological evaluation of any patient presenting with schizophrenia-like symptoms.

Some entities in the differential diagnosis can be detected by history or examination, while others require laboratory assessment. Although the extent of laboratory testing needed to exclude alternative diagnoses may be controversial, given that medical and neurological conditions that present with psychosis are uncommon and may declare themselves on history and physical examination during follow-up, early detection and treatment of these conditions are likely to reduce morbidity and possibly mortality. The workup for a patient presenting with new-onset psychosis should include a complete history (including family history); physical and neurological examinations; a blood sample for laboratory assessment of electrolyte, glucose, albumin, BUN, and calcium levels; HIV and VDRL/FTA testing (in patients who may be at risk); erythrocyte sedimentation level (to screen for inflammatory processes); and thyroid function tests.

Clinicians should consider obtaining either a ceruloplasmin plasma level or a slit-lamp examination (looking for Kaiser-Fleischer rings) to address the relatively low probability of early (i.e., highly treatable) Wilson's disease, which may present with or without early evidence of the characteristic movement disorder. Urine should be collected for routine analysis and toxicology screen. A CT or MR scan of the head, principally for the evaluation of possibly 'silent' mass lesions of the frontal and temporal lobe, should be obtained. Specific historical or physical examination findings may lead to additional tests such as serum B_{12} and folate levels, heavy metal levels, a lumbar puncture, or an electroencephalogram.

Etiology and pathophysiology

The etiology of schizophrenia remains uncertain, though great strides have been made in recent years. As noted previously, current data suggest that schizophrenia is a heterogeneous neurodevelopmental disorder related to genetic susceptibility and early brain insults that appear to contribute to the core clinical features of the disorder and lead to progressive, endogenous neurotoxic injury in some patients. Findings emerging from basic neuroscience research, genetic studies, and clinical schizophrenia research may explain key increases in risk for the disorder, critical changes in neurotransmitter function, and fundamental mechanisms underlying neuronal injury. However, the variety of clinical presentations (within and between subjects) and highly variable biological characteristics complicate the search for etiology. A number of etiologic factors may work together to produce schizophrenia, or, alternatively, make variable contributions in different individuals to produce variable forms of the disorder.

This complexity reflects the limitations of diagnostic criteria that are set, as with many medical disorders, without knowledge about etiology. The advantage of standardized operational diagnostic criteria (like the DSM system) is that they at least allow the high levels of agreement that are essential to replicate studies of pathophysiologic and etiologic mechanisms. However, given the limitation that it is difficult to say that one definition of schizophrenia has greater validity than others, some investigators have suggested that a flexible polydiagnostic approach be adopted for biological research paradigms. Using this approach, diagnoses and analyses can be made using multiple criterion systems. One structured interview, the Diagnostic Interview for Genetic Studies (DIGS), was constructed to offer just such a state-of-the-art diagnostic assessment for schizophrenia, based on several diagnostic systems (e.g., DSM, ICD, RDC).

This section reviews several important lines of research on the etiology and pathophysiology of schizophrenia. A wealth of important findings from structural neuroimaging (e.g., enlarged cerebral ventricles, reduced gray matter volumes, functional neuroimaging (e.g., reduced frontal activation during demand conditions, so-called hypofrontality), neuropsychology (e.g., prominent impairments in medial temporal lobe functions, attentional impairments, and impairment in working memory function), eye tracking studies (e.g., abnormalities suggesting frontal lobe impairments), and post-mortem studies (e.g., changes to cingulate cortex, hippocampus, parahippocampal gyrus and entorhinal cortex) are not reviewed here, but the interested reader is referred to references listed at the end of this chapter.

Genetic factors

A series of findings confirming a higher risk for psychotic disorders in families where another member has already been affected have provided strong support for the idea that schizophrenia and related disorders cluster in families. The pattern of familial transmission, especially for schizophrenia itself, strongly supports a genetic component to the risk of developing the illness. Key observations come from studies of monozygotic twins (showing a 45% concordance rate for schizophrenia in monozygotic twins vs. a 15% concordance rate in dizygotic twins), from adoption studies where the influence of genetic and at least some environmental factors can be distinguished, and from family studies (showing higher rates of schizophrenia in first-degree versus second-degree relatives of those diagnosed with the disorder).

Family studies demonstrate an increased risk of developing schizophrenia when raised by parents who have the disorder. However, this familial risk could be related to genetic factors, psychosocial factors, or intrauterine environmental effects. Adoption or foster rearing studies provide a means of separating the psychosocial effects of being raised by a parent(s) with schizophrenia from genetic effects on the risk of developing the disorder. The results of the first study of this kind (conducted in Oregon by Heston and colleagues), a group of important adoption studies in Denmark (a collaboration between American [Kety, Rosenthal, and Wender] and Danish investigators [Schulsinger, Welner, and Jacobsen]) using national registers for both psychiatric illness and adoption, and a Finnish adoption study all support an important role for congenital factors (genetic or intrauterine). The work by Kety and colleagues included a comparison of maternal and paternal half-siblings, providing evidence that genetic factors were stronger contributors to the risk of developing schizophrenia than intrauterine environment.

Gottesman has articulated the concept of increasing genetic risk as individuals share increasing amounts of genetic material with the affected relative(s) (Fig. 13.2). Kendler and colleagues have interpreted the results of their family studies of psychiatric illness to suggest that what is transmitted in families is not the schizophrenic syndrome per se, but a more general vulnerability to the entire group of nonaffective psychoses, including schizophrenia, delusional disorder, schizophreniform disorder, schizoaffective disorder, and atypical psychosis.

The search for genetic factors has advanced substantially in recent years with the discovery of specific genes associated with schizophrenia. Chumakov and colleagues have shown that a newly identified gene on chromosome 13q34, labeled G72, is associated with increased incidence of schizophrenia. This gene interacts with the gene for D-amino acid deoxylase (DAAO) and thereby affects glutaminergic signaling through the N-methyl D-aspartate (NMDA) receptor pathway (more on this pathway below). These findings were

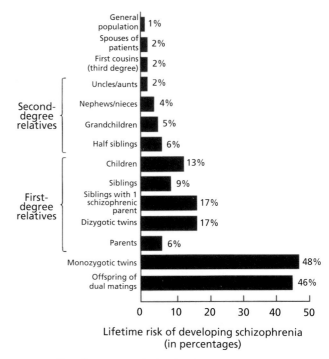

Fig. 13.2 Grand average risks for developing schizophrenia show that the degree of risk is strongly associated with the degree of genetic relatedness (compiled from family and twin studies conducted in European populations between 1920 and 1987). From *Schizophrenia genesis: the origins of madness* by Irving I Gottesman. © 1991 by Irving I Gottesman. Used with permission of Worth Publishers.

consistent in both French-Canadian and Russian population samples. Linkage analyses performed by several groups on chromosome 13 markers (based in the nearby 13q32 region) have found markers associated with schizophrenia; Faraone and colleagues found such associations in a large sample of American veterans, consistent across ethnic boundaries. In addition, the genes for dysbindin and neuregulin—proteins that may also affect the NMDA receptor system—have recently been found to influence susceptibility to schizophrenia. A possible association has been reported with the nicotinic alpha-7 receptor gene. Genetic associations can be determined in a variety of ways, including for example comparisons of single nucleotide polymorphisms (SNPs), which are mapped to known locations on a given chromosome. By tracking the distribution of known SNPs, chromosomal regions can be identified that contain candidate genes, to varying degrees of statistical strength.

The significant risk of the transmission of schizophrenia within families is important information for couples planning to have children when one or both of the partners have a family history of psychosis. For some time physicians and genetic counselors have been trained to provide couples with important information about the familial transmission of medical disorders such as sickle cell anemia, allowing adequate planning and preparation to precede the birth of an affected child. More recently, researchers and genetic counselors have applied the additional knowledge gleaned from studies of the familial transmission of psychiatric disorders to the field of genetic counseling. Discussed in detail in Chapter 24, psychiatric genetic counseling presents unique challenges but offers families important information from a wealth of well-designed studies. Of note, the risk of a child developing schizophrenia is around 10% when one parent has schizophrenia but rises to more than 40% when both parents are affected.

In line with the high risk of comorbid depression in patients with schizophrenia, genetic studies have found that depression (but not mania) also clusters in families with schizophrenia. Conversely, patients with depression do not have familial clustering of schizophrenia. This may be a function of the more heterogeneous nature of depression, which can be caused by multiple biologic and environmental factors, some of which occur in schizophrenia. It is worth noting that twin studies have strongly supported the diagnostic and familial separation of schizophrenia and bipolar disorder; however, there are fewer data available regarding delusional disorder and the other nonaffective psychoses.

Early brain injury

A growing understanding of normal maturational processes in the brain has led to important hypotheses regarding specific disruptions in the normal brain cell migration and organization that occurs during the second trimester *in utero*. A disruption in these normal developmental events has been proposed to explain post-mortem findings of abnormal patterns of cellular orientation, abnormal cell counts, other abnormal morphological features, and reduced gray matter (cell body) volume on magnetic resonance imaging of the brains of patients with schizophrenia.

Several studies have reported that patients with schizophrenia have a higher chance of being born to mothers exposed to influenza in the second trimester; however, this association has not been consistently replicated. Other developmental events in the second trimester include the migration and organization of cells forming the ridges that constitute permanent fingertip patterns. While these patterns are normally almost identical in monozygotic twins, researchers have found that twins who are discordant for schizophrenia show significant differences in these patterns. In line with neurodevelopmental hypotheses, other studies have suggested that patients with schizophrenia may have been subjected to a higher rate of perinatal complications — e.g. neonatal hypoxia — than matched controls. Such obstetric complications seem to be more common in patients who do not have a family history for the disorder. However, these findings remain nonspecific associations only (i.e., no causality has been established).

Olney and colleagues recently reported that even modest exposure to agents such as ethanol during the critical brain maturational period of synaptogenesis (e.g., third trimester in humans) can lead to the apoptotic cell death of NMDA glutamate receptor-bearing neurons in several brain regions. This finding may help to explain observations of increased prevalence of psychiatric disorders such as schizophrenia in the offspring of alcoholic mothers. Discussed below, there is growing interest in the potential role of NMDA glutamate receptor hypofunction in schizophrenia and other psychotic disorders.

Synergistic dysfunction in neurotransmitter systems

Early models of neurotransmitter dysfunction in schizophrenia, which focussed primarily on dopamine hyperactivity, are giving way to a more complex model of brain dysfunction involving multiple neurotransmitter pathways. The hypothesis that a primary disturbance of dopamine neurotransmitter systems is responsible for symptoms of schizophrenia is supported by several key observations, including: (1) effective antipsychotic medications block dopamine receptors and their clinical potency is often related to the ability to block those receptors, (2) indirect measures of dopamine activity in the brain are related to levels of psychosis before, during, and on withdrawal of treatment, (3) drugs that increase dopamine transmission increase psychosis, and (4) increased dopamine receptor concentrations have been found in never-treated patients with schizophrenia. However, initial versions of the "dopamine hypothesis" are unable to explain early structural changes in specific brain regions, the reason for a dissociation between the temporal onset of those changes and symptom onset, the progressively deteriorating course that afflicts some patients (and characterized the disorder prior to the availability of antipsychotic medications), and the ability of early and effective treatment to beneficially alter long-term course.

The understanding of dysfunction in dopamine systems in the brain is changing. For example, animal studies have shown that (1) the sensory-gating properties of dopaminergic neurons are region-specific (for example, dopaminergic neurons in the anterior dorsal striatum are involved in sensory latent inhibition whereas those in the posterior dorsal striatum are not); and that (2) neonatal hypoxia, implicated as a contributing factor in schizophrenia (see above), causes a *decrease* in stress-induced dopamine release in specific brain areas. Data such as these suggest a region-specific pattern of dopamine dysfunction in schizophrenia, with hyperfunction in some areas and hypofunction in others. An emerging model implicates hypofunction of glutamate systems as an important pathological factor, interacting with changes in dopamine neurotransmission.

Post-mortem data have shown alterations in glutamate

receptor density and composition in several key brain areas. Central to this line of research is the NMDA receptor hypofunction (NRH) hypothesis. This hypothesis focuses on the NMDA subtype of the glutamate receptor, which can be effectively blocked by a number of agents including ketamine and phencyclidine (PCP) to produce an animal and human experimental model of NRH. These drugs also produce a relatively complete clinical model of schizophrenia when administered to humans, including positive, negative, disorganized, and cognitive symptoms (in comparison to drugs like amphetamine and LSD). NRH that is sufficiently prolonged and/or pronounced is now known to produce excitotoxic brain injury in an anatomic distribution that resembles the distribution of brain injury found in schizophrenia. However, this mechanism for neurotoxicity is not active until puberty, consistent with the observation that the psychotomimetic effects of NMDA antagonists are relatively absent in children and begin to occur in adolescents, and consistent with the predominantly young adult age-of-onset of schizophrenia.

NRH-induced neurotoxicity seems to require simultaneous activation of several neurotransmitter systems. Recent data suggest that NMDA receptors on GABAergic, serotonergic, and noradrenergic neurons maintain tonic inhibitory control over a multitude of excitatory pathways. Loss of inhibitory control results in prolonged excitation that can lead to "excitotoxic" neuronal damage. NMDA blockade has been shown to increase dopamine release in the mesolimbic system, and the action of antipsychotic drugs at the dopamine D2 receptor has recently been found to enhance functioning of the NMDA receptor. Recent evidence suggests that dopamine receptors regulate NMDA receptors in multiple brain systems, suggesting a relationship between dopamine dysfunction and NRH-induced abnormalities.

In utero damage to the brain, leading to schizophrenia, might be produced by viral infection, ethanol or other mechanisms, some of which are known to target NMDA receptor-bearing GABAergic neurons. The NRH hypothesis predicts that *in utero* damage to NMDA receptors and/or GABAergic neurons would lead to an NRH-equivalent condition with latent psychotogenic potential that would not manifest itself until adolescence. Interestingly, investigators have reported defects in GABAergic markers in post-mortem samples of patients with schizophrenia. Subsequent activation of NRH-induced neurotoxic mechanisms could produce the pattern of structural brain changes found in neuroimaging and post-mortem studies, involving neuronal damage in cingulate cortex, hippocampus, parahippocampal gyrus, and entorhinal cortex.

A number of specific pharmacologic agents can block the NRH-related circuit required for both psychosis and neurotoxicity. These include first- and second-generation antipsychotic medications (see below), providing an expanded explanation for their acute antipsychotic effects and a new

and powerful explanation for the observation that early treatment with these medications may prevent long-term clinical deterioration. The NRH hypothesis also has implications for previous work suggesting that a relative failure of those brain circuits providing a gate or filter for sensorimotor pathways—previously seen as primarily a function of dopamine—leads to a flood of unmodulated input (e.g., hallucinations). The NRH hypothesis increases the complexity of this gating hypothesis by suggesting a mechanism whereby several different cortical input paths could be disinhibited by the state of NRH. Overall, the NRH hypothesis offers a substantial amount of preclinical and clinical supporting data and a powerful explanatory capacity to incorporate various lines of experimental evidence.

Treatment

Few points are certain about the pre-modern history of treatments for conditions like schizophrenia and related disorders, except that this history probably extends back as far as humans have attempted to care for others with disease and dysfunction. Treatments have included an often bizarre array of physical and pharmacologic approaches. The past century has witnessed a revolution in the treatment of these disorders with the advent of relatively effective pharmacologic therapies for psychosis, which are now the principal mode of treatment. Surgical procedures have transformed from trephining to more modern procedures that involve relatively specific brain structures and are guided by sophisticated structural and/or functional neuroimaging procedures. So-called psychosurgery is currently used very rarely. Other procedures from the last century include insulin coma and early convulsive therapy, the latter evolving into current techniques for the safe and effective application of electroconvulsive therapy (ECT; see Chapter 23). Schizophrenia and associated disorders are considered indications for the use of ECT, particularly in the setting of catatonia, prominent affective symptoms, a prior ECT response, or poor drug response. Further research is warranted to more clearly define indications, particularly the relative risks and benefits of ECT compared with drug therapy.

The mainstay of effective treatment for schizophrenia and related disorders is antipsychotic medication. Medications account for therapeutic improvement during acute treatment and prevent relapse during maintenance treatment. The efficacy of antipsychotic therapy for the treatment of psychotic symptoms during acute exacerbations of illness is firmly established by a large number of randomized-assignment, placebo-controlled clinical trials. Antipsychotic pharmacotherapy plays a critical role in the treatment of hospitalized patients and outpatient treatment of acutely ill and stabilized patients. Antipsychotic medication appears to effectively treat up to 80% of patients with schizophrenia, targeting primarily positive and disorganized symptoms.

TABLE 13.7	Cumulative relapse risk in schizophrenia after continued vs. discontinued neuroleptic treatment*			
	Time at risk (mo)	Continued treatment	Discontinued treatment	Ratio
	0–3	3.8 ± 2.7 (26)	49.5 ± 1.2 (173)	12.9
	3–6	17.4 ± 4.0 (402)	55.8 ± 7.4 (1254)	3.2
	6.5–12	22.6 ± 3.5 (450)	62.1 ± 4.5 (639)	2.7
	18–24	28.5 ± 3.6 (247)	54.0 + 6.1 (281)	1.9

* Data are given as relapse risk ± SD (total number of subjects studied), weighted by the number of subjects per study based on data of Gilbert *et al.* The overall weighted mean ratio of the within-study difference in relapse risk was 5.78 ± 7.12.
From Baldessarini, RJ and Viguera, AC (1995) Neuroleptic withdrawal in schizophrenic patients, *Arch Gen Psychiatry* 52:189–192. Copyright © 1995, American Medical Association. All rights reserved. Reprinted by permission.

Most antipsychotic medications, with the exception of some second-generation drugs (discussed below), are less helpful or even counter-productive for the negative and cognitive symptoms of schizophrenia.

The efficacy of antipsychotic medications for the prevention of psychotic relapse following acute treatment is also clearly established. The prescription of, and adherence to, effective maintenance doses of antipsychotic medication is the most important determinant of patients' relative risk of relapse following successful acute treatment (Table 13.7). While individual variations in illness course suggest that some patients may not require continuous prophylactic treatment, there is still no clinical means of predicting who will or will not relapse after treatment discontinuation. The average rate of psychotic relapse in placebo-treated patients in remission or partial remission appears to be approximately 60% within one year, with no evidence that overall rates of relapse change appreciably in the second or third year. Unfortunately, medication side effects, a lack of knowledge about the long-term adverse consequences of under-treatment, and an illness-related loss of insight into the need for treatment can all undermine adherence to treatment. Long-acting depot antipsychotic medication can address some adherence issues, but attention to the unpleasant subjective effects and neurologic side effects of these medications is critical to maintaining an effective relationship with the patient. The recent availability of long-acting injectable second-generation antipsychotics may improve adherence to treatment while minimizing the unpleasant side effects associated with first-generation antipsychotics. Long-acting medications are not a substitute for personalized care, and clinical research has helped to define the primary importance of forming a strong treatment alliance with patients and their families, facilitating medication adherence and treatment follow-up.

Even with medication adherence and excellent follow-up, many patients experience psychotic relapse or symptom exacerbations that may be most safely treated in the hospital, usually on a well-staffed locked psychiatric unit. The major indications for hospitalization are usually disorder-related episodes of dangerousness to self or others, or a temporary state of severe disability that compromises the patient's capacity to provide food, shelter or adequate clothing. The decision to hospitalize a patient is best made in consultation with a psychiatrist with expertise in the hospital management of patients with psychotic disorders, optimally the treating psychiatrist. This individual can also assist in decisions about the capacity of the patient to be treated on a voluntary (versus involuntary) basis, providing expertise on the safest and most expeditious means of getting the patient out of danger and into a safer setting. The majority of patients can be treated and stabilized during a relatively brief hospitalization, often lasting 1–2 weeks, that reflects the onset of antipsychotic medication effects.

The treatment alliance

The treatment alliance is based on the patient's fundamental belief that the clinician is there to provide help. To achieve a strong treatment alliance, clinicians must build rapport with their patients through a commitment to educating the patient about their condition and its treatment. Busy primary care providers can receive some assistance with this goal through the use of written materials from sources such as the National Institute of Mental Health, the National Alliance for the Mentally Ill, and local and state departments of mental health. This treatment alliance should be explained to patients and conducted as a cooperative relationship where the clinician brings expertise on the disorder and its treatment to the patient, and the patient brings expertise on their own experience and treatment responses to the clinician. Patients should be provided with as much information as they can understand, based on their clinical condition.

The important point is that these patients may be

psychotic but they are not necessarily incompetent, unreasonable, incomprehensible or irrational, and an effective working relationship should not be excluded from an effective treatment plan. Simply prescribing medications, monitoring side effects, and leaving the relationship to someone else (i.e., the nurse, psychologist, social worker, or other ancillary staff) provide a less effective level of care, analogous to prescribing insulin to diabetic patients without personally providing at least some instruction about the role of insulin in their illness and its overall management.

- The treatment alliance should be explained to patients and conducted as a cooperative relationship where the clinician brings expertise on the disorder and its treatment to the patient, and the patient brings expertise on their own experience and treatment responses to the clinician.
- Patients should be provided as much information as they can understand, based on their clinical condition.
- An important point is that patients with schizophrenia may be psychotic but they are not necessarily incompetent, unreasonable, incomprehensible or irrational, and an effective working relationship with them cannot be excluded from an effective treatment plan.
- Simply prescribing medication, monitoring side effects, and leaving the relationship to someone else (i.e., the nurse, psychologist, social worker or other ancillary staff) provide a less effective level of care, analogous to prescribing insulin to diabetic patients without personally providing instruction about the role of insulin in their illness and its overall management.

Specific impediments to the treatment alliance and an understanding of the illness and its treatment can be found within each symptom grouping discussed previously. An initial approach to each is outlined below, but the management of these problems is ultimately guided by the clinician's judgment about how best to strengthen the alliance with individual patients. While some patients may appear to only slowly or minimally engage in the alliance and setbacks may be encountered during periods of illness exacerbation, steady, unpressured effort from a clinician who remains comfortable with the patient is usually rewarded. Families should also be included in this process of education and alliance to the greatest extent possible (e.g., meeting with the family may be problematic when chronic paranoid delusions regarding them could jeopardize the alliance with the patient). Including families provides support to both the patient and family, brings valuable data and extra partners

into the clinician's care of the patient, and can further ensure medication adherence.

Patients with positive psychotic symptoms may have delusions or hallucinations whose content impinges on an effective relationship with the clinician or others (e.g., a delusion that the clinician aims to harm them). This possibility should be directly addressed in an interview, and if found, directly and matter-of-factly countered. Most helpful are simple statements indicating the clinician's belief that these ideas, while very real for the patient, are part of a brain illness interfering with the patient's perceptions. When it is likely to be accepted, the clinician should make an offer to work together with the patient to help sort out those perceptions that are distorted by the illness from those that are accurate, studiously avoiding the impression that he or she is belittling or devaluing the patient's experience. Avolition and ambivalence can be equally devastating to the therapeutic alliance. Persistent efforts to engage and educate the patient, combined with gentle encouragement, are the best approach.

Disorganization and cognitive impairment can also seriously undermine an educational program, but this should not be considered a justification to forgo the effort to provide education. Rather, such patients require extra time from the clinical staff along with straightforward, clear explanations in plain language, making sure that the patient understands each step of the conversation. A large number of patients can be helped to understand even difficult issues such as the risk-benefit balance concerning adverse events such as tardive dyskinesia and weight gain during treatment with antipsychotic medications, making reasonable decisions and giving well-informed consent when provided with the facts. These discussions can initially be spread out over several visits and should then be repeated over multiple visits, reinforcing the initial information and adding additional information as understanding permits.

First-generation ("typical") agents

From their introduction into practice in the 1950s until quite recently, first-generation or "typical" antipsychotic medications, also referred to as "neuroleptics" or "major tranquilizers," were essentially the only available choice for the pharmacologic treatment of psychotic disorders. Despite their capacity to produce a number of important side effects, including the common extrapyramidal symptoms that define their "typicality" (see Chapter 22), the clear efficacy of these agents for the treatment of positive symptoms and disorganization was rapidly recognized and widespread treatment instituted.

Individual first-generation antipsychotic medications are generally considered to be equally effective when given at equipotent doses. There is no reason for concomitant therapy with more than one first-generation antipsychotic medication, and the potential for additional problematic side effects (discussed below) suggests a relative contraindication. Exceptions to this rule occur during the transition from one antipsychotic to another and for the brief management of psychotic exacerbations where a single agent may lack sufficient sedative effect (e.g., use of an adjunctive small nighttime dose of a more sedating antipsychotic during primary treatment with haloperidol). Individual medications have been characterized as "low potency" and "high potency," with an inverse relationship to the effective acute treatment dose. Significant inter-individual differences in absorption, metabolism, and effects on sites of action produce substantial inter-individual differences in clinically effective doses, underscoring the importance of individual dose titration. Important ethnic differences in drug metabolism have been identified (e.g., a higher rate of side effects and relatively higher plasma antipsychotic levels for a given dose in Han Chinese individuals). Another important example is found in the growing elderly population of patients where age-related declines in the capacity to metabolize drugs lead to lower effective doses and a lower dose threshold for the development of many problematic side effects (see Chapter 26).

The important differences among individual typical antipsychotic agents are found with respect to side effects and mainly include varying levels of sedation and autonomic and neurologic side effects. In general, lower potency typical antipsychotic agents (e.g., substituted phenothiazines) tend to be associated with more sedation, more weight gain with some associated metabolic risk (e.g., increased risk of diabetes mellitus and dyslipidemia), and more autonomic and other unwanted side effects than higher potency agents (e.g., the butyrophenone, haloperidol). On the other hand, the higher potency agents are more likely than low-potency agents to cause extrapyramidal and other neurologic symptoms at clinically effective doses; "extrapyramidal" symptoms refer to parkinsonism, akathisia, dyskinesias (acute and tardive), and dystonias (acute and tardive). Both parkinsonism and akathisia are associated with important behavioral and/or emotional effects. Considerable research has found that both side effects can mimic primary symptoms of schizophrenia and adversely affect therapeutic outcome, in a generally dose-dependent manner. Akathisia, defined as a subjective desire to move with or without objective motor signs, is a particularly unpleasant side effect of typical antipsychotic medications, with an average prevalence estimate of 20%. Akathisia is also associated with higher doses of antipsychotic medications and may have a major impact on treatment adherence and treatment outcome. Parkinsonism and akathisia remain under-recognized side effects of antipsychotic therapy that, either directly or as a stress or cue for additional symptoms, account for higher levels of psychopathology in affected patients.

The tardive (i.e., late-onset) variant of dyskinesia is relatively common (approximately 20% average prevalence and

- Individual antipsychotic agents differ with respect to side effects, mainly varying levels of sedation, autonomic and neurologic side effects.
- In general, lower potency first-generation antipsychotic agents (e.g., substituted phenothiazines) tend to cause more sedation, more autonomic and other unwanted side effects than higher potency agents (e.g., the butyrophenone, haloperidol).
- The higher potency agents are more likely than low-potency agents to cause extrapyramidal and other neurologic symptoms at clinically effective doses.
- While sedation is sometimes tolerated during acute treatment (less often during maintenance), autonomic side effects are generally problematic and unwanted (e.g., dry mouth, accommodation disturbance), and poorly tolerated or even contraindicated in the elderly (e.g., constipation, tachycardia, hypotension).
- The CNS consequences of anticholinergic effects, prominent with lower potency agents, include impairment in memory and learning that is detectable in young subjects and becomes even more pronounced in the elderly.
- Anticholinergic effects are an important reason to avoid low-potency agents in the elderly, if not in all patients, many of whom already suffer some degree of disorder-related cognitive impairment.
- The general rule that a past therapeutic response to a specific agent suggests using it again is a good one except when applied to aging patients or those with impaired metabolic capacity (e.g., competing drugs, hepatic injury) who may have previously tolerated a particular agent or combination but are now less able to do so.

4–5% average annual incidence), with variable degrees of resolution and persistence. While sedation is sometimes tolerated during acute treatment (less often during maintenance), autonomic side effects are generally problematic (e.g., dry mouth, accommodation disturbance), and poorly tolerated or even contraindicated in the elderly (e.g., constipation, tachycardia, hypotension). Further, the CNS consequences of anticholinergic effects, prominent with lower potency typical agents, include impairment in memory and learning that is detectable in young subjects and may become even more pronounced in the elderly. This is an important reason to avoid low-potency typical agents in the elderly, many of whom already suffer some degree of disorder-related cognitive impairment. The general rule that a past therapeutic response to a specific agent suggests using it again is a good one except when applied to aging patients or those with impaired capacity to metabolize a drug (e.g., competing drugs, hepatic injury) who may have previously tolerated a particular agent or combination but are now less able to do so.

- Even experts trained to make such discriminations cannot separate some negative symptoms of schizophrenia from parkinsonism, meaning, in short, that treatment-induced parkinsonism associated with higher doses of antipsychotic medications appears to worsen some negative symptoms.
- Akathisia, defined as a subjective desire to move with or without objective motor signs, is a common and unpleasant side effect of typical antipsychotic medications, with an average prevalence estimate of 20%.
- Akathisia is also associated with higher doses of antipsychotic medications and may have a major impact on treatment compliance and treatment outcome.
- Some investigators have found that patients with akathisia have more positive psychotic symptoms and a poor positive psychotic symptom response during acute treatment, independent of the success or failure of akathisia treatment with benztropine mesylate.
- Akathisia has been more consistently related to anxiety and depression during both acute and maintenance haloperidol treatment. This is consistent with subjective descriptions of akathisia and with an early observation that akathisia may be mistaken for agitated depression.
- Parkinsonism and akathisia remain under-recognized side effects of antipsychotic therapy that, either directly or as a stress or cue for additional symptoms, account for higher levels of psychopathology in affected patients.

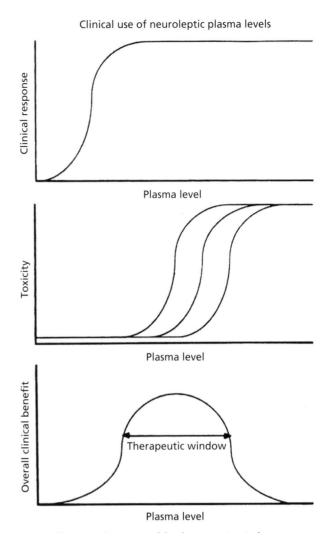

Fig. 13.3 Theoretical concept of the therapeutic window produced by the difference between plasma level producing clinical effect and plasma level producing toxic side effects. From Marder, SR, Davis, JM, and Janicak, PG (eds) (1993) *Clinical Use of Neuroleptic Plasma Levels*, Washington, DC, American Psychiatric Press, www.appi.org. Reprinted by permission.

The high-potency first-generation antipsychotic medications haloperidol and fluphenazine are available as long-acting depot injections (2–4-week dosing intervals). This route of drug delivery can improve relapse prevention, largely but perhaps not entirely explained by improved treatment adherence. Haloperidol and fluphenazine have received the greatest amount of investigation concerning the relationship between plasma levels and clinical response. When appropriate assays and consultant guidance are available, plasma levels may guide dose selection in patients who fail to respond adequately to conventional dose titration.

First-generation antipsychotics have long been thought to control psychosis through a single mechanism: blockade of the dopamine D2 receptor (sometimes referred to as the "neuroleptic receptor"). Second-generation agents had been presumed by many to work through more complex mechanisms, though recent analyses suggest that they probably exert their antipsychotic effect through D2 blockade as well (see below). A phenomenon termed the neuroleptic threshold has gained substantial recognition. The neuroleptic threshold model is based, in part, on the *in vivo* neuroimag-

ing observation that at approximately 70% striatal D2 receptor occupancy, the antipsychotic action of the drug is effectively maximized and further dose increase leads to the onset of extrapyramidal symptoms. Consequently, a "therapeutic window" of treatment exists, as the onset of extrapyramidal side effects generally occurs at doses just above the maximum clinically required (Fig. 13.3). This phenomenon can be quite useful, as doses can be increased gradually while monitoring for the emergence of EPS (e.g., starting at 2 mg/day of haloperidol and increasing by 2 mg every other day), stopping at the first indication of EPS. There is good evidence from clinical studies and positron emission tomography studies to support this approach to optimizing the therapeutic response; however, some evidence suggests that akathisia may be more difficult to avoid than parkinsonism during treatment with typical antipsychotics. Data suggest that D2 blockade may be optimized at doses equivalent to, or even below, approximately 5 mg/day of haloperidol. In general, acute treatment studies have suggested that doses equivalent to oral haloperidol at greater than 10 mg/day offer no additional benefits and an increased incidence of side effects.

Second-generation ("atypical") agents

Rapidly replacing the "typical" antipsychotics as first-line agents, the second-generation or "atypical" antipsychotics all share the characteristic of having more limited extrapyramidal side effects at clinically effective doses, although individual agents vary in the extent to which they avoid this group of adverse events. The currently marketed second-generation antipsychotic medications are clozapine, risperidone, olanzapine, quetiapine, ziprasidone, and aripiprazole.

The first marketed second-generation antipsychotic medication was clozapine. Clozapine was initially introduced in the 1960s, but it was withdrawn from the market for several years as a result of incidents of fatal agranulocytosis (see below). Clozapine is unique even among the second-generation agents, as it is primarily indicated for (and approved by the FDA for) the management of treatment-resistant schizophrenia. There is some consensus that "treatment-resistant" patients are defined as patients having an inadequate response to two previous trials of first- or second-generation antipsychotic medications of adequate dose and duration (see below). Clozapine has been demonstrated to produce improvements in symptoms in approximately 30% of treatment-resistant patients, with as many as 60% improving when treatment is continued for 12 months, offering an important and well-established option for those patients who fail other therapy. More recently, clozapine has been noted by the FDA to reduce the risk of suicide in treated patients.

Clozapine is not a first-line treatment for schizophrenia because of the occurrence of agranulocytosis in approximately 1% of patients (in contrast to 1 out of 2,000 patients treated with first-generation antipsychotics). Monitoring white cell counts is mandatory for the duration of treatment, for the first six months on a weekly basis and thereafter reduced in frequency based on established protocols. Clozapine also carries a dose-dependent risk of inducing seizures and is associated rarely with eosinophilic myocarditis. Additional potentially troublesome side effects include orthostatic hypotension, tachycardia, sialorrhea, sedation, weight gain, and an increased risk of dyslipidemia and hyperglycemia, including type 2 diabetes mellitus.

In the past decade, risperidone, olanzapine, quetiapine, ziprasidone, and (most recently) aripiprazole have been introduced. These agents have similar efficacy with differences in side-effect profiles. A meta-analysis of extensive patient data performed by Leucht and colleagues has shown that second-generation agents generally afford a 30% lower risk of EPS than first-generation agents. Clozapine, quetiapine, and aripiprazole carry less risk of prolactin elevation, as well. Increases in plasma prolactin are most commonly asymptomatic, but they may present with sexual dysfunction, galactorrhea, and amenorrhea. Though currently unclear, there may also be an association between prolactin elevation and osteoporosis.

The efficacy of second-generation agents in treating psychotic symptoms tends to be equal to that of first-generation agents. A pivotal short-term treatment trial for risperidone demonstrated efficacy superior to that of haloperidol, and similar superiority to haloperidol was demonstrated for relapse prevention in a recent well-designed maintenance treatment study. It remains to be seen whether other newer agents will demonstrate similar superiority to haloperidol, with most meta-analyses indicating similar effect sizes for positive symptom efficacy across all the post-clozapine second-generation agents. The newer agents differ from clozapine in that they do not appear to share clozapine's unique effectiveness for treatment-resistant patients or the risk of agranulocytosis. Otherwise, no single drug has been shown to be substantially superior to the others in its antipsychotic efficacy. The choice between the newer second-generation drugs should therefore largely be made on the basis of tolerability and side-effect profile. One important risk that varies by drug is weight gain and related metabolic disturbances (see Medical comorbidities below).

The mechanism of action of second-generation antipsychotics has been the subject of much debate. In addition to the D2 receptor, second-generation agents bind to varying degrees to the dopamine D4 receptor, the serotonin 5HT2 and 5HT4 receptors, and to a lesser extent, to noradrenergic receptors. Competing theories have suggested that a ratio of 5HT2 to D2 receptor affinity or D4 to D2 receptor affinity is important for either efficacy or reductions in the risk of extrapyramidal side effects or both. Kapur and Seeman have recently argued that second-generation agents exert their therapeutic effects exclusively via D2 receptors (just like first-generation agents). The apparent lower affinity of some agents for the D2 receptor results from rapid dissociation from the receptor after binding, which may create the appearance of lower affinity in standard *in vitro* tests. This model is supported by rapid *in vivo* measurement of D2 occupancy via positron emission tomography, which shows, for example, that quetiapine occupies 65% of D2 receptors two hours after administration (roughly comparable to haloperidol) vs. only 20% 10 hours later. An agent in use in Europe, amisulpride, provides an "atypical" antipsychotic effect—plus, reports suggest, improved treatment of negative symptoms—despite binding primarily to D2 and D3 receptors. Notably, the latest second-generation agent approved in the United States, aripiprazole, may function as a partial agonist at the D2 receptor.

In addition to side-effect profile, general considerations for all second-generation agents include the issue of concomitant use of other antipsychotics, initiation of treatment, order of use, and cost-effectiveness. There are no data to support the addition of a second antipsychotic medication to ongoing treatment with a second-generation agent, and the proposed mechanism of action for these drugs suggests that concomitant treatment—particularly with a first-generation agent—may compromise their "atypical" side-effect profile. Nonetheless, it is prudent to continue previous antipsychotic therapy for a brief period during the initial titration of any second-generation drug. Ideally, the replacing agent should be gradually introduced during the gradual discontinuation of the previous second-generation drug. There are limited data to guide the timing of such overlapping titrations. In addition, a second antipsychotic agent can sometimes be used in lieu of a benzodiazepine (see below) for the brief management of psychotic exacerbations where the primary antipsychotic agent may lack sufficient sedative effect (e.g., use of an adjunctive small nighttime dose of a more sedating antipsychotic during primary treatment with a less sedating agent). Clinical vigilance and judgment should be applied to any period of medication change.

Use of adjunctive medications

A number of psychotropic medications have been used adjunctively in the treatment of schizophrenia, often with little convincing, controlled data about their efficacy for this indication. In particular, mood stabilizers (see Chapter 8), including lithium, valproate, carbamazepine, and several other agents, have often been used to reduce agitation in psychotic patients. Recent data suggest that other antiepileptic medications may be used to augment antipsychotic treatment. The use of these augmenting agents, while promising, awaits further confirmatory data.

In general, adjunctive psychotropic medications can be very useful for treating symptoms that are not responsive to, or perhaps caused by, the primary antipsychotic medication. It is always important to consider the possibility that an antipsychotic agent may be contributing in some way to problematic symptoms. Symptoms like agitation or insomnia may be symptoms of disease that persist because of inadequate dosing or response; conversely, they may reflect akathisia, a side effect of the antipsychotic itself.

It is preferable to optimize treatment with the primary antipsychotic medication, even considering a change in the primary agent, prior to the addition of second (or third) agents. The common indications for adding adjunctive medications are listed in Box 13.3.

BOX 13.3

Common indications for adding adjunctive medications

1 For the treatment of acute dystonic reactions, anticholinergic agents (e.g., benztropine, trihexyphenidyl and diphenhydramine) are highly effective first choices and may not be needed chronically insofar as dystonias are more common early (first ten days) in the treatment course.

2 For the treatment of drug-induced parkinsonism, anticholinergic medications and amantadine can be used (with attention to additional unwanted effects), although an antipsychotic dose decrease, when feasible, is preferred.

3 For the treatment of akathisia, beta-blockers (e.g., propranolol), benzodiazepines (e.g., lorazepam), amantadine and anticholinergics are often effective, but again an antipsychotic dose decrease, when feasible, may produce the desired effect.

4 The treatment of agitation and/or insomnia is less straightforward, as such symptoms may reflect overall exacerbation of illness-related symptoms, suggesting the utility of a dose increase or the temporary addition of a benzodiazepine, or they may reflect akathisia related to treatment with a high-potency agent or higher doses in general.

5 For the treatment of persistent or emergent depression, tricyclic antidepressants and selective serotonin reuptake inhibitors have been used effectively. (The latter have been used for both depression and emergent obsessive-compulsive symptoms on clozapine.) Overall response rates may be lower in schizophrenia than in primary affective disorders, however.

6 For the treatment of mood instability or the appearance of "manic" symptoms in patients with schizophrenia, lithium, valproic acid, and carbamazepine have been used adjunctively with an antipsychotic medication. However, relatively little well-controlled data exist to guide clinical practice in this indication.

CONSIDER CONSULTATION WHEN...

- Initial evaluation, diagnosis, and treatment plan are needed for first onset of illness or initial clinical presentation in the treatment setting.
- Patient presents with new onset suicidal/dangerous ideation or behavior.
- Patient is not responding adequately to first-line treatment plans.
- Patient requires hospitalization.
- Patient is experiencing substantial weight gain and/or metabolic abnormalities associated with treatment.

TABLE 13.8

Features suggesting good and poor prognoses in schizophrenia

Good	Poor
Late onset	Early onset
Obvious precipitating factors	No precipitating factors
Acute onset	Insidious onset
Good premorbid social, sexual, and work history	Poor premorbid social, sexual, and work history
Affective symptoms (especially depression)	Withdrawn, autistic behavior
Paranoid or catatonic features	Undifferentiated or disorganized features
Married	Unmarried, divorced, or widowed
Family history of mood disorders	Family history of schizophrenia
Good support system	Poor support system
Undulating course	Chronic course
Positive symptoms	Negative symptoms
	Neurological signs and symptoms
	History of perinatal trauma
	No remission in three years
	Numerous relapses

Adapted from Cancro, R and Lehmann, HE: Schizophrenia: clinical features, in Sadock, BJ and Sadock, VA (eds) (2000) *Kaplan & Sadock's Comprehensive Textbook of Psychiatry/VII*, Philadelphia, Lippincott Williams & Wilkins, page 1197. Used with permission.

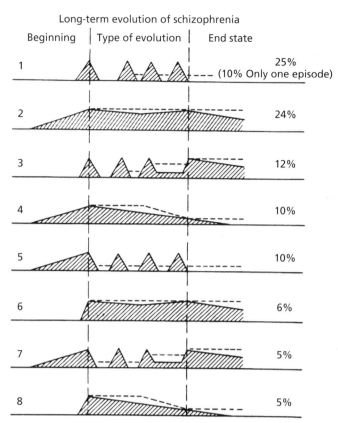

Fig. 13.4 Schematic representations of the different types of long-term courses of schizophrenia. (Average follow-up 36.9 years, n=228. Dotted line represents alternative forms of evolution within the same type.)
From Ciompi, L, Miller, NE, and Cohen, GD (eds) (1987) *Schizophrenia and Aging*, New York, Guilford Press. Reprinted by permission.

Prognosis, course, and comorbidities

Prognosis and disease course

The prognosis for individual patients with schizophrenia is a complex function of (1) specific illness-related impairments suffered by the individual (e.g., some impairments have long-lasting consequences such as school failure or job and insurance loss), (2) the patient's pattern of remission, persistence or worsening over time (i.e., illness course), (3) treatment factors (e.g., antipsychotic medication), and (4) harmful prognosis-altering factors (Table 13.8). Overall, the course of illness in patients with schizophrenia is generally chronic with highly variable patterns of exacerbation and remission (Fig. 13.4). The variable clinical course associated with schizophrenia has led to some debate about overall rates of remission or deterioration. There is some evidence that the frequency of progressively deteriorating outcomes may have diminished in recent decades. Treatment with antipsychotic medication may partly explain the apparent re-

duction in very poor outcomes since the advent of neuroleptic treatment in the late 1950s.

Psychiatric, social, and behavioral comorbidities

Multiple hospitalizations have a profoundly disruptive and long-lasting effect on the social and occupational functioning of patients. The risk of exacerbation and repeated hospitalization in patients with schizophrenia is inversely related to adequate treatment with antipsychotic medication.

Morbidity is further enhanced by the loss of medical benefits and poor self-care that often go along with psychosis. Patients with schizophrenia also have a high rate of depression that adds to overall morbidity. The lifetime risk of a major depressive episode occurring secondary to schizophrenia has been estimated to be as high as 60%. Further, it has been suggested that patients with negative symptoms may be at even greater risk for depression—though this can be a confusing phenomenon, as there is a great deal of overlap between the clinical signs of depression and negative symptoms. Beyond increased morbidity, schizophrenia has been found to be associated with an increased mortality rate, which is partially explained by increased rates of completed suicide (up to 10% of patients die by suicide). Although the prediction of suicide in an individual patient is impossible, a number of factors confer increased risk: (1) male gender; (2) white race; (3) social isolation; (4) depression; (5) sense of hopelessness; (6) past history of suicide attempts; (7) family history of suicide; (8) unmarried status; (9) unemployed status; (10) deteriorating health with a high level of premorbid functioning; (11) recent loss or rejection; (12) parental loss during childhood; (13) limited external support; (14) family stress or instability; (15) use of alcohol or illicit drugs. Additional increases in morbidity and mortality are related to medical illnesses, which are discussed below.

Another important factor in the prediction of illness course is substance abuse and dependence. Lifetime risk of comorbidity for alcohol and/or drug abuse and dependence in patients with schizophrenia is approximately 50%. This problem has been associated with increased rates of violence and suicide, non-adherence with treatment, psychotic exacerbation, antipsychotic treatment refractoriness, hospitalization, tardive dyskinesia and homelessness. However, treatment of a substance use disorder can reverse the adverse effects on overall prognosis.

Nicotine use is particularly common in patients with schizophrenia. These individuals have the highest rate of smoking of any psychiatric population and have three to four times the rate of smoking found in the general population. They also tend to be heavy smokers and to smoke "high-tar" cigarettes; indeed, studies have shown that this population tends to smoke in ways that maximize their intake of nicotine. There are a number of possible physiologic explanations for the heavy nicotine use associated with schizophrenia. Nicotine increases dopaminergic activity in the prefrontal cortex and nucleus accumbens, which might reduce negative symptoms. Smoking reduces blood levels of antipsychotic medications by up to 50%, likely by induction of specific liver enzymes; patients may therefore be self-treating antipsychotic side effects by smoking.

Recent studies have also implicated specific nicotinic receptors in the pathophysiology of schizophrenia. Data by Leonard and colleagues have suggested that the nicotinic alpha-7 receptor may have a role in the "sensory gating" abnormality found in 85% of schizophrenia patients. Normal individuals demonstrate decreased response to an auditory stimulus that is preceded by a matching stimulus; schizophrenia patients tend to show impairment in this inhibition, indicating a deficit in "sensory gating." Interestingly, 50% of the first-degree relatives of patients with schizophrenia show similar inhibitory deficits, suggesting a possible predisposing genetic factor independent of the mechanisms discussed previously. Generally speaking, smoking cessation techniques can be effective in patients with schizophre-

nia, but relapse rates are even larger than those in the general population, and many experience strong withdrawal symptoms (e.g., craving, anxiety) when they attempt to quit smoking.

Despite public perception, violence and homicide do not appear to be more common in people with schizophrenia. Risk factors for violence in the hospital are low (subtherapeutic) plasma levels of antipsychotic medication, higher levels of overall psychosis, and a past history of violence. Contrary to persistent myth, psychotic patients are more likely to be the victims of violence than the perpetrators.

Medical comorbidities

Patients with schizophrenia often have poor health and unhealthy lifestyles and consequently are at risk for common physical illnesses and increased mortality. In fact, life expectancies for patients with schizophrenia are 57 years for men and 65 years for women—20% shorter than the general population. While factors contributing to this lower life expectancy include markedly increased risks for suicide as well as infectious and respiratory diseases, cardiovascular mortality is the major contributor to excess mortality in schizophrenia. In addition, patients with schizophrenia suffer from impaired insight, lack of resources (i.e., access to medical care), lower medication and treatment compliance and more psychosocial stress, all of which can compound medical problems.

Patients with schizophrenia have 1.6 times the death rate of the general population; 38% of the excess death is associated with suicide and homicide, while the other 62% results from "natural" causes. Patients with schizophrenia are about twice as likely to die from CVD as people from the general population. Such high risks of death from CVD are likely a result of the higher rates of obesity, lipid abnormalities, diabetes, hypertension, physical inactivity, and smoking. Obesity (predominantly abdominal adiposity), lipid abnormalities, hypertension, and impaired glucose tolerance can occur together as the "metabolic syndrome" (also known as "insulin resistance syndrome" or "syndrome X"). Patients with psychotic disorders—in part because of lifestyle changes and in part because of the effects of medications—are at increased risk for various components of this syndrome, beginning with increased adiposity.

Clinicians might be able to manage some of the CVD risk associated with schizophrenia through their choice of antipsychotic treatment. Short-term weight gain data supplied by manufacturers indicates that the second-generation antipsychotic medications (aripiprazole, olanzapine, quetiapine, risperidone and ziprasidone) are associated with clinically significant weight gain (defined by the FDA as >7%) compared to placebo, although rates vary greatly among medications. Aripiprazole, risperidone, and ziprasidone treatment are associated with approximately twice the placebo-associated incidence of weight gain, quetiapine approximately three times the incidence, and olanzapine with approximately ten times the placebo-associated incidence of weight gain during short-term trials. Long-term data indicate that ziprasidone- and aripiprazole-induced weight gain remain limited to approximately 1 kg over the first year of treatment, similar to the weight gain profile of high-potency typical antipsychotics like haloperidol, while quetiapine and risperidone are associated with approximately 2–3 kg increases over the same one-year period. The mean weight gain associated with olanzapine treatment at commonly used antipsychotic doses exceeds 10 kg during the first year of exposure. While antipsychotic drugs are typically associated with weight gain, clozapine and olanzapine are the most problematic.

The overall management of schizophrenia requires effective treatment of psychosis and non-psychotic symptoms (e.g., affective symptoms, cognitive impairment, anxiety) and the prevention of relapse. Effective treatment is defined by efficacy and tolerability, so clinicians should aim to maximize each while recognizing that individual patients may require different solutions to achieve the best balance between sometimes competing considerations. Effective treatment can include the use of clozapine for selected patients with refractory schizophrenia, despite some of the adverse events that can be associated with this agent. Considering the chronic nature of schizophrenia and the associated need for chronic use of medications to treat symptoms and prevent relapse, it is critical that clinicians aim to minimize antipsychotic associated adverse events, particularly those that can contribute to significant increases in medical comorbidity and medical mortality. The selection of antipsychotic treatment can play a role in risk management. In addition, clinicians can attempt to assist patients with schizophrenia in managing medical risk factors for CVD and other morbidities through patient education and assistance with dietary choices, and by encouraging smoking cessation. Careful monitoring for medical complications such as weight gain, hypertension, lipid abnormalities, and other medical morbidity should lead to early detection of disease, appropriate use of medical specialists, judicious use of concomitant medications, and ongoing critical review of appropriate psychotropic choices.

Schizophreniform disorder and brief psychotic disorder

These diagnoses are applied when a patient's clinical picture is fully consistent with schizophrenia, but symptoms have not been present long enough to justify the official diagnosis. The simplest way to remember these disorders is by the duration requirements: brief psychotic disorder applies to symptoms that have been present for more than one day and less than one month, and schizophreniform disorder applies

to symptoms present for longer than one month but less than six months.

The DSM-IV criteria for brief psychotic disorder are listed in Box 13.4, with associated features listed in Table 13.9. DSM-IV criteria for schizophreniform disorder are listed in Box 13.5, with associated features listed in Table 13.10.

> **Box 13.4 Brief psychotic disorder**
>
> A. Presence of one (or more) of the following symptoms:
> - delusions
> - hallucinations
> - disorganized speech (e.g., frequent derailment or incoherence)
> - grossly disorganized or catatonic behavior.
> **Note:** Do not include a symptom if it is a culturally sanctioned response pattern.
>
> B. Duration of an episode of the disturbance is at least one day but less than one month, with eventual full return to premorbid level of functioning.
>
> C. The disturbance is not better accounted for by a mood disorder with psychotic features, schizoaffective disorder, or schizophrenia and is not due to the direct physiological effects of a substance (e.g., a drug of abuse, a medication) or a general medical condition.
>
> *Specify* if:
> - *with marked stressor(s)* (brief reactive psychosis): if symptoms occur shortly after and apparently in response to events that, singly or together, would be markedly stressful to almost anyone in similar circumstances in the person's culture
> - *without marked stressor(s):* if psychotic symptoms do *not* occur shortly after, or are not apparently in response to events that, singly or together, would be markedly stressful to almost anyone in similar circumstances in the person's culture
> - *with postpartum onset:* if onset within four weeks postpartum.
> *From American Psychiatric Association (2000) Diagnostic and Statistical Manual of Mental Disorders, 4th Edition, Text Revision, Washington, D.C., American Psychiatric Association.*

Schizoaffective disorder

Schizoaffective disorder is a relatively controversial diagnosis that has changed considerably over the years. The simplest description of this disorder is that it is an independent combination of schizophrenia-like psychotic symptoms and affective symptoms. The symptoms may be unipolar (depressive) or bipolar. The term "schizoaffective" was coined by Jacob Kasinian in 1933; patients diagnosed using his original criteria would today be considered to have

Table 13.9 Brief psychotic disorder

Discriminating features

1   One (or more) of the following symptoms are present:
    - delusions
    - hallucinations
    - disorganized speech (e.g., frequent derailment or incoherence)
    - grossly disorganized or catatonic behaviour.
2   The duration of the disturbance is at least one day but less than one month.

Consistent features

1   Not due to the effects of substance use or general medical conditions.
2   Not accounted for by another psychotic disorder, such as schizophrenia or schizoaffective disorder.
3   Not accounted for by a major affective disorder.

Variable features

1   Presence of marked stressors triggering the disturbance.
2   Postpartum onset.
3   Cultural sanction of the response pattern (note that cultural acceptance of the behavior generally precludes the diagnosis of brief psychotic disorder).

Table 13.10 Schizophreniform disorder

Discriminating features

1   Two (or more) of the following, each present for a significant portion of time during a one-month period (or less if successfully treated):
    - delusions
    - hallucinations
    - disorganized speech (e.g., frequent derailment or incoherence)
    - grossly disorganized or catatonic behavior
    - negative symptoms, i.e., affective flattening, alogia, or avolition.
2   One or more major areas of functioning are markedly below the level achieved prior to the onset.
3   Continuous signs of the disturbance persist for at least one month but for less than six months.

Consistent features

1   Not due to the effects of substance use or general medical conditions.
2   Not accounted for by major affective disorder.

Variable features

1   Inappropriate affect.
2   Anhedonia.
3   Dysphoric mood.
4   Disturbances in sleep pattern.
5   Abnormalities of psychomotor activity.
6   Difficulty concentrating.
7   Cognitive dysfunction.
8   Confused or disoriented.
9   Lack of insight.
10 Depersonalization, derealization, and somatic concerns.

Box 13.5 Schizophreniform disorder

A. Criteria A, D, and E of schizophrenia are met.

B. An episode of the disorder (including prodromal, active, and residual phases) lasts at least one month but less than six months. (When the diagnosis must be made without waiting for recovery, it should be qualified as "Provisional.")

Adapted from American Psychiatric Association (2000) Diagnostic and Statistical Manual of Mental Disorders; 4th Edition, Text Revision, Washington, D.C., American Psychiatric Association.

purely affective disorders. DSM-II considered schizoaffective disorder as a subtype of schizophrenia. In DSM-III, it became a "psychotic disorder not elsewhere classified," and in DSM-IV, schizoaffective disorder was given full standing as a separate and uniquely defined psychotic disorder in the schizophrenia-like family. The DSM-IV criteria for schizoaffective disorder are listed in Box 13.6, with associated features listed in Table 13.11. With each classification change came substantial changes in the diagnostic criteria, confounding efforts to study the disorder over time.

The controversy surrounding schizoaffective disorder has resulted from the difficulty that investigators have had in

establishing the validity of the diagnosis. To date, there are still scant data to support the validity of this disorder, in part because shifting criteria have made it difficult to study. Skeptics' concerns are amplified by the relative vagueness of the current criteria—particularly the requirement that affective symptoms are present for a "substantial portion" of the duration of illness, leaving the definition of what constitutes "substantial" open to unguided interpretation. While some data have suggested that patients with this diagnosis may have an overall prognosis intermediate between those of schizophrenia and affective disorders, other data have suggested that patients with "depressive type" schizoaffective disorder have a disease course similar to patients with pure schizophrenia, whereas those with "bipolar type" schizoaffective disorder have a course more akin to bipolar disorder. These latter data cast further doubt on the validity of schizoaffective disorder as a unique entity.

With its current classification as a separate schizophrenia-spectrum disorder, schizoaffective disorder has been diag-

Box 13.6 Schizoaffective disorder

A. An uninterrupted period of illness during which, at some time, there is either a major depressive episode, a manic episode, or a mixed episode concurrent with symptoms that meet criterion A for schizophrenia.
Note: the major depressive episode must include criterion A1: depressed mood.
B. During the same period of illness, there have been delusions or hallucinations for at least two weeks in the absence of prominent mood symptoms.
C. Symptoms that meet criteria for a mood episode are present for a substantial portion of the total duration of the active and residual periods of the illness.
D. The disturbance is not due to the direct physiological effects of a substance (e.g., a drug of abuse, a medication) or a general medical condition.
Specify type:
Bipolar type: if the disturbance includes a manic or a mixed episode (or a manic or a mixed episode and major depressive episodes)
Depressive type: if the disturbance only includes major depressive episodes.
From American Psychiatric Association (2000) Diagnostic and Statistical Manual of Mental Disorders, 4th Edition, Text Revision, Washington, D.C., American Psychiatric Association.

Table 13.11 Schizoaffective disorder

Discriminating features

1 An uninterrupted period of illness including:
  • a major depressive, manic, or mixed episode.
  • symptoms meeting criterion A for schizophrenia.
2 During this period of illness, delusions or hallucinations occur for at least two weeks in the absence of prominent mood symptoms.

Consistent features

1 Not due to the effects of substance use or general medical conditions.
2 If a major depressive episode is present, it must include depressed mood as a symptom.

Variable features

1 Manic symptoms.
2 Depressive symptoms.
3 Mixed affective symptoms.
4 Inappropriate affect.
5 Abnormalities in psychomotor activity.
6 Lack of insight.
7 Cognitive dysfunction.
8 Confused or disoriented.
9 Difficulty concentrating.
10 Depersonalization, derealization, and somatic concerns.

nosed with increased frequency. Unfortunately, given the careful chronological history required to make the diagnosis—which is not always available, particularly during an initial assessment—it seems to be often used as a "compromise" diagnosis for patients who present with a confusing mixture of psychotic and affective symptoms. (Given the prevalence of depression among patients with schizophrenia, discussed previously, this can happen quite often.) Further research is required to establish the validity—or lack thereof—of schizoaffective disorder and to further specify its diagnostic criteria. At this time, the pharmacological treatments for the psychotic component of schizoaffective

Box 13.7 Delusional disorder

A. Nonbizarre delusions (i.e., involving situations that occur in real life, such as being followed, poisoned, infected, loved at a distance, or deceived by spouse or lover, or having a disease) of at least one month's duration.
B. Criterion A for schizophrenia has never been met.
Note: tactile and olfactory hallucinations may be present in delusional disorder if they are related to the delusional theme.
C. Apart from the impact of the delusion(s) or its ramifications, functioning is not markedly impaired and behavior is not obviously odd or bizarre.
D. If mood episodes have occurred concurrently with delusions, their total duration has been brief relative to the duration of the delusional periods.
E. The disturbance is not due to the direct physiological effects of a substance (e.g., a drug of abuse, a medication) or a general medical condition.

Specify type (the following types are assigned based on the predominant delusional theme):
• *Erotomanic type*: delusions that another person, usually of higher status, is in love with the individual.
• *Grandiose type*: delusions of inflated worth, power, knowledge, identity, or special relationship to a deity or famous person.
• *Jealous type*: delusions that the individual's sexual partner is unfaithful.
• *Persecutory type*: delusions that the person (or someone to whom the person is close) is being malevolently treated in some way.
• *Somatic type*: delusions that the person has some physical defect or general medical condition.
• *Mixed type*: delusions characteristic of more than one of the above types but no one theme predominates.
• *Unspecified type.*
From American Psychiatric Association (2000) Diagnostic and Statistical Manual of Mental Disorders, 4th Edition, Text Revision, Washington, D.C., American Psychiatric Association.

Table 13.12 Delusional disorder

Discriminating features

1 Nonbizarre delusions of at least one month's duration.
2 Apart from the impact of the delusion(s), functioning is not markedly impaired and behavior is not obviously odd or bizarre.

Consistent features

1 If tactile and olfactory hallucinations are present, they are related to the delusional theme.
2 If mood episodes have occurred concurrently, their total duration has been brief relative to the duration of the delusional periods.
3 The disturbance is not due to the effects of substance use or medical condition.

Variable features

1 Delusions that another person, usually of higher status, is in love with the individual.
2 Delusions of inflated worth, power, knowledge, identity, or special relationship to a deity or famous person.
3 Delusions that the individual's sexual partner is unfaithful.
4 Delusions that the person (or someone to whom the person is close) is being malevolently treated in some way.
5 Delusions that the person has some physical defect or general medical condition.

disorder appear to be essentially the same as those for schizophrenia (the same antipsychotic medications discussed previously), plus either an antidepressant or a mood stabilizer for the depressive or bipolar subtypes, respectively (see Chapter 8).

Delusional disorder

Delusional disorder has been reported to have a generally later age of illness onset (35–45 years) and to occur in both males and females (with conflicting data regarding more common occurrence in one gender over the other). The DSM-IV criteria for delusional disorder are listed in Box 13.7 and associated features are listed in Table 13.12.

Summary

This chapter has reviewed current information on the epidemiology, course, symptom definitions, diagnoses, etiology, pathophysiology, and treatment for schizophrenia and related disorders. The details provide the primary care clinician, psychiatrists, and others with practical information

bearing on the evaluation, diagnosis, and treatment of patients with these disorders. An increased understanding of current clinical perspectives and research on schizophrenia and delusional disorder sharpens diagnostic and symptom recognition skills, promotes early identification of concurrent medical conditions, and clarifies the approach to solving clinical management problems. The overall goal is to strengthen the working relationship between primary care clinicians and psychiatrists in the management of patients with psychotic disorders.

Annotated bibliography

American Psychiatric Association (2000) *Diagnostic and Statistical Manual of Mental Disorders*, 4th Edition, Text Revision. Washington, DC, American Psychiatric Association.
This book provides the currently used diagnostic criteria for schizophrenia and delusional disorder, including a general description of the disorders, their symptoms, course, associated features, and differential diagnosis.

Andreasen, NC (1993) Diagnosis and Classification of Schizophrenia, *Schizophr Bull* 19: 199–214.
This article provides background concerning the diagnostic and classification systems applied to schizophrenia.

Casey, DE, Haupt, DW, Newcomer, JW, Henderson, DC, Sernyak, MJ, Davidson, M, Lindenmayer, JP, Manoukian, SV, Banerji, MA, Lebovitz, HE, and Hennekens, CH (2004) Antipsychotic-induced weight gain and metabolic abnormalities: implications for increased mortality in patients with schizophrenia, *J Clin Psychiatry* 65 (Suppl 7): 4–18.
A comprehensive review of the role of weight gain and associated metabolic abnormalities in the excess mortality of schizophrenia.

Cloninger, CR (2002) The discovery of susceptibility genes for mental disorders. *Proc Natl Acad Sc* 99(21): 13365–13367.
This review article provides a useful synopsis of recent findings regarding the genetic basis of schizophrenia.

Egan, MF and Hyde, TM: Schizophrenia: Neurobiology in Sadock, BJ and Sadock, VA (eds) (2000) *Comprehensive Textbook of Psychiatry*, 7th Edition, Chapter 12.4, pp. 1129–1147, Philadelphia, Lippincott Williams & Wilkins.
This chapter provides a useful overview of the varied lines of research into the etiology of schizophrenia, including genetic and environmental factors, neuroanatomy, and neurotransmitter systems.

Gottesman, II (1991) *Schizophrenia Genesis: The Origins of Madness*, New York, W.H. Freeman & Company.
This book is a very readable text, aimed at a sophisticated lay reader, and covers the history of the disorder called schizophrenia. There is a detailed discussion of genetic and some environmental insults, moving clinical anecdotes, and a discussion of some of the important social policy issues related to the disorder.

Kapur, S and Seeman, P (2001) Does fast dissociation from the dopamine D2 receptor explain the action of atypical antipsychotics?: A new hypothesis, *Am J Psychiatry* 158(3): 360–369.
This is a key article describing the primacy of the dopamine D2 receptor in the pathophysiology and pharmacotherapy of schizophrenia. It includes concise and compelling evidence that previous theories involving other receptor systems are not consistent with the current data.

CHAPTER 14

Alcoholism and Drug Use Disorders

Wilson M. Compton, MD

Introduction

Extreme, end-stage cases of addiction are unfortunately common (see Case 14.1). They are readily diagnosed by clinicians and by most reasonable people. On the other hand, milder cases of alcoholism and other addictions are some of the most frequently overlooked medical disorders. Even the most competent clinician may miss these cases because the chief complaint is apparently unrelated to substance abuse. The chief complaint to the primary care physician is usually a non-specific medical complication of the substance use. Headaches, gastrointestinal complaints, and accidents are some of the most common reasons for consultation; each may be a symptom of a substance abuse problem.

Why is it so difficult to diagnose substance abuse problems in the primary care setting? Often the answer is that the presenting physical problem is easily treated and responds to short-term care. By focusing on the immediate issues and ignoring the underlying addiction, the physician avoids painful confrontation with the patient. And, indeed, substance abuse disorders are often subtle and hard to detect in their earliest forms. Nevertheless, if a substance abuse problem is not recognized and addressed, the chances for further complications are high.

The lack of insight that many substance abusers have concerning their own substance use patterns contributes to the underdiagnosis of addiction. Perhaps the most difficult aspect of recognizing and treating these disorders is the baffling and complex presentation in the face of massive denial by the patient. That is, patients in the earlier stages of addiction rarely recognize the impact of the disease on their lives and on those around them. Frequent statements include: "I'm still working—it hasn't hurt my job. I can't be an addict." Or "I can quit any time. I just don't want to right now." So how do competent clinicians diagnose these disorders, and what can primary care physicians do about them? Patients often minimize or ignore early warning signs; thus the primary care physician's role is most important for such people. Developing techniques to evaluate and treat patients with substance use disorders represents a challenging (and rewarding) clinical task. The goal of this chapter is to provide ways to recognize and treat addictions including alcoholism in their early forms where intervention and treatment are most critical.

Diagnosis

Alcoholism and other drug use disorders are behavioral diseases that have the (obvious) necessary component of substance consumption. In addition, for a substance use disorder to be diagnosable there must be evidence of problems resulting from the consumption. The types of problems vary considerably, but it is important to keep in mind several concepts: (1) the progressive nature of substance depend-

---

Jane C injects heroin 4–5 times a day, starting early in the morning and continuing throughout the day. She wakes each day with jitteriness, anxiety, runny nose, and abdominal cramping. She has been hospitalized for dermal abscesses and hepatitis. She feels unable to function without heroin and has lost all contact with her children because they have given up on her. She has been unable to stop using opioids for longer than a few weeks despite multiple attempts. This inability to control her use of heroin persists in spite of the fact that she has been in multiple treatment programs, both for detoxification and for rehabilitation. Her physicians are frustrated with her care, and she seems destined for an early heroin-related demise.

CASE 14.1

ence; (2) the stereotyped and consistent manifestations of the severe forms of substance dependence; (3) substance dependence can affect all aspects of human existence (physical, psychological, emotional, familial, legal, employment, spiritual); and (4) the pharmacology of different substances explains some of the variation in addictive potential and withdrawal severity.

Alcoholism as a term originated in the mid-19th century, but descriptions of problems from alcohol consumption date from antiquity. The first writings to describe alcoholism as a disease are from the early 19th century, and by the end of that century several facilities had been established for the treatment of alcoholics. In fact, the *Journal of Inebriety* was started in 1876 based on the explicit idea that drunkenness was a mental disease. In the modern era perhaps the best-known descriptions of alcoholism as a disease have been written by Jellinek, whose writings helped convince the medical community of the usefulness of the disease model of alcoholism. He described the symptoms and signs of alcoholism and emphasized the chronic, progressive course of the syndrome. His detailed analyses of the differences between men and women in symptoms and course remain a major contribution to the clinical understanding of these difficult conditions.

In the mid-1970s, Edwards and Gross described the "dependence syndrome," which emphasized symptoms of loss of control over alcohol in addition to tolerance and withdrawal. This approach to the diagnosis of alcoholism was adopted in the *International Classification of Diseases—Tenth Edition* (ICD-10) and the American Psychiatric Association's *Diagnostic and Statistical Manual for Mental Disorders*, Third Edition—Revised (DSM-III-R). Although the precise criteria vary between these systems, the essential concepts persist in current nosology (DSM-IV-TR). The approach has been applied to other substance dependence syndromes as well, so that a single set of criteria is used for all substances in DSM-IV-TR and ICD-10. The basic concepts include the following:

- *Loss of control over substance use* seen in the inability to quit or cut down, excessive time spent in activities surrounding substance use, the way non-substance related activities are reduced, continued substance use despite significant problems, and using more of a substance than intended.
- *Physiological symptoms of dependence*, such as tolerance (needing more or responding less to the same dosages), typical withdrawal symptoms (varies depending on the substance), and use of a substance to avoid withdrawal.
- *Significant problems from substance use*, including problems with physical health, psychological health, the legal system, employment, and social relationships.
- *Feeling dependent on a substance*, including cravings or urges to use, and inability to function without substance use.

DSM-IV defines substance dependence as three or more symptoms (from a list of seven) occurring within a one-year period (see Box 14.1 for details). Substance abuse is defined as a residual category for people who have certain social or legal problems resulting from substance use but not enough of the dependence symptoms to meet criteria for that disorder. People can abuse or be dependent on several substances at the same time, and according to DSM-IV-TR, each of these diagnoses would be made separately. Because each particular substance has unique associated problems, it is important to list all of the individual diagnoses. That way, communication with other physicians is facilitated, and the physician's own charts become a clearer record of the clinical presentation. The features of substance dependence are listed in Table 14.1.

DIAGNOSTIC CRITERIA

Box 14.1 Substance dependence and abuse

Substance dependence

A maladaptive pattern of substance use, leading to clinically significant impairment or distress, as manifested by three (or more) of the following, occurring at any time in the same 12-month period:

1. tolerance, as defined by either of the following:
   - a need for markedly increased amounts of the substance to achieve intoxication or desired effect
   - markedly diminished effect with continued use of the same amount of the substance;
2. withdrawal, as manifested by either of the following:
   - the characteristic withdrawal for the substance
   - the same (or a closely related) substance is taken to relieve or avoid withdrawal symptoms;
3. the substance is often taken in larger amounts or over a longer period than was intended
4. there is a persistent desire or unsuccessful efforts to cut down or control substance use
5. a great deal of time is spent in activities necessary to obtain the substance (e.g., visiting multiple doctors or driving long distances), use the substance (e.g., chain-smoking), or recover from its effects
6. important social, occupational, or recreational activities are given up or reduced because of substance use
7. the substance use is continued despite knowledge of having a persistent or recurrent physical or psychological problem that is likely to have been caused or exacerbated by the substance (e.g., current cocaine use despite recognition of cocaine-induced depression, or continued drinking despite recognition that an ulcer was made worse by alcohol consumption).

Specify if:
- *with physiological dependence*: evidence of tolerance or withdrawal (i.e., either item 1 or 2 is present)
- *without physiological dependence*: no evidence of tolerance or withdrawal (i.e., neither item 1 nor 2 is present)

Course specifiers (see DSM-IV-TR for definitions):
- *early full remission*
- *early partial remission*
- *sustained full remission*
- *sustained partial remission*
- *on agonist therapy*
- *in a controlled environment.*

Substance abuse

A maladaptive pattern of substance use leading to clinically significant impairment or distress, as manifested by one (or more) of the following, occurring within a 12-month period:
- recurrent substance use resulting in a failure to fulfill major role obligations at work, school, or home (e.g., repeated absences or poor work performance related to substance use; substance-related absences, suspensions, or expulsions from school; neglect of children or household)
- recurrent substance use in situations in which it is physically hazardous (e.g., driving an automobile or operating a machine when impaired by substance use)
- recurrent substance-related legal problems (e.g., arrests for substance-related disorderly conduct)
- continued substance use despite having persistent or recurrent social or interpersonal problems caused or exacerbated by the effects of the substance (e.g., arguments with spouse about consequences of intoxication, physical fights)

The symptoms have never met the criteria for substance dependence for this class of substance.
Modified from American Psychiatric Association (2000) Diagnostic and Statistical Manual of Mental Disorders, 4th Edition, Text Revision, Washington, D.C., American Psychiatric Association.

Table 14.1 Substance dependence

Discriminating features

1 Continued use of a substance despite significant problems.
2 Repeated self-administration of a substance.
3 Evidence of loss of control over substance use.

Consistent features

1 Chronic relapsing course.
2 Multiple social, psychological, and physical complications.
3 Craving for the substance is common.

Variable features

1 Physiological signs and symptoms (tolerance and withdrawal).
2 Psychiatric comorbidity, especially antisocial personality disorder and mood disorders.
3 Family history of substance-related problems.

increasing in prevalence across the Midwest and East, especially in rural areas, and an epidemic of oxycodone abuse has also been described in certain areas of the country. The complete list of typically abused substances is long (Table 14.2), and relatively new substances, such as MDMA (produced illicitly as one of the famous "club drugs") and fentanyl (developed by a pharmaceutical company), have been added recently. Pharmacological principles are important in understanding the abuse potential of various substances: (1) rapid onset is generally associated with abuse potential—thus, injection and smokable forms of a drug are generally more addictive than an oral form; and (2) short half-life is generally associated with abuse potential.

Focusing on substances that have the greatest public health concern, five main categories are covered in this

Which substances should the primary care physician know about? As mentioned previously, despite the common approach to the diagnosis of addiction, each substance has distinct characteristics. Because they may sometimes play a role in access to certain substances, physicians should be particularly aware of the patterns of abuse and addiction to opioid analgesics, sedative-hypnotics, and stimulants. Evidence of the increasing prevalence of problems associated with these prescription agents, especially opioid analgesic agents, makes this an urgent matter. In addition, for nearly all communities, alcohol and nicotine addiction are the disorders associated with the highest morbidity and mortality. Particular communities may also face other, unique challenges. For example, use of amphetamines has recently been

TABLE 14.2 List of typically abused substances

Alcohol	
Cannabinoids:	marijuana, hashish
Hallucinogens and dissociative drugs:	LSD, mescaline, peyote, psilocybin, PCP
Inhalants (solvents and other):	glue, toluene, gasoline, paint, nitrous oxide, amyl nitrate
Nicotine:	cigarettes, cigars, tobacco
Opioids:	codeine, Darvon, Demerol, Dilaudid, heroin, methadone, morphine, oxycodone, Oxycontin, Percodan, Talwin, Vicodin
Sedatives:	barbiturates, benzodiazepines
Stimulants:	amphetamines, cocaine (including "crack")

chapter: nicotine, alcohol, opioids, cocaine/stimulants, and cannabinoids. Other categories of substances are mentioned briefly because of their importance to certain groups of patients.

Because tobacco is its principal vehicle for administration, nicotine is the most common and most destructive single substance of abuse. Nicotine binds to a large family of receptors that are widely distributed throughout the brain and body. Chronic nicotine exposure appears to increase receptor expression and decreases the drug's effects, perhaps explaining some of the tolerance seen with chronic exposure to nicotine. The physical destructiveness of nicotine in its tobacco form is well known to physicians and includes mouth, larynx, and lung cancers, emphysema, vascular diseases, and a variety of other conditions. The addictive potential of nicotine is also familiar to physicians who have become frustrated in attempts to get patients to quit smoking. This addictive potential has been shown conclusively in animal and clinical models. No diagnosis of tobacco abuse is made, but the usual criteria for tobacco dependence are used.

Alcohol (ethanol) is responsible for thousands of injuries and deaths in every region of the country each year. It is a readily available drug, which after consumption is present at high concentrations in the body. These high concentrations explain the large variety of neurophysiological effects. For example, alcohol perturbs multiple cellular processes, altering second messenger systems and ion channels playing prominent roles in central nervous system function. Symptoms of alcoholism (i.e., alcohol dependence), in addition to those part of the general substance dependence syndrome described above, include blackouts (anterograde amnesia), benders, and drinking of non-beverage alcohol. Alcohol withdrawal is a typical reason for medical consultation and is discussed in some detail below.

Opioids include an important group of analgesic agents derived from the sap of the opium poppy and chemically related synthetic compounds. Multiple opioid receptors have been found in the central nervous system, and each of these receptors is associated with specific drug effects. Most prominent in the addictive properties of opioids is the mu receptor, which is primarily responsible for the analgesic effects of the drugs and mediates most of their reinforcing (i.e., addictive) actions. Routes of administration include by mouth, injection, and smoking. Opioid use disorders include abuse, dependence, withdrawal, and overdose. These conditions have been recognized and studied for decades. Opioid dependence usually involves significant tolerance and withdrawal symptoms, but all of the other symptoms of dependence may also be present. People who become dependent on heroin (the classic street opioid) generally begin use in their late teens or early twenties but do not seek treatment for many years. Progression of symptoms may be dependent on the context of opioid use, as documented by Robins in the very low rates of continued opioid dependence among opioid-addicted Vietnam veterans returning to the United States. Of note, abuse of prescription opioids (such as oxycodone, hydrocodone, and others) has been increasing markedly over the past decade and may represent a novel pathway into opioid addiction. For instance, it has long been recognized that heroin addicts use prescription opioids as an alternative to heroin, but recent studies have demonstrated that significant numbers of people develop abuse and dependence on prescription opioids without use of heroin. This is an increasing public health concern and requires physicians to balance the need for appropriate pain control with the risk of iatrogenic addiction as they treat patients with chronic pain conditions.

Cocaine and stimulants such as amphetamine have been among the most significant illicit drugs of abuse in the past two decades with the dissemination of the "crack" (smokable base) form of cocaine and the recent upsurge in methamphetamine abuse. Both of these agents are very addictive; this addictive potential seems to be related to their prominent ability to increase transmission of dopamine in key central reward circuits of the brain. Cocaine acts on dopamine neurons primarily by blocking reabsorption of dopamine released by pre-synaptic neurons. Amphetamine also inhibits dopamine uptake and causes an increase in dopamine release. Thus, both agents markedly increase the amount of dopamine available in the synaptic cleft, and with chronic administration, significant changes in receptor activity and transmission occur. Because of rapid absorption, the smokable forms of these substances are particularly addictive. Further, many people are less reluctant to smoke substances than to inject them, yet the addictive potential of the smokable forms is quite similar to injectable ones. Dependence on cocaine and stimulants have the usual symptoms, except that the withdrawal syndrome is mild and has quite non-specific symptoms of poor concentration, disrupted sleep pattern, depression, appetite change, craving, and restlessness. The progression of the dependence syndrome seems to be more rapid for these substances than for alcohol or opioids such that the time from first use to entry into treatment is shorter for cocaine than for these other substances.

Cannabis is generally administered by smoking but can be taken orally. Cannabis receptors were discovered approximately ten years ago, and the function of these receptors is under intensive study. For example, cannabis CB1 receptors are common in many sites of the central nervous system, but CB2 receptors are primarily found in peripheral tissues. A specific CB2 receptor agonist has demonstrated an impact on neuropathic pain in animal models without the side effects associated with opioids. Further work with the cannabinoid system has demonstrated potential utility in obesity because of an impact on feeding behaviors. In terms of the substance abuse and dependence potential, cannabis use disorders have been shown by Compton and colleagues to be common and increasing in prevalence in the United States over the past decade. Furthermore, the increases may result from marked increases in the potency of cannabis during the same time period. Cannabis abuse and dependence are prevalent in about 1.5% of the overall adult population but, like other substances, rates are particularly elevated among young adults. Withdrawal symptoms from cannabis, if any, are generally mild; they include sleep disturbance, impaired concentration, irritability or anxiety, and craving for the drug. Psychosis has also been described as a rare complication of cannabis use.

There are many other psychoactive substances. As new therapeutic agents are introduced and as the drug-using public develops tastes for different substances, the profile of substances abused in a given community may change. Thus, it is important that physicians remain up to date concerning the substances that are common in their own community. This can be accomplished through discussion with colleagues concerning agents identified in emergency room patients in specific communities. In addition, local and national sources of data exist such as the National Institute on Drug Abuse Community Epidemiology Workgroup and the Substance Abuse and Mental Health Services Administration Drug Abuse Warning Network survey, both of which present early indications of newly prevalent substances. At present other substances include the following:

- Sedative/hypnotics (primarily benzodiazepines and barbiturates) are commonly prescribed and are usually taken without significant symptoms of abuse or dependence. Barbiturates historically were the prototype for these agents, but prescriptions for barbiturates have been replaced with benzodiazepines that have a much wider margin of safety in overdose and have less potential for abuse. Both benzodiazepines and barbiturates enhance the inhibitory tone of the central nervous system by amplifying the flow of chloride ions through GABA-A receptors. Withdrawal symptoms are similar to those of alcohol and can be fatal in the most extreme cases. Agents with short half-lives are the most likely to produce significant withdrawal. Also, abuse potential varies among the benzodiazepines; diazepam is the most popular among substance abusers.
- Hallucinogens (LSD, psilocybin, etc.) are usually taken orally, but some preparations may be taken intranasally, injected, or absorbed through mucous membranes. Tolerance develops very quickly and daily use is uncommon. Dependence is unusual. Overdose/intoxication is marked by agitation, perceptual distortions, frank hallucinations (especially visual), and severe anxiety. Flashbacks may occur chronically.
- Phencyclidine has gained in popularity in certain areas again. The usual route of administration is by smoking, but it is sometimes taken orally, by injection, or intranasally. Acute effects include nystagmus (especially

vertical nystagmus), disinhibition, analgesia, flushing, diaphoresis, disorientation, and disorganized violent attacks. It has been reported to precipitate chronic psychosis.
- Hydrocarbon inhalants are numerous in type and include toluene, gasoline, and paint thinner. The effects of these substances are short-lived (i.e., about 30 minutes) and include ataxia, euphoria, and sometimes hallucinations. Significant neurological damage is seen in chronic abusers. A full dependence syndrome is unusual, but progression to other substances is common. An association of inhalant use with future injection drug use has been hypothesized by Compton and colleagues.
- With other agents (steroids, amyl nitrite, etc.) the bottom line is "if it has a significant acute CNS effect, someone will abuse it." Most of these other agents would not be expected to lead to a dependence syndrome.

Natural history

The course of alcoholism and other addictions has been described by many authors on the basis of retrospective analysis, but only a few have examined these conditions prospectively and most of these have focused primarily on alcoholism, not on other substances. Published longitudinal studies have included (among others) samples from a variety of settings: prisoners, outpatients, inpatients, and college students.

Despite different samples, different definitions of alcoholism/addiction and different lengths of follow-up, several important characteristics emerge from these studies. A small but significant percentage of addicts remit each year, no matter the sample source. Return to controlled substance use (mostly shown for drinking) seems to be rare and primarily limited to mild cases at baseline. The onset of addiction is generally insidious, and the course and symptoms vary between men and women. Women seem to begin substance use at a later age, have more varied courses and may have a more rapid progression of symptoms. In general, alcoholism and other addictions fit the pattern of chronic, relapsing disorders. Periods of remission may last for varying times, and outcome can be expected to include relapse in the majority of cases.

Differential diagnosis

Substance use disorders are fairly straightforward and have clearly operationalized criteria, thus differential diagnosis is not difficult. Screening for primary and secondary psychiatric conditions is important. That is, patients with other psychiatric symptoms are at particularly high risk of having substance abuse problems, and patients with substance use disorders are at similarly high risk of having additional psychiatric disorders. When substance abuse is suspected, it is reasonable to consider carefully whether other psychiatric conditions, such as depression, anxiety or personality disorders, are present. Similarly, when psychiatric symptoms are detected, it is critical that substance abuse be considered as part of the differential diagnosis. Screening for additional substance use problems is also important when one disorder is suspected.

What tools can help primary care physicians screen for alcoholism and other addictions? Several have been described in the literature and have been used extensively during the past two decades. Commonly used screening instruments include the Michigan Alcohol Screening Test (MAST), and a related drug abuse instrument called the Drug Abuse Screening Test (DAST), and the Alcohol Use Disorders Identification Test (AUDIT) developed by Babor and a group from the World Health Organization. The MAST

and DAST are similar to each other in that they both were developed by Skinner, are self-administered by respondents, and have been shown to identify most people with substance problems. Those scoring positive on three or more items on either of these tests need further evaluation for possible substance abuse problems, and those scoring positive on five or more items have a high likelihood of having a substance use disorder. The AUDIT is a short screening test for alcoholism with very good sensitivity and specificity. As shown in Table 14.3, the AUDIT consists of ten items. A score of eight means there is a possible alcohol disorder, and a score of ten or greater is indicative of a probable disorder. A complementary clinical screening evaluation can also be used. This clinical scale includes liver enzyme functioning (GGT), history of head injury and accidents, and coded results of physical

TABLE 14.3

WHO Alcohol Use Disorders Identification Test (AUDIT)

1. How often do you have a drink containing alcohol?
(0) Never
(1) Monthly or less
(2) 2–4 times a month
(3) 2–3 times a week
(4) 4 or more times a week
2. How many drinks containing alcohol do you have on a typical day when you are drinking?
(0) 1 or 2
(1) 3 or 4
(2) 5 or 6
(3) 7, 8, or 9
(4) 10 or more
3. How often do you have six or more drinks on one occasion?
(0) Never
(1) < monthly
(2) Monthly
(3) Weekly
(4) Daily or almost daily
4. How often during the last year have you found that you were not able to stop drinking once you had started?
(0) Never
(1) < monthly
(2) Monthly
(3) Weekly
(4) Daily or almost daily
5. How often during the last year have you failed to do what was normally expected of you because of drinking?
(0) Never
(1) < monthly
(2) Monthly
(3) Weekly
(4) Daily or almost daily

6. How often during the last year have you needed a first drink in the morning to get yourself going after a heavy drinking session?
(0) Never
(1) < monthly
(2) Monthly
(3) Weekly
(4) Daily or almost daily
7. How often during the last year have you had a feeling of guilt or remorse after drinking?
(0) Never
(1) < monthly
(2) Monthly
(3) Weekly
(4) Daily or almost daily
8. How often during the last year have you been unable to remember what happened the night before because you had been drinking?
(0) Never
(1) < monthly
(2) Monthly
(3) Weekly
(4) Daily or almost daily
9. Have you or someone else been injured as a result of your drinking?
(0) Never
(1) < monthly
(2) Monthly
(3) Weekly
(4) Daily or almost daily
10. Has a relative or friend or a doctor or another health worker been concerned about your drinking or suggested you cut down?
(0) No
(2) Yes, but not in the last year
(4) Yes, during the last year

From Babor, TF et al. (1992) AUDIT—the Alcohol Use Disorders Identification Test: guidelines for use in primary health care, Geneva, World Health Organization Programme on Substance Abuse.

exam. These screening instruments can be used in a variety of inpatient and outpatient settings. They may be particularly appropriate for evaluation of new outpatients.

When incorporating questions concerning substance abuse into an examination, it is important to keep in mind communication techniques that help improve accurate reporting by the patient of substance use and substance-related symptoms (see Box 14.2), that is, ways to reduce "denial." First and foremost, it is important to ask detailed and direct questions. Other techniques should be considered in the context of particular clinical settings. In general, it is appropriate to assume that the behavior is present and to avoid undue confrontation (balanced with the need to clarify responses). Assuming the behavior means asking "What drugs have you ever taken to feel better, more alert or high?" instead of "Have you ever used drugs to feel better, more alert or high?" Using these techniques, many "unexpected" cases of addiction are discovered.

BOX 14.2

Clinical interviewing techniques to improve accuracy of reporting of substance abuse

Communicate an expectation for accurate information.
Provide assurance of confidentiality by asking
    questions in private.
Show empathy.
Assume behavior and ask for details.
Avoid undue confrontation but clarify responses.
Avoid moralistic or threatening overtones.
Integrate information from different sources.

Epidemiology and pathophysiology

According to numerous studies, rates of substance use and related disorders remain very high, especially in young segments of the population. Understanding the rates of alcoholism and other addictions among different groups gives an important insight into the places where prevention (both primary and secondary) is most needed. Although the rates of alcoholism and illicit substance abuse vary across studies (perhaps based on different samples, diagnostic instruments, and different diagnostic criteria), associations with certain "risk factors" are consistent. For example, in a large number of epidemiological samples strong associations have been found between male gender and substance abuse and between antisocial personality disorder and substance abuse.

According to recent studies of the general population, nicotine dependence is the most common of all substance use disorders. Up to 25% of the adult population is currently addicted to nicotine. The rate among women in the past few

---

KEY CLINICAL QUESTIONS AND WHAT THEY UNLOCK

- *For which patients should addictions be considered?*
  Although addictions most commonly begin during adolescence or early adult life, they may be seen in all ages, all socioeconomic and ethnic groups, and both sexes. The types and patterns of addiction vary in different groups but all are at some risk. This is the reason why physicians should become comfortable asking patients about addictions, even when they are not explicitly expected.

- *Few patients in the early stages of addiction volunteer for intervention or treatment. Why should primary care physicians care about this?*
  The very conditions that primary care physicians attend are often negatively impacted by substance use. Diabetes, depression, heart disease, HIV, hypertension, and renal failure are all often complicated by addiction. Treatment of the co-occurring addiction may have a positive impact on the primary medical illness. Because of their unique relationship to patients, physicians, especially those in primary care, can have a major impact on their patients' addictive behaviors and, forthright, non-judgmental discussion is a key ingredient.

- *Since addictions are more common in younger age groups, what about older patients?*
  Although addictions begin in the youngest ages, they can persist for decades. Given the variable nature of complications from addictions, even older patients should be screened for addiction and interventions planned accordingly.

- *How often should drug testing be used in people who are trying to quit substance use?*
  Drug testing is useful in several ways for the management of addiction. For patients who admit using one substance, use of additional, clinically relevant substances is sometimes uncovered with a drug screen. For those who are in recovery, periodic testing encourages honesty about behavior. Because embarrassment about relapse is frequent with resulting verbal denial of drug use, drug testing can be very helpful in providing an early warning of behavior change.

---

decades has nearly equaled that of men (seen indirectly in the higher rates of lung cancer among women). Alcohol dependence (alcoholism) is the next most common substance use disorder with a past year prevalence of 8.5% according to the National Epidemiologic Survey on Alcohol and Related Conditions (NESARC). Alcohol disorders are more common among men than women and tend to run in families (though the inheritance pattern is somewhat uncertain). Other substance abuse and dependence is less common—about 2.0% past year prevalence according to the NESARC. Like alcohol, other substance abuse and dependence is more common among younger age groups and men.

The association of substance use disorders with other psychiatric conditions (e.g., antisocial personality disorder, depression, anxiety, schizophrenia) is complex. Comorbidities are extremely common with an excess of substance use disorders found among people with other psychiatric conditions and excess of other psychiatric conditions found in people diagnosed with substance use disorders being well documented. Recently, for example, Grant and colleagues reported high rates of independent mood and anxiety disorders among people with substance use disorders, especially drug use disorders.

Psychosocial research into drug abuse has been extensive, and some of the most important findings have been the relationship of low social conformity, emotional distress, and poor academic performance to future drug use and drug problems. A relationship between preexisting conduct problems and substance abuse has also been found. Other work has shown a consistent relationship of attitudes towards drug use and rates of consumption. In these studies, an increase in use of drugs by adolescents is inversely correlated with perceptions of the harmfulness of the drug and with disapproval of drug use. In contrast, perceived availability of drugs is not highly correlated with rates of drug use. This implies that interventions designed to affect attitudes towards drugs may be particularly important in drug prevention programs.

HIV risk behaviors are more common among people with substance abuse and dependence. These include both the obvious injection behaviors and sexual risk behaviors. Heavy substance abusers may trade sex for drugs or may engage in prostitution in order to make money to support a drug habit. Use of safer sex techniques is unfortunately not the norm. In addition, use of psychoactive substances reduces inhibitions and impairs judgment. Heavy alcohol users and other substance abusers engage in more risky sexual behaviors than other people. Furthermore, increased HIV risk behaviors may be even more common among substance abusers with co-occurring psychiatric conditions such as antisocial personality disorder.

Genetic epidemiology

Family, twin, and adoption studies have provided evidence for a genetic component to addictions. For example, family studies have shown much higher than expected rates of alcoholism among the relatives of alcoholics. Of course, familial clustering does not prove a genetic component to the inheritance of alcoholism. Adoption studies have generally shown that alcoholism and drug addiction in offspring is predicted by alcoholism among biological, but not adoptive, relatives. One study showed some evidence that drug misuse also was associated with alcoholism in biological relatives. Another study showed a tendency for antisocial behavior to be inherited by a subgroup of adoptees of alcoholics; otherwise

no other psychiatric conditions were consistently seen to coexist with alcoholism.

Twin studies have shown an excess of alcoholism and drug addiction in the co-twins of monozygotic (MZ) twins compared with dizygotic (DZ) twins. Most recently, twin studies have demonstrated that there are both common and specific genetic factors important in the inheritance of addictions. This means that there is a genetic predisposition to addictions in general as well as predisposition to addiction to particular substances.

Currently, major projects supported by the National Institute on Drug Abuse and the National Institute on Alcoholism and Alcohol Abuse are under way to determine the genetic basis for addictions through the molecular genetic study of twins, adoptees, and high-risk families. These projects are based on the longstanding observation that alcoholism and other addictions run in families and have a strong genetic component. Thus, the acceptance of the familial/genetic nature of addictions has led to studies that may be able to uncover specific causes of these devastating conditions. One promising approach is the candidate gene study, where specific alleles are tested for association with the substance use phenotype. Using these techniques, several promising genetic locations have been identified where specific genetic variants may be responsible for some of the risk of addiction.

Pathophysiology

Animal and behavioral models of addiction have begun to unravel the underlying brain mechanisms of reward and reinforcement (which are key components of addiction) and thus may provide evidence about the etiology of addictive behavior. The circuitry and neurochemistry of the brain reward system is complex and primarily involves the mesolimbic and mesocortical dopamine pathways. Investigation of the brain mechanisms of reward are based on the demonstration of the ability to addict animals to various illicit substances and has provided some of the strongest evidence of the external validity of addiction. No longer can simple morality be invoked to explain addictive behavior. Furthermore, as major progress has been made to unravel the brain reward systems, it has allowed investigators to begin to integrate basic science and clinical medicine in a way that has not been possible in other areas of psychiatry.

Why is pathophysiology important since the precise mechanisms of action have not yet been determined? The cause of substance dependence is unknown, but examples of compulsive use of abusable substances by animals has allowed extensive laboratory manipulation and evaluation of brain structures thought to be important in addictive behavior. New treatments are likely to be based on this understanding of the pathophysiology of addiction. The most important system in animal models of the brain reward and reinforcement circuitry involves the ventral tegmental area—nucleus accumbens dopamine pathways. A consistent body of evidence indicates that these pathways are at the core of the brain reward system and are impacted by all the common substances of abuse. In addition, receptors for most abused substances have been identified and represent an important area of investigation in psychiatric research.

Treatment issues

Alcoholism and other addictions fit the pattern of chronic, relapsing disorders. Many factors influence the prognosis such as co-occurring psychiatric illness, environmentally limited substance use, severity of symptoms, age of onset of symptoms, and duration of dependence. Thus, a successful (though hardly ideal) outcome may include extending the time to next relapse, reducing the severity of the dependence syndrome, or reducing complications. The clinical goal is total abstinence because there is little evidence that return to controlled substance use is feasible and progression of symptoms with continued use is the rule. However, knowing that relapse is common, especially in the first few months of sobriety, helps clinicians avoid becoming angry when patients do relapse. The trick is to remain empathic, though firm, with patients who have relapsed. Thus, one of the goals for physicians caring for patients struggling with addiction is to remain consistent about treatment goals while communicating an understanding of the difficulties inherent in changing addictive behaviors.

It may be helpful to consider some of the basic principles of addiction treatment, as many of the concepts are applicable across the various substances. According to the National Institute on Drug Abuse (NIDA), the scientific literature supports 13 principles essential to effective drug treatment:

1 No single treatment is appropriate for all individuals. Matching treatment settings, interventions, and services to each patient's problems and needs is critical.

2 Treatment needs to be readily available. Treatment applicants can be lost if treatment is not immediately available or readily accessible.

3 Effective treatment attends to multiple needs of the individual, not just his or her drug use. Treatment must address the individual's drug use and associated medical, psychological, social, vocational, and legal problems.

4 At different times during treatment, a patient may develop a need for medical services, family therapy, vocational rehabilitation, and social and legal services.

5 Remaining in treatment for an adequate period of time is critical for treatment effectiveness. The time depends on an individual's needs. For most patients, the threshold for significant improvement is reached at about 3 months into treatment. Additional treatment can produce further progress. Programs should include strategies to prevent patients from leaving treatment prematurely.

6 Individual or group counseling and other behavioral therapies are critical components of effective treatment for addiction. In therapy, patients address motivation, build skills to resist drug use, replace drug-using activities with constructive and rewarding non-drug-using activities, and improve problem-solving abilities. Behavioral therapy also facilitates interpersonal relationships.

7 Medication is an important element of treatment for many patients, especially when combined with counseling and other behavioral therapies. Methadone and buprenorphine help people addicted to opioids stabilize their lives and reduce drug use. Naltrexone is effective for some opioid addicts and some patients with alcohol dependence. Nicotine patches or gum, or an oral medication, such as buproprion, can help people addicted to nicotine.

8 Addicted or drug-abusing individuals with coexisting mental disorders should have both disorders treated in an integrated way.

9 Medical detoxification is only the first stage of addiction treatment and by itself does little to change long-term drug use. Medical detoxification manages the acute physical symptoms of withdrawal. For some individuals, it is a precursor to effective drug addiction treatment.

10 Treatment does not need to be voluntary to be effective. Sanctions or enticements by the family, employment setting, or criminal justice system can significantly increase treatment entry, retention, and success.

11 Possible drug use during treatment must be monitored continuously. Monitoring a patient's drug and alcohol use during treatment, such as through urinalysis, can help the patient withstand urges to use drugs. Such monitoring also can provide early evidence of drug use so that treatment can be adjusted.

12 Treatment programs should provide assessment for HIV and AIDS, hepatitis B and C, tuberculosis and other infectious diseases, and counseling to help patients modify or change behaviors that place them or others at risk of infection. Counseling can help patients avoid high-risk behavior and help people who are already infected manage their illness.

13 Recovery from drug addiction can be a long-term process and often requires multiple episodes of treatment. As with other chronic illnesses, relapses can occur during or after successful treatment episodes. Participation in self-help support programs during and following treatment often helps maintain abstinence.

The primary care physician's role in the treatment of patients with substance abuse depends on where the patient is identified. For example, a comatose patient with an opioid overdose has a medical emergency that requires immediate assistance; a chronic alcoholic with long-standing, severe drinking patterns needs a prompt (24–48 hours) evaluation;

and a nicotine addict with no current medical emergencies who requests help to quit smoking requires an outpatient appointment (preferably within one week).

In order to perform appropriate triage of patients, it is useful to consider when and how to interact with treatment programs, hospitals, and community support systems such as Alcoholics Anonymous (AA). Medical emergencies directly attributable to substance use itself include overdose, severe alcohol or sedative/hypnotic withdrawal, and idiosyncratic reactions. Medical complications of substance use represent the other main category of medical care and include such conditions as intracranial bleed or myocardial infarction from cocaine, chronic obstructive pulmonary disease or lung cancer from tobacco, cirrhosis of the liver or cardiomyopathy from alcohol, or HIV infection from injection drug use. The treatment and evaluation of these conditions is beyond the scope of this chapter, and interested readers are referred to the *Comprehensive Textbook of Substance Abuse* listed in the Annotated bibliography.

Overdose/intoxication

Most substances can be dangerous when consumed in large quantities. Symptoms of alcohol (and other sedative/hypnotic) overdose and intoxication include agitation, nystagmus, uncoordinated speech and ambulation, and impairment on tests of cognitive functioning. In extreme cases, overdose can be fatal. Opioid overdose can be a medical emergency. Symptoms include small pupils, somnolence, uncoordinated gait, coma, and poor respiration. Death usually occurs from respiratory depression. Overdose is easily treated with naloxone (a potent opioid receptor antagonist). Symptoms of cocaine and other stimulant overdose and intoxication include tachycardia, arrhythmias, hypertension, tremor, paranoid psychosis, psychomotor agitation, mood elevation (or sometimes irritability). Overdose can be fatal.

Withdrawal treatment/detoxification

Detoxification from addictive substances is one of the foremost areas in which physicians are expected to provide care for substance abusers. The assessment and treatment of alcohol, opioid, and other withdrawal syndromes is therefore discussed in some detail. When considering treatment options, the first step is careful assessment of the patient's physical and mental condition. Once the severity of the withdrawal syndrome is assessed, treatment options are considered. In general, for mild cases with few symptoms, observation is all that is needed. Perhaps the most important task is to identify when a substance was last used. If more than four half-lives have passed since the last consumption without significant symptoms, no severe withdrawal is anticipated. On the other hand, if the last dose was only a few

hours prior to evaluation, the prognosis is much more uncertain. When considering medications to treat withdrawal, it is important to consider cross-tolerance with the substance being detoxified and the relative half-life of the medication. It is thus generally recommended that long-acting agents be used, that they be gradually tapered, and that careful clinical monitoring and judgment be utilized in all cases in which medications are required for acute detoxification.

Alcohol withdrawal symptoms include four major types. Acute withdrawal symptoms begin 4–8 hours after the last drink and peak within 48–72 hours. Symptoms include tremor, diaphoresis, nausea, headache, and diarrhea. Alcoholic hallucinosis, which includes auditory and/or visual hallucinations without disorientation, starts 4–24 hours after the last drink. Generally, the hallucinations subside within a few days but rarely persist for weeks or months. Alcohol withdrawal seizures that are generalized tonic-clonic seizures typically occur 12–48 hours after the last drink. They seem to be more common among people with any history of prior seizures and people who have had multiple detoxifications in the past. Thus, treatment recommendations include consideration of a brief course of an antiepileptic medication in high-risk patients. Delirium tremens (DTs) or alcohol withdrawal delirium is rare and usually follows the other withdrawal symptoms. More likely to occur in seriously debilitated patients and those with an intercurrent medical condition, DTs usually begin 24–72 hours after the last drink. The syndrome is characterized by delirium (waxing and waning level of consciousness, disorientation, hallucinations, delusions) with severe tremors and autonomic instability (elevated temperature, blood pressure, pulse, and respirations). The mortality rate is up to 15%.

One reliable way to evaluate patients with alcohol withdrawal is to administer the Clinical Institute Withdrawal Assessment for Alcohol, Revised (CIWA-AR). As shown in Table 14.4, this instrument provides scores ranging from 0 to 67 based on clinical items rated to assess the severity of alcohol withdrawal.

As shown in the flow sheet in Box 14.3, triage of patients at risk for alcohol withdrawal can be standardized. For patients with significant withdrawal symptoms who are not at particularly high risk of seizures (based on no prior clinical history of seizures and fewer than four previous medical detoxifications), benzodiazepines are the treatment of choice because of the high therapeutic safety index of these agents. Long-acting benzodiazepines are usually used because they are cross-tolerant with the abused substance and have a good safety profile. In patients with significantly impaired liver function, use of lorazepam or oxazepam is recommended to avoid risk of over-sedation. These are the only benzodiazepines that do not undergo oxidative metabolism, which is reduced in the face of impaired liver function. Treatment is usually begun with 'as needed' dosing based on clinical rating of withdrawal symptoms. Dosages of medication are

TABLE 14.4

Addiction Research Foundation — Clinical Institute Withdrawal Assessment for Alcohol (CIWA-AR)

Nausea and vomiting — Ask "Do you feel sick to your stomach? Have you vomited?" and observe.
0 no nausea and no vomiting
1 mild nausea with no vomiting
2
3
4 intermittent nausea with dry heaves
5
6
7 constant nausea, frequent dry heaves and vomiting

Tremor — Observe arms extended and fingers spread apart.
0 no tremor
1 not visible, but can be felt fingertip to fingertip
2
3
4 moderate, with patient's arms extended
5
6
7 severe, even with arms not extended

Paroxysmal sweats — Observe.
0 no sweat visible
1 barely perceptible sweating, palms moist
2
3
4 beads of sweat obvious on forehead
5
6
7 drenching sweats

Anxiety — Ask "Do you feel nervous?" and observe.
0 no anxiety
1 mildly anxious
2
3
4 moderately anxious, or guarded, so anxiety is inferred
5
6
7 equivalent to acute panic states as seen in severe delirium or acute schizophrenic reactions

Agitation — Observe.
0 normal activity
1 somewhat more than normal activity
2
3
4 moderately fidgety and restless
5
6
7 paces back and forth during most of the interview, or constantly thrashes about

Tactile disturbances — Ask "Have you any itching, pins and needles sensations, any burning, any numbness or do you feel bugs crawling on or under your skin?" and observe.
0 none
1 very mild itching, pins and needles, burning or numbness
2 mild itching, pins and needles, burning or numbness
3 moderate itching, pins and needles, burning or numbness
4 moderately severe hallucinations
5 severe hallucinations
6 extremely severe hallucinations
7 continuous hallucinations

Auditory disturbances — Ask "Are you more aware of sounds around you? Are they harsh? Do they frighten you? Are you hearing anything that is disturbing to you? Are you hearing things you know are not there?" Observe.
0 not present
1 very mild harshness or ability to frighten
2 mild harshness or ability to frighten
3 moderate harshness or ability to frighten
4 moderately severe hallucinations
5 severe hallucinations
6 extremely severe hallucinations
7 continuous hallucinations

Visual disturbances — Ask "Does the light appear to be too bright? Is its color different? Does it hurt your eyes? Are you seeing anything that is disturbing to you? Are you seeing things you know are not there?" and observe.
0 not present
1 very mild sensitivity
2 mild sensitivity
3 moderate sensitivity
4 moderately severe hallucinations
5 severe hallucinations
6 extremely severe hallucinations
7 continuous hallucinations

Headache, fullness in head — Ask "Does your head feel different? Does it feel like there is a band around your head?" Do not rate for dizziness or lightheadedness. Otherwise, rate severity.
0 not present
1 very mild
2 mild
3 moderate
4 moderately severe
5 severe
6 very severe
7 extremely severe

Orientation and clouding of sensorium — Ask "What day is this? Where are you? Who are you?"
0 oriented and can do serial additions
1 cannot do serial additions or is uncertain about date
2 disoriented for date by no more than two calendar days
3 disoriented for date by more than two calendar days
4 disoriented for place and/or person

increased until withdrawal symptoms are controlled. If a patient becomes somnolent, the dosage is reduced. After the first 24 hours, the dose is reduced by 25–50% each day. With this rapid taper, detoxification can be completed in 2–5 days. It is important to note that this rapid taper does not necessarily prevent development of DTs. If such a severe withdrawal syndrome develops, high-dose intravenous benzodiazepines are often required, and monitoring in an intensive care unit is indicated because supportive measures (i.e., intravenous fluids, cardiac monitoring, etc.) are needed. In all cases of alcohol detoxification, high doses of B vitamins should be administered, especially thiamine, to reduce the risk of peripheral neuropathy and the Wernicke-Korsakoff syndrome (see Chapter 11).

BOX 14.3

Alcohol withdrawal treatment algorithm

1 Treat all patients with withdrawal symptoms with high doses of B vitamins, especially thiamine.
2 Is the CIWA-AR* score greater than 10?
　Yes: Does the patient have significant liver pathology?
　　Yes: Use benzodiazepines that are not oxidatively metabolized such as oxazepam or lorazepam for detoxification.
　　No: Use benzodiazepines with a long half-life such as diazepam or chlordiazepoxide for detoxification.
　No: Observe without sedative medications.
*Clinical Institute Withdrawal Assessment for Alcohol, Revised.

Nicotine withdrawal follows quickly after the last use of tobacco because of the short half-life of nicotine (2–4 hours). Symptoms include irritability, restlessness, poor concentration, increased appetite, depression, anxiety, poor sleep, and craving for tobacco. These symptoms are not medically serious but can lead to relapse. Most symptoms resolve within several days, but some (appetite increase, depression, craving) may last for months or years. Use of topical nicotine transdermal patches has been shown to reduce symptoms of withdrawal and relapse to tobacco among patients in behavioral treatment programs.

Opioid withdrawal has a well-described course and symptom profile. The first symptoms generally begin within 8–12 hours after the last dose of a short-acting opioid (later with a long-acting agent) and include restlessness, pupil dilation, yawning, lacrimation, rhinorrhea, diaphoresis, and/or poor sleep. Within 24–48 hours nausea, vomiting, chills, muscle pain, abdominal cramps, diarrhea, tremor, mild tachycardia, and increased blood pressure develop. Rarely, unstable blood pressure and pulse become clinically significant. Untreated, symptoms will subside within 4–7 days. Opioid detoxification can most easily be accomplished with a long-acting opioid agent such as buprenorphine or methadone. The initial dose is based on severity of withdrawal symptoms and is reduced over a 7–10 day period. Alternatively, clonidine (an alpha-2 agonist) has been shown to be effective in ameliorating some of the symptoms of opioid withdrawal. If clonidine is used, monitoring of blood pressure is warranted and additional medications for specific symptoms may be needed such as a benzodiazepine for agitation, poor sleep, and restlessness, and an antiemetic for nausea. Of interest, lofexidine, a medication with alpha-2 agonist effects similar to clonidine, is currently approved for use in other countries and is currently under investigation in the United States. Lofexidine appears to have the same ability to reduce opioid withdrawal symptoms as clonidine without lowering blood pressure.

Cocaine and other stimulants generally have non-specific withdrawal symptoms that do not require medical intervention. Withdrawal from chronic cannabis consumption is not clearly associated with specific withdrawal symptoms although some patients report craving, changes in sleep pattern and appetite, irritability, and impaired concentration. For hallucinogens, phencyclidine, and inhalants, no particular withdrawal syndromes have been noted.

Urine drug testing

Clinicians often ask when urine drug testing is useful. For patients admitted to an emergency room after accidents or injuries, drug testing should always be considered. The evaluation of unconscious patients or those with new onset psychiatric symptoms also should include drug testing. In an outpatient setting, urine drug testing can be useful in the initial assessment of patients with a "history of" illicit substance abuse for uncovering recent substance use that may be otherwise denied by the patient. Patients should be informed that urine drug testing will be obtained before asking about substance use to enhance the self-report of such use. Routinely obtaining urine specimens from patients recently sober is also advised to detect early substance use, which may otherwise be denied. That way, such use can be discussed before a long-term pattern is established. On the other hand, there are severe limitations to urine drug screening. All abusable substances (with the exception of cannabinoids) can only be detected for 24 to 72 hours after last ingestion. Even cannabinoids are routinely detected for only one to two weeks unless particularly sensitive tests are used or if the use has been particularly heavy and chronic. Thus, only very recent substance use is detected.

Treatment of addiction

The mainstay of substance abuse and dependence treatment is psychosocial rehabilitation. This general label includes community support treatments (AA and other 12-Step groups), specific relapse prevention behavioral therapies, family therapies, psychoeducation, and supportive individual therapies. AA is by far the most common treatment approach to alcoholism (and probably for other addictions as well), but there is little data regarding the effectiveness of AA. What is certainly true is that as free support groups for people with addictions, AA (and other 12-Step groups) offer fellowship in times of need and have been life-saving for many people. Clinicians should be aware of where and when meetings are held in their communities so that referral of appropriate individuals can be made. Which patients are "appropriate" for referral remains uncertain, however. Many clinicians refer all addicted patients to AA groups, although additional treatment referral to professional programs may be warranted in more severe cases, especially those with intercurrent medical or psychiatric disorders.

Medications for addictions

Psychological treatments are often combined with pharmacological therapies. For some alcoholic patients, disulfiram (Antabuse) is recommended, although evidence indicates that the effects of this agent are primarily psychological because the dose does not matter much and only the most motivated patients do well—patients who would likely do well on no medication. About a decade ago, Volpicelli and O'Malley showed that naltrexone can be helpful in the treatment of alcoholism when used in combination with traditional alcohol rehabilitation treatment. This finding supports the validity of the disease model because naltraxone is a mu opioid receptor blocker and therefore is a treatment regimen with theoretically based ties to the brain reward mechanisms. A second medication, acamprosate, has just been approved for use in the United States to prevent alcohol relapse. Acamprosate is an amino acid analog and has been shown to significantly enhance abstinence in several studies when combined with behavioral approaches. In contrast, no antidepressants have been shown to be consistently helpful in reducing alcohol consumption in human trials (though they may be helpful in treating co-occurring depressive syndromes).

Nicotine dependence is often treated with transdermal nicotine replacement. Such treatment, combined with behavioral psychotherapies, is more useful than placebo, but the relapse rate remains high even in the best prognostic groups. Treatment of co-occurring depression or anxiety may improve the outcome of nicotine dependence. Another pharmacotherapeutic approach to treating nicotine dependence is buproprion. For maximum benefit, this agent should be started approximately two weeks prior to smoking cessation. This agent, which is well known as an antidepressant, has been shown to be helpful for smoking cessation whether or not co-occurring depression is present.

Opioid dependence has been treated most successfully with long-term methadone substitution therapy. With such treatment, the psychosocial and medical complications of illicit opioid addiction are ameliorated. Unfortunately, it is not clear how long patients should be maintained on methadone, and some long-term studies have indicated significant relapse rates upon discontinuation of methadone even after many years of treatment. If methadone maintenance is requested, it is important that the methadone be administered appropriately. For the most part, this means using adequately high doses to produce significant tolerance to the effects of opioids. Programs that use lower doses have much higher rates of illicit opioid use in their patients compared to programs administering high doses. The purported mechanism of this improved outcome for high-dose programs is that additional doses of opioids (i.e., those ingested illicitly) do not produce any euphoria because of the significant tolerance. Thus, patients quickly learn not use opioids illicitly. In contrast, low methadone doses block withdrawal symptoms but do not prevent euphoria with additional doses of opioids. Patients will continue to use opioids illicitly.

Naltrexone, a potent and orally active opioid receptor antagonist, has been helpful in the treatment of many narcotic addicts. Naltrexone has a long half-life and so can be administered three times a week in a supervised setting. Such dosing completely blocks effects of opioids, and thus illicit use is curtailed because no euphoria is obtained even with high doses. Naltrexone has been most widely used in the treatment of addicted physicians who are exposed to opioids in the workplace and are at risk of job loss if they do not follow treatment recommendations. Otherwise, most opioid addicts do not volunteer for naltrexone treatment.

A recent advance in the treatment of opioid addiction is the approval of buprenorphine for prescription by physicians outside the methadone system of care. Two forms of buprenorphine are currently available: parenteral and sublingual. Oral route of administration is not feasible because of marked first-pass liver metabolism. The sublingual form is also available in a combined form with naloxone (Narcan); this combination reduces the possibility of diversion and use as an injected drug. Naloxone is not active as an opioid receptor blocker when given sublingually (or orally), but when the medication is injected, naloxone precipitates opioid withdrawal. According to clinical trials, buprenorphine appears to be safe and effective when administered daily or even when administered three times a week. Johnson and colleagues, for example, showed that buprenorphine, levomethadyl acetate, and high-dose methadone are all more effective than low-dose methadone in the treatment of opioid dependence.

No medications have proven consistently helpful in the treatment of cocaine, stimulants or other addictions not discussed above. Although several agents (e.g., desipramine, fluoxetine, and amantadine) appeared promising after initial trials, larger and more comprehensive studies have failed to demonstrate consistent treatment effects. Trials of antidepressants, dopamine agonists and antagonists have all been disappointing. Despite these results, ongoing studies of other agents continue. For example, recent reports of the potential efficacy of disulfiram for cocaine dependence, even in the absence of alcohol consumption, show the potential for novel agents in the treatment of cocaine disorders.

Conclusions

The epitome of the medical approach to any disorder is to diagnose the illness, plan treatment, and predict outcome. As explicated by Guze, applying the medical model to addiction psychiatry implies that the "concepts, strategies, and jargon of general medicine are applied to psychiatric disorders: diagnosis, differential diagnosis, etiology, pathogenesis, treatment, natural history, epidemiology, complications, and so on." Like all other medical specialties, evidence regarding treatment does not necessarily have to go hand in hand with knowledge of pathophysiology, and novel approaches are always acceptable if based on available evidence. Differential diagnosis is a key component in the medical approach because it forces the clinician to weigh possible explanations for a given patient's symptoms/signs and is based on a general understanding that variability of presentation is usual for virtually all illnesses.

Although the precise pathophysiology of addiction has not yet been elucidated, significant clues to the brain mechanisms involved in reward and reinforcement have allowed significant insight into the connection between basic brain mechanisms and pathological behavior. Similarly, the commonality of these conditions and their familial nature have been demonstrated through many studies. Furthermore, alcoholism and other addictions have been recognized as the underlying cause of severe medical conditions for centuries. Yet, in subtle forms, these conditions are often unrecognized by competent clinicians. Using appropriate screening instruments, such as the MAST, DAST, and AUDIT, clinicians can increase the identification of these patients. In fact, perhaps the most important way to improve recognition of these disorders is to routinely ask all patients about their substance use in ways that enhance reporting of substance use.

Case 14.2 is typical in many ways of those that confront primary care physicians. Little direct evidence is presented to indicate that alcoholism was the underlying condition, although several clues might have been recognized. These clues include unresponsive hypertension, history of injuries, attending a doctor's appointment smelling of alcohol, and mild elevation of GGT. The physician's first question about consuming "a lot of alcohol" was structured in such a way that the patient could easily deny any problems because it lacked precision and a non-objective approach. Use of collateral informants was most helpful in eliciting the history and a "happy ending" has been posited.

Once identified, substance abuse disorders should be managed forthrightly and non-judgmentally, keeping in mind their chronic relapsing nature. Certain substance-related conditions, such as overdoses, head injury, and delirium, represent medical emergencies. Medical complications of chronic substance use warrant careful consideration, though the most important treatment of these medical complications is total abstinence. Physicians are also asked to intervene in withdrawal syndromes; these syndromes generally require medical intervention, though recent practices have shown that many can be managed safely in the outpatient setting with proper supervision.

Treatment of the dependence syndrome itself is a more complicated matter. Total abstinence must always be considered the goal even though relapses are usually encountered. The primary care physician should consider various levels of treatment from a simple referral to community support (e.g., AA) to referral to a full treatment program. It is important to become familiar with local resources. Referral phone numbers for AA are almost always in the phone book, and most communities have a variety of substance abuse programs. Medications can also be used to treat addictions. Buprenorphine has recently been approved by the FDA for treatment of opioid addiction as has acamprosate for the treatment of alcohol dependence. Disulfiram for alcoholism, and

---

Jim has been treated for hypertension for many years by his primary care physician. He has required multiple medications and has had only a moderate reduction in blood pressure despite "triple therapy." Jim is divorced but has had consistent employment. He has had several injuries requiring sutures and once came to a doctor's appointment with alcohol on his breath. Physical exam was unremarkable except for obesity, which made evaluation of liver size impossible. Routine laboratory evaluation was unremarkable, except that GGT was at the upper end of the normal range.

When asked if he "drank a lot," Jim said "no." Yet, on further evaluation, including interview with Jim's children, a 20-year history of heavy alcohol consumption was revealed, along with evidence of continued use despite family problems, two arrests for driving while intoxicated, and frequently drinking more than intended. With careful questioning and open discussion of the signs and symptoms, Jim agreed to attend an outpatient treatment program. Interestingly, once sober, Jim's hypertension was controlled with propranolol alone.

CASE 14.2

The evaluation and management of substance abusers

- Drug use disorders are very common but are often overlooked by physicians and patients until they have severe consequences.
- Physicians should incorporate routine questioning about substance use patterns into every new patient evaluation.
- Current diagnostic practice is to diagnose dependence or abuse for each appropriate substance separately.
- Overlap of substance abuse with psychiatric symptoms is common, and patients with psychiatric symptoms may have an underlying addiction.
- Nearly all addictions present with symptoms of tolerance, loss of control over use of the substance, and evidence that the substance has become an increasingly important part of one's life.
- Common illicit substances vary from community to community so clinicians should keep up with local drug use patterns.
- Patients with medical conditions like diabetes mellitus or hypertension that are unresponsive to usual therapies or who are non-compliant may be substance abusers.
- Self-administered and clinical screening questionnaires for alcoholism and drug abuse are easy to use and can be incorporated into usual practice.
- Screening instruments do not take the place of careful and thorough history and physical examination of patients with substance abuse.
- Community support such as Alcoholics Anonymous is important for short and long-term sobriety for many patients.
- New medications for addiction include buprenorphine for opioid addiction.
- Two consistent themes emerge when discussing drug abuse: (1) clinical presentations are similar no matter which substance is considered, and (2) differences exist among the various substances.
- Relapses are common, though not universal, especially in the first few months of sobriety.
- There are substantial limitations to urine drug screening. Only very recent substance use (24–72 hours after ingestion) is detectable for most abusable substances, and a limited number of substances are included in most tests.
- Avoiding anger in dealing with substance-abusing patients is sometimes difficult.
- HIV risk behaviors of substance abusers include increased sexually risky behaviors as well as needle use behaviors.

naltrexone or methadone for opioid addiction have been used for over 20 years. For the past 10 years, naltrexone has been approved by the FDA for the treatment of alcoholism as well; it has been demonstrated to be a useful adjunct to psychological treatment. Similarly, nicotine replacement therapy and buproprion as an adjunct to behavior therapies for nicotine addiction have been shown to be helpful. Other medications have shown promise in the treatment of addictions, and major medication development programs are currently under way at the National Institutes of Health for all addictions.

Finally, many substance-abusing patients test limits, and primary care physicians need practice dealing directly with non-compliance with recommendations. Finding ways to motivate patients at various stages of addiction to change their behaviors is challenging but very rewarding. Understanding the long-term outcome and finding creative ways to intervene are the goals for treatment.

CONSIDER CONSULTATION WHEN...

- The patient is noncompliant with the treatment regimen or relapses.
- The patient's substance use has led to potentially life-threatening complications.
- The patient has significant psychiatric symptoms in addition to substance abuse.
- The family is overwhelmed by the patient's behavior.
- The patient has complicated withdrawal symptoms, possibly including seizures and/or delirium.

Annotated bibliography

Galanter, M and Kleber, HD (eds) (2004) *Textbook of Substance Abuse Treatment*, 3rd Edition, American Psychiatric Press, Inc. *This textbook provides a thorough review of all treatment modalities for alcoholism and other addictions. The writing is clear and all major treatment modalities are reviewed.*

Goodwin, DW (2000) *Alcoholism: The Facts*, 3rd Edition, Oxford University Press. *This text on alcoholism is written in a readable and upbeat manner. Given the target of the book is alcoholic patients and their families, the writing style is essential and is generally well received. It provides a wealth of information, including descriptions of social, psychological, and medical components of alcoholism.*

Lowinson, JH, Ruiz, P, Millman, RB, and Langrod, JG (eds) (2004) *Substance Abuse—A Comprehensive Textbook*, 4th Edition, Lippincott, Williams and Wilkins. *A weighty tome, the Comprehensive Textbook is the standard review text for psychiatrists preparing for addiction subspecialty examinations. Topics are covered in great depth, and this text is appropriate for the serious student of addiction.*

Miller, WR, Rollnick, S, and Conforti, K (2002) *Motivational Interviewing, Second Edition: Preparing People for Change*, Guilford Press.

Motivational interviewing has been shown to be effective as a brief intervention for alcoholism and certain other addictions. These techniques may be useful for physicians who are working to enhance a variety of health behaviors. This book in previous editions has become a standard for the field.

Shuckit, MA (1999) *Drug and Alcohol Abuse: A Clinical Guide to Diagnosis and Treatment*, 5th Edition, Kluwer Academic/ Plenum Publishers.

This text is written for students and clinicians, especially those handling emergency problems. It provides a clinically oriented guide and an introduction to both clinical pharmacology and management for addictions.

CHAPTER 15

Eating Disorders: Bulimia Nervosa and Anorexia Nervosa

Richard W. Hudgens, MD

Introduction

The family physician is likely to diagnose and treat patients with eating disorders. Three eating disorders—bulimia nervosa (BN), anorexia nervosa (AN), and binge eating disorder (BED)—are commonly seen by psychiatrists. These three disorders are marked by maladaptive eating behavior; maladaptive beliefs concerning eating, body shape, and weight; and an array of psychological symptoms like depression, anxiety, obsessions, and compulsions. The family practitioner may be the only physician the patient regularly sees and needs to grow skilled in recognizing these often hidden syndromes and in caring for less severe cases. Obesity, not classified as either a psychiatric illness or an eating disorder, should also be discussed in any textbook regardless of specialty, since this chronic and increasingly prevalent disorder dominates the landscape of all medicine.

These four disorders share a common feature: disruption of the processes maintaining balance between caloric intake and expenditure. This disruption can be caused by primary disorders of gastrointestinal, endocrine, and CNS mechanisms controlling hunger and satiety or by psychopathological processes so strong that they drive behaviors overriding those homeostatic mechanisms. From the interaction of these complex factors proceeds much suffering.

The present chapter discusses bulimia nervosa and anorexia nervosa. The following chapter deals with binge eating disorder and obesity.

Bulimia nervosa

Historical recognition of the syndrome

Binges of eating—the consumption of large amounts of food in a short period of time—have been described for centuries and are sometimes associated with psychopathology. The Old English word *bulimy* meant "a morbid hunger" and was derived from words of Greek origin meaning "ox-hunger." Compensatory behaviors to avoid discomfort or obesity also have an ancient history, from sybarites of the Roman Empire vomiting to make room for more food, to a significant proportion of young women with anorexia nervosa whose restriction of food intake is at times interrupted by bouts of gorging on food and who overcompensate by vomiting, excessive exercising, or the inappropriate use of laxatives and diuretics.

In the second half of the 20th century, bulimia came chiefly to mean binge-eating followed by purging and was recognized as a phenomenon that could occur in the presence of various psychiatric disorders or in the absence of any other disorder at all. By the 1970s psychiatric investigators regarded bulimia as the chief symptom of a syndrome occurring in people without anorexia nervosa and marked by food-binging, a feeling of loss of control over eating binges, compensatory behaviors, and preoccupation with food, weight, and body image. It was termed bulimia nervosa and was recognized to be often comorbid with other psychiatric disorders.

Diagnosing bulimia nervosa

History

BN is common, occurring in American women at an incidence ranging from about 2% in the general population to as high as 10% in surveys of college women. Questions directed toward uncovering bulimic behavior should be part of routine medical history-taking, whatever the reason the patient is seeing a doctor. It is predominantly a disorder of adolescent girls and young women and should especially be investigated in these groups.

The typical patient rarely presents to the family physician complaining about bulimia. Patients with bulimia are embarrassed about their food-binging and compensatory behavior, especially vomiting, laxative abuse, and consumption of diet pills. They are much more likely to complain spontaneously of anxiety, depression, and the inability to lose weight. The physician must take the initiative to ask about binging, purging, and excessive exercising. When discovered, patients often express hating having bulimia, wanting to get rid of it, but feeling that the process is beyond control. Moreover, fearing obesity, patients are usually ambivalent about abandoning compensatory behaviors. These young women typically say they have a low opinion of themselves, and when asked why, they say things like, "I'm too fat," "My rear is too big," "My face looks like a chipmunk." Dissatisfaction with size and shape can trump all positive attributes and dominate the picture of low self-esteem.

The physician should elicit details regarding the patient's behavior, as these offer clues to severity and guides to treatment. How often does the patient binge on food? What types of food are eaten, how much, and under what circumstances? What thoughts, emotions, and physical sensations does the patient experience during and after a binge? What compensatory behaviors does the patient employ, why those methods, and what is the extent of them? In what ways has the patient tried to control the process and with what success? Binging is more likely to occur when the patient is alone, anxious or depressed, and stressed; when high-calorie foods are available; and after fasting (even for part of a day) in an attempt at weight control. Episodes of drinking and recreational drug use, also often concealed, are common triggers of binging as well.

Compensatory behavior is triggered by a feeling of abdominal fullness and by the emotion of self-disgust, driving an urgent need to get rid of the food ingested and avoid additional pounds. Vomiting, if it occurs soon enough after the food binge, is the favored and a more efficient way to block calories than exercising, diuretics, or laxatives. But even with vomiting after each meal, it is estimated that less than half the food is regurgitated.

Symptoms of bulimia loom largest among the patient's concerns whatever the initial desire to conceal it. But bulimia may be only part of an underlying disorder. The physician should inquire about symptoms of major depression, generalized anxiety disorder, obsessive compulsive disorder, and substance abuse. When any of these is present, the bulimia will not come under satisfactory control unless the comorbid disorder is dealt with, and sometimes not even then.

Physical and laboratory examinations

The appearance of patients with BN gives no clue to the disorder. Weight is usually normal or moderately above normal. There may or may not be erosion of tooth enamel, redness of oral mucosa, enlargement of parotid and submaxillary salivary glands, and calluses on the dorsal surfaces of the fingers—all stigmata of self-induced vomiting. Serum potassium may be low if the patient is abusing laxatives or vomiting. Other less common electrolyte derangements and serious complications of purging are discussed in the section on medical consequences of BN and AN.

Mental status

During the initial examination, patients often exhibit anxiety, depressed mood, and preoccupation with food, eating, weight, and physical appearance. Once the diagnosis has been brought to light, denial of the problem is not typical, since each common feature of BN—binging, purging, and emotional distress at loss of control—is part of the patient's complaints. But regardless of awareness of the syndrome and the suffering caused by it, the patient may be reluctant to give it up, fearing fatness more than the illness itself. Substance abuse, often present, may be concealed or made light of. Distortion of body image, often present to an extreme degree in AN, is less prominent in BN.

Course and outcome

Clues to cause

Family and twin studies strongly suggest a genetic contribution to susceptibility for AN and BN, irrespective of the presence or absence of other psychiatric illnesses. This finding

DIAGNOSIS

Table 15.1 Bulimia nervosa

Discriminating features

1 Persistent and recurrent binge-eating in the absence of low weight.
2 Inappropriate compensatory behavior—fasting, purging, excessive exercise—in the absence of low weight.

Consistent features

1 Feeling of loss of control over binge-eating.
2 Preoccupation with food, weight, and body shape.
3 Extreme psychological or physical discomfort after binge-eating.
4 Rebound binging after fasting.

Variable features

1 Young and female.
2 Comorbid with other psychiatric disorders and substance abuse.
3 Physical signs of self-induced vomiting.
4 Amenorrhea.
5 Electrolyte abnormalities.

Box 15.1 Bulimia nervosa

A. Recurrent episodes of binge-eating. An episode of binge-eating is characterized by both of the following:
  - eating, in a discrete period of time (e.g., within any two-hour period) an amount of food that is definitely larger than most people would eat during a similar period of time and under similar circumstances
  - a sense of lack of control over eating during the episode (e.g., a feeling that one cannot stop eating or control what or how much one is eating).

B. Recurrent inappropriate compensatory behavior in order to prevent weight gain, such as self-induced vomiting; misuse of laxatives, diuretics, enemas, or other medications; fasting; or excessive exercise.

C. The binge-eating and inappropriate compensatory behaviors both occur, on average, at least twice a week for three months.

D. Self-evaluation is unduly influenced by body shape and weight.

E. The disturbance does not occur exclusively during episodes of anorexia nervosa.

Specify type:
  - *Purging type:* during the current episode of bulimia nervosa, the person has regularly engaged in self-induced vomiting or the misuse of laxatives, diuretics, or enemas.
  - *Nonpurging type:* during the current episode of bulimia nervosa, the person has used other inappropriate compensatory behaviors, such as fasting or excessive exercise, but has not regularly engaged in self-induced vomiting or the misuse of diuretics, laxatives, or enemas.

From American Psychiatric Association (2000) Diagnostic and Statistical Manual of Mental Disorders, 4th Edition, Text Revision, Washington, D.C., American Psychiatric Association.

---

has helped to stimulate current investigations searching for chronic or intermittent disruptions of CNS processes governing appetite regulation. No specific biologic risk factors have been found.

In the US and Western Europe, BN is most commonly reported among white teenage girls and young women of middle to upper social class, the group which most prizes thinness and abhors excessive weight. This may reflect selection bias, since women from economically privileged groups are more likely to seek treatment. Lately, increasing numbers are being reported among African American girls and women. BN (and the milder occasional habit of purging and exercising after big meals) may be driven in part by culturally influenced notions of beauty. Pressure on girls to be thin may come from parents, peers, magazines, movies, TV, and now even from websites promoting anorexia and bulimia as ways of life, not illnesses.

Patients with BN have an increased prevalence of major depressive disorder, bipolar disorder, obsessive-compulsive disorder, and substance abuse among their relatives. These same syndromes often appear in the patients themselves, sometimes even preceding the onset of bulimia, which may then justifiably be regarded as a symptom of the underlying illness. Weight-conscious young women who develop major depressive disorder, for example, may find their anxiety, fear of fatness, and low self-esteem exaggerated by that illness, leading them to maladaptive eating and weight-control behaviors.

Natural history

BN, whether or not it is comorbid with another psychiatric disorder, typically begins in the teens or twenties. In severe cases, bouts of overeating, followed by compensatory actions to eliminate or burn off calories, accelerate in frequency and intensity, worsening as, for example, eating follows vomiting and vomiting follows eating in rapid succession, perhaps many times a day. The patient becomes trapped in this cycle, a cycle that can come to dominate every aspect of the patient's life. Factors associated with poorest prognosis include frequent episodes of binging and compensatory behavior, lower than normal weight, and duration of bulimia for more than a couple of years.

Over time, binging and compensatory behavior diminish in people with less severe cases of the syndrome. Whether the patient is treated or not, the best outcome occurs in those who had good personal adjustment before bulimia began and who are free of concurrent psychiatric illness, including substance abuse. In patients burdened with additional psychiatric disorders, bulimia may disappear when those illnesses are controlled, but even then it may acquire a life of its own, a behavior driven by anxiety that is hard to completely shake. In a significant minority of people with BN, symptoms smolder for years to a mild degree, regardless of the presence or absence of comorbid psychiatric disorders.

Complications

BN, even if unaccompanied by other disorders, can interfere with all aspects of life—school, work, and personal relationships. It is always accompanied by varying degrees of anxiety, predilection to worsening with normal life stressors, expenditure of time in unhealthy compensatory behaviors, and varying degrees of deception to conceal the behavior from other people. These complications finally drive patients to seek help. Through their concern with controlling their weight and appearance, they have become slaves of the very methods they use to pursue that goal.

Medical complications of BN are rarer than in AN. Tooth enamel is eroded over time by acid from the stomach; the esophagus may bleed or even rupture from the trauma of violent episodes of vomiting; vomiting and laxative abuse may leading to life-threatening hypokalemia; and emetine poisoning of the myocardium can occur if large amounts of ipecac are used to induce vomiting. Over-the-counter or illegal appetite-suppressing drugs can cause agitation and, like hypokalemia, can cause fatal cardiac conduction disturbances.

Treatment

General principles

Goals of treatment for BN include the establishment of healthy eating patterns, elimination of fasting as a means of weight control, avoidance of alcohol and recreational drugs, and simultaneous treatment of comorbid psychiatric disorders. Many people tell of having gone through a bulimic phase and having dealt with it successfully, never having sought professional help.

Insofar as lay-run weight-control programs promote good eating habits and avoidance of fasting (which increases the risk of food-binging), they may be useful, and some overweight people with BN find their way into these programs. There are enthusiastic endorsements of their effectiveness, but no research data are available on the usefulness of this approach.

Psychotherapy

It is not the milder and transient cases of BN that commonly come to the attention of the family doctor. People presenting for help have usually tried treating themselves and become frustrated and discouraged by lack of success. For those patients, individual or group psychotherapy guiding a systematic attack on the bulimic behavior is the treatment most associated with long-term success. This therapy can be carried out by any well-trained health professional. A series of frequent sessions should explore the patient's emotions and beliefs about weight, appearance, self-worth, and interaction with important people in her life, currently or in the past. Understanding an apparent psychological basis for bulimia can help the therapist and patient challenge the poor self-image and negative expectations that drive some of the maladaptive behavior. These principles have been incorporated into specific psychotherapies including cognitive-behavioral therapy and interpersonal therapy (discussed in the following chapter in relationship to binge eating disorder), which have both shown more promise for sustained control of the binge-purge cycle than has the use of medica-

tion alone. It follows that the soundest therapeutic approach to BN should deal with both cognitive-behavioral and interpersonal issues.

Behavior change is also promoted by education about nutrition and by guiding the patient in establishing healthy eating habits, which must include avoidance of the fasting and restrictive dieting that lead to food-binging. Part of behavioral control is the avoidance of triggers that lead to binging, for example, availability of excessive amounts of high-calorie food and the use of alcohol or recreational drugs. In recent years manuals for therapists and patients have become available which outline this systematic cognitive-behavioral approach.

Medication

Medication has been helpful in treating people who have BN. Reports from as long ago as the 1960s describe improvement in bulimic behavior when antidepressants are given, even in the absence of depression. When BN is comorbid with illnesses such as major depressive disorder, obsessive-compulsive disorder, panic disorder, or generalized anxiety disorder, medication is indicated. Antidepressants are the first choice, especially the serotonin reuptake inhibitors (SSRIs) as they target symptoms of depression, anxiety, and obsessionality that often accompany bulimia nervosa. Also, the SSRIs seldom increase appetite, in contrast to the tertiary tricyclic antidepressants amitriptyline and imipramine or the monoamine oxidase inhibitor phenelzine.

Chronic use of benzodiazepines for anxiety is not recommended, because patients become habituated to them and may begin a cycle of dose escalation. When antipsychotic drugs are used, either to treat delusions and hallucinations associated with comorbid psychotic disorders or as an adjunct to SSRIs in the treatment of resistant obsessions and compulsions, it is wise to use drugs that do not increase appetite or are associated with marked weight gain. The latter is especially a problem with olanzapine, risperidone, and clozapine, and less so with some of the older "typical" medium-potency antipsychotics like thiothixene and trifluoperazine. Recently, psychiatrists have begun using aripiprazole and ziprasidone, the most weight-neutral new generation antipsychotic medications yet developed. No research data on their use in bulimia are available at this time.

Reports are emerging on the use of the antiepileptic drug topiramate in patients with BN. For several years, it has been given to some patients with affective disorders as a secondary mood stabilizer. Topiramate reduces appetite, unlike the other mood stabilizing antiepileptics, and is sometimes employed as a bedtime medication for people who awaken in the night and attack the refrigerator. Its usefulness in BN has not been convincingly demonstrated, unlike the antidepressant drugs.

When BN is associated with substance abuse, the substance abuse must be confronted directly by the physician. It can acquire a life of its own, independent of the eating disorder, and become the most destructive factor in a patient's life. Referral to treatment programs and to recovery groups such as Alcoholics Anonymous (AA) and Narcotics Anonymous (NA) should be prompt.

Role of the primary physician

Most people who suffer from BN, even those who have failed self-help methods, do not need to see a psychiatrist. If the primary physician is willing to prescribe and monitor the use of medication, when indicated, and work with a therapist who employs a systematic cognitive and behavioral approach that targets the symptoms and behaviors, a successful outcome can be expected in most cases. Referral to a psychiatrist is warranted for treatment-resistant cases. Typically these include patients with duration of illness of more than two years, very underweight patients, patients who are actively suicidal, and those with significant complications resulting from comorbid disorders.

Anorexia nervosa

Historical recognition of the syndrome

AN is self-starvation accomplished by restricted eating and often accompanied by purging as well. Over 90% of cases present in teenagers or young women. Patients with AN maintain unduly low weight and an implacable refusal to gain or maintain normal weight. They have an intense fear of obesity and a distorted perception of themselves as fat or bloated. In severe cases, AN can lead to death by starvation or suicide. AN has a higher mortality rate than any other psychiatric disorder. (The DSM-IV criteria for AN gives as an example "weight loss leading to maintenance of body weight less than 85% of that expected." This figure serves as a practical guideline for the clinician, but should not be interpreted rigidly.)

Case reports of a disorder resembling AN appeared in Britain in the 1600s. These cases were recognized as different from cachexia secondary to infection or cancer. The full syndrome was first described in France in the 1860s and 1870s. Aware of the irrational thinking that accompanied the disorder, Marce called it a "hypochondriacal delusion" in 1860. Fear of fatness was not mentioned in the 19th-century accounts of the illness, but neither was that feature said to be absent. The consensus is that the thin-is-beautiful notion is a 20th-century phenomenon influencing the thought content characteristic of the syndrome, at least in Europe and North America. Some case reports from Asia have noted the absence of this feature. By the middle of the 20th century, AN was clearly distinguished from other disorders, including the rare Simmond's cachexia, a wasting disorder that fol-

Bulimia nervosa

- Food-binging and purging, usually by vomiting, occur in as many as 2% of Americans. Patients may not volunteer that they engage in such behavior; the physician must ask about it.
- Teenage girls and young women of middle or higher social strata—those who prize thinness most—are the Americans most at risk for BN and AN.
- Patients with BN feel out of control and ashamed of binging and purging.
- Fasting is bad whether it occurs in people with BN or in those who are obese. It is a common trigger for uncontrolled food-binging.
- BN often occurs with another psychiatric disorder, especially major depression, obsessive-compulsive disorder, generalized anxiety disorder, and substance abuse, which must also be treated.
- Cognitive-behavioral psychotherapy and interpersonal psychotherapy offer the most promise in achieving and maintaining the chief goals of treatment: establishment of healthy eating behavior and elimination of fasting as a means of weight control.
- Antidepressant medications are useful in treating BN. Selective serotonin reuptake inhibitors (SSRIs) decrease obsessions and seldom increase appetite. Therefore, they are the first choice for pharmacologic treatment.

lows infarction of the pituitary, with which it was confused for a time.

Diagnosing anorexia nervosa

History

A new case of AN usually involves a teenage girl who begins to diet in response to the belief that she is fat, whether she is or not. When she reaches her target weight she continues to diet, sometimes to emaciation, with the fear that if she stops, she will lose control and rebound into obesity. She typically underestimates the extent of her thinness, despite confrontation by others and the evidence of her own eyes when she looks in a mirror. Her body image is distorted to an extent that sometimes seems delusional.

In the restrictive subtype of AN, patients achieve and maintain weight loss by eating tiny amounts of food and seldom or never purge. In the binge-eating/purging subtype, patients also habitually eat little, but regularly binge on food as hunger recurs, then engage in the compensatory behaviors discussed in the section on bulimia nervosa, especially vomiting after eating. Compulsive exercising is common in both the restrictive and binge/purge subtypes. Despite their frail appearance, these young women may deny being fatigued until advanced stages of emaciation.

Similarly, they often describe their appetites as good until they become severely weak.

Patients' preoccupation with food can lead to great attention to nutrition and cooking. They may prepare food for others, which they themselves take pride in not eating. They may shoplift items they do not need, including food they do not eat. They may hoard food, hiding it until it rots. Conversations with anorectic women often circle back again and again to food-related subjects, regardless of what they talk about at the beginning of the conversation.

The history of AN in males, who comprise only 5–10% of cases, is similar to that in women. The average age of onset is mid-teens, and the same attitudes about food and weight are present. Like girls with anorexia nervosa, these boys engage in excessive exercise. But the pursuit of thinness is at variance with society's ideal of a male body type. Some of these boys become body-builders and bypass the risks of starvation.

Most challenging are the cases of "older" anorectics, both those whose illness begins in the mid-twenties or later and those whose illness begins earlier but persists untreated into adulthood. These patients are more guarded than teenagers about revealing items in their history that would betray the diagnosis, and they are better able to resist coercion into treatment. They come to physicians complaining of gastrointestinal or other physical symptoms but flatly lie in response to questions about anorectic behavior and fear of fatness. The history has in effect gone underground, as patients fear that revealing it may threaten their control over maintenance of thinness. For adults with AN as well as for adolescents, a separate history should be obtained from an informant.

DIAGNOSIS

Table 15.2 Anorexia nervosa

Discriminating features

1 Refusal to maintain minimal body weight.
2 Absence of medical illness to explain weight loss.
3 Denial of seriousness of weight loss.

Consistent features

1 Amenorrhea.
2 Intense fear of weight gain.
3 Preoccupation with food and weight.
4 Disturbance in perception of own shape and weight.

Variable features

1 Begins in women under 20.
2 Absence of fatigue despite weight loss.
3 Rigid perfectionism and obsessionality.
4 Food binging and purging.
5 Starvation and its complications.
6 Withholding or lying about history.
7 Hoarding of food.

Physical and laboratory examinations

The appearance of patients with severe AN is striking. They are invariably compared with concentration camp survivors, but they have a degree of energy that is surprising. The skin is characteristically dry and sometimes yellowish in color. Scalp hair is brittle, and there may be fine hair, lanugo, over the body. Temperature, heart rate, and blood pressure are low. As in BN, frequent self-induced vomiting can cause calluses on the dorsal surfaces of knuckles and fingers, enlargement of salivary glands, redness of gums and palate, and erosion of tooth enamel.

The routine battery of laboratory tests is not likely to help in diagnosis. A minority have high serum bicarbonate and low potassium, hallmarks of vomiting and laxative abuse. If starvation proceeds to dangerous levels there are other findings, discussed below in the section on medical complications.

Mental status

By the time most patients see a physician their families may be in turmoil and the emotion displayed by the patient may be anger directed toward "interfering" relatives. Most people with AN are stubbornly resistant to handing over any measure of control to others, especially to physicians who want them to gain weight.

As long as restricting or purging behavior is allowed, the patient may deny depression or anxiety, but express a horror of fatness. Conversation betrays a preoccupation with food, eating, and appearance. Given enough time to talk about life issues, the patient may reveal a host of worries beneath a façade of cheerful unconcern. Rigid perfectionism and a need to be in control in many areas besides weight may be evident, as well as despair of ever being adequate.

Course and outcome

Clues to cause

Speculations about cause, previously discussed in the section on bulimia nervosa, apply as well to anorexia nervosa. There are additional considerations in AN because of the conspicuous degree of weight loss.

By the time a patient enters treatment, preoccupation with food, eating, and body image is already apparent. Considerable family turmoil has often been generated by the patient's alarming condition and refusal to stop losing weight. Some have proposed that family conflict and issues of perfectionism and control precede the illness and are causative. This hypothesis has not been proven, but regardless of etiologic importance, these issues are significant because they complicate treatment and must be addressed. Numerous biologic studies of AN have demonstrated derangements in major endocrine systems and disturbances—confirmed or inferred—in some neurotransmitter systems. However, star-

Box 15.2 Anorexia navosa

A. Refusal to maintain body weight at or above a minimally normal weight for age and height (e.g., weight loss leading to maintenance of body weight less than 85% of that expected, or failure to make expected weight gain during period of growth, leading to body weight less than 85% of that expected).

B. Intense fear of gaining weight or becoming fat, even though underweight.

C. Disturbance in the way in which one's body weight or shape is experienced, undue influence of body weight or shape on self-evaluation, or denial of the seriousness of the current low body weight.

D. In postmenarcheal females, amenorrhea, i.e., the absence of at least three consecutive menstrual cycles. (A woman is considered to have amenorrhea if her periods occur only following hormones, e.g. estrogen, administration.)

Specify type:

- *Restricting type:* during the current episode of anorexia nervosa, the person has not regularly engaged in binge-eating or purging behavior (i.e., self-induced vomiting or the misuse of laxatives, diuretics, or enemas).
- *Binge-eating/purging type:* during the current episode of anorexia nervosa, the person has regularly engaged in binge-eating or purging behavior (i.e., self-induced vomiting, or the misuse of laxatives, diuretics, or enemas).

From American Psychiatric Association (2000) Diagnostic and Statistical Manual of Mental Disorders, 4th Edition, Text Revision, Washington, D.C., American Psychiatric Association.

---

vation from other causes produces similar changes. Definite biologic precursors to AN have not yet been found.

The peculiarities of eating behavior and suppression of reproductive function, with amenorrhea sometimes preceding weight loss, have directed attention to the hypothalamus and its involvement in the pituitary-gonadal system and role in hunger and satiety. But dysfunction predictive of eating disorders or trait markers for them has not been discovered. Studies of hunger and satiety leave many questions unanswered: lack of appetite is not the main drive for fasting in anorexia nervosa, and binge eating often occurs in the absence of hunger.

Natural history

AN usually begins during the teen years, and its onset is rare after age 25. Although it can be a devastating, sometimes fatal, illness, most people recover from AN. Follow-up studies reveal full or partial recovery in over half of subjects. Some patients who recover and never have AN again later develop other psychiatric disorders, including depression, alcohol or drug dependence, anxiety disorder, panic disorder and obsessive-compulsive disorder (OCD).

One-fourth to one-half of patients with AN continue to suffer from the illness with varying degrees of severity, even after treatment, and it may run a fluctuating course throughout the lives. In follow-up studies of more than 20 years, mortality rates are between 10% and 20%. The majority of deaths result from complications of starvation, and most of the rest from suicide. The latter observation serves as a warning that concurrent depression must be treated aggressively.

Poorer long-term outcome is predicted by late onset of the illness (after age 20), late entry into treatment, persistence of the illness for more than two years, extremely low weight at the beginning of treatment, purging as a significant means of weight control, poor premorbid psychological adjustment, and drug or alcohol abuse. Studies over the span of the 20th century do not show an improvement in overall outcome for recent decades.

Complications

Severe AN interrupts life. Damage occurs in family and other personal relationships, in school, and in work. This usually occurs during the teen years, a time of particular vulnerability because progress should be taking place in all those areas.

Medical complications stem from purging behavior, starvation, and treatment of starvation. Purging—vomiting, enemas, and laxative abuse—can lead to low potassium, sodium, magnesium, phosphate, and chloride levels. Hypokalemia may lead to cardiac arrhythmia and disorders of conduction. Severe hyponatremia, or its too-rapid correction, can lead to coma and death. In some cases with severe dehydration resulting from vomiting or abuse of laxatives and diuretics, secondary aldosteronism develops. Hypokalemia and metabolic alkalosis can occur. By contrast, metabolic acidosis can develop if enemas and laxative abuse are dominant, flushing alkaline fluids from the colon. The risks of esophageal rupture from vomiting and emetine poisoning of heart muscle from ipecac have been mentioned above.

Consequences of starvation include muscle wasting, weakness, lowered levels of reproductive hormones with consequent amenorrhea, delayed gastric emptying, low serum protein, edema, high plasma cortical levels, osteoporosis (which may not be corrected even after nutritional recovery), hypotension, and bradycardia.

Whenever possible, patients should accomplish refeeding by feeding themselves. The restoration of nutrition carries risks of its own, especially when tube feeding, intravenous glucose, or intravenous total parenteral nutrition (TPN) is employed and when nutritional restoration is too rapid. For example, in a starved patient, the sudden influx of a large glucose load can lead to a deficiency of phosphate that may be severe enough to result in fatal encephalopathy. Rapid refeeding by tube can lead to aspiration, acute pancreatitis, and dilation or rupture of the stomach. Occasionally, a patient with AN who is finally coming to treatment thus dies of the consequences of refeeding.

Treatment

General principles

As with BN, there is a spectrum of severity associated with AN. Some teenagers and young adults go through an episode of AN without becoming dangerously underweight and never consult a doctor. Physicians see the sicker patients. Restoration and maintenance of normal weight through proper eating is a primary goal of treatment. This cannot be achieved unless there is reduction of the patient's psychological discomfort. Anxiety about losing control over weight-maintenance may make a patient reluctant to enter treatment. This fear becomes even more intense as weight starts to increase.

Hospital treatment: psychological, nutritional, medical

Patients with more severe cases of AN may not gain weight unless they are hospitalized. Hospitalization is especially necessary if the patient is cachectic. Medical complications can be best addressed in a hospital; patients are more likely to begin eating properly in a controlled environment; and psychotherapy and the administration of medication can be initiated more intensively. The process of virtually coerced weight gain and concomitant reduction of fear can be aborted by premature discharge. In the 1970s, inpatient stays of two months or longer for patients with AN were not unusual. Those days are gone forever. Residential treatment facilities and partial hospital programs provide less intense care, but successful treatment of people with severe AN remains one of the great challenges of psychiatry.

The previous discussion regarding psychotherapy and pharmacotherapy in the section on BN applies as well to AN. Several additional points should be made about the treatment of AN. First, because family members are usually alarmed by the physical state of many patients—most of whom are teenage girls living at home—the family's participation in the treatment program is essential. Second, since the mid-20th century patients hospitalized for the treatment of severe anorexia nervosa are usually treated with antidepressant, antipsychotic or anxiolytic drugs, including those that increase appetite. None has been shown to be effective in promoting normalization of eating and weight in the acute phase, although specific agents may be appropriately prescribed for treatment of symptoms of depression, obsessions, and severe anxiety, as well as for the occasional patient with delusions. Finally, because severe depression in anorectic patients leads to prolonged anorexia and sometimes to suicide, electroconvulsive therapy (ECT) should be considered in persistently depressed patients when pharmacotherapy has failed. No controlled studies have been published, but anecdotal reports of its effectiveness and safety are encouraging.

Whether or not the patient is treated in the hospital, the methods for achieving nutritional goals remain the same: regularly scheduled meals, vitamin and mineral supplements as indicated, and avoidance of fasting, binging, purging, alcohol, recreational drugs, and excessive exercise. It is helpful to prescribe ahead of time the type and amount of food to be eaten, in conformity with guidelines of nutritional specialists. In this way the patient is relieved of burdensome decisions about what and how much to eat. Weight goals should be set at the beginning of treatment, as well as the expected rate of weight gain, often from two to three pounds per week.

Patients commonly resist weight gain. In the beginning they may develop peripheral edema, caused by rehydration in the presence of low serum protein. They quickly feel full because gastric emptying is delayed in people who have been starving. Their abdomens may protrude. This bloating distresses them greatly. It may be necessary to keep patients within sight for an hour or longer after each meal to keep them from vomiting. When hospital treatment programs need to coerce weight gain because of life-threatening circumstances, privileges like visitors, telephone, recreation, and ultimate discharge can be made contingent on achieving food intake and weight goals. Tube feeding is occasionally necessary if patients absolutely refuse to eat, but intravenous total parenteral nutrition is a last resort and should be used only when tube feeding is contraindicated.

From the above discussion it should be clear why adults with AN are so much harder to treat than adolescents. The physician cannot force them to stay in treatment programs involuntarily unless a court can be convinced that they are an immediate danger to themselves, which is not usually the case. Indeed, the physician cannot make a minor child or adolescent stay in the hospital either, unless parents are in agreement with the treatment plan and resist their child's pleas for escape from treatment.

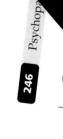

Outpatient treatment: psychological, nutritional, medical

The principles discussed for the treatment of AN in the hospital apply as well to outpatient treatment. Psychotherapy should employ the elements of both cognitive-behavioral and interpersonal psychotherapy as well as attention to nutrition. Family therapy has been shown to be effective in younger patients, with whom the family is usually closely involved. Pharmacotherapy addresses the symptoms of depression, obsessions, and anxiety. As in BN, fearful obsessions seem to drive the maladaptive behavior in many patients with AN. SSRI antidepressants are the first choice for medical treatment of these symptoms, and there are encouraging reports that the SSRI fluoxetine reduces the incidence of relapse.

Role of the primary physician

In new and less severe cases of AN, that is, subsyndromal cases where weight loss has not yet become extreme, the primary physician, often a pediatrician, can manage the case when willing to assume that responsibility. This physician must arrange referral to a professional who will work with the patient and family in psychotherapy, and to a nutritionist. The primary physician should keep track of the patient's nutritional progress.

As noted in the section on [...] cated to treat depression, anxi[...] tical matter, the only psychi[...] physicians are comfortable p[...] and anxiolytics, and the latt[...] short-term treatment in AN[...] physicians do not venture b[...] they try, usually an SSRI. Wh[...] another class of drug) is called for, most primary care phys[...] cians find it helpful to consult a specialist knowledgeable about the treatment of eating disorders.

Ideally psychiatrists should be involved in cases of AN, especially if the illness progresses beyond a few months or to extreme weight loss, or is accompanied by severe depression. Many AN patients, no matter how sick, will not agree to see a psychiatrist with any degree of consistency and comply with treatment. The primary physician may hospitalize severely anorectic patients at times of nutritional deterioration, patching up the situation, making a psychiatric referral in vain, and waiting for the next crisis. In the most severe and chronic cases, the patients' implacable opposition toward treatment and their resistance, even hostility, to those who want to help them, wear everyone down. Fortunately, the majority of patients with AN have a better prognosis.

CONSIDER CONSULTATION WHEN...

- Patients with BN or AN do not begin to improve after two months of treatment.
- Hospitalization for AN is required because of medical complications, including starvation, the risk of suicide, or failure of outpatient treatment.

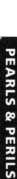

Anorexia nervosa

PEARLS & PERILS

- Complete evaluation for AN should include an interview of a knowledgeable informant.
- The self-destructive behavior in AN is driven by obsessive fear of becoming fat, not by poor appetite.
- Long-term mortality from AN is 10% to 20% in chronic cases. Death is almost always from either starvation or suicide.
- The restoration of normal weight is only the first of treatment goals. Without reduction in obsessive fear of fatness and other psychiatric symptoms, starvation will recur.
- Major depressive disorder in patients with AN should be treated vigorously with medication or ECT, as well as psychotherapy.
- Rapid refeeding in starvation, especially intravenously or by tube, can be dangerous, even fatal. If at all possible, it is best for the patients to feed themselves.
- The older the patient with AN, the more successfully she hides her history and evades treatment. Young teenagers with cooperative parents are the least problematic.

KEY CLINICAL QUESTIONS AND WHAT THEY UNLOCK

- *What things about yourself cause you the most worry, unhappiness, or dissatisfaction?*
  This can uncover preoccupation with shape and weight, as well as binge-eating.
- *What are all the ways you use to lose weight and to keep weight off? How well are those methods working?*
  This can uncover self-induced vomiting and other compensatory behaviors.
- *What are your hopes, plans, and goals for yourself in the near future and in the long run? What are the roadblocks in the way of achieving those goals?*
  This can uncover issues of poor self-esteem, depression, and loss of control over the eating disorder, offer insight into the illness, and suggest guidelines for determining the success of treatment.
- *How often do you think about suicide?*

...nt depression is very common and can ...tate interventions such as antidepressant ...rmacotherapy and emergent hospitalization.
...low often do you use alcohol? Amphetamines? Cocaine? Other illicit drugs?
Although less common than depression, substance abuse markedly complicates the course and treatment, particularly the use of stimulants to suppress appetite. Urine drug screens for illicit drugs may be useful.

- *What does the patient weigh?*
  The answer to this question helps separate anorexia nervosa, associated with a substantially increased risk of mortality, from other psychiatric disorders. Weight is also critical to treatment planning—marked weight loss and malnutrition may require hospitalization. It is sometimes difficult to formulate a treatment plan that incorporates good nutrition and weight gain/stabilization without producing an adversarial relationship. A consistent weighing approach can be critical to obtaining accurate weights—patients with anorexia nervosa can deceive themselves and others.

- *What is the patient's fluid and electrolyte status?*
  Dehydration and disturbances of electrolytes can complicate management of eating disorders.

Annotated bibliography

Bliss, EL and Branch, CCH (1960) *Anorexia Nervosa: its history, psychology, and biology*, New York, Hoeber.
An old text, included here because of excellent case descriptions.

Fairburn, CG and Brownell, KD (eds) (2002) *Eating Disorders and Obesity: a comprehensive handbook*, 2nd Edition, New York, Guilford Press.
Broad, and with the most current information.

Fairburn, CG and Harrison, PJ (2003) Eating Disorders, *Lancet* 361: 407–416.
Outstanding brief summary of current knowledge. Large bibliography through 2002.

Marce, L-V: Note on a form of hypochondriacal delusion consecutive to the dyspepsias and principally characterized by refusal of food (1860). Translated from French by Blewett, A and Bottero, A (1994) *History of Psychiatry*, 5: 273–283.
The first comprehensive description of anorexia nervosa, published a decade before rival accounts and emphasizing the irrational cognitions accompanying the disorder.

Mehler, PS and Andersen, AE (eds) (1999) *Eating Disorders: a guide to medical care and complications*, Baltimore, Johns Hopkins University Press.
This text deals with the medical issues that are a constant concern.

CHAPTER 16

Obesity and Binge Eating Disorder

Anja Hilbert, PhD, Andrea B. Schnur, BA, and Denise E. Wilfley, PhD

Overview

At the time of writing, about 30% of American adults are obese, and prevalence rates are rising. Obesity is a major cause for morbidity and mortality, substantially increasing the risk for diseases such as hypertension, diabetes, and cardiovascular disease. Not surprisingly, health care services, e.g., visits to doctors or outpatient clinics, are frequently utilized by obese patients. Obesity has proven difficult to treat, with high relapse rates after behavioral and pharmacological weight loss treatments. Even moderate amounts of sustained weight loss (10%) decrease the severity of obesity-associated risk factors and significantly improve health and well-being.

Although not characteristically a psychiatric condition, obesity is associated with an elevated risk for comorbid psychiatric disorders, especially binge eating disorder (BED), which may complicate the management of obesity. BED is a clinical eating disorder usually co-occurring with, yet distinct from, obesity. Compared with obese individuals without BED, individuals with BED may have increased psychiatric comorbidity, present with more medical complaints, and have greater impairments in psychosocial functioning and overall quality of life. For these reasons, special care appears indicated for obese patients with BED. This chapter reviews clinically relevant research on the development, characteristics, and treatment of adult obesity and binge eating disorder.

Classification, clinical description, and etiology of obesity

Classification

Obesity refers to an excess of body fat. It is determined by the body mass index (BMI), calculated by dividing weight (in kilograms) by height (in meters) squared. According to guidelines by the National Heart, Lung, and Blood Institute, which are consistent with recommendations by the World Health Organization, overweight is defined as a BMI of $25–29.9\,\mathrm{kg/m^2}$ and obesity as a BMI of $30\,\mathrm{kg/m^2}$ or greater. BMI of $30–34.9\,\mathrm{kg/m^2}$ is classified as class I obesity, $35–39.9\,\mathrm{kg/m^2}$ as class II obesity, and $40\,\mathrm{kg/m^2}$ or more as class III or extreme obesity. BMI is a useful indicator for assessing an individual's relative disease risk, with higher classes of obesity indicating greater health risks.

DIAGNOSIS

Table 16.1 Obesity

Discriminating features

1 BMI* > 30 kg/m²:
   - class I obesity: BMI 30–34.9 kg/m²
   - class II obesity: BMI 35–39.9 kg/m²
   - class III (extreme) obesity: BMI > 40 kg/m².

Consistent features

1 Abdominal adiposity:
   - in men, waist circumference >102 cm (>40 in)
   - in women, waist circumference >88 cm (>35 in).
2 Increased risk for morbidity and mortality.

Variable features

1 Presence of medical complications, e.g., metabolic syndrome.
2 Presence of comorbid psychopathology.
3 Psychosocial impairment.
4 Etiological factors (i.e., genetic, drug-induced, psychological).
5 Readiness for change.
* BMI indicates body mass index.

While BMI is a useful measure in terms of predicting morbidity and mortality, it does not capture body composition (fat mass vs. lean, or fat-free, mass), and thus may incorrectly classify some individuals as obese (i.e., those with increased muscle mass) or non-obese (i.e., those with a high percentage of body fat but of average weight). Independent of BMI, body fat distribution is an important indicator of disease risk: central adiposity is a risk factor for cardiovascular disease, type 2 diabetes, and stroke, while peripheral obesity is associated with risk for less serious conditions such as varicose veins and joint-skeletal problems. Abdominal adiposity, which is correlated with a waist circumference of >102 cm (>40 in) for men and >88 cm (>35 in) for women, or a waist/hip circumference ratio of >1.0, can be used to identify obesity-related disease risk in adults with a BMI of 25–34.9 kg/m². Methods of circumference measurement (e.g., measuring tape) are useful for determining abdominal adiposity in clinical practice.

Epidemiology

Recent data from the National Health and Nutrition Examination Survey (NHANES 1999–2000) estimate that 30% of adults in the United States are obese and that 64% are either overweight or obese. While the percentage of individuals considered overweight but not obese has remained fairly stable over the past four decades, rising by about 4%, rates of obesity in the United States have more than doubled since 1960. Considered a global epidemic, obesity is common in industrialized countries but is also rising in developing countries, often coexisting with undernutrition. Throughout the world, the prevalence of obesity increases with age, although less common after age 70, and is elevated in females. In the United States, obesity occurs more frequently in individuals belonging to lower socioeconomic classes than in those of higher socioeconomic status. African-American and Hispanic women are particularly vulnerable to obesity, and Native Americans have a high prevalence of obesity across both sexes. Consequently, prevention and early intervention are especially imperative in these high-risk populations.

Medical complications

Obesity is a chronic condition, associated with increased morbidity and mortality. Research has indicated strong links between obesity and an increased risk of hypertension, dyslipidemia, type 2 diabetes, coronary heart disease, stroke, gallbladder disease, osteoarthritis, sleep apnea, respiratory abnormalities, and certain types of cancer (colon, breast, prostate, and endometrial). Abdominal adiposity is indicative of an increased risk for type 2 diabetes and coronary heart disease; for example, metabolic syndrome, a clustering of metabolic risk factors (hyperinsulinemia, glucose intolerance, dyslipidemia, and hypertension), is associated with high amounts of abdominal adipose tissue. In women, obesity is also associated with menstrual irregularity and amenorrhea, impaired fertility, and increased risk of complications during pregnancy. Overall, mortality is markedly increased for obese individuals, particularly for those with class III obesity, and is modestly increased for overweight but not obese individuals.

Psychological and social correlates

Obesity is associated with psychological and social problems, as well as with an increased risk for comorbid psychiatric disorders. Psychosocial functioning is decreased in the obese. Obese individuals frequently suffer from lower self-esteem and a more negative body image than their normal-weight counterparts. For example, they may be more dissatisfied and preoccupied with their physical appearance and more likely to avoid social situations because of body-related concerns. Obesity confers negative consequences not only on psychosocial but also on physical aspects of quality of life, e.g., impairment of daily life routines through limited mobility. Furthermore, obesity increases the likelihood of experiencing discrimination in a variety of settings: it is associated with disadvantages in employment, education, renting a residence, and getting married. Pervasive societal attitudes stigmatizing obese individuals as "lazy," "stupid," "cheats," and "ugly" may contribute to this discrimination. Unfortunately, obese patients frequently feel that they are treated disrespectfully by health care professionals, among whom negative stereotypes of obesity are common. Consequently, obese individuals may be hesitant to seek health care, which precludes early detection of medical problems and thus may contribute to an exacerbation of health care costs. Obesity also burdens society at large, with related health care and lost productivity costs amounting to nearly $100 billion per year.

Comorbid psychiatric psychopathology, e.g., depressive symptomatology, has been shown to be more prevalent in obese individuals seeking weight loss treatment than in normal-weight individuals. Binge eating disorder, characterized by recurrent binge eating in the absence of regular use of inappropriate compensatory behaviors (described below), frequently occurs in obese individuals. Another eating-related syndrome, night eating syndrome (NES), has established links with obesity. NES combines symptoms of disordered eating, sleep, and mood. It is characterized by a delay in onset of appetite in the morning (morning anorexia), followed by overeating at night (evening hyperphagia). In contrast to obese individuals without NES, individuals with NES consume most of their daily caloric intake in snacks after the last evening meal (between 8 pm and 6 am), frequently during nightly awakenings. Related to insomnia, individuals with NES display lower mood than individuals without NES but, unlike many depressed people, experience a drop rather than improvement in mood during the evening. NES is currently understood as a disorder of biological rhythm intensified in response to stress. While rare in the general population, NES is more common among obese people; initial findings suggest that 10–25% of obese individuals seeking weight loss treatment may suffer from NES. In need of further empirical evidence, NES is currently not included in the *Diagnostic and Statistical Manual of Mental Disorders* (DSM-IV).

Etiology

Obesity is best understood as a multifactorial condition resulting from genetic, environmental, and behavioral factors. Adoption, twin, and family studies have established the heritability of body weight, with genetic factors explaining 30–70% of the variance in BMI. Individuals with a family history of obesity have 2–3 times greater risk of developing obesity than the general population. The genetic basis for obesity is corroborated by molecular genetic research. Six single gene defects have been identified as accounting for a small portion of obesity cases, e.g., mutations in the gene encoding leptin on chromosome 7. Most cases of obesity are potentially influenced by a large number of genes, located on all human chromosomes except chromosome Y. A criticism of this genetic research is that it narrowly focuses on a few aspects of obesity phenotypes (e.g., excess of body mass or percent body fat) and misses other genetically based phenotypes relevant to obesity, e.g., behavioral phenotypes.

Behavioral phenotypes such as eating behavior (e.g., strong preferences for dietary fat), physical activity, and mood (e.g., depression) have a considerable genetic component. The relationship between genes and their behavioral phenotypes is largely unknown. Nevertheless, integration of molecular genetic research with an understanding of metabolic pathways regulating energy expenditure and food intake may contribute to the development of effective approaches for the treatment and prevention of obesity.

A discussion of new findings involving leptin serves to illustrate clinical applications of molecular research. Hypothalamic pathways of energy metabolism, which are the best studied pathways for the regulation of energy intake and expenditure, are controlled by leptin. Leptin, a protein hormone, suppresses food intake and stimulates energy expenditure. It is primarily produced by adipocytes in white fat tissue. Secreted into the circulation, leptin acts on specific brain areas through the leptin receptor. Neuronal hypothalamic targets of leptin, including proopiomelanocortin and neuropeptide y/agouti-related peptide neurons, exert opposing effects on energy balance and are reciprocally regulated by changes in fat stores. Although most obese individuals have normal genetic sequences for leptin and its receptor, observations of decreased leptin concentrations in cerebrospinal fluid led to the suggestion that obese individuals may be resistant to leptin. Initial studies suggest that recombinant human leptin may potentially be effective for treatment of leptin-deficient patients, as well as for enhancing weight loss outcome in overweight people without mutations in the leptin gene. Likewise, melanocortin, β_3-adrenergic, and cholecystokinin receptor agonists are currently being explored for potential use in pharmacological treatment of obesity.

While genes determine who in a given population is susceptible to obesity, environmental factors are responsible for their expression. Much of the recent rise in obesity has been attributed to a "toxic environment," in which high-fat, high-calorie foods are often the most inexpensive and accessible options available, especially in the form of fast food. Furthermore, billions of dollars are spent each year on advertising unhealthy foods and beverages, resulting in constant reminders of their palatability. Portion sizes have markedly increased in the past several decades. In addition, energy-saving devices such as elevators, automobiles, and computers are commonplace and may facilitate a sedentary lifestyle.

Although the environment is likely to fuel the obesity epidemic, the interaction between environmental factors and behavior is not clear. Despite increased use of low-calorie and low-fat products, daily calorie consumption has increased over past decades. It has been argued that a decline in non-leisure physical activity (e.g., occupational or household activity) and an increase in sedentary leisure activities (e.g., television viewing) have especially contributed to reduced energy expenditure over the last few decades, likely leading to a positive energy balance. A consistently positive energy balance, even if the differences between energy intake and energy expenditure are very minor, can lead to large changes in body fat mass over time. For example, for the average non-obese adult, a daily ingestion of only 150 calories more than expended, the caloric equivalent of 12 oz of soda, could result in the accumulation of approximately 12 lbs of adipose tissue in one year. The effects of a small energy surplus on body weight is especially relevant in view of increasing portion sizes, as experimental studies support the fact that people tend to eat more if larger portion sizes are offered. Paradoxically, the decrease in smoking over the past several decades may be partly responsible for the rise in obesity, as smoking cessation is often accompanied by weight gain.

Another etiological factor, especially relevant to psychiatric populations, is drug-induced weight gain. In particular, many antipsychotic (e.g., thioridazine, olanzapine, chlorpromazine, risperidone and clozapine), antimanic (e.g., lithium, valproic acid, carbamazepine), and antidepressant medications (e.g., tricyclics such as amitriptyline, the monoamine oxidase inhibitor [MAOI] phenelzine) induce weight gain.

Treatment of obesity

Treatment of obesity is aimed at improving health and well-being. Although losing weight is probably the most emphasized approach for the treatment of obesity, it is important to note that weight loss is only one means by which these aims can be reached. For example, physical activity is effective in improving both health and psychological well-being and also reduces the risk of disorders commonly associated with obesity. However, there is convincing evidence that even a modest weight loss of 5–10% of initial body weight significantly reduces health risks and improves health and well-being (e.g., mood, psychosocial functioning, and quality of life) in obese patients, at least in the short term. Body image can also be improved through weight loss, although it may be adversely affected by weight regain.

CONSIDER CONSULTATION WHEN...

- BMI* > 40 kg/m², or >35 kg/m² with comorbidity.
- Medical conditions requiring specialized care are present (e.g., coronary artery disease).
- Patient exhibits comorbid psychopathology (e.g., binge eating disorder, depression).
- Quality of life is drastically impaired.
- * BMI indicates body mass index.

To date, a variety of treatment approaches for obesity is available, including behavioral weight loss treatments (BWL), pharmacotherapy, surgery, and combinations of these approaches. BWL treatment represents the first-line treatment for obesity. According to the guidelines of the National Institutes of Health, weight loss through BWL is indicated for obese patients with a BMI > 30 kg/m², as well as for overweight patients with medical comorbidities. Pharmacotherapy should be considered only for patients not responding to BWL treatment (i.e., weight loss <1 lb after six months of BWL treatment). Pharmacotherapy may be used in obese patients with a BMI > 30 kg/m², and in patients with a BMI of 27–29.9 kg/m² and comorbid medical disorders. Weight loss surgery should be reserved for patients with a BMI > 40 kg/m² and for patients who have a BMI of 35–39.9 kg/m² with comorbid medical disorders for whom other treatment options have failed. Of note, weight loss is not indicated for overweight patients at low risk; rather, these patients should be counseled about possible lifestyle changes in order to maintain weight and to prevent further weight gain. Further, weight loss is not indicated for pregnant or lactating women, individuals with uncontrolled psychiatric disorders (e.g., active substance use disorder), individuals with anorexia nervosa or bulimia nervosa, or individuals whose medical condition does not allow for caloric restriction.

Behavioral weight loss treatment

Behavioral weight loss (BWL) treatment is presently considered the standard treatment for obesity. BWL treatment primarily aims to modify eating habits and physical activity, emphasizing behavior change in order to restrict energy intake and to increase energy expenditure. The aim is to obtain a negative energy balance, thereby facilitating weight loss. A number of cognitive and behavioral strategies are employed to induce behavior change, e.g., goal setting of calorie intake, physical activity, and weight loss; self-monitoring of food intake and physical activity; and problem-solving regarding barriers to change.

BWL programs are typically administered on a group basis; user-friendly manuals for health-care practitioners are available. Duration of treatment ranges from four to six months of weekly sessions. Once the patient achieves the target weight loss, weight maintenance needs to be prioritized. Weight maintenance requires continued care in which the described behavioral principles are applied for sustaining weight loss, and relapse prevention training is provided. Extended treatment contact, e.g., via telephone, email, or clinic visits, has been shown to enhance maintenance of weight loss. Additional social support (e.g., self-help groups) may facilitate weight maintenance.

BWL treatment typically emphasizes moderate caloric restriction (1,200–1,500 kcal per day), but has also utilized very-low-calorie diets (VLCDs) of 800 kcal or fewer. VLCD initially produces faster weight loss than moderate caloric restriction, but weight regain usually occurs more rapidly, resulting in a net weight loss equivalent to that produced with moderate caloric restriction. Therefore, severe caloric restriction is not recommended as a dietary regimen. Low-carbohydrate diets (high-fat, high-protein) are currently popular (e.g., Atkins diet) and also show promising results for more rapid initial weight loss than standard BWL treatment, although net weight loss appears to be equivalent with longer durations of treatment. However, the long-term efficacy and safety of low-carbohydrate diets are not sufficiently established (e.g., risk of kidney disease from high-protein intake). Presently, low-fat, high-carbohydrate diets derived from the food guide pyramid are the most well-established dietary regimens (see Fig. 16.1).

Beyond caloric restriction, the achievement of a negative energy balance is facilitated by physical activity. While physical activity alone has only a minor effect on initial weight loss, it has consistently been shown to prevent or delay weight regain and is thus critical for effective maintenance of weight loss. BWL treatments focus on promoting lifestyle physical activity. In the lifestyle physical activity approach, patients are encouraged to change a sedentary lifestyle by integrating more physical activity into their daily lives through routines at home and at work, for example, by using stairs instead of the elevator or walking to work or to

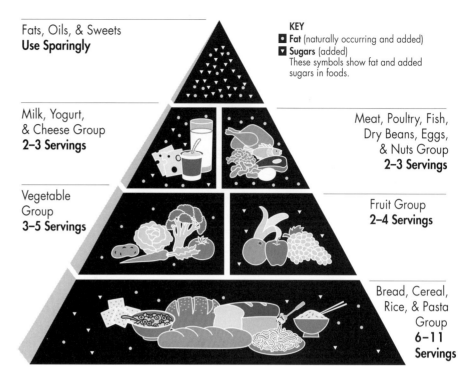

KEY
- **Fat** (naturally occurring and added)
- **Sugars** (added)
  These symbols show fat and added sugars in foods.

Fats, Oils, & Sweets
Use Sparingly

Milk, Yogurt,
& Cheese Group
2–3 Servings

Meat, Poultry, Fish,
Dry Beans, Eggs,
& Nuts Group
2–3 Servings

Vegetable
Group
3–5 Servings

Fruit Group
2–4 Servings

Bread, Cereal,
Rice, & Pasta
Group
**6–11
Servings**

Fig. 16.1 United States Department of Agriculture and United States Department of Health and Human Services Food Guide Pyramid. From the United States Department of Agriculture website <http://www.usda.gov>.

the store. Lifestyle physical activity is as effective as traditional exercise training (e.g., formal aerobics classes) in improving activity levels, cardiopulmonary fitness, blood pressure, and body composition. Furthermore, it may be more suitable for patients who dislike vigorous activity or who lack time to exercise. Current physical activity guidelines recommend that patients accumulate at least 30 minutes of moderate-intensity lifestyle or formal activity (e.g., brisk walking, cycling) on most days of the week. For safety purposes, patients should slowly increase activity levels until the recommended amount is accrued. Home-based training, such as home treadmill use, may improve adherence to structured exercise routines, however, data are mixed regarding its benefit over on-site activity (e.g., in health clubs).

With 4–6 months of treatment duration, BWL treatment generally produces an average weight loss of 7–10% of initial body weight. BWL treatment also significantly improves depression, self-esteem, body image, and interpersonal functioning. However, a criticism of BWL is that short-term weight loss is typically not well maintained in the long term without ongoing clinical contact. At one-year follow-up, approximately one-third of lost weight is regained. For most but not all patients, lost weight is gradually regained over time. The long-term effects of BWL treatment on psychosocial outcomes, such as quality of life or depression, are not clear. Predictors of successful weight loss consist of early weight loss and compliance with self-monitoring during

BWL treatment. There is also encouraging data suggesting better weight maintenance with longer-term care.

Pharmacological treatment

Pharmacotherapy has been used to treat obesity since the early 20th century, but public interest was stimulated in 1992 with the introduction of the combination drug fenfluramine/phentermine (Pondimin, and Adipex or Fastin, respectively). This drug produced sustained weight loss but was taken off the market after reports of primary pulmonary hypertension and valvular heart disease surfaced. Currently, two medications, sibutramine and orlistat, are approved by the Food and Drug Administration (FDA) for long-term use of up to two years. Their use is only recommended in conjunction with BWL treatment, producing a 5–20 lbs greater weight loss than BWL treatment alone. Further, weight-loss medications have been found to facilitate long-term maintenance of weight loss. However, regaining weight is common following discontinuation of medication.

Sibutramine (Meridia), an appetite suppressant, inhibits the reuptake of serotonin and norepinephrine. In conjunction with a lifestyle modification program, sibutramine produces weight loss of about 5–8% of initial body weight over six months, compared to 4% produced by sibutramine alone, and 1–4% produced by placebo. Over the long term, sibutramine has proven effective in helping sustain weight loss, both when prescribed during or following BWL treatment.

In addition to its weight loss effects, sibutramine has been associated with improvements in triglycerides and high-density lipoprotein (HDL) cholesterol. Higher doses of sibutramine induce greater weight loss (4% weight loss with 5 mg, 6% with 10 mg, or 7% with 15 mg after six months of treatment), and standard dosing of 10 mg once daily can be increased to 15 mg in the absence of adequate initial weight loss. Adverse effects lead to discontinuation in approximately 9% of patients and include constipation, dry mouth, headaches, insomnia, and, in some cases, increased blood pressure. Sibutramine is not recommended for patients taking serotonergic agents (e.g., fluoxetine, fluvoxamine, paroxetine) or MAOIs; those with poorly controlled hypertension, a history of coronary artery disease, congestive heart disease, arrhythmia, stroke, severe renal or hepatic impairment, or seizures; or for women who are breast-feeding or pregnant.

Orlistat (Xenical) reduces fat absorption from the intestines by binding to gastrointestinal lipases. Standard intake of 120 mg of orlistat within one hour after meals leads to excretion of approximately one-third of ingested dietary fat in the stool. In conjunction with a low-calorie diet, 120 mg daily of orlistat results in a weight loss of about 9% of initial body weight after the first year vs. approximately 6% among those treated with 30 mg of orlistat, 7% among those treated with 60 mg of orlistat, and 6% among those treated with placebo. Over the second year of use, it has been shown to facilitate weight maintenance. Furthermore, when prescribed following dietary management, orlistat results in significantly less weight regain than placebo. It has also been shown to reduce LDL cholesterol independent of reductions induced by weight loss. Adverse effects include mild to moderate gastrointestinal symptoms (e.g., flatulence at discharge, steatorrhea, fecal urgency, fecal incontinence, oily spotting, increased frequency of defecation), which generally lessen after twelve weeks of treatment, but may lead to increased discontinuation of the treatment (approximately 9%). Orlistat also limits the absorption of fat-soluble vitamins, thus multivitamin supplementation is recommended. Orlistat is not advisable for pregnant or breast-feeding women or for patients with chronic malabsorption or cholestasis.

Topiramate (Topamax), an anticonvulsant, is being evaluated at the time of writing for the treatment of obesity. One randomized controlled trial has shown its efficacy over placebo (5–6% weight loss with topiramate, dose dependent, vs. 3% weight loss with placebo). Another longer-term trial replicated these findings over one year (7–9.7% weight loss with topiramate, dose-dependent, vs 1.7% weight loss with placebo). Further research is needed to determine its long-term efficacy and safety.

Several over-the-counter drugs touting weight-loss effects are also available (e.g., chitosan, chromium picolinate, and conjugated linoleic acid), but their efficacy and safety are not sufficiently documented. The ephedrine (ephedra or ma huang) and caffeine combination (guarana, kola nut), found in many herbal weight-loss products, induces greater weight loss than placebo for up to one year. However, because of the risk of harmful effects, e.g., hypertension, tachycardia, and stroke, the Food and Drug Administration has issued a rule prohibiting the sale of products containing ephedrine and has warned consumers using and buying ephedra products.

Surgical treatment

At the time of writing bariatric surgery is the only treatment shown to be effective in the long-term management of extreme obesity. As a result of weight loss through bariatric surgery, obesity-related comorbidity remits or improves (e.g., type 2 diabetes, metabolic syndrome [hyperinsulinemia, hypertension, glucose intolerance, and dyslipidemia], sleep apnea, asthma, daytime sleepiness, infertility), and disease risk is lowered (e.g., for cardiovascular disease). Psychosocial outcomes, such as depressive symptoms, self-esteem, body image, and quality of life, are also likely to be improved.

Nevertheless, expected benefits and risks of bariatric surgery need to be carefully weighed for each individual patient. Bariatric surgery carries with it a roughly 2% mortality risk, a risk of short-term complications (e.g., peritonitis, anastomotic leaks) and long-term complications (e.g., cholelithiasis, vitamin and mineral deficiencies), and continued medical monitoring is required thereafter. Eating habits are fundamentally changed; for example, patients with restricted gastric capacity are no longer able to eat more than a limited amount of food at one time, and therefore need to eat several small meals per day. However, despite the limitations imposed by surgery, some patients manage to eat in a way that maintains their preoperative weight. An average of 20–30% of patients who undergo bariatric surgery are unimproved in the long term. Surgery is not indicated in patients with uncontrolled psychiatric diseases (for psychological assessment, see Practice Guidelines for Obesity and BED-Assessment, later in this chapter), in patients who are unable to understand the impact of the procedure or in patients who report being unable to comply with procedural requirements.

Bariatric surgery achieves its effects by limiting the stomach's capacity (restrictive procedures) and/or inhibiting absorption of ingested nutrients (malabsorptive procedures). The most common surgical procedures are Roux-en-Y gastric bypass (RYGB), gastric banding, and vertical banded gastroplasty (VBG) (for illustrations, see http://www.niddk.nih.gov/health/nutrit/pubs/gastric/gastricsurgery.htm).

RYGB combines a restrictive and malabsorptive approach. A small gastric pouch beneath the esophagus is created to which a section of the small intestine is attached ("Roux limb"), forming a y-shape with the remaining portion of the small intestines. This allows food to bypass the lower portion of the stomach, the duodenum, and the first portion of the jejunum, thus reducing caloric absorption. RYGB is currently considered the gold standard in weight loss surgery, with approximately 65% of excess weight lost after two years and 50–60% after 5–14 years. RYGB carries a 3–20% risk of major complications, including pulmonary embolus, gastrointestinal leak, and anastomotic stricture in the short term, and hernia, ulcers, and bowel obstructions in the long term. Wound-related complications can be reduced by laparoscopic operation. A common nutritional complication, encountered by over 50% of patients undergoing RYGB, is the dumping syndrome, consisting of nausea, flushing, lightheadedness, and diarrhea that occurs after consumption of high-sugar liquid meal (e.g., ice cream). Multivitamin and mineral supplementation is recommended.

Adjustable gastric banding, a restrictive procedure, places an inflatable silicone band below the esophagus in order to form a small gastric pouch with an adjustable outlet (LAP-BAND). The operation is mainly performed laparoscopically. Unlike RYGB and VBG, gastric banding is reversible, and the size of the outlet can be adjusted according to patients' needs by inflating or deflating the band. Gastric banding results in a loss of about 40–60% of excess body weight after three to five years. Operative mortality is rare, and major complications are usually uncommon. However, high failure rates have occasionally been reported, with a significant number of patients (<13%) requiring band removal as a result of inadequate weight loss or complications such as band slippage, leakage from the inflatable silicone ring or infection. Other complications include solid food intolerance, stomach perforation, intra-abdominal infection, and pulmonary embolism.

VBG, formerly the most commonly performed surgical procedure for obesity, limits gastric capacity by creating a small vertically stapled pouch below the esophagus. A band of nonexpandable synthetic material placed around the distal portion of the pouch limits its opening to the stomach. VBG results in a 30–50% loss of excess weight three to five years postsurgery, with decreasing success rates over time. VBG carries a risk of complications (<15%), including leaks or tearing at the surgical site, wound infection, band erosion, ulcer formation, vomiting, subphrenic abscess formation, and stomal obstruction. Multivitamin supplementation is recommended.

Classification, clinical description, and etiology of binge eating disorder

Classification

Binge eating disorder (BED) is an eating disorder that is prevalent in a subset of the obese population. BED is included in the DSM-IV as a provisional diagnosis in need of further study and is currently classified as an Eating Disorder

PEARLS & PERILS

- Currently, about 30% of American adults are obese, and 64% are overweight or obese.
- Rates of obesity increase with age, and are higher in females, minority populations, and groups with lower socioeconomic status.
- Obesity is associated with medical complications such as coronary heart disease, type 2 diabetes, and certain types of cancer. It is also associated with negative psychosocial outcomes such as reduced quality of life, disadvantages in employment, education, and marriage.
- The development and maintenance of obesity is caused by an interaction of genetic, environmental, and behavioral factors.
- Behavioral weight loss (BWL) treatment is the standard treatment for obesity. As a second step, pharmacological treatments may be added to BWL if BMI* > 30 kg/m², or > 27 kg/m² with comorbid medical conditions. Surgical treatments are indicated for individuals with a BMI > 40 kg/m², or a BMI > 35 kg/m² with comorbid medical conditions when other treatments have failed.

*BMI indicates body mass index.

KEY CLINICAL QUESTIONS AND WHAT THEY UNLOCK

- *Was the patient obese as a child?*
  Since childhood obesity is a negative prognostic indicator for psychosocial and medical outcomes, patients with childhood onset of obesity may need additional assessment and specialized care.
- *Does the patient have medical conditions that may have contributed to the development of obesity?*
  Medical conditions contributing to the development of obesity (e.g., hypothyroidism) require adequate treatment.
- *Does the patient have characteristics associated with the development of other medical disease?*
  If premorbid disease characteristics are present (e.g., pre-diabetes), consider whether weight loss alone will be sufficient for prevention of full-syndromal disease development.
- *Has the patient attempted to lose weight in the past?*
  If the patient has failed at weight loss attempts in the past, pharmacotherapy or surgical treatment may be indicated.
- *Is the patient's weight gain associated with the use of medications that may have contributed to the problem?*
  In case of drug-induced weight gain, consider replacement or adjusting dosage.
- *Does the patient have comorbid psychiatric conditions?*
  For obese patients with comorbid psychopathology (e.g., binge eating disorder), a stepped care approach may be considered.

Not Otherwise Specified (EDNOS). BED is characterized by the consumption of large amounts of food in a discrete period of time with an accompanying sense of loss of control and in the absence of regular use of inappropriate compensatory behaviors aimed at preventing weight gain. The disorder has established links with obesity, making it a complex problem with psychological and medical sequelae. However, it should be noted that a substantial portion (35–40%) of individuals with BED do not meet the criteria for obesity.

BOX 16.1

Research criteria for binge eating disorder

A. Recurrent episodes of binge eating. An episode of binge eating is characterized by both of the following:
  • eating, in a discrete period of time (e.g., within any two-hour period), an amount of food that is definitely larger than most people would eat in a similar period of time under similar circumstances
  • a sense of lack of control over eating during the episode (e.g., a feeling that one cannot stop eating or control what or how much one is eating).

B. The binge eating episodes are associated with three (or more) of the following:
  • eating much more rapidly than normal
  • eating until feeling uncomfortably full
  • eating large amounts of food when not feeling physically hungry
  • eating alone because of being embarrassed by how much one is eating
  • feeling disgusted with oneself, depressed, or very guilty after overeating.

C. Marked distress regarding binge eating is present.

D. The binge eating occurs, on average, at least two days a week for six months.

E. The binge eating is not associated with the regular use of inappropriate compensatory behaviors (e.g., purging, fasting, excessive exercise) and does not occur exclusively during the course of anorexia nervosa or bulimia nervosa.

From American Psychiatric Association (2000) Diagnostic and Statistical Manual of Mental Disorders, 4th edition, Text Revision, Washington, D.C., American Psychiatric Association.

Epidemiology

Binge eating disorder is the most prevalent eating disorder, with rates ranging from 2–3% of the adult population, approximately 8% of the overweight population in community samples, and more than 25% of the severely obese weight-loss treatment-seeking population. BED is common in both men and women (3:2 female to male ratio) and in minorities, particularly African-American and Hispanic individuals.

DIAGNOSIS

Table 16.2 Binge eating disorder

Discriminating features

1. Recurrent binge eating with an accompanying sense of loss of control and in the absence of regular inappropriate compensatory behaviors aimed to prevent weight gain.

Consistent features

1. Overevaluation of shape and weight.
2. Moderate dietary restraint.
3. Impaired psychosocial functioning.
4. Overweight.

Variable features

1. Co-occuring Axis I and/or Axis II psychiatric disorders.
2. Comorbid obesity.
3. Medical conditions associated with obesity.

Medical complications

Overall, obese individuals with BED exhibit the same types and rates of medical comorbidities as obese individuals without BED. They, however, self-report poorer physical health status and present with more medical complaints, such as greater sleep disturbance and neck, shoulder, back, and muscle pain, than the non-BED obese.

Psychological and social correlates

Individuals with BED suffer from higher eating disorder and general psychopathology than individuals without BED. They display more chaotic eating patterns and greater disinhibition and emotional eating. They also exhibit more shape and weight concerns as well as overevaluation of shape and weight than individuals without BED. Individuals with BED suffer from lower self-esteem, greater interpersonal problems, and more impairment in work and social functioning than obese individuals without BED. BED is further associated with increased rates of DSM-IV psychiatric disorders, most prominently Axis I mood disorders, anxiety disorders, and substance abuse disorders, and Axis II personality disorders.

Etiology and course

Emerging evidence has revealed the following risk factors for BED: adverse childhood experiences (e.g., sexual or physical abuse, bullying); family problems and psychopathology (e.g., parental psychiatric disorder, parental criticism, lack of affection, underinvolvement or overprotection); and repeated exposure to teasing and negative comments about eating, shape, and weight. Negative self-evaluations and childhood obesity also increase the risk for later development of BED. Furthermore, the genetic basis for BED is currently being investigated (e.g., mutations in the melanocortin-4 receptor gene).

Two subtypes of BED have been identified based on the pattern of onset: those whose binge eating precedes their first dieting attempt and those whose dieting precedes their binge eating. Those who report binge eating prior to their first attempt at dieting report an earlier onset of BED (childhood or adolescence) than those whose first dieting attempt preceded their binge eating (early adulthood). These individuals also may show higher levels of eating disorder and general psychopathology. The course of BED is controversial because of ambiguity regarding stability of the disorder and rates of spontaneous remission. Some studies show persistence of BED symptomatology, while others suggest a tendency of remission over time. In clinical settings, patients with BED often report a long history of the illness. Thus, it is plausible that BED has a fluctuating course, marked by intermittent remission and resurgence of symptoms. Future studies will help to clarify the natural course of BED.

Treatment of binge eating disorder

BED's distinctive combination of eating disorder, comorbid psychiatric disturbance, impairment in psychosocial functioning, and obesity poses a challenge to clinicians wanting to treat the psychological and/or medical symptoms associated with the disorder. Currently, a stepped-care approach is recommended, with medical urgency of weight loss, degree of psychopathology, patient preference, and available resources determining the order and type of treatment. In obese patients with BED who present with eating disorder and general psychopathology, evidence-based psychotherapy (e.g., cognitive-behavioral therapy, interpersonal psychotherapy) may represent the first step of treatment that can, as a second step, be augmented by weight loss treatment. However, with high medical comorbidity, weight loss treatment represents the first-line treatment that, if necessary, can be supplemented by psychotherapy. Normal or overweight patients with BED who do not exhibit other evidence of eating disorders or general psychopathology may first be treated with self-help approaches before psychotherapy warrants consideration.

Psychotherapy

Cognitive-behavioral therapy
Cognitive-behavioral therapy (CBT) is the best established treatment for BED. Adapted from CBT for bulimia nervosa, CBT for BED focuses on normalization of eating patterns and relief of distress associated with binge eating, but it is not specifically aimed at weight loss. CBT for BED progresses through three distinct stages, usually over twenty sessions, and is applicable in individual and group formats. Sessions are structured and problem-oriented.

During stage one, overall chaotic eating habits are normalized through the introduction of a regular pattern of eating (e.g., three planned meals, two planned snacks), and through use of self-monitoring of food intake and nutritional counseling. Calorie-counting may help patients to establish healthy restraint over eating. Patients are encouraged to weigh themselves weekly and to engage in regular physical activity, both to balance energy intake and expenditure and to promote active stress management. During this initial stage, patients are taught techniques to avoid binge eating, such as planning behavior that is incompatible with binge eating (i.e., taking a walk) and avoiding foods that typically trigger binges. Further, information is provided on healthy body weight regulation, the adverse effects of dieting, and the causes and consequences of binge eating and obesity.

During stage two, the focus of treatment is on identification and modification of dysfunctional thoughts and beliefs about dieting, shape, and weight. Main therapeutic techniques include self-monitoring of negative thoughts and cognitive restructuring. Patients are also taught problem-solving skills in order to cope with specific problems rather than using binge eating for the solution of such problems. At this stage of treatment, typical "trigger" foods are reincorporated into planned meals and snacks. Unrealistic weight-loss goals and perceived failures regarding eating and weight are also the focus of cognitive interventions. Furthermore, psychoeducation focuses on the psychosocial consequences of being obese in a weight-conscious society.

In the third stage of treatment, the focus is on maintenance of change. Strategies for preventing or dealing with relapse are devised, and the patient is encouraged to develop realistic expectations concerning potential setbacks. Therapeutic work focuses on patient acceptance of a larger-than-average body size that may not be easily modified.

CBT for BED typically results in an 80–95% reduction in binge frequency, with approximately 50% of patients achieving abstinence from binge eating at post-treatment. Changes are largely maintained in the long term, with a slight decline in recovery and abstinence rates at follow-up, but frequency of binge eating remaining significantly below pretreatment levels. CBT results in modest but significant decreases in BMI, with patients who are abstinent from binge eating tending to lose the most weight (approximately 5 lbs), and those who are no longer recovered tending to gain weight. Furthermore, abstinence is associated with better maintenance of weight loss and significantly improves weight loss outcome in subsequent BWL treatment, thus advocating a stepped care approach. Usually, CBT is highly acceptable to patients. Greater binge frequency prior to treatment seems to predict poor outcome, possibly indicating a longer duration of treatment in these patients. In addition, greater interpersonal problems and younger age at pretreatment predict lower likelihood of abstinence.

Interpersonal psychotherapy

Interpersonal psychotherapy (IPT) makes the basic assumption that binge eating occurs in an interpersonal context and that current interpersonal relationships have an impact on treatment outcome. Therefore, IPT for BED focuses on identifying and changing the interpersonal context in which the disorder developed and/or is currently maintained. Like CBT, IPT for BED progresses through three stages, lasts approximately twenty sessions, and can be applied to both individual and group formats.

The first stage of treatment focuses on problem identification. The therapist provides and explains the diagnosis of BED to the patient and then describes the nature and rationale of IPT. The interpersonal inventory is conducted, the goal of which is to identify the interpersonal problem areas associated with the onset and/or maintenance of binge eating. This entails reviewing past and present relationships and evaluating interpersonal precipitants to specific episodes of binge eating. Four areas of interpersonal problems exist: unresolved grief because of a loss of a person or relationship; interpersonal role disputes, referring to conflicts with family members or other significant people that arise from differing expectations about the relationship; role transitions or difficulties associated with a change in life status, such as moving, changing jobs, marrying, or getting divorced; and interpersonal deficits, applying to patients who are socially isolated or are in chronically unsatisfying relationships. Collaboratively, therapist and patient select interpersonal problem areas contributing to BED and set up goals for treatment.

The second phase of IPT focuses on developing and implementing strategies to resolve the identified interpersonal problems. This involves illuminating connections between interpersonal events and resulting eating disorder symptoms. Further, the patient is encouraged to identify and manage negative mood states associated with interpersonal problem areas. Therapeutic techniques that may be utilized include exploratory techniques for clarification, encouragement of affect, and communication analysis.

In the final stage of treatment, the goal is to consolidate work the patient has done thus far and outline areas for remaining work. The patient is educated about the end of treatment as a time for potential grieving and is encouraged to identify and verbalize associated emotions. Progress is reviewed in order to foster feelings of accomplishment and competence. Further, the patient is advised to identify areas and warning signs of anticipated relapse. Finally, a specific plan is devised for continued work after treatment is terminated.

IPT has proven as effective as CBT for the treatment of BED. At post-treatment, binge frequency is reduced by about 90%, with about 60% of patients abstinent from binge eating and approximately 70% recovered from a clinically significant eating disorder at one-year follow-up. Improvement is also evident in eating disorder and general psychopathology. These gains are maintained over one year following treatment, with binge frequency remaining significantly lower than baseline and recovery and abstinence rates remaining only slightly lower than those seen at post-treatment. As with CBT, IPT participants who achieve abstinence following treatment can expect a modest weight loss. IPT is similarly acceptable to patients, and dropout rates are low. Greater severity of binge eating and greater interpersonal problems at baseline predict a lower likelihood of abstinence following IPT treatment; thus, such patients may require a different, combination, or augmented treatment approach.

Behavioral weight loss and self-help treatment

As opposed to CBT and IPT, both of which involve specialist care (e.g., through trained therapists), BWL and self-help treatments can be administered by non-mental health professionals such as nurses and dietitians. Furthermore, BWL and self-help treatments are more disseminable and less costly than specialist treatments such as CBT and IPT.

A few studies have addressed the short-term effects of BWL in obese patients with BED. Given the link between dieting and the onset of bulimia nervosa (See Chapter 15), it was argued that dietary treatment might trigger or exacerbate binge eating in obese patients with BED. On the contrary, moderate caloric restriction within BWL treatment was found to decrease binge eating in the short term. Initial findings suggest that BWL treatment is as effective as CBT in improving the specific and general psychopathology associated with BED, although CBT appears to produce better maintenance of change in eating disorder symptomatology than BWL treatment. Long-term effects of BWL treatment on binge eating remain unknown, and some studies suggest that individuals with BED regain weight faster following BWL than those without BED.

Self-help treatments for BED are typically manual-based forms of CBT for BED, and are applied in both guided (i.e., a book used in conjunction with guidance from a health care professional) and unguided formats (i.e., a book used by the individual alone). Both guided and unguided self-help have been found to be effective in reducing binge eating and related psychopathology in the short term, and initial evidence suggests long-term effectiveness. Future research may establish self-help as a viable treatment option for BED.

Novelty treatments that have not yet been established for the treatment of BED include dialectical behavior therapy and appetite awareness training. Dialectical behavior therapy, which focuses on affect regulation, has been shown to result in high abstinence rates at post-treatment and short-term follow-up and may prove effective after further evaluation. Appetite awareness training is a brief intervention designed to enhance eating in response to hunger and satiety, and to reduce eating in response to environmental or affective cues. Appetite awareness training shows initial efficacy in reducing binge eating.

Pharmacological and surgical treatment

Appetite suppressants (d-fenfluramine and sibutramine), antidepressants (tricyclics and selective serotonin reuptake inhibitors [SSRIs]), and anticonvulsants have been evaluated for their efficacy in reducing both weight and binge frequency in BED. However, they are not yet approved for the treatment of BED and long-term outcomes are unknown. In recent trials, the appetite suppressant sibutramine has been found to be useful in reducing weight, binge frequency, and general psychopathology among obese individuals with BED in the short term.

Evidence is mixed as to whether antidepressant treatment of BED produces greater reductions in binge frequency and weight than those produced by placebo; the tricyclics desipramine and imipramine and the SSRIs fluvoxamine, fluoxetine, and sertraline have not yet shown consistent benefit over placebo. There is little consistent evidence that adding antidepressant medication to CBT enhances a reduction of binge eating, while CBT alone appears superior to antidepressants for reducing eating disorder symptomatology. However, adding antidepressants to CBT has shown benefit in lessening depressive symptomatology, and thus they may be indicated when pronounced depressive symptomatology is present. Anticonvulsant medications, particularly topiramate (Topamax), have also shown promise in decreasing binge frequency and weight in some individuals with BED in the short term.

PEARLS & PERILS

- BED is associated with overweight and obesity, although it may also be seen in normal-weight individuals.
- Cognitive-behavioral therapy and interpersonal psychotherapy have demonstrated the most robust long-term treatment outcomes.
- According to a stepped care model, obese patients with BED with high eating disorder and general psychopathology may benefit from evidence-based psychotherapy as the first step of treatment that later may be augmented by weight loss treatment. For BED patients with extreme obesity or high medical comorbidity, weight loss treatment represents the first step of treatment that may be supplemented by evidence-based psychotherapy.

KEY CLINICAL QUESTIONS AND WHAT THEY UNLOCK

Screening for BED should focus on forms of overeating and loss of control, weight loss attempts, and extreme compensatory behaviors aimed at preventing weight gain, and shape and weight concerns; questionnaires and interviews are available.

- *How severe is the binge eating behavior?*
  Treatment duration may increase with severity of binge eating problems.
- *Is the patient depressed?*
  Comorbid depression may indicate the necessity for specialist treatment with or without additional antidepressant medication.
- *How old is the patient? Does the patient have problems with his or her relationships with friends, family, and coworkers?*
  Older patients may have better outcome in cognitive-behavioral therapy than in interpersonal psychotherapy, while individuals with high interpersonal distress may have better weight loss outcome in interpersonal psychotherapy.
- *Did the patient have difficulties with binge eating prior to his or her first attempt at dieting?*
  If binge eating preceded the first attempt at dieting, the patient is likely at increased risk for additional psychiatric disturbances requiring specialist care.

Concerning surgical weight loss treatment, BED may be a negative outcome predictor. Eating disorder symptomatology may persist after bariatric surgery, and individuals with BED report greater weight gain at long-term follow-up than those without BED.

Practice guidelines for obesity and BED

The reception of the patient

The reception of the patient requires environmental preparations and a sensitive stance towards the psychological suffering associated with obesity and BED from any health care practitioner having patient contact. Environmental conditions include easily accessible locations (e.g., locations on the first floor or elevators, broad doorways, spacious facilities); suitable furniture (e.g., chairs without arms); and special or adapted large-size equipment (e.g., measuring tape, scales measuring weight >400 lbs, extra-large gowns). Sensitivity towards obesity- and BED-related distress is advisable; patients often suffer from feelings of failure, shame, embarrassment, and guilt about body weight, shape, and binge eating. In addition, obesity-related discrimination likely worsens these feelings.

It is recommended that health care providers adopt a nonjudgmental stance towards obesity. Further, confronting a patient about his or her obesity, binge eating, and their impacts on health may result in resistance to treatment and intensify feelings of helplessness. Also, simple advice-giving ignoring the complexity of obesity and BED, but typically provided in many health care settings, will likely be ineffective (e.g., bare advice to lose weight). Techniques founded in CBT are helpful for addressing these challenges and promoting health behavior change in patients with obesity and/or BED (see below).

Assessment

Assessment should include a comprehensive medical history including a history specific to overweight issues, physical examination, and laboratory tests for medical conditions. In addition, weight, height, and waist circumference should be measured. Calculators and tables are available for quick calculations of BMI. BMI and waist circumference allow for determination of disease risk based on classification of obesity. It is important to ensure that the patient is currently receiving appropriate preventive and curative medical care (e.g., gynecological care) because patients may be hesitant to seek treatment.

Since a subset of obese patients exhibit binge eating problems, careful screening of eating pathology by practitioners is indicated. Assessment of binge eating focuses on forms of overeating and loss of control; weight loss attempts and extreme compensatory behaviors aimed at preventing weight gain (e.g., dieting, purging, use of diet pills, excessive exercising); and shape and weight concerns. Useful assessments include the Eating Disorder Examination Questionnaire (EDE-Q), a self-report questionnaire assessing the frequency of key eating disorder behaviors and other eating disorder psychopathology, and the Questionnaire for Eating and Weight Patterns (QEWP), a brief self-report scale focusing specifically on diagnostic criteria for BED. It should be noted, however, that self-report measures do not usually provide as reliable and valid information as structured clinical interviews such as the Eating Disorder Examination (EDE).

Promoting health behavior change

CBT provides useful techniques for moving patients toward behavior change. Some of these techniques have been operationalized in motivational interviewing, which takes into account that patients vary in the degree to which they are ready to change their behavior. Motivation for change needs to be assessed and, often, enhanced. Thus, motivational enhancement is undertaken by focusing on discrepancies between the patient's current behavior and goals, for example, increasing the patient's awareness of the consequences of his/her behavior (e.g., even small amounts of energy intake exceeding expenditure lead to increasing body weight over the long term) and contrasting these consequences with his/her goals (e.g., improved health). Further, ambivalence to change, which frequently interferes with treatment success at any stage, needs to be identified and addressed (e.g., asking the patient to identify advantages and disadvantages of a problem behavior such as overeating). Examples of motivational interviewing techniques and helpful questions for counseling obese patients are presented in Table 16.3.

As is the case with any other medical intervention, a collaborative and supportive relationship between practitioner and patient appears most promising for treatment success. This rapport may be established through reflective listening and asking open-ended questions. Further, the patient's problem (e.g., obesity and/or BED) should be addressed respectfully, acknowledging the patient's individual suffering. The practitioner may focus on understanding rather than arguing against the patient's views, which will likely lead to resistance.

Psychoeducation on the nature of obesity and/or BED should be provided by sharing the provider's concerns, rather than by presenting possible outcomes in a confrontational or threatening way (e.g., health risks of obesity). Effective psychoeducation requires the use of language that the patient will understand. The Internet may also be a useful source of patient information (see http://www.nhlbi.nih.gov/health/public/heart/obesity/lose_wt/index.htm; http://www.niddk.nih.gov/health/nutrit/pubs/unders.htm and binge.htm). In addition, outlining treatment options is indispensable. Hence, it should be acknowledged that although the patient is responsible for change, the practitioner might facilitate the process.

In weight loss counseling for obese patients, the emphasis is on health behavior change concerning eating and activity patterns; weight loss and maintenance are regarded as outcomes of successful implementation of both. The practitioner should educate the patient about healthy weight loss and emphasize the health benefits from even modest weight loss (or maintained body weight) and increased activity. When indicated, reasonable weight loss goals may be established collaboratively (e.g., 10% reduction of initial body weight in six months of weight-loss treatment). Many obese patients have unrealistically high weight-loss goals, and perceived failure may undermine motivation for long-term weight management.

Conclusion

Obesity and BED are major health problems associated with increased morbidity and mortality risks. Since treatment of obesity and BED is a complex challenge, prevention and early intervention should become a priority. In a preventive effort, public health efforts should focus on changing the "toxic" environment, for example, by enhancing opportunities for physical activity; promoting healthy eating by subsidizing

TABLE 16.3 Motivational interviewing techniques for obesity and sample questions

Techniques	Sample questions
Ask open-ended questions	"How are you feeling today?"
Obtain permission to speak about obesity	"Would you mind spending a few minutes talking about your weight and how you feel it is affecting your health?"
Assess readiness to change	"How do you feel about your weight?" "How ready are you to change your eating behavior?" "How ready are you to change your physical activity?"
Enhance readiness for change	"Your weight is within the range considered obese. Is there anything that you would like to know about obesity?" "Is there anything that you like about your weight?" "Would you like to share some of these things with me?" "What are the things that you don't like about your weight?" "What concerns do you have about your weight?"
Provide information about obesity in a nonthreatening way and ask for the patient's understanding	"Obesity increases the risk for certain medical problems, e.g., hypertension, stroke, diabetes, cancer, respiratory diseases, gallbladder disease. That does not mean that you necessarily will develop these diseases, but it does mean that you are at a higher risk for developing these diseases than a normal-weight person. What do you think about this?"
Share your concerns with the patient	"I am concerned that your eating and physical activity behaviors are negatively impacting your health." "I am concerned that your weight will continue to rise and will aggravate your diabetes."
Provide support for health behavior change	"Here are some options for change: learning ways to restrict energy intake and increase energy expenditure (behavioral weight loss) is the standard weight-loss treatment. It would be indicated in your case. Other options, e.g., medicines or weight loss surgery, are not indicated for you." "Balancing your eating and activity patterns can help you maintain your weight and improve your health." "What do you think would work best for you?" "What eating- and activity-related behaviors would you like to change?" "What would be your overall goals for treatment?" "What benefits do you expect from weight loss?" "Research has shown that a modest 5–10% reduction of body weight significantly reduces health risks and improves health."

the sale of healthy foods and appropriate portion sizes, e.g., in work and school environments; and by improving health education about behaviors leading to weight gain, binge eating, and obesity in a destigmatizing way. Efforts at early intervention may include counseling any overweight patient at low medical risk about possible lifestyle changes for weight maintenance and/or prevention of further weight gain. Early intervention is also imperative in overweight children and adolescents in order to prevent adult obesity and eating disorders. Children of obese parents may be at increased risk for obesity and eating disorders, and special attention is warranted by health care practitioners to assure that these children learn healthy eating behaviors and are sufficiently active.

Obesity and BED represent challenges to practitioners wishing to treat these conditions and associated medical and/or psychological disturbances. However, by receiving adequate treatment, many patients with obesity and/or BED are able to make significant and sustained improvements on overall health and well-being.

Annotated bibliography

Devlin, MJ, Yanovski, SZ, and Wilson, GT (2000) Obesity: What mental health professionals need to know, *Am J Psychiatry* 157:854–866.
This article provides a comprehensive overview of pathogenesis and treatment of obesity, tailored especially to the mental health professional diagnosing and treating obese patients.

Fairburn, CG and Brownell, KD (eds) (2002) *Eating Disorders and Obesity: A Comprehensive Handbook,* 2nd Edition, New York, Guilford Press.
An invaluable textbook providing state-of-the-art information on most relevant aspects of eating disorders and obesity. Includes comprehensive and reader-friendly chapters from renowned experts in both fields.

National Institutes of Health (1998) Clinical guidelines on the identification, evaluation, and treatment of overweight and obesity in adults: The evidence report, *Obes Res* 6(Suppl 2):51S–209S.
An excellent resource for practitioners focusing on diagnosis and evidence-based treatments for obesity.

Wilfley, DE, Wilson, GT, and Agras, WS (2003) The clinical significance of binge eating disorder. *Int J Eat Disord* 34(Suppl):S96–S106.
A critique of the literature on binge eating disorder, focusing on key features distinguishing it as an eating disorder of clinical severity.

Wilson, GT and Fairburn, CG: Eating disorders, in Nathan, PE and Gorman, JM (eds) (2002) *A Guide To Treatments That Work*, 2nd Edition, New York, Oxford University Press, 559–592.
Comprehensively reviews outcome research for anorexia nervosa, bulimia nervosa, and binge eating disorder, focusing on randomized controlled trials.

Author note

This work was supported by grant 5R01MH064153–03 from the National Institutes of Health, Bethesda, MD.

CHAPTER 17

Somatoform Disorders

Carol S. North, MD

Clinical relevance: importance and scope of the problem

Somatoform disorders present some of the most confusing and difficult problems in the practice of medicine. Somatoform disorders often go unrecognized in clinical practice, even by very experienced physicians and psychiatrists. Nonrecognition of somatoform disorders results in unnecessary medical and surgical procedures, patient dissatisfaction with medical care, and frustration of physicians. With some basic background and vigilance, most of these problems can be circumvented.

This chapter defines somatoform disorders, points out clinical indicators to alert the physician to the presence of these disorders, explains how to recognize and diagnose them, and describes their management. Because somatization disorder and conversion disorder are the most prevalent somatoform disorders and because they are the best understood of this set of disorders, this chapter focuses on these two disorders.

History of somatization and conversion disorders

Hysteria, the precursor to somatization disorder, was well known by the ancient Egyptians long before the time of Hippocrates. Hysteria was thought to be caused by a wandering uterus, hence the name hysteria, derived from the Latin word for uterus. The association of the uterus with hysteria may have sprung from the observations that this is predominantly a disorder of women and that gynecological symptoms, such as menstrual and reproductive complaints, are central to the clinical presentation.

In the 9th century, hysteria was conceptualized as a purely physical disorder. However, by the Middle Ages hysteria was viewed not as a medical condition but as a spiritual disorder of evil and demonic possession. In the 17th century, the English physician Sydenham reawakened medical interest in hysteria. Sydenham observed that hysteria could simulate almost any medical disease. More than a century ago, Briquet provided the first systematic description of hysteria with a series of 430 cases that he studied for a decade. He observed that dramatic and medically unexplained complaints were characteristic features of the disorder and that patients with these complaints were extremely impressionable and emotionally labile. He described hysteria as a serious illness with devastating effects on patients and their families. Briquet and his contemporaries, Reynolds and Charcot, classified hysteria as a disorder of the central nervous system. Although Briquet recommended the term *hysteria* be dropped because of its pejorative connotations, the condition's name was not changed until almost a century later.

Kraepelin, another contemporary of Briquet, also studied patients with hysteria. His observations showed that the characteristic features of the disorder included tendency to exaggerate, emotional instability, and severe social disability. His patients also complained of hallucinations. Around the turn of the century, Janet, Savill, Breuer, and Freud's patients with hysteria exhibited dual personalities, a popular new trend in psychiatric circles. As discussed in the Special Issues section, patients with somatization disorder are often captured by "trendy" new psychiatric or medical illnesses.

In the first half of the 20th century, the concept of hysteria focused on the histrionic personality traits associated with the disorder, submerging the characteristic unexplained medical traits. However, in the 1960s and 1970s researchers at Washington University in St Louis revived hysteria as a "medical model" syndrome, defining it on the basis of multiple unexplained medical complaints in multiple organ systems; the histrionic personality components were considered secondary. Criteria for the diagnosis proposed in the classic work of Perley and Guze required the presence of

261

at least 25 of 59 possible medically unexplained symptom complaints in at least nine of ten possible symptom groups. In honor of the first systematic observer of hysteria, Guze in 1970 suggested the name Briquet's syndrome for the disorder. This name gained popularity in many sectors, but was not universally embraced.

Current official criteria for psychiatric disorders published by the American Psychiatric Association grew out of original criteria established by research efforts of the Washington University group in the 1970s. These official criteria use the term somatization disorder in place of the older term hysteria. This new name follows the tradition of defining the disorder based on multiple unexplained somatic complaints. Although the criteria for Briquet's syndrome describe a more cohesive disorder that is more relevant to epidemiological research than the criteria for somatization disorder, in clinical practice the less cumbersome somatization disorder criteria are used in making the diagnosis.

Sigmund Freud originated the term *conversion*, applying it to symptoms he viewed as resulting from substitution of somatic symptoms for repressed emotions. According to the Freudian theory of conversion, mental conflicts are converted into physical and mental symptoms through unconscious mechanisms of symbolism (the symptom serves as a symbol of the conflict) or primary gain (that is, the desire to enact the patient role). Conversion symptoms were recognized as part of hysteria until 1980, when conversion and somatization were separated into distinct categories in DSM-III. At that juncture, somatization disorder followed the Washington University group's model of a polysomatoform disorder, and conversion disorder continued with Freudian concepts of psychological conflicts manifesting as somatic phenomena. Somatization disorder has been well validated as a diagnosis through studies that have defined core symptoms, delineated the syndrome from other disorders, documented familial aggregation, and demonstrated stability of diagnosis on follow-up examinations. Such studies have yet to be completed for conversion disorder.

Somatization disorder

Diagnosis

According to the DSM-IV-TR criteria, patients with somatization disorder have a history of significant symptoms in at least the following four categories: pain, gastrointestinal symptoms, sexual symptoms, and pseudoneurological symptoms (see Box 17.1 and Table 17.1). To qualify as significant, each symptom must be medically unexplained; this includes known effects of drugs or alcohol to which the individual was exposed. When a related medical condition is present, a symptom qualifies only if it, or the social or occupational impairment it causes, is in excess of that expected from the degree of the associated medical condition. By definition, somatization disorder must begin by age 30. Any

Box 17.1 Somatization disorder

A. A history of many physical complaints beginning before age 30 that occur over a period of several years and result in treatment being sought or significant impairment in social, occupational, or other important areas of functioning.

B. Each of the following criteria must have been met, with individual symptoms occurring at any time during the course of the disturbance:
   * *four pain symptoms*: a history of pain related to at least four different sites or functions (e.g., head, abdomen, back, joints, extremities, chest, rectum, during menstruation, during sexual intercourse, or during urination)
   * *two gastrointestinal symptoms*: a history of at least two gastrointestinal symptoms other than pain (e.g., nausea, bloating, vomiting other than during pregnancy, diarrhea, or intolerance of several different foods)
   * *one sexual symptom*: a history of at least one sexual or reproductive symptom other than pain (e.g., sexual indifference, erectile or ejaculatory dysfunction, irregular menses, excessive menstrual bleeding, vomiting throughout pregnancy)
   * *one pseudoneurological symptom*: a history of at least one symptom or deficit suggesting a neurological condition not limited to pain (conversion symptoms such as impaired coordination or balance, paralysis or localized weakness, difficulty swallowing or lump in throat, aphonia, urinary retention, hallucinations, loss of touch or pain sensation, double vision, blindness, deafness, seizures; dissociative symptoms such as amnesia; or loss of consciousness other than fainting).

C. Either (1) or (2):
   (1) after appropriate investigation, each of the symptoms in criterion B cannot be fully explained by a known general medical condition or the direct effects of a substance (e.g., a drug of abuse, a medication)
   (2) when there is a related general medical condition, the physical complaints or resulting social or occupational impairment are in excess of what would be expected from the history, physical examination, or laboratory findings.

D. The symptoms are not intentionally produced or feigned (as in factitious disorder or malingering).
From American Psychiatric Association (2000) Diagnostic and Statistical Manual of Mental Disorders, 4th Edition, Text Revision, Washington, D.C. American Psychiatric Association.

Table 17.1 Somatization disorder

Discriminating features

1 Medically unexplained somatic complaints in four or more organ systems:
   - four or more pain symptoms (e.g., back, joint, extremity, rectal, chest, head pain, or dysmenorrhea)
   - two or more gastrointestinal symptoms (e.g., nausea, vomiting, diarrhea, or abdominal bloating)
   - one or more sexual symptoms (e.g., dyspareunia, anorgasmia, menstrual complaints, or sexual indifference)
   - one or more pseudoneurological symptoms (e.g., paralysis, pseudoseizures, aphonia, blindness, deafness, diplopia, or amnesia).

Consistent features

1 More than 95% of cases are women.
2 Onset is usually in adolescence to early adulthood but must begin before age 30 by definition.
3 Tends to be a chronic condition.
4 Multiple psychosocial and interpersonal problems.

Variable features

1 Patients often have psychological complaints, but they may refuse all consideration of psychological problems.
2 Sometimes complicated by substance abuse (including iatrogenic).
3 Spouses often have drug or alcohol abuse, antisocial personalities, and physical abusiveness.

patient with a new onset of multiple medically unexplained somatic complaints in the fourth decade of life or older should be considered undiagnosed until a medical evaluation indicates otherwise.

Patients with somatization disorder often display histrionic (dramatic) behaviors. The current definition of somatization disorder, departing from its historical roots in hysteria, does not require a hysterical presentation, nor is such a presentation pathognomonic of this disorder. Some patients may assume the apparent opposite emotional stance, expressing inappropriate indifference in the face of seemingly tragic and overwhelming medical events, a sign termed *la belle indifférence*. For example, a patient may describe vomiting buckets of blood until passing out with no trace of emotional concern.

The speech of patients with somatization disorder tends to be circumstantial and vague, which presents difficulties in eliciting a medical history. Descriptions of symptoms are often dramatic, exaggerated, and extremely colorful, with sometimes bizarre and even outlandish examples. For example, one patient described her menstrual pain as rivers of fire

in her belly and stated that it was so severe she had to double over to crawl to the toilet. Another patient reported that her headache was so severe that it felt like a bomb had blown off the top of her head. A patient diagnosed with mitral valve prolapse reported that when she felt upset she had "leaking" in her chest.

Certain red flags in the medical history should alert the physician to the possibility of somatization disorder. A complicated medical history with multiple diagnoses, multiple failed treatments, and an associated voluminous medical record is often the first clue. There are a number of other features, none of which are pathognomonic by themselves but when combined with other clues should also alert the physician. These include multiple allergies or medication intolerances. One patient reported that she was allergic to every antibiotic and painkiller ever made. She said that when she was given intravenous penicillin on two occasions, it caused a cardiac arrest; both times she was revived by the heroics of a cardiopulmonary resuscitation team. Neither episode was documented in her medical record. Other features include complaints of many disorders (often disorders that have been popularized in the media) for which no well-integrated structural or pathophysiological models are known or for which the patient does not fit the definition of the syndrome. Examples of these disorders include chronic fatigue syndrome, fibromyalgia, hypoglycemia, chronic pain syndromes, temporomandibular joint syndrome, premenstrual syndrome, reflex sympathetic dystrophy, tension headache or migraine, irritable bowel syndrome, atypical chest pain, and multiple environmental allergies ("allergic to everything").

The family history often reveals further evidence, such as somatization disorder, antisocial personality disorder, criminality (for example, a prison history), and substance abuse in family members. Although not diagnostic, such information can alert the physician to search for further data supporting the diagnosis of somatization disorder. The social history may also provide clues to the diagnosis. Childhood histories of abuse and dysfunctional or substance-abusing family backgrounds arc commonly described. These patients often live with or marry people who are alcoholic or antisocial. The school or work history may be characterized by excessive disruptions because of medical problems and interpersonal difficulties. Despite this, if the employer is sympathetic and the patient does good work when she is healthy, she may have a long and seemingly stable history with that employer.

Patients with somatization disorder are characteristically unreliable historians, not usually providing sufficient detail about their extensive medical history in the initial medical visit to allow the physician to make a diagnosis of somatization disorder. When presenting to a medical specialist, they may focus on their chief complaint and downplay or even entirely omit mention of their extensive symptoms in other multiple organ systems. Therefore, it is important to persist in tracking down medical records and to obtain additional history from others who know the patient. Making the diagnosis may require the accumulation of symptoms over time, since the patient may voice new symptom complaints to the physician as her symptom focus changes and evolves. Combining the patient's complaints elicited over time with those documented by other sources is often necessary to establish the diagnosis with confidence.

KEY CLINICAL QUESTIONS AND WHAT THEY UNLOCK

- *How can these patients be readily identified?*
  A big, fat chart is the first clue to the complicated medical histories characteristic of these patients. After that, detailed documentation of multiple complaints that are medically unexplained is required, and patients are often not reliable enough to provide this in a single interview.
- *What if the physician suspects that the patient may have somatization disorder but can not elicit the history of multiple medically unexplained complaints needed for the diagnosis?*
  The physician can gather medical records from other treating physicians, obtain collaborative information about "hypochondriac" behaviors from family members, and directly observe and document the patient's protean patterns of presentation of complaints over time in support of the diagnosis.
- *Should the physician try to get rid of these patients?*
  The goal is not to refer these patients to psychiatrists (unless there are significant psychiatric complaints), but to work with patients in the medical setting where their medical complaints are appropriately managed (see general treatment strategies), sometimes with psychiatric consultation if the patient is willing.

Natural history

Although by definition, somatization disorder must begin before age 30, it typically begins in the decade after puberty. The disorder is a chronic, lifelong condition with fluctuations in symptom severity. Prolonged, complete remissions rarely occur. On follow-up examination after several years, 90% of women with the disorder still meet criteria for the diagnosis, and few new diagnoses are found to explain the symptoms. However, men meeting criteria for somatization disorder have a greater likelihood of subsequently being diagnosed with a medical disorder that explains the symptoms.

Social complications of somatization disorder include marital difficulties (which are often associated with sexual symptoms), occupational impairment, parenting problems, and multiple social problems such as stormy interpersonal relationships, legal problems related to divorce and other interpersonal problems, and family difficulties. Patients

with somatization disorder report being confined to bed an average of seven days out of each month. An area of special concern for medical professionals is these patients' pattern of extensive use of medical services that results in unnecessary multiple medical and surgical procedures and treatments, thereby increasing the risk for complications and additional morbidity as well as opportunities for claims of medical damages. Smith and colleagues at the University of Arkansas demonstrated that patients with somatization disorder seek health care excessively and at considerable expense, generating costs as much as nine times greater than other medical patients.

Suicide attempts are common in somatization disorder. In one sample, 51% of patients with somatization disorder had made suicide attempts. Completed suicide is fortunately not a common outcome of somatization disorder, but risk increases when comorbid substance abuse is present. However, in any disorder in which suicidal gestures are encountered, some gestures have the potential to result in unanticipated death. All suicide attempts, whether medically serious or trivial, are socially disruptive to families and other contacts of these patients.

Differential diagnosis

Somatization disorder is most often confused with medical conditions. Indicators of somatization disorder in the medical history include distribution of complaints in multiple organ systems and a lack of evidence of medically or structurally documented abnormalities or laboratory indicators over years of evaluation. Somatization disorder baffles physicians, as documented by a study by Tomasson and colleagues demonstrating that, despite lack of medical documentation, 86% of patients received other (a mean of 2.8) medical diagnoses.

In addition to medically undocumented somatoform symptoms of multiple medical disorders that patients do not really have, somatization disorder also produces "psychoform" symptoms of various psychiatric disorders that may be a result of somatization disorder and not necessarily another psychiatric disorder. Two-thirds of all patients with somatization disorder complain of current psychological symptoms. In fact, psychological symptoms are the most common main symptom complaint in somatization disorder, occurring in 25% of cases. More than one-half of all patients with somatization disorder report prior treatment for psychiatric symptoms.

The most common psychological symptoms expressed by patients with somatization disorder are anxiety and depression. People who have somatization disorder report more depressive symptoms than do patients without somatization disorder who actually meet full criteria for major depression. Sometimes the distinction of somatization disorder from depressive and anxiety disorders can be quite problematic. Criterion symptoms of major depression—mood disturbance, hopelessness, suicidality, and vegetative symptoms such as fatigue and appetite disturbance—also serve as criterion symptoms of Briquet's syndrome and are highly prevalent in somatization disorder. Conversely, patients with depressive disorders often report some hypochondriacal and somatic symptoms.

Depressed patients without somatization disorder may demonstrate several somatic complaints that are temporally associated with the depressive episode. However, depression in the absence of somatization disorder does not produce the multiple symptoms in multiple organ systems that are the hallmark features of somatization disorder. Patients experiencing a major depressive episode usually describe the mood disorder as a distinct change from how they usually feel; this is very different from the worsening of the usual state described by patients with somatization disorder.

Anxiety disorders generate many somatic symptoms, especially cardiorespiratory symptoms (for example, palpitations, shortness of breath, and dizziness). Somatization disorder symptoms are differentiated from anxiety disorders by the multiple organ systems chronically involved in somatization disorder. Symptoms of panic disorder occur by definition during panic attacks; in somatization disorder they must also occur at other times to be counted toward the diagnosis.

Patients with somatization disorder often complain of psychotic symptoms such as hallucinations, and for this reason somatization disorder is sometimes confused with psychotic disorders. However, the psychotic-like symptoms of somatization disorder differ qualitatively from the stereotypical voices associated with schizophrenia, which talk to each other or engage in a running commentary. Visual hallucinations of sexual or sexually symbolic objects and cartoon figures, such as snakes, little naked (sometimes green) men running across the room, and monkeys on motorcycles, are more characteristic of the pseudopsychotic symptoms of somatization disorder. Voices telling the person to harm someone she despises or would like to harm are also uncharacteristic of schizophrenia. Patients with somatization disorder may report episodes of physical hyperactivity and other manic-like symptoms, such as jitteriness, distractibility, sexual promiscuity, and excessive spending of money; however, on closer examination these symptoms do not fit the characteristic episodic nature of bipolar disorder and therefore this diagnosis is not warranted.

Patients with somatization disorder studied in academic centers almost always meet criteria for one or more other psychiatric syndromes. The somatization disorder usually precedes the onset of other psychiatric disorders, which by definition makes somatization disorder the primary diagnosis. At times, it is difficult even for the well-trained psychiatrist to distinguish between the symptoms of somatization disorder mimicking those of other disorders.

However, in primary care settings the rates of psychiatric comorbidity may be somewhat lower.

Drug and alcohol use disorders are commonly comorbid with somatization disorder. Most patients with somatization disorder also meet criteria for a personality disorder, and some experts feel that somatization disorder arises from a personality pathology. Pennebaker and Watson argue that somatization disorder belongs not on Axis I where it is currently classified, but on Axis II with the personality disorders.

Genetics and family history

Somatization disorder is a familial disorder, especially in women. It runs in affected families along with male-dominant antisocial personality disorder. Patients with somatization disorder have first-degree male relatives with elevated rates of antisocial personality disorder and, through the association with antisocial personality disorder, alcoholism. Female relatives of women with somatization disorder have increased rates of somatization disorder and also of antisocial personality disorder. A complication to understanding the relationship of these two disorders in families is the phenomenon of assortative mating. Women with somatization disorder tend to pair off with men who are antisocial and alcoholic, adding these conditions to the family illness pattern.

The familial associations of somatization disorder described in family studies have been confirmed by twin studies providing even more evidence of a genetic link. Torgerson showed that concordance rates of somatization are nearly three times higher in monozygotic twins (29%) than in dizygotic twins (10%). Adoption studies have provided the most compelling evidence of genetic contribution to the familial association of somatization disorder and antisocial personality disorder. Adopted offspring of biological parents with antisocial behavior studied by Cadoret and colleagues showed much higher rates of somatoform symptoms and diagnoses of somatization disorder than did adoptees without antisocial biological parentage.

Somatization and antisocial personality disorders are associated within individuals as well. Rates of antisocial personality disorder in women with somatization disorder may be as high as 25%. People with antisocial personality disorder also have more somatoform symptom complaints than do people without this disorder.

Epidemiology

Somatization disorder is not one of the most prevalent psychiatric disorders, occurring in 1 of 50 women in the general population. In certain settings it is much more prevalent; somatization disorder occurs in 9% of medical and surgical inpatients, 10% of psychiatric inpatients, 17% of patients with irritable bowel syndrome, 27% of women undergoing hysterectomies for noncancerous indications, 26% of first-degree female relatives of patients with somatization disorder, and 41% of female felons. Tertiary medical settings attract patients with somatization disorder, who gravitate toward centers of medical expertise as they search for answers for multiple medically unexplained symptom complaints. Somatization disorder is also more prevalent among lesser educated populations.

Somatization disorder is almost exclusively a women's disorder, although it is well documented to occur rarely in men. When somatization disorder occurs in men, it is considered to be a more severe condition than in women, as shown by its higher comorbidity rates of alcoholism and depression.

Conversion disorder

Diagnosis

The hallmark of conversion disorder is the presence of one or more symptoms or deficits relating to voluntary motor or sensory function (see Box 17.2 and Table 17.2). The symptoms may suggest a general medical condition, but classically the symptoms are "pseudoneurological," suggesting illnesses such as multiple sclerosis or seizure disorder. Symptoms of conversion disorder are by definition medically unexplained, and they either cause significant social or occupational impairment or warrant medical evaluation. The following four types of conversion symptoms are recognized: (1) symptoms with motor deficit (for example, paralysis or weakness of a limb, difficulty walking because of weakness or balance problems, aphonia, and urinary retention); (2) symptoms with sensory deficit (such as numbness, blindness, tunnel vision, deafness, and hallucinations); (3) seizures or convulsions; and (4) mixed symptom types. The most common main complaints documented in patients with conversion disorder are numbness, aphonia, ataxia, fits, paralysis, and blindness.

The Washington University group suggested that the presence of pseudoneurological symptoms defines conversion disorder in atheoretical terms without the need to invoke the role of psychological mechanisms in the etiology or pathogenesis of the disorder. Established criteria of the American Psychiatric Association, however, require documentation of psychological factors associated with the onset or exacerbation of symptoms, such as emotional conflicts and stressors. An example of psychological factors associated with conversion symptoms is the case of a woman who, after her husband told her he was going to leave her, woke up the next morning to find herself paralyzed from the waist down. A problem with this requirement is that it is difficult to operationalize psychological factors into objective measures, and therefore no data are available to support this

Box 17.2 Conversion disorder

A. One or more symptoms or deficits affecting voluntary motor or sensory function that suggest a neurological or other general medical condition.

B. Psychological factors are judged to be associated with the symptom or deficit because the initiation or exacerbation of the symptom or deficit is preceded by conflicts or other stressors.

C. The symptom or deficit is not intentionally produced or feigned (as in factitious disorder or malingering).

D. The symptom or deficit cannot, after appropriate investigation, be fully explained by a general medical condition, or by the direct effects of a substance, or as a culturally sanctioned behavior or experience.

E. The symptom or deficit causes clinically significant distress or impairment in social, occupational, or other important areas of functioning or warrants medical evaluation.

F. The symptom or deficit is not limited to pain or sexual dysfunction, does not occur exclusively during the course of somatization disorder, and is not better accounted for by another mental disorder.

Specify type of symptom or deficit:
- with motor symptom or deficit
- with sensory symptom or deficit
- with seizures or convulsions
- with mixed presentation.

From American Psychiatric Association (2000) Diagnostic and Statistical Manual of Mental Disorders, 4th Edition, Text Revision, Washington, D.C., American Psychiatric Association.

requirement in the criteria. A creative physician could always hypothesize a connection between personal events and pseudoneurological symptoms.

Natural history

Conversion disorder can begin at any age, although its onset is most often between the ages of 10 and 35. The onset of conversion symptoms in middle age or later should raise the serious possibility of an occult neurological or general medical source for the symptoms. A sizable proportion of patients with conversion disorder (20–30%) are later found to have a medical illness that, in retrospect, accounts for the symptoms. Approximately one-third to one-half of patients who do not have somatization disorder but have symptoms diagnosed as conversion are later found to have a documented neurological disease. In contrast, only 10% of patients with somatization disorder who have conversion symptoms are found to have a medical illness that explains the symptoms.

Table 17.2 Conversion disorder

Discriminating features

1 One or more pseudoneurological symptoms relating to voluntary sensory or motor function.
2 The four types of symptoms are motor deficit, sensory deficit, seizures or convulsions, and mixed types.
3 Differentiated from somatization disorder by lack of many symptoms in many organ systems.

Consistent features

1 Men more often have conversion disorder than somatization disorder (but women predominate in both disorders).
2 Onset usually age 10 to 35, but it may begin at any age.
3 Isolated conversion symptoms are rare in the absence of another medical or psychiatric disorder. (Look for other disorders when considering a diagnosis of conversion disorder.)

Variable features

1 20–30% of patients are found to have a medical illness that explains the symptoms.
2 Prognosis for individual symptoms is favorable, but long-term prognosis is for recurrence of same or new symptoms.
3 Onset of symptoms in middle age or later greatly increases chance for medical explanation. (Look carefully for other illnesses and continue to look over time.)
4 Somatization disorder and antisocial personality are common comorbid conditions.

The long-term prognosis of conversion disorder is poor, with two-thirds or more of all patients remaining symptomatic at follow-up examinations an average of six years later. Other conversion symptoms, as well as additional psychiatric problems, commonly develop even though the original conversion symptom may have disappeared.

The extreme degree of social and occupational disability that is characteristic of somatization disorder is not necessarily associated with conversion disorder. The prognosis of conversion disorder tends to follow that of the comorbid psychiatric disorder, with patients who have somatization disorder faring the worst. Compensation and other psychosocial factors, including monetary or legal compensation factors and interpersonal conflict, are often apparent in the individual's current situation. Compensation factors are more common in male patients with conversion symptoms, and they may be important in assessing conversion in military and criminal justice settings.

The prognosis for specific conversion symptoms is relatively favorable, with recovery typically within two weeks.

Two-thirds of individual conversion symptoms are absent at follow-up examinations an average of six years later. However, symptom recurrence is common, occurring at a rate of 20% to 25% within one year. Favorable prognosis of conversion symptoms is associated with acute onset, an identifiable associated precipitating stressor, brief duration of symptoms before treatment, and high intelligence. Conversion symptoms with the poorest outcomes include pseudoseizures and conversion tremors.

Isolated conversion symptoms in the absence of another disorder, psychiatric or physical, are uncommon, and those unassociated with a psychiatric disorder are much more likely to be found later to have a specific medical illness that explains the symptom. Therefore, the old term *conversion reaction* is now a useless diagnosis and in fact potentially dangerous if it leads the physician to abandon further medical work-up. In cases of apparent isolated conversion symptoms without overt evidence of a major psychiatric disorder, physicians are encouraged to resist the temptation to attribute the symptom to psychological processes. Although it is frustrating for physicians to deal with unexplained phenomena such as this, nothing is gained by making unwarranted assumptions about etiology or diagnosis. To make premature and arbitrary conclusions about the etiology of isolated conversion symptoms only invites the passage of time to prove a conclusion wrong. Instead, the physician must learn to accept uncertainty.

Differential diagnosis

In conversion disorder, as in somatization disorder, the main differentiation to be made is from medical (predominantly neurological) disorders. This process is similar to the differentiation of somatization symptoms from medically based symptoms. Conversion syndromes are commonly seen in patients with a variety of documented neurological conditions, including seizure disorders, head injuries, central nervous system tumors, frontal lobe lesions, cerebrovascular accidents, acute encephalitis, delirium, Klinefelter's syndrome, and multiple sclerosis.

Somatization disorder is differentiated from conversion disorder by the greater number of symptoms and their wide range of distribution in different organ systems. The most common psychiatric diagnosis in patients with conversion symptoms is somatization disorder. More than one-half of the inpatients with conversion symptoms on neurology wards have been found to qualify for a diagnosis of somatization disorder. Conversion disorder is also associated with the diagnosis of antisocial personality disorder. More than one-third of general medical patients with conversion disorder meet criteria for somatization disorder or antisocial personality.

Depressive syndromes have also been found in association with conversion. However, closer examination has revealed that this depression is usually secondary depression in individuals with preexisting somatization disorder or antisocial personality disorder. There is little evidence of association of conversion disorder and primary mood disorder. Therefore the physician is cautioned to persist in screening for other psychiatric disorders even when depression is recognized, because there is usually another important diagnosis (somatization disorder or antisocial personality disorder) lurking behind the scenes.

Genetics and family history

Little is known about family transmission of conversion disorder. An isolated study of familial psychiatric illness found considerable diagnostic heterogeneity, a reflection of the fact that patients with conversion disorder are probably not a homogenous group. The known comorbidity of somatization disorder and antisocial personality disorder with conversion might suggest the presence of somatization disorder and antisocial personality disorder in relatives of patients with these comorbid disorders, although not necessarily in relatives of patients without them.

Epidemiology

Conversion symptoms are relatively prevalent. It has been estimated that up to 25% of hospital inpatients have had conversion symptoms at some time, and around 10% of psychiatric consultations on general hospital medical and surgical inpatients are for conversion symptoms. Conversion disorder is more prevalent in women than men, with 75–90% of cases occurring in women. Conversion disorder is more common in lesser educated, lower socioeconomic populations.

Other somatoform disorders

Other somatoform disorders include hypochondriasis, pain disorder, body dysmorphic disorder, somatoform disorder not otherwise specified (NOS), and undifferentiated somatization disorder (a category of somatoform symptoms not meeting criteria for any of the other somatoform diagnoses). Few published data are available on these other somatoform disorders, and therefore little can be said about their natural history, genetic and familial patterns, epidemiology, and treatment.

Hypochondriasis is defined by a period of at least six months of preoccupation with having a serious disease, and it represent the misinterpretation of bodily symptoms despite appropriate medical evaluation and reassurance. The term *hypochondria* has carried multiple meanings in modern as well as historical cultures, and therefore it is an imprecise term that may encompass a wide variety of contexts. The focus of body dysmorphic disorder is an imagined defect in a person's physical appearance that is accompanied by marked and excessive concern about slight physical anomalies such as an excessively large nose, asymmetry of physical features, dissatisfaction with the alignment of one's teeth, or a woman's preoccupation with the size of her breasts (either too small or too large). The category of somatoform disorder NOS includes somatoform disorders of sufficient severity that fail to meet criteria for other established somatoform disorders. Included in this category is pseudocyesis, a false belief of being pregnant without supporting objective physical signs such as enlarged abdomen, disappearance of menstruation, breast engorgement, and fetal movements.

Hypochondriacal disorders, body dysmorphic disorders, and other somatoform disorders may have psychotic or delusional features, invoking differential diagnosis that includes delusional disorder (somatic type), chronic schizophrenia, or obsessive-compulsive disorder.

Pathophysiology

The pathophysiology of somatoform disorders is unknown. The lack of known pathology for these disorders may lead physicians to dismiss patients with these disorders as playing games—simulating and pretending illness that they do not have. It is important for the physician to recognize that although these patients do not have the serious medical illnesses their symptoms suggest, somatoform disorders are often severely disabling illnesses with considerable personal suffering and emotional anguish. These are serious disorders requiring specific responses from the physician.

Treatment

Brown and Smith (1988) observed, "The first major obstacle in dealing with somatization disorder patients is making the diagnosis." Somatization disorder is especially vexing and perplexing to the physician if it is not recognized, and it may lead to considerable medical morbidity. Because of somatization disorder's proclivity to mimic medical conditions and the fact that it is often seen by nonpsychiatric physicians, all clinicians must be remain alert to the possibility of the condition (see *Pearls & Perils*). Although making the diagnosis can be somewhat laborious, the amount of guidance the diagnosis can give physicians dealing with these often difficult cases makes the effort worthwhile.

Psychiatric consultation

Busy physicians may become disheartened by their limited ability to help patients with somatization disorder, in part because of the magnitude of difficulties they have experienced with such patients in the past and the tremendous amount of physicians' time that they can absorb. A common automatic response is to refer the patient to a mental health

Diagnosis of somatoform disorders

- The classic features of somatization disorder are a complicated medical history with multiple diagnoses, multiple failed treatments, and a voluminous medical record.
- Any patient with new onset of multiple medically unexplained somatic complaints in the fourth decade or older should be assumed to have an organic condition until medical evaluation documents otherwise.
- The depression described by patients with somatization disorder is a worsening of their usual state, as opposed to the distinct change from usual feelings described by patients without somatization disorder who are experiencing a major depressive episode.
- Pseudoneurological symptoms are characteristic of patients with conversion disorder, who do not display the multiple somatoform symptoms in multiple organ systems characteristic of somatization disorder.

professional as quickly as possible. Patients with somatization disorder may resist seeing a psychiatrist because of the implication that "it's all in my head." Psychiatric consultation is useful only when it is acceptable to the patient, and consultation is preferable to a transfer out of the provider's practice, which patients may perceive as a personal rejection.

Patients with somatization disorder who also have psychological symptoms may gravitate to psychiatric care on their own, but this is not often the case. Some patients may blame any emotional difficulties they experience on the medical problem they believe they have, contending that if the physician could just find and fix the medical problem there would be no basis for the emotional response. ("If the pain would just go away then I wouldn't be so depressed!") When the patient rejects psychiatric care, the total burden of care rests with nonpsychiatric physicians. If the primary physician is vigilant for this disorder and can make the diagnosis, the patient can often be managed effectively without psychiatric referral.

General treatment strategies

Few empirical data exist on the most effective treatment of somatoform disorders, and no prospective treatment trials have been reported in the literature. However, a general consensus on medical model treatment principles in the literature can guide the physician. In one of the few systematic studies examining treatment practices related to patients with somatization disorder, Smith and colleagues reported that psychiatric consultation to confirm the diagnosis and recommend conservative treatment reduced health-care

expenditures without adversely affecting health status or patient satisfaction with health care.

Treatment recommendations are similar for all the somatoform disorders and are modeled on established principles of treatment for somatization disorder. The most important role of the physician in managing somatization disorder is orchestration of treatment. This includes physician rather than patient initiation of all referrals to medical specialists, informing consulted medical specialists of the patient's somatoform disorder, and discouraging unnecessary procedures and treatments. Because patients with somatization disorder tend to consult large numbers of specialists for extensive complaints in multiple organ systems, careful central management of their overall treatment plan can protect them from unnecessary treatments and procedures, dangerous treatment interactions and other iatrogenic complications, and gradual removal of all expendable body organs over time. If at all possible, referrals for specialty care should be made by one primary physician, who might in some cases be the patient's psychiatrist. This practice also allows the physician to set limits on the doctor-shopping to which these patients are prone.

The goal of treatment of somatization disorder is not to cure it (as a cure is not known) but to manage the illness and prevent complications. The first principle in treating these patients invokes the portion of the Hippocratic oath that says, "do no harm." The physician's natural tendency is to want to do something for the patient, when in actuality it is often more beneficial for these patients to avoid "doing" for them.

The ultimate goal is not to remove all sources of the patient's discomfort (which is impossible) but to aim for the patient to be able to live with her symptoms, avoiding temptation to regard them as serious or requiring emergency or surgical intervention. In order to achieve these ends, it is necessary to develop a lasting, empathetic relationship with the patient. Genuine and compassionate interest by the physician helps patients with somatization disorder bond within the physician-patient relationship. The best strategy is to give the patient regular outpatient appointments so she does not have to generate symptom complaints to be seen, thus avoiding the reinforcement of somatoform symptoms in the physician-patient relationship. It is recommended that a physical examination be performed at medical appointments, because this demonstrates the physician's caring concern and interest, as well as a desire to understand what the patient perceives as her real problem. This strategy naturally directs the physician to listen to the patient's complaints and examine her instead of proceeding directly to extensive medical evaluations and procedures.

When no medical explanation can be found for a given symptom with the treatment plan described in this chapter, the patient is reassured that the physician has paid serious attention to the symptom and found that there is no medically worrisome cause for it; furthermore, she sees that the physician will continue to monitor for signs of serious disease. Often this is enough to satisfy the patient. Despite this, some patients are more demanding and insist on further evaluation and may threaten to find a "more expert" physician who by virtue of superior medical skill will find the cause of the symptoms. On one hand, it is undesirable for the physician to feel manipulated into performing further tests or procedures by pressure from the patient, but on the other hand there is value in trying to retain these patients in the practice to prevent them from shopping for another physician who will perform unnecessary tests and procedures. If the physician who understands somatization disorder does not treat the patient, another physician who does not recognize the disorder will do so.

In spite of these considerations, physicians are ultimately advised not to compromise the standard of care to satisfy these patients' demands. When the patient threatens to change physicians, the clinician can acknowledge to the patient that she has the power to terminate the relationship along with the opinion that this would be a regrettable error. Experience has shown that few patients change physicians as a result of the physician's consistency in following the principles of management outlined here, and many patients feel more comfortable with physicians who set clear limits.

Eventually the unnecessary costs and risks associated with exhaustive medical evaluations of all symptoms should become apparent to the physician treating somatization disorder, and a decision made to limit more extensive evaluation to situations when objective physical findings are present or when the history is compellingly suggestive of a medical disorder. When this judgment becomes difficult, the problem may be resolved by discussing the case with a trusted colleague rather than defaulting by ordering more tests. These decisions must also be balanced with continuing awareness that patients with somatoform disorders are not immune to developing other medical conditions. The physician must maintain vigilance for other treatable medical problems when presented with objective signs or otherwise convincing clinical pictures. Unfortunately, when these patients become medically ill, the differentiation of a somatoform disorder from medical symptoms sometimes becomes even more difficult.

Physicians are discouraged from telling patients, "It's all in your head." It is more helpful to become comfortable with the uncertainty of medically unexplained somatic symptoms, offering to patients the honest conclusion of "I don't know what is causing the symptoms." Both the physician and the patient may be comforted by the fact that additional time may clarify the origin of the symptoms. However, when time does not provide answers, the physician is left without an explanation for the patient about her symptoms. Admitting to a lack of an explanation is preferable to telling the patient that she is imagining the symptom (which she may

not be if an occult medical cause exists). This strategy allows the physician to offer potential options for treatment of psychiatric comorbidity or for palliative relief of distress, including several classes of medications, such as antidepressants, antianxiety agents, and sedative agents, which are sometimes beneficial. Caveats in the use of these agents in patients with somatoform disorders are discussed later in this chapter.

PEARLS & PERILS

Management of somatoform disorders

- The goal of treatment of somatoform disorders is not to cure but to manage the illness and prevent complications.
- Effective management requires orchestration of treatment by the patient's primary physician, whether that person is a psychiatrist, family physician, or other medical specialist. Orchestration of treatment includes initiation of all referrals to medical specialists, informing the patient's medical specialists of the somatoform disorder, and discouraging unnecessary procedures and treatments.
- The quality of the relationship between the primary physician and the patient is critical to the management of somatization disorder. Regularly scheduled office visits, physical examinations, and listening to the patient's complaints in a sympathetic but nonreactive manner are key elements.
- Physicians treating patients with somatoform disorders are advised to avoid proceeding to invasive treatments and procedures unless sufficient objective evidence warrants such action. These patients complain vociferously of many symptoms, underscoring the value of resisting the temptation to act on the magnitude of specific complaints unless objective indicators are present. (However, this is not to imply that these patients cannot develop serious illness; a physician must not dismiss complaints without a reasonable effort to substantiate or rule out documentable medical illness.)
- Patients with somatoform disorders are at increased risk for substance abuse, both iatrogenic and illicit. Therefore, caution is indicated when prescribing potentially abusable substances for these patients who tend to elicit prescriptions with their often vocal complaints of insomnia, anxiety, depression, or pain.
- Although suicide gestures are common in somatization disorder, completed suicide is rare.

Behavioral management

Somatoform behavior is encouraged by environmental reinforcement, such as attention for fainting spells by the family who gather at her side and rush her to the emergency room; similarly, symptoms can be attenuated or extinguished by removal of such rewards. The family can be advised to monitor the effects of their own behaviors on the patient's response. Excessive inquiry by the physician into symptoms at appointments encourages patients to focus on symptoms and is therefore best avoided.

Although attention to symptoms can encourage more symptoms, some attention to symptoms can be a useful tool. Because these patients often feel that physicians do not understand them or respond appropriately to their distress, allowing them to ventilate their difficulties helps to strengthen the rapport with the physician. Thus, physicians are advised to listen to complaints but to refrain from responding to them with further medical work-ups if there are no objective signs.

Over time, the physician may begin to inquire into the patient's social and interpersonal difficulties, which conveys to the patient that the most important and interesting aspect of her is not her symptoms. The additional concern and support for the patient demonstrated by inquiry into her psychosocial life also helps her begin to discuss her psychosocial problems, which are almost invariably part of the disorder and its sequelae. This in turn provides opportunities for supportive psychotherapy and guidance in practical problem-solving. As the physician-patient relationship grows more secure, the patient's dependence on the relationship enhances the physician's leverage in working with the patient to change her behavior. Leading the patient to work on real interpersonal difficulties and other psychosocial problems is more productive than attention to a litany of somatoform symptoms generated at repeated office visits. These excessive symptom complaints can be managed positively with praise given to the patient for endurance of her symptoms.

It is important for the physician to realize that because these patients' lives revolve so heavily around their symptoms, providing care can become excessively demanding if special attention is not paid to the physician-patient relationship from the start. Therefore, getting the diagnosis right and then setting limits and boundaries in advance is a healthy medical practice that protects physicians from personal encroachment by patient demands. These limits build patient perceptions of professionalism and competence of the physician and a sense of security in a relationship with well-defined boundaries. Patients who call often between appointments can be informed that the general office policy limits phone calls to one per week unless it is a bona fide emergency. Patients may test limits early in the relationship, but once the limits are defined for them, they can often respect them.

In the inpatient setting, behavioral shaping of somatoform and conversion syndromes by reward contingency and redirection may hasten improvement. At the start, all the patient's hospital privileges are removed with the explanation that she must maintain total bed rest to avoid worsening her condition. She is told that as she shows signs of clinical improvement she will gain privileges that are appropriate for each level of function achieved. This positive framework helps redirect the patient from perceiving the program as punishment and reacting angrily toward the physician. It also allows patients with conversion symptoms to "save face" as symptoms are confronted not directly but rather allowed to resolve in the overt context of healing and improved functioning. Placebos such as saline injections intended to encourage these suggestible patients to believe they are recovering may have dramatic immediate effects, but their use is discouraged because of the dishonesty required to administer them and because in the long run they reinforce patients' concepts of themselves as medically ill.

Patients with somatization disorder can behave seductively toward physicians, who need to be especially cognizant of professionalism and boundaries with these patients. Social physical contact other than a handshake is not recommended, especially early in the relationship. Use of the patient's title and last name (for example, Mrs Smith) helps maintain appropriate distance. When patients cross boundaries (such as trying to hug, kiss, or sexually touch the physician), such incidents are best handled by prohibiting further boundary violations, discussing the incident with another professional, and documenting the consultation. Referral to another physician may be necessary if the issue cannot be resolved relatively quickly.

The practice of confronting patients directly about the reality of their symptoms is generally not recommended, nor is presenting them with the diagnosis of a somatoform disorder, a difficult concept for patients to understand. The suggestion that the symptoms are not "real" alienates the patient and results in an unnecessarily adversarial relationship, with the patient believing that the physician does not know what he or she is talking about. Patients interpret such confrontations as implying that the physician thinks they are either crazy or lying, with neither concept perceived by patients as respectful. It is not useful to argue whether the symptoms are "real;" it is more helpful to recognize that the patient's pain seems real to her.

Psychotherapy

Patients with somatoform disorders typically develop little insight over time. Insight-oriented and expressive psychotherapies are usually ineffective. There is no evidence to suggest that hypnosis, sodium amytal interviews, or other techniques aimed at helping the patient remember, relive, abreact, or work through alleged traumas and connect to their emotions are helpful. Patients with somatization disorder already rely too heavily on emotional responses and need no further encouragement of this behavior. Such techniques may in fact be harmful by allowing patients to focus therapeutic attention away from the behaviors and problems at hand, blame others for their problems, and avoid working to find genuine solutions.

At best, patients with exceptional verbal abilities can achieve improved insight into the mind-body connection of stress and physical symptoms. Patients may accept the suggestion that responses to stress and pressure influence normal human physiology and can generate symptoms in many people. Physicians can help patients with somatization disorder learn that their headaches do not necessarily indicate that they have a brain tumor or anything else seriously wrong. Sometimes these normalizing explanations for symptoms elicit reactions of genuine relief.

A useful technique is to explain that such symptoms may continue to bother people for a while or from time to time and to predict that this will probably be the case for the patient's current symptoms. Sometimes the patient wants to "prove" the physician wrong, and the symptoms will disappear altogether. Conversely, if the patient continues to be symptomatic, the physician can help the patient remember the earlier prediction that this might happen. Behavioral change in these patients is typically gradual, proceeding over months and possibly years. Over the long haul, the best strategy is empathetic engagement coupled with helping patients appreciate the natural association of increased physical symptoms with stressful times.

Psychiatric symptoms and psychotropic medications

Symptoms of other psychiatric disorders routinely reported by patients with somatization disorder may complicate treatment if they are not recognized within the context of somatization disorder. The most difficult aspect of these commonly reported psychoform symptoms is that they provide a smokescreen for the treatment of the primary disorder (somatization disorder) if they become the focus of treatment. Complaints of anxiety and panic symptoms may invite physicians to prescribe benzodiazepines, and pain complaints may lead to the use of narcotics. Patients with somatization disorder are at greatly increased risk of abusing these medications, which therefore should be limited and closely monitored. Psychiatrists treating these patients may have to detoxify them from benzodiazepines and pain medications prescribed by other physicians who, not suspecting somatization disorder, may have inadvertently contributed to iatrogenic drug dependence. Buspirone, a nonaddictive antianxiety agent, can sometimes be useful for management of anxiety. Additionally, the sedating properties of antihistamines such as hydroxyzine can aid in the management of insomnia and daytime anxiety, which often trouble these patients.

Patients with somatization disorder who require abusable substances such as benzodiazepines or narcotics for documented medical conditions should be carefully monitored.

Counting the prescribed pills can avoid escalations of dosage to which these patients are prone. Before prescribing abusable drugs, physicians should assess substance abuse history and document the findings in the chart. Ground rules need to be established at the outset, and the patient should be advised that the abusable medication is a short-term remedy only and that dosage increases will not be forthcoming. When informed of the abuse potential of benzodiazepines, many patients minimize their use or even avoid taking them at all. Although it may be tempting to prescribe antipsychotic agents for anxiety or insomnia when benzodiazepines are not a reasonable choice—especially when patients complain of psychotic-like symptoms—antipsychotic medications are not a good choice because of the potential for the development of tardive dyskinesia, a potentially irreversible syndrome, and other serious side effects.

Unfortunately there is no available medication specific for the treatment of somatization disorder. A useful philosophy is to encourage patients to deal with their emotional symptoms without resorting to pharmacological solutions whenever possible.

Because a goal in treating somatization disorder is simplification of the medication regimen, the physician should avoid puritanical wishes to immediately remove all seemingly unnecessary or harmful medications. Initially, patients can be reassured that medications they need will not be withdrawn. Whereas the virtue of removing unnecessary and excessively complex medications is valued, the abrupt discontinuation of one or more medications can be problematic because of the well-known physical, as well as psychological, withdrawal effects of stopping benzodiazepines and antidepressants.

Treatment of comorbid psychiatric disorders

Admissions to psychiatric facilities for patients with somatization disorder are usually the result of complaints of depression or suicidality. Patients with somatization disorder commonly experience an improvement within a few hours or days of being on the ward and away from the interpersonal and other psychosocial precipitants of their symptoms, even if they have had no specific treatment for their depressive symptoms. This phenomenon supports the decision to wait two or three days before prescribing antidepressant medication. Otherwise, clinical improvement may be incorrectly attributed to the medication.

Little is known about the epidemiology and management of major depression in relation to somatoform disorders. Somatization disorder patients meeting full criteria for major depression may benefit from the usual treatments for major depression. However, physicians are cautioned not to treat depressive symptoms without first establishing a definite diagnosis of major depression. For patients with somatization disorder who develop major depressive features, treatment of the depression may improve the somatoform symptoms as the depressive episode resolves. Good choices for antidepressants in these patients are serotonin-selective reuptake inhibitors such as fluoxetine, paroxetine, and sertraline because of a low risk profile (compared with tricyclic antidepressants) in this patient population prone to overdose in suicide gestures. The generally lower side-effect profiles of these agents are also preferable, as patients with somatization disorder tend to tolerate medication side effects poorly. This latter problem advocates for the practice of starting psychotropic medications for these patients at low doses and increasing them slowly.

Antidepressant medications are also used in the treatment of chronic pain syndromes and for symptoms of irritable bowel syndrome, which are prevalent in these patients. Relief may be obtained at doses lower than those required to achieve antidepressant efficacy.

Suicide threats and attempts, even in patients with somatization disorder who rarely carry them to completion, must be taken seriously and dealt with carefully and vigorously, either by hospitalization or by close watch at home. If it can be determined that the suicidal crisis is related to an interpersonal problem that passed quickly, the patient should be encouraged to state how things have changed and to demonstrate ways she could handle her difficulties without resorting to suicide. This critical information must be documented in the chart. However, in the event that the patient cannot do this, she may require brief hospitalization while the interpersonal problem is being resolved. Restriction of privileges or seclusion administered nonpunitively ("for your own good" or "for your safety") after suicidal gestures can dramatically reduce further suicidality.

Special issues

Media attention and patient contact with disease-specific self-help groups such as those for chronic fatigue syndrome and for environmental allergies are on the rise and are thought to reinforce patients' medical appraisals of their symptoms. Patients with these syndromes may reorganize their lives and their identities around their alleged illness, pursuing activities related to it with all-consuming vigor. These patients also visit alternative medical care providers such as homeopaths and natural healers whose professional sanctioning of symptoms may further entrench patients' erroneous convictions of serious medical disease.

Dissociative identity disorder (DID), formerly known as multiple personality disorder, is a popular forum for such disease-related activities in patients with somatization disorder. A recent increase in reported cases of MPD to epidemic proportions has been attributed in part to spread through popular medical opinion and through the media. Most patients with DID have been documented to meet criteria for somatization disorder, a diagnosis that can account for

the symptoms of DID. A more recent phenomenon closely allied with DID is the dramatic increase in accusations of childhood sexual molestation at the hands of family members and, more dramatically, of satanic ritual abuse. These accusations often arise in therapy designed to recover childhood memories of abuse. This entity tends to afflict the patients with somatization disorder who are also diagnosed with DID, and it also tends to be uncovered by the same therapists who have an interest in DID.

Conclusion

This chapter reviewed the somatoform disorders with focus on the most prevalent and best understood diagnoses of somatization disorder and conversion disorder. Somatoform disorders have earned a reputation for being difficult to treat, but most of the difficulty lies with the lack of recognition of the disorder and failure to apply established principles of treatment. The goals of physicians treating patients with somatoform disorders are to orchestrate treatment, prevent complications resulting from unnecessary medical procedures and tests, and assist the patient in navigating through the interpersonal and other psychosocial problems that are inherent to these disorders.

CONSIDER CONSULTATION WHEN...

- Somatization disorder is suspected.
- There are multiple unexplained medical complaints.
- There are medically unexplained neurological complaints.
- The patient demands additional evaluations or treatments when the medical situation does not warrant them.
- The medical history, symptoms, and signs do not add up.

Annotated bibliography

Andreasen, NC and Black, DW (2001) Somatoform and related disorders in *Introductory Textbook of Psychiatry*, Edition 32, Washington, D.C., American Psychiatric Press.
This text, designed for medical students, is useful for all clinicians, as well as mental health and non-mental health professionals, to achieve a basic and practical understanding of psychiatric disorders, their diagnosis, natural history, and treatment. The chapter on somatoform disorders provides complete information on the subject.

Goodwin, IM and Guze, SB (1989) Hysteria (somatization disorder), in *Psychiatric Diagnosis*, Edition 4, New York, Oxford University Press.
This chapter provides physicians with an understanding of the diagnosis of somatoform disorders. This is achieved through atheoretical descriptions of these disorders without hypotheses about etiology, which have not been documented in these disorders. In particular these disorders are described in terms of the core symptoms that define them, delineation from other disorders (exclusion criteria), family studies, and follow-up studies.

Othmer, E (ed.) (1988) Somatization disorder, *Psychiatr Ann* 18:330–362.

This special issue of this journal contains several seminal articles describing somatization disorder in general practice, guiding the physician on detection, diagnosis, and management of this disorder. It further updates the physician with data relating to comorbid diagnoses and its presentation in the general medical setting.

Smith, GR Jr, Monson, RA, and Ray DC (1986) Psychiatric consultation in somatization disorder, *N Engl J Med* 314: 1407–1413.

This concise article describes essential features of management of somatization disorder for the primary care physician and demonstrates benefit of this method on both patient satisfaction and dramatic savings in medical care costs.

CHAPTER 18

Dissociative Disorders, Factitious Disorders, and Malingering

Carol S. North, MD and Sean H. Yutzy, MD

Introduction

This chapter covers two categories of psychiatric disorders: dissociative disorders and factitious disorders. These disorders are alike in that, in contrast to malingering, the alleged motivation for creation of the symptoms is not within conscious control. In other words, the motivation for both disorders is said to be unconscious. They are also alike in that little systematic information exists about either of them. These two categories of disorders differ in definition: dissociation is a *subjectively* reported perceptual disruption of an individual's experience of self and/or environment, whereas factitious disorders manifest *objective* medical findings that are fabricated by physical manipulation.

Dissociative disorders

Perspective on dissociative disorders

Dissociation remains poorly understood despite a recent upsurge in the amount of published literature on the topic. The principal diagnosis in the category of dissociative disorders is dissociative identity disorder, formerly termed multiple personality disorder (MPD). Dissociative identity disorder is perhaps the most controversial disorder in psychiatry. It has divided the mental health field into polarized groups of enthusiastic believers and vocal skeptics. Reasonable professionals find their limits of credibility stretched by claims that multiple people can exist within one person, a situation not mitigated by the flamboyant symptom displays of patients with dissociative identity disorder. Chaos surrounds the occurrence of dissociative disorders in clinical settings and stems from staff division, the patient acting out, and a lack of unified and scientifically based clinical direction regarding the proper care for these patients.

The paucity of systematic study of dissociation has yielded little empirical information. The field has advanced largely on anecdotal experience, poorly conceived studies, and polemical arguments that form the bulk of the published literature. Published investigations to date have suffered from a lack of adequate controls, selection bias, biased ascertainment, unwarranted conclusions from data, and a failure to address the most critical questions. Studies to validate dissociative identity disorder according to well-established traditions in medicine and psychiatry have not been performed, and therefore the diagnosis has not been scientifically validated.

During the latter part of the 20th century, an American epidemic of dissociative identity disorder captivated the attention of both public and professional audiences. Record numbers of patients claimed to have the disorder, and increasing numbers of professionals devoted interest to it. As a result, the mental health field saw burgeoning numbers of patients with these complaints and an expanding professional literature regarding these disorders. The unprecedented rapid growth of this topic has outstripped available empirical evidence, leaving physicians to face clinical dilemmas with little informed direction. This chapter provides information to help the physician sort through the morass of published literature and point to some practical ways of understanding and managing this confusing set of disorders in routine clinical practice. It will draw on available data and on the experience of medical model psychiatric professionals in dealing with these patients to address diagnostic and treatment issues. Limitations of the published literature will be identified.

History of dissociative disorders

The popularity and recognition of dissociative disorders has waxed and waned throughout medical history. Although the basic core manifestations of dissociation have remained constant, conceptualizations of the phenomenon have varied through different periods of time. Dissociation was first recognized in ancient Egypt, taking the form of spirit possession. In the Christian Bible, Jesus cast off evil spirits from a man named Legion whom some modern authorities believe was afflicted with multiple personalities. Such conceptualization of an association between dissociation and spirit possession persisted into the 1600s, 1700s, and 1800s. Several case reports of multiple personalities written during these centuries described prominent conversion features such as amnesia, paralysis, and aphonia. In the mid-1800s, the phenomenon of exorcism of evil spirits evolved into "animal magnetism" and the practice of mesmerism. These practices were forerunners of modern hypnosis.

The rapid rise in the popularity of hypnotism near the end of the nineteenth century was paralleled by the rise in popularity of multiple personality syndromes. This trend was met with a backlash of professional criticism and skepticism about therapists creating cases by suggestion and about patients beguiling their therapists by faking and acting out parts of separate personalities. Curiously, the majority of the reported cases of dissociative identity disorder were concentrated in the United States and were contributed by a small cluster of authors who cross-referenced each other extensively.

In the first half of the twentieth century, attention to dissociative disorders diminished to their near extinction. Throughout this period, dissociation was considered part of the syndrome of hysteria, now known as somatization disorder. It was not until the late 1960s that dissociation was separated from hysteria and given its own category in official diagnostic nomenclatures. Since then dissociative disorders have developed a large following of believers who maintain that they are common and underrecognized. In the early to mid-1970s, the average number of publications in the scientific literature regarding dissociative disorders began a steady increase from less than a handful per year to as many as sixty per year in the early 1990s, thereafter declining.

With the dramatization of famous cases in movies such as *The Three Faces of Eve* and *Sybil*, dissociative identity disorder erupted into an epidemic in the 1980s and 1990s, which played prominently in national magazines and on television talk shows. A parallel rise in professional interest in the disorder produced accelerating numbers of diagnosed cases and a proliferation of reports in the literature. A professional society dedicated to the study and further recognition of dissociative disorders, the International Society for the Study of Dissociation, was formed in 1984 and acquired thousands of members in a short time. The tide of popularity of multiple personalities seems to have turned in the early to mid-1990s, as the dramatic rise in cases dropped off as quickly as it had increased to less than ten per year by the turn of the current

century. The current trend in the professional literature is the conceptualization of dissociation as a post-traumatic phenomenon, with de-emphasis of the more extreme occurrence of multiple personalities.

The case described in *Sybil* was the first to draw widespread attention to the connection between childhood abuse and dissociative identity disorder, paralleling national attention to issues of child abuse in the same time period. In recent decades, dissociation has come to be more closely tied with a history of child abuse or other personal trauma, which has gained popular acceptance as causal to the disorder. This interesting theory is based largely on subjectively reported data and association rather than empirical evidence of causality.

Clinical features

The essential feature describing dissociative disorders is a disrupted integration of the mental functions of consciousness, identity, perception of the environment, and memory. The anchor diagnosis in this group of disorders is dissociative identity disorder. It is the best studied of these disorders and is by far the most represented in the literature on dissociation. Therefore, this section focuses on the diagnosis of dissociative identity disorder. Other dissociative disorders, including dissociative amnesia, dissociative fugue, and depersonalization syndrome, are discussed briefly.

Although the clinical features of dissociative disorders have been well described in a voluminous literature, an underrecognized but vital aspect of the presentation is the polysymptomatic nature of the clinical presentation. This aspect of the presentation creates issues in differential diagnosis and separation from other known disorders required for validation of diagnosis. Other related polysymptomatic disorders include somatoform disorders and personality disorders. Dissociative phenomena continue to be blurred with somatization, conversion, and post-traumatic conditions in the current literature.

Diagnosis

Dissociative identity disorder

Established diagnostic criteria for dissociative identity disorder are vague and allow opportunities for many different clinical presentations to qualify for the diagnosis. Essentially all that is required for the diagnosis is the display of two or more personalities (or "personality states") that have amnesia for each other and take control of the body at different times. Additionally, symptoms cannot be explained by the use of a substance such as alcohol or a known medical condition such as temporal lobe epilepsy (Box 18.1 and Table 18.1). In this context, *personality* is defined as an enduring pattern of behaviors that remains consistent across a wide range of situations and environments. "Personality states" are

Dissociative Disorders, Factitious Disorders, and Malingering   **277**

distinguished from complete personalities by their narrower range of occurrence, which is a vague qualifier to an intrinsically vague concept and an apparent oxymoron because "personality" refers to stable personal traits and "states" refers to unstable characteristics.

DIAGNOSTIC CRITERIA

Box 18.1 Dissociative identity disorder

A. The presence of two or more distinct identities or personality states (each with its own relatively enduring pattern of perceiving, relating to, and thinking about the environment and self).

B. At least two of these identities or personality states recurrently take control of the person's behavior.

C. Inability to recall important personal information that is too extensive to be explained by ordinary forgetfulness.

D. The disturbance is not due to the direct physiological effects of a substance (e.g., blackouts or chaotic behavior during alcohol intoxication) or a general medical condition (e.g., complex partial seizures). Note: in children, the symptoms are not attributable to imaginary playmates or other fantasy play.

From American Psychiatric Association (2000) Diagnostic and Statistical Manual of Mental Disorders, 4th Edition, Text Revision, Washington, D.C., American Psychiatric Association.

DIAGNOSIS

Table 18.1 Dissociative identity disorder

Discriminating features

1 Two or more distinct personalities take control of the person.
2 Amnesia between personalities.
3 Not explained by substance abuse or medical condition.

Consistent features

1 Vast majority of cases are young women.
2 Rarely a freestanding condition; 2–4 other diagnoses are common.
3 Comorbid somatization and borderline personality (women), antisocial personality (men).
4 Multiple symptoms in multiple organ systems are classic features, as are multiple diagnoses and multiple failed treatments.

Variable features

1 Substance use disorder is common.

Although the previously mentioned criteria are all that are technically needed for the diagnosis of dissociative identity disorder, the vagueness of these criteria has led experts in

the field to identify additional "core" features without concluding that the symptoms really fit the syndrome as intended by the definition (Box 18.2).

BOX 18.2

Additional symptoms of dissociative identity disorder

1 Time distortion or time lapses.
2 Report of behavioral episodes (of alternate personalities) by others that the individual does not recall.
3 Notable changes in behavior associated with the use of a different name.
4 Severe headaches associated with blackouts, seizures, dreams, visions, or voices (presumably switches between personalities).
5 Use of "we" to refer to self in conversation.
6 Discovery of writings, drawings, or new articles of clothing in the patient's possession that are not recognized by the patient.
7 Appearance of personalities with hypnosis.
8 Hearing internal voices.

The diagnosis of dissociative identity disorder has not been validated by the five-phase process of Robins and Guze that is patterned after the medical criteria of Sydenham. This process includes clinical description of the syndrome, delineation from other psychiatric disorders, family studies, follow-up studies to ascertain stability of the diagnosis over time, and laboratory studies to define unique objective characteristics of the syndrome. In particular, studies to delineate dissociative identity disorder from other psychiatric disorders, as well as family studies and follow-up studies, are lacking. However, such investigations are feasible. Therefore, the remainder of the discussion of dissociative disorders proceeds with the recognition that these syndromes do not yet constitute validated diagnoses.

Other dissociative disorders

Dissociative amnesia, formerly termed psychogenic amnesia, is defined as a loss of memory for important personal information that is too extensive to be explained by ordinary forgetfulness and that occurs in the context of traumatic or stressful events or psychological conflicts. A dissociative fugue is characterized by sudden, unexpected travel from usual surroundings with no recollection of the person's autobiographical past. The individual presents with confusion about personal identity or may even adopt a totally new identity with complete amnesia for the former one. The new personality usually is more gregarious and uninhibited than the individual's usual character and shows no overt evidence of psychiatric illness aside from the identity switch. Lack of memory for the fugue state after recovering from it is characteristically reported. Depersonalization disorder is the experience of one or more episodes of prominent feelings of detachment from oneself, as if an outside observer of one's body or mind, or in a dream. However, contact with reality is intact.

These dissociative disorders are diagnosed only when symptoms are significantly distressing or impair an individual's ability to function in social, occupational, or other important areas of life; they do not constitute separate diagnoses if they are part of dissociative identity disorder. By definition, dissociative disorders are not diagnosed if the symptoms occur only as part of another psychiatric disturbance such as post-traumatic stress disorder (PTSD), somatization disorder, or schizophrenia or if the symptoms are caused by a neurological or other medical condition (such as head trauma or seizure disorder) or by the effects of a substance (such as alcohol or prescription or illicit drugs).

Natural history

Ninety percent of patients with dissociative identity disorder are women. Women with this disorder most often come to the attention of professionals in the mental health system; men with this disorder usually receive attention through the criminal system. Age of diagnosis is typically in the third and fourth decades, and the average time between symptom onset and diagnosis of dissociative identity disorder is said to be 6–7 years. The onset of dissociative symptoms may be associated with stressful or traumatic situational difficulties.

Popular professional belief maintains that although dissociative identity disorder is seldom recognized until adulthood, its origins may typically occur between the ages of five and ten years. However, these claims are based on information retrospectively reported, often in the context of trying to connect the first onset of dissociative symptoms to alleged childhood molestation. Although as many as 96–98% of cases of dissociative identity disorder have been reported to have been preceded by a history of childhood sexual abuse, no methodologically adequate studies are available to document or refute such claims. Regardless, childhood sexual and physical abuse histories are commonly reported by these patients, often in graphic detail.

Dissociative symptoms often (but not always) appear to arise in the context of hypnosis, hypnotherapy, or guided imagery therapy. However, given the amount of media information and endorsement widely available, dissociation can occur outside of any therapeutic context.

Although high-functioning patients occasionally have been described in the literature, patients with dissociative disorders may be severely disabled. Little is known about the long-term prognosis, but the comorbid disorders that usually accompany dissociative disorders (see the section on differential diagnosis) are chronic and disabling conditions with typically poor outcomes that indicate a guarded overall prognosis. The ultimate prognosis is thought to depend on the presence or absence of such comorbid disorders. Overall improvement may be evident during middle age, which is also the documented course for the common comorbid diagnoses regardless of the presence or absence of dissociative disorder. Recurrent episodes may occur during particularly stressful or traumatic periods of the individual's life.

Differential diagnosis

Dissociative disorders must be differentiated from medical conditions, particularly neurological conditions such as head injuries, and from the effects of psychoactive substances that can lead to memory impairment (see Chapter 14). Unlike dissociative disorders, head injuries tend to produce circumscribed, retrograde memory loss typically involving the period directly before the injury. Similarly, electroconvulsive therapy produces immediate, temporary retrograde memory impairment with occasional brief difficulty in generating new memories. In contrast, dissociative memory difficulties are typically anterograde (that is, the memory loss is restricted to a circumscribed period following a traumatic event) and are very specific to certain time periods surrounding personally traumatic events and to specified content such as an inability to recall certain personal information (such as name, address, current employment, or family). Characteristic dissociative complaints include an inability to recall memories before a certain age and sometimes amnesia for an entire childhood. Similarly, patients may claim to lack any memory for a specific time period such as between 6 and 12 years of age or throughout a period of alleged childhood incest experiences. Amnesia of medical origin is not generally reversible, in contrast with the sometimes dramatic and sudden return of memories with dissociative amnesia, often in a flood of visualizations and flashbacks (especially when aided by hypnosis or guided imagery).

Dissociative fugues must also be differentiated from complex partial seizures. With the latter, patients may wander, exhibit semipurposeful behavior, and display amnesia. Distinguishing features of seizure disorders are characteristic auras, motor abnormalities, stereotyped behaviors, perceptual alterations, postictal phenomena, and abnormal electroencephalographic findings that evolve over time. True seizure episodes are brief, typically lasting less than five minutes and sometimes less than one minute, whereas dissociative episodes may last hours to days or sometimes periods of weeks or longer.

Dissociative identity disorder has been compared with syphilis in its proclivity to simulate a wide array of medical and psychiatric conditions. Patients with dissociation may report multiple unexplained medical symptoms in multiple organ systems that are indistinguishable from the pattern of patients with somatization disorder (see Chapter 17). Of the patients with dissociative identity disorder, 80–100% have been found to qualify for a diagnosis of somatization disorder. Conversion symptoms, including florid presentations such as limb paralysis and pseudoseizures, are common.

Elaborate diagnostic comorbidity is a consistent feature of dissociative identity disorder; therefore, it has been characterized as a polysymptomatic, polysyndromic condition. The average patient with this disorder meets criteria for three or four additional psychiatric disorders. Severe depression is present in 70–100% of these patients, and approximately 75% of the patients also report "high periods." Anxiety symptoms and panic attacks are prominent complaints. Psychotic symptoms are reported by at least 90% of patients, and they tend to report more psychotic symptoms than do patients with documented schizophrenia. Although patients with dissociative identity disorder do not develop schizophrenia, about one-half receive this diagnosis in error during the course of their treatment.

Personality disorders have been diagnosed in 69–84% of patients with dissociative identity disorder. The most prevalent Axis II disorder is borderline personality, with one-half of patients meeting criteria for this disorder. The next most prevalent personality disorder is antisocial personality, with one-fourth to one-half of cases meeting criteria. Patients with dissociative disorders often have significant impulse control problems. Eating disorders, particularly bulimia, are commonly associated. At least one-half of patients develop comorbid substance abuse.

Considerable disagreement surrounds the classification of the many comorbid conditions for which patients with dissociative identity disorder technically meet criteria. Some experts maintain that dissociative identity disorder is the superordinate condition and subsumes all the (extensive) comorbid psychopathology. Others argue that the other psychiatric disorders are relevant, perhaps even more relevant than the dissociative identity disorder in terms of course, prognosis, and treatment. Our view is that dissociative identity disorder is most likely an epiphenomenon or a severity marker of comorbid diagnoses, most commonly somatization disorder and borderline personality disorder in women and antisocial personality disorder in men. An advantage of the multiaxial classification scheme of psychiatric disorders is that it allows diagnosis of all relevant disorders, which facilitates the management of dissociative identity disorder within its larger and important multidiagnostic context.

Dissociative disorders must be differentiated from malingering, in which an individual may feign loss of self-identity, amnesia for certain actions, and lack of responsibility for actions of an alternate personality. For example, an individual might purposely enact a dissociative fugue with the clear intent to escape personal troubles such as legal action, financial consequences of bad debts, or military duty. In a famous case, the Hillside Strangler (Kenneth Bianchi) faked dissociative identity disorder skillfully enough to convince several experts. He used this disorder in court as a defense for his serial murders but ultimately failed.

The nature of the diagnostic criteria makes an accurate diagnosis of "real" dissociative syndromes a formidable challenge and hence renders the distinction between real and feigned dissociations virtually impossible. Hypnosis and amytal interview do not distinguish dissociative disorders from malingering, which may be successfully maintained even during these maneuvers. Although there is no simple technique to distinguish the two disorders, this task may be aided by identifying other signs of dissociative disorders (such as polysomatoform symptoms, suicide gestures, self-mutilation, childhood amnesia, and dissociative symptoms preexisting the current situation) that support the diagnosis.

Diagnosistic issues related to dissociative disorders

- Multiple symptoms of multiple disorders are a consistent feature of dissociative identity disorder. Patients with this disorder report many unexplained medical symptoms in many organ systems, as well as symptoms of other psychiatric diagnoses.
- Dissociative identity disorder almost never occurs in the absence of psychiatric comorbidity. The average patient with this disorder meets the criteria for 2–4 other psychiatric diagnoses.
- Somatization disorder and borderline personality disorder are common coexisting disorders; in men antisocial personality disorder is especially common.

PEARLS & PERILS

Genetics and family history

Genetic transmission of dissociative identity disorder has not been established. No family studies (actual examination of family members) have been done. Family history studies (asking patients about their relatives) provide imprecise evidence through secondhand information from the patients. Such studies suggest an increase in reported dissociative disorders among first-degree relatives of patients with dissociative identity disorder. One study found that the majority of parents of adolescents with the disorder have high rates of dissociative problems themselves. Children of patients with dissociative identity disorder have been reported to have frequent and severe psychiatric problems, including anxiety disorders, conduct disorders, learning disorders, and attention deficit disorders.

Many patients with a dissociative disorder have alcoholic family members, including at least one-third of fathers in one series. Because of the overwhelming comorbidity of somatization disorder and borderline personality disorder in patients with dissociative disorders, diagnoses of substance abuse, somatoform disorders, and antisocial and other personality disorders are not unexpected in family members. This array of psychiatric disorders in families would predict increased vulnerability for exposure to violent trauma and child abuse in the family environment. General experience with these families has identified dysfunctional patterns with authoritarian and excessively strict parenting, extreme fundamentalist religiosity, and patterns of child abuse and neglect.

Epidemiology

Just half a century ago, dissociative identity disorder was thought to be so rare that it was considered nonexistent or extinct. However, the 1980s and 1990s witnessed a precipitous and exponential increase in reported cases, appropriately labeled an epidemic. In part, this increase in cases may stem from heightened public and professional awareness of the disorder leading to increased diagnosis. Alternatively, increased symptom reports by highly suggestible individuals may be influenced by therapists or popular sources of information.

The prevalence of dissociative identity disorder has not been adequately established in the general population. Depending on the definition used, the prevalence of dissociative identity disorder has been estimated to be between 1% and 5%, but "florid" cases are thought to be limited to 1 of every 500 people. Methodological problems, including an inadequate definition of the disorder and biased ascertainment of cases, render existing estimates unreliable. Various reports have found dissociative identity disorder to be quite prevalent in selected populations such as prostitutes (5%), psychiatric inpatients (13%), forensic patients (39%), and exotic dancers (50%).

Proponents of the validity of dissociative identity disorder claim that the disorder continues to be grossly underdiagnosed because of lack of professional awareness and general closed-mindedness. Others, however, believe that the disorder is wildly overdiagnosed by a subset of physicians and that highly suggestible individuals are vulnerable to developing symptoms of the disorder through iatrogenesis. Until more specific and reliable criteria for dissociative identity disorder are available and applied to systematically selected and representative population samples, meaningful population estimates of prevalence cannot be established.

Pathophysiology

The pathophysiology of dissociative disorders is unknown. Claims have been made regarding physiologic differences associated with different personalities, including reports of distinct responses of different personality states to alcohol, food, and allergens; differences in visual acuity and dominant handedness; and changes in handwriting styles. These claims, however, are subjective reports lacking objective verification. More objectively defined differences in respiration, heart rate, blood pressure, skin conductance, visual evoked potentials, and brain wave activity have been documented; these have been interpreted as physiological manifestations of switching personalities. Such changes, however, may represent ordinary fluctuations of normal physiological mechanisms in association with changes in emotional state that are not unique to dissociation and have been measured in other psychiatric disorders—including disorders commonly associated with dissociative disorders.

Psychological testing for dissociative identity disorder reveals characteristic profiles. Hypnotizability and suggestibility have been documented in patients with dissociative disorders through standardized tests. The typical Minnesota Multiphasic Personality Inventory (MMPI) profile in these patients shows validity scales consistent with exaggeration of disease, faking symptoms, complaint of extreme distress, and plea for help. The MMPI clinical scales show elevations of all complaint areas to pathological extremes, the highest clinical subscale being "schizophrenia," which does not measure schizophrenia in these patients but rather mirrors the common misdiagnosis of this disorder in them. (Only the masculinity–femininity scale is not elevated, tending to be low in women, which reflects stereotypical feminine interests and dependency.) Therefore, these patients complain that everything is wrong with them psychologically and physically. The MMPI profiles of patients with somatization disorder or histrionic personality and those of patients with borderline personality disorder show patterns that are indistinguishable from those of patients with dissociative identity disorder. All of these disorders are characterized by exaggerations of disease and extremely high rates of symptom complaints across the clinical scales.

Treatment

Proponents of the diagnosis of dissociative identity disorder argue that because the presentation of the disorder is often covert, concerted efforts to elicit it are necessary to allow proper treatment. A long list of symptoms containing features of practically every psychiatric disorder has been compiled to alert consideration of this diagnosis. No studies have documented that such techniques identify cases fitting established diagnostic criteria, and this practice has been criticized for its potential to overdiagnose dissociation. Unfortunately, in the zeal to uncover cases of dissociation, other important diagnoses may be overlooked. Because dissociative identity disorder rarely occurs in the absence of comorbid psychiatric disorders, especially somatization disorder and borderline personality disorder, exclusive focus on dissociative disorders obscures these other important disorders, which bears directly on treatment and outcome. Therefore, the first consideration when embarking on the treatment of dissociative disorders is to complete the psychiatric evaluation so that the important comorbid disorders –perhaps the only important disorders—are not left unaddressed.

Traditional treatment of dissociative identity disorder rests on helping the patient fuse the personalities into one—the "host" personality, or the individual who existed before allegedly breaking into two or more personalities. The prolonged treatment with intensive psychotherapy recommended by proponents of this diagnosis includes encouraging and assisting patients to recall traumatic memories, usually memories of sexual molestation during childhood. This process is often aided by hypnotic techniques to help patients learn about and fuse their personalities.

Champions of dissociative identity disorder treatment reason that successful treatment proves that the cause of the syndrome is the splitting of the consciousness into individual personalities, allegedly as a result of traumatic experiences, especially chronic abuse. Treatment outcomes do not validate diagnoses, however. Further, no controlled outcome studies of dissociative identity disorder are available to demonstrate effectiveness of such treatment methods.

Because individuals with dissociative disorders have been shown to be highly suggestible, caution is urged in efforts to help these individuals recover "lost" memories to avoid creation of false memories. Reports of recovered memories of sexual or physical abuse in childhood that had been forgotten are presently the subject of heated controversy and suspicion. While some clinicians feel that experiences of childhood abuse are grossly underreported because of a lack of professional recognition and undue skepticism, others assert that such instances are overreported and that many are iatrogenically induced by therapy or media influences. No reliable methods are available to differentiate recovered memories of actual childhood events from implanted memories, and therefore caution is recommended in interpreting such claims. The entire concept of memory repression has been challenged as being a theoretical construct whose very existence is untestable.

Caution is urged to avoid creating additional alternate personalities in these highly suggestible patients. Hypnosis and/or intensive psychotherapy that focuses on the different personalities typically yields increasing numbers of new personalities that evolve during the therapeutic process. The most expedient recommendation is avoidance of hypnosis altogether in these patients.

Even successful fusion of the personalities does not result in remission and elimination of psychiatric disability; many problems remain. These remaining problems include serious comorbid disorders (somatization disorder and borderline, antisocial, and other personality disorders) that are themselves disabling and require a great deal of time and skill to manage. It has been said by Kluft that "treatment of

MPD [multiple personality disorder] leaves one with single personality disorder, the state at which most patients enter treatment." Continued therapy is routinely recommended for at least one to two years and sometimes up to five or six years after successful fusion of the personalities. Although favorable treatment outcomes have been documented in anecdotal cases and small series of patients, common experience holds that relapse is characteristic, even among those whose personalities are apparently fused.

We recommend a diametrically opposite treatment approach. Instead of interpreting the multiple and often exotic psychiatric and somatoform symptoms exhibited by these patients as evidence of switching personalities, physicians are directed to recognize these symptoms as ordinary, typical symptoms of documented comorbid psychiatric disorders (usually somatization disorder and borderline and antisocial personality disorders). This orientation helps the physician steer through the smokescreen of dissociative symptoms while maintaining the perspective of the overall clinical picture of familiar and well-validated disorders. Physicians are reminded to remain focused on treating the comorbid psychiatric disorders, dealing with dissociative symptoms as they occur in this context. Principles delineated in other chapters of this volume regarding the treatment of somatization disorder and personality disorders are relevant for the treatment of dissociative disorders and should be followed in managing patients with these comorbid disorders—regardless of the bizarre and extreme presentations of the dissociative symptoms encountered.

Contrary to the opinions of proponents of dissociative identity disorder, we believe that the diagnosis and treatment of dissociation does not require any special background in the recognition of dissociation or in the performance of complicated procedures for fusing personalities. We believe that professionals trained in medical model psychiatry and proficient in routine management of somatization disorder and personality disorders are best equipped to manage dissociative disorders through well-established procedures for the treatment of these associated conditions.

A protocol of "benign neglect" for selected symptoms, which has been successfully applied in the treatment of somatization disorder, also has been invoked as a helpful treatment for patients with dissociative identity disorder. This does not imply neglect of the patient, but rather directing professional attention to or away from selected aspects of the patient's presentation—a form of behavioral management that steers the patient's elaboration of the illness toward healthier behaviors. Successful treatment of dissociative identity disorder with these methods has been documented by Coryell, Fahy and colleagues, Cutler and Reed, and Kohlenberg. These authors ignore the dissociative symptoms and focus therapeutic attention on encouraging patients to cope with life's difficulties and solve their interpersonal and other psychosocial difficulties without relying on dissociation.

Once therapy for the comorbid disorders is under way, some dissociative symptoms may remain to be managed. Skeptics encourage confronting the patient and forbidding him or her to discuss dissociative symptoms in a behavioral program that directly discourages displays of dissociative symptoms and rewards efforts focused on resolving situational problems. Although anecdotal reports have described effective use of this method, such confrontational techniques carry the risk of alienating the patient, as well as some of the patient's social supports who may also be invested in the patient's dissociation.

A less confrontational approach establishes therapeutic engagement of the patient by first obtaining a history of dissociative symptoms (such as the names and descriptions of all the alternate personalities) and then informing the patient gently that, although he or she may experience different personalities, these personalities represent different aspects of one person with different feelings, urges, and behavior patterns. The patient is then encouraged to begin accepting these aspects as part of his or her personality and to become involved in the process of starting to solve problems and learning better ways to cope. Over time, the complaints of multiple personalities and the associated constellation of symptoms can begin to fade as the patient obtains positive attention for responsible behaviors and begins to enjoy the fruits of achieving mastery over problem areas of life.

Patients with dissociative disorders may have had previous treatment that encouraged them to recall previous traumas such as childhood molestation for the purpose of confronting and psychologically working through the trauma. Such work may have occurred in "survivor group" settings that encourage patients to further entrench themselves in the victimization role. Although issues of victimization cannot be ignored, therapy must balance resolution of traumatic experiences with helping the patient emerge from the victim role and develop an increasing sense of self-reliance and control over destiny.

Therapy with dissociative disorder patients can be extremely demanding, frustrating, and even harrowing, partly because these patients can be skillful at carving deep divisions between caregivers. Differences of opinion among mental health professionals regarding the existence of dissociative identity disorder and the interpretation of its symptoms provide fertile ground for manipulative behaviors to create havoc in the treatment team. Satisfactory management demands obtaining the agreement of the entire treatment team and establishing firm boundaries early in the treatment process.

Patients with dissociative disorders often display suicidal and self-destructive behaviors, such as self-mutilation by cutting themselves with razor blades, burning themselves with cigarettes, or inserting sharp or caustic substances into the vagina. These behaviors are also exhibited by patients with severe borderline personality disorder. In environments that provide attention and positive rewards for these behaviors, the behaviors can escalate to chronic suicidality, frequent suicide gestures, and preoccupation with self-mutilation. A united treatment team can respond to such behaviors by discouraging repetition and setting limits, helping the patient find more appropriate ways to deal with conflicts and meet personal goals.

No medications have been documented to be of specific value for the treatment of dissociation. When a diagnosis of major depressive disorder can be made (often a difficult distinction in these polysymptomatic patients), antidepressant medication may be appropriate for treating the depression. Serotonin-selective reuptake inhibitors are safer than tricyclic antidepressants in these often impulsive, self-destructive individuals who are prone to overdoses. Complaints of anxiety may tempt the physician to prescribe benzodiazepines, but caution is recommended in prescribing abusable medications in dissociative patients because of their high risk for abuse and dependence. Complete evaluation of these patients must always include attention to possible substance abuse disorders because of the high rates of such disorders in dissociative identity disorders. Chemical dependency treatment may be indicated if substance abuse is present. Although patients with dissociative disorders often complain of psychotic-like symptoms, these patients are not considered to be psychotic. Antipsychotic medications are not generally indicated for the treatment of dissociative disorders, especially when the potential for irreversible involuntary movement disorders such as tardive dyskinesia and other potentially serious side effects are considered.

Treatment of dissociative disorders

PEARLS & PERILS

- Make sure the psychiatric evaluation is complete.
- The central tasks of management are to diagnose and treat the coexisting disorders, which are likely to be more relevant than the dissociative disorder for designing treatment and establishing prognosis.
- Physicians and other caregivers are cautioned not to get lost in the smokescreen of dissociative, psychiatric, and medical symptoms, but to remain focused on the overall clinical picture, which includes remaining oriented to the more relevant coexisting disorders.
- Established treatments for coexisting disorders (e.g., somatization disorder and borderline personality disorder) are relevant for the treatment of patients with dissociative disorders and should be followed, regardless of the extreme or bizarre presentation of dissociation.

Special issues in dissociation

A recent trend in popular mental health and self-help circles is the identification of a childhood history of satanic cult abuse. Many therapists who diagnose and treat large numbers of patients with dissociative identity disorder are also involved with helping patients recover memories of satanic cult abuse, and many of the patients at risk for dissociative identity disorder are also at risk for developing these recovered memories. A popular genre of self-help books on uncovering forgotten childhood memories of abuse and satanic ritual abuse has spread these ideas and has provided often-recommended reading to accompany child abuse survivor therapy. Patients exposed to this material through books, the media, other patients, or therapist suggestion and encouragement may describe macabre stories of extreme abuse at the hands of a satanic cult, often with stereotypical content involving ritualistic sexual torture, impregnation of young girls and sacrifice of the fetus, the importation of babies from third-world countries for sacrificial rituals, and the consumption of blood, urine, and human flesh—stories that push the outer boundaries of believability for most professionals.

Therapeutic recommendations by some proponents of dissociative disorders include blaming family members, particularly parents, for the abuse. Formal accusations against family members and the termination of family contact by such patients has led affected families to band together into a national group, the False Memory Syndrome Foundation. This group allows families to deny these accusations formally, recover from alleged damages to their families and community reputations, support one another in trying to regain contact with their loved ones, and advocate against therapy designed to recover such memories.

When managing patients who have allegations of sexual abuse based on recovered memories, it is recommended that physicians maintain a neutral stance, neither accepting the claims uncritically nor rejecting them outright. It is not the physician's role to be a detective, and further exploration of the memory (via hypnosis, guided imagery, or amobarbital) without external validation does not enhance the validity of the memory as a reflection of past events. Physicians should maintain the perspective of the overall clinical picture, diagnose and treat relevant comorbid disorders, and help patients learn to cope with and solve interpersonal difficulties and other psychosocial dilemmas that are almost invariably present.

Physicians and mental health professionals are encouraged to maintain an atheoretical stance on the etiology of the psychopathology of dissociative disorders. Childhood abuse has no more been shown to be a cause of dissociative disorders than it has been shown to be the etiological basis of somatization disorder or borderline personality disorder, which are conditions that also are associated with childhood abuse. Maintaining such an agnostic stance enables physicians to proceed with treatment unencumbered by preconceived notions of the need to resolve childhood abuse issues in order to cure the disorder.

Factitious disorders

Perspective on factitious disorders

The intentional production or feigning of physical or psychological signs or symptoms without an external incentive (Box 18.3 and Table 18.2) is indicative of some of the most interesting illnesses in psychiatry with their bizarre, colorful, dramatic, dangerous, and frustrating presentations. It is easy to appreciate the physician's (and the public's) fascination in trying to understand the following behavior(s)/claim:

> Self-destructiveness in injecting oneself with parrot feces, the grandiosity of claiming to be an oceanographic physicist working with Jacques Cousteau, the passivity of submitting to 48 lumbar punctures, the skill to stop breathing to unconsciousness, and the wanderlust for 423 admissions. (Pankratz, 1981)

Unfortunately, scientific understanding of these disorders is still in its infancy because of numerous issues: (1) evolving conceptualization of the disorder, (2) changing descriptions of "typical patient" profiles, (3) difficulties inherent in establishing the diagnosis, (4) infrequent case identification, (5) difficulties in delimitation from comorbid illness, (6) lack of significant follow-up studies, (7) lack of significant family studies, and (8) problematic management issues (such as patients providing misleading information, refusing treatment and failing to follow up). All of these factors preclude scientific validation of the diagnosis. The entire literature on factitious disorder consists of approximately 1000–2000 case reports, several collected series, several retrospective record reviews, anecdotal reports of treatment (single-case), and a substantial amount of academic review papers considering theoretical aspects. Nonetheless, few if any authors doubt the existence of the phenomenon and that the patients suffer.

Box 18.3 Factitious disorder

DIAGNOSTIC CRITERIA

A. Intentional production or feigning of physical or psychological signs or symptoms.

B. The motivation for the behavior is to assume the sick role.

C. External incentives for the behavior (such as economic gain, avoiding legal responsibility, or improving physical well-being, as in malingering) are absent.

Code based on type:

- with predominantly psychological signs and symptoms: if psychological signs and symptoms predominate in the clinical presentation
- with predominantly physical signs and symptoms: if physical signs and symptoms predominate in the clinical presentation
- with combined psychological and physical signs and symptoms: if both psychological and physical signs and symptoms are present but neither predominates in the clinical presentation.

From American Psychiatric Association (2000) Diagnostic and Statistical Manual of Mental Disorders, 4th Edition, Text Revision, Washington, D.C., American Psychiatric Association.

History of factitious disorder

Although Munchausen's syndrome is the most commonly described manifestation of factitious disorder, it appears to represent only the most extreme (and notorious) form of what is in all likelihood an uncommon phenomenon. The first known medical description of factitious illness was by Chowne in 1843 as cited in Enoch and Trethowan. Chowne identified a man with "great bodily weakness and depression," which was attributed to "an irritable testicle." Unilateral orchiectomy provided the man with some relief, but the relief was only temporary, and it was decided that the other testicle had to be removed.

In 1951, Asher borrowed the name *Munchausen* and applied it to patients who demonstrated pathological lying (pseudologia fantastica) and wandering (peregrination).

DIAGNOSIS

Table 18.2 Factitious disorder

Discriminating features

1 Intentional production or feigning of physical or psychological signs or symptoms.
2 Motivation is to assume the sick role.
3 No secondary gain evident.

Consistent features

1 Intentionality is apparent (e.g., injecting feces, ingesting phenolphthalein).
2 Factitious disorder by proxy involves inflicting factitious symptoms on another (typically the patient's own child).

Variable features

1 May include psychiatric as well as physical scenarios.
2 Patients with Munchausen's syndrome demonstrate extreme peregrination and repetitive visits to multiple medical centers.
3 Patients produce simple to complicated and imaginative syndromes.
4 Many patients work in the health care field.

The name was taken from Rudolf Eric Raspe's book, *Baron Munchausen's Narrative of His Marvelous Travels and Campaigns in Russia,* because of the colorful accounts and peregrinations of Baron Karl Friedrich Hieronymous von Munchausen. The Baron, a former calvary officer in the Russian army, had a reputation for being a raconteur of outrageous stories and wandering to find audiences.

Asher's eponym was subsequently faulted by Spiro because the term *Munchausen's syndrome* was "too closely associated with lying, swindling, and the negative connotations of these behaviors." Additionally, the label was considered to be a misnomer according to Nadelson because Baron von Munchausen was not known for seeking medical attention or for engaging in self-destructive acts. In 1988, Patterson wrote that there was no evidence that Baron von Munchausen believed his stories or was trying to deceive his listeners. It appeared that Raspe alone benefitted financially from his book, and Baron von Munchausen was embarrassed as well as resentful of the unwanted fame it brought him. Nevertheless, Munchausen's syndrome remained the selected nomenclature because, as Nadelson wrote, "The Baron's name is a more charming, evocative, antique, and noble reference and makes a more mouthfilling phrase."

Numerous other pseudoscientific appellations have been applied to patients who exhibit signs or symptoms of Munchausen's syndrome, including "hospital hobos," "hospital addicts," "metabolic malingerers," and "peregrinating problem patients." In 1968, Spiro proffered the term *chronic factitious symptomatology,* which was in part included in the DSM-III in 1980.

Asher was more successful with his original descriptions of these patients and captured the essence of their medical presentation, which warrants repeating:

> The patient showing the syndrome is admitted to the hospital with apparent acute illness supported by a plausible and dramatic history. Usually his story is largely made up of falsehoods; he is found to have attended, and deceived, an astounding number of hospitals; and he nearly always discharges himself against advice, after quarreling violently with both doctors and nurses. A large number of abdominal scars is particularly characteristic of this condition (Asher, 1951).

Asher went on to describe several well-known varieties that resemble organic emergencies:

1 The acute abdominal type (laparotomaphilia migrans), which is the most common. Some of the patients have had surgery so often that the development of genuine intestinal obstructions from adhesions may confuse the picture.

2 The hemorrhagic type, who specializes in bleeding from the lungs or stomach or from other blood loss. These types are colloquially known as "haemoptysis merchants," and "haematemesis merchants."

3 The neurologic type, who has a paroxysmal headache, loss of consciousness, or peculiar fits.

Subsequent to Asher's description of Munchausen's syndrome, a disproportionate amount of the literature focused on an evolving profile of the typical patient with factitious disorder as mostly male with a history of antisocial behavior (with or without criminality), multisystem complaints, substance abuse, and drifting behavior with numerous hospitalizations. Interestingly, contemporaneous with early descriptions were a small number of reports identifying a different type of patient—young, geographically stable women. These early reports were supported by the case series (collected from interview and hospital records) reported by Carney and by Reich and Gottfried. Together, both series contained a total of 65 women (76 patients total) who were mostly young female nonwanderers. Reich and Gottfried opined that approximately 90% of the patients with factitious disorder would not fit the typical profile of (male) Munchausen's syndrome.

In 1976, Sneed and Bell applied the term dauphin of Munchausen's to a case in which a mother was suspected of conspiring with a ten-year-old boy to present factitious recurrent urinary calculi. In 1977, Meadow applied the term Munchausen by proxy to an individual who fabricates signs or symptoms of illness in another person with the intention of indirectly assuming the sick role (Box 18.4). The term was usually applied to a parent-child interaction in which the parent assumes the sick role indirectly through the child. The

child was not diagnosed with factitious disorder unless he or she was part of the conspiracy.

The literature has described two other potential variants of factitious disorder, but no distinct patient profile has emerged. These labels are factitious disorder with predominantly psychological symptoms and factitious disorder with combined psychological and physical symptoms. In 1980, DSM-III formally codified factitious disorders. Establishing criteria facilitated the development of a conceptual framework for all the "simulating" disorders: malingering, factitious disorder, and somatoform disorders. This paradigm was based on ascertaining whether a symptom was voluntarily or involuntarily produced and whether it originated consciously or unconsciously. A simulating spectrum model could be established with malingering (voluntarily produced symptoms consciously constructed) at one end and somatoform disorders (involuntarily produced symptoms unconsciously constructed) at the other. Factitious disorder would be placed between the poles because symptoms are voluntarily produced but unconsciously constructed (a nebulous concept at best).

In 1985, Jonas and Pope advocated avoiding the conundrum of attempting to ascertain voluntary control and consciousness of symptoms in favor of focusing on objective features. In particular, they suggested that studies "using modern diagnostic criteria, might assess the demographics, associated phenomenology, biological findings (if any), family history, treatment response, and long-term outcome of a cohort of patients presenting particularly clear-cut factitious signs or symptoms."

Clinical features

Diagnosis

Although the diagnostic criteria for factitious disorder (see Box 18.3 and Table 18.2) remain controversial and unvalidated, sufficient overlapping descriptive case material on factitious disorder with predominantly physical signs and symptoms exists to provide guidance to the physician in recognizing these patients. In what appears to be the more severe form, physicians would expect to find some (or all) of the following features: pseudologia fantastica, peregrination (wandering), antisocial behavior, substance abuse, an extraordinarily complex medical history with an above-average level of medical knowledge, and chaotic hospital course.

Pseudologia fantastica is probably the most commonly identified facet of this illness and refers to the generation of innumerable fabrications that involve both medical information and life history. The descriptions are dramatic, flamboyant, plausible, intriguing, and almost always untrue. According to Asher, patients with this disorder "lie for the sake of lying." Peregrination is often uncovered in patients who choose to divulge information about their multiple medical hospitalizations and treatment in various regions or states. Some patients eagerly describe prior extensive medical and surgical procedures but refuse to identify or allow contact with the health care providers. These patients may demonstrate a particular symptom and deny prior evaluation and/or treatment, but a physical examination reveals numerous surgical scars and other evidence, such as bus tickets or suitcases, that suggests traveling.

Antisocial tendencies are commonly described in these individuals but usually take the form of minor antisocial acts such as vagrancy, peace disturbance, petty theft, and misdemeanor drug transgressions. Substance abuse is a common problem, but these individuals are not often described as dependent.

The medical knowledge exhibited by these individuals can be astounding. At initial presentation, some can provide their diagnosis, the founder of the disease, and the "classic" description of their illness. While discussing their evaluation, they may directly and without deviation provide the information necessary to drive the medical decision algorithm. Even when patients do not intentionally attempt to demonstrate medical knowledge, the physician may be alerted to this issue when the patient asks for certain medications by generic name or seems to be familiar with the hospital routine after a brief stay. A noteworthy clinical point is the common incongruence between what the patient describes as extremely serious medical illness and a lack of appropriate concern demonstrated by the patient (for example, an inpatient calmly relates the presence of gross blood in the saliva and urine (from a surreptitious finger stick) but vigorously complains about the smoking restrictions in the hospital).

Chaotic hospitalizations are the rule with these patients. Their hospital stays begin quietly as the initial work-up proceeds. However, as the final laboratory work is processed or as the wound heals, the patient may begin to evolve "new symptoms." Additionally, the patient may develop difficulties with the hospital staff regarding policies and procedures. At this juncture these patients often sign out of the hospital against medical advice.

In the apparently "less severely ill" female patients with factitious disorder, the absence of the more flamboyant features may prove particularly troublesome in establishing the diagnosis. In Reich and Gottfried's large outpatient series of patients with factitious disorder, pseudologia fantastica or peregrinations were not described but rather single body system complaint(s) with fewer hospitalizations. These authors collected and described a number of presentations (with etiologies) of factitious illness, including: (1) sepsis (introduction of contaminant), (2) failure of wound healing (introduction of a foreign body or manipulation), (3) fever (manipulation of thermometer), (4) metabolic disturbance (such as diuretics), (5) inappropriate use of indicated or surreptitious illicit substances (such as insulin), (6) frankly simulated history and signs of illness, and (7) surreptitious introduction of blood to body cavities, secretions, and excretions.

Wallach identified a number of common illnesses associated with factitious disorder, as well as a lengthy list of uncommonly produced illnesses. Although space does not permit lengthy review, the identification of several of these serves the purpose of educating the physician about the extraordinary interventions these patients undertake to remain in the sick role. These include simulation of pheochromocytoma by self-injection of metaraminol, isoproterenol hydrochloride, or epinephrine (along with addition of epinephrine to the urine); pancytopenia by the ingestion of alkylating agents; and liver disease precipitated by hypervitaminosis A or by excessive ingestion of retinol.

Two final remarks about these patients are warranted. First, a significant number of patients with identified factitious disorder with physical symptoms worked in the health care field. Aduan and colleagues reported a series of 13 patients with self-induced infections; 10 of these patients were nurses. In the Reich and Gottfried series, 28 of 39 patients worked in the health care field. Finally, physicians should be aware that the only limitations to a factitious complaint are the patient's intelligence, motivation, and ingenuity.

Rosenberg reviewed 117 well-documented cases collected from the literature that were considered to represent the phenomenon of factitious disorder by proxy. Rosenberg found that 98% of the perpetrators were the biological mothers (producing symptoms in their children) and estimated the mortality rate at 9%. The factitious symptoms represented a wide variety of body system(s) dysfunctions, including bleeding (44%), seizures (42%), central nervous system (CNS) depression (19%), apnea (15%), hematuria (13%), diarrhea (11%), vomiting (10%), fever (10%), rash (9%), hemoptysis (3%), and upper respiratory tract abnormalities (1%). (The percentages add up to more than 100% because of multiple factitious symptoms.)

The clinical features of both factitious disorder with predominantly psychological symptoms and factitious disorder with combined psychological and physical symptoms have not been adequately described.

Natural history

The natural course of factitious disorders is unknown.

Differential diagnosis

The possibility that a physical illness is causing the sign(s) and/or symptom(s) must be thoroughly evaluated first. A number of common medical illnesses that often manifest as vague motor or sensory symptoms (such as multiple sclerosis, acute intermittent porphyria, systemic lupus erythematosus) must be considered. Occasionally, serious thought is given to truncating the medical evaluation of "difficult patients," but a thorough assessment should be completed before psychiatric intervention. Mood and psychotic disorders can occasionally present with somatic symptomatology but are usually easily excluded by a complete review of the case history and consideration of the diagnostic criteria.

A confident diagnosis of factitious disorder requires excluding other simulating disorders. Although somatization (involuntary production) is almost always part of a general differential, the voluntary production of a symptom is rarely considered. In an attempt to determine the voluntary and conscious production of a symptom, the physician usually must change his role to a more investigative stance. This change may require a range of new behaviors, including multiple interviews with the patient, increased observation of the patient, additional laboratory evaluation, interview of collateral sources, and possibly a room search. All of these activities are undertaken in the best interest of the patient to answer the diagnostic issue. Finally, potential external incentives ("secondary gain") should be reviewed to facilitate the exclusion of malingering.

The presence of factitious disorder does not prevent patients from developing physical illness as a result of previous actions (such as bowel obstruction from adhesions or endocarditis). It also does not prevent the occurrence of "natural" medical illness.

Genetics and family history

The genetics and family history of factitious disorder are unknown.

Epidemiology

The epidemiology of factitious disorder is unknown.

Pathophysiology

The pathophysiology of factitious disorder is unknown.

PEARLS & PERILS

Factitious disorders

- Factitious disorder is rare. Physicians should focus on a thorough evaluation of the complaint(s) with the expectation that a good history, physical examination, and laboratory tests will be helpful and may detect unexpected pathology in addition to factitious complaints.
- Although patterns of presentation have been proposed, each patient will have distinctive features and generalization across patients is difficult.
- Factitious disorder is associated with dramatic, flamboyant fabrications that seem plausible, at least initially.
- Patients with factitious disorder are likely to wander from hospital to hospital. Sustaining a therapeutic relationship between caregivers and patient is difficult.
- Patients with factitious disorder often have substantial knowledge of medicine and many have connections to the health care field.
- Factitious disorder by proxy can be a form of abuse/neglect.

Treatment

Once the diagnosis of factitious disorder has been established, most experts suggest consultation with psychiatrists. Unfortunately, no controlled trials regarding the psychiatric/medical management of these patients have been conducted. Treatment recommendations identified in the literature are based on case reports involving one or two patients. In fact, the core issue of how patients should be confronted has not been settled. Stone advocated vigorous confrontation at an early stage of treatment. Hollender and Hersh suggested that both the primary physician and the psychiatrist be involved in the confrontation. According to Eisendrath, Ford suggested that confrontation be performed in a manner that is neither hostile nor punitive, with the primary care physician and the psychiatrist both continuing to treat the patient. Some authors have suggested that patients should not be confronted at all. Physicians should be prepared for the possibility that patients may sign out of the hospital against medical advice. Should the patient be engaged for treatment, controlled trial data do not support any particular form of psychiatric intervention.

Malingering

Perspectives on the label

Malingering is listed in the DSM-IV-TR, but neither as a mental illness nor a mental disorder. It is listed under the section entitled, "Other conditions that may be the focus of clinical

DSM-IV-TR definition of malingering

The essential feature of malingering is the intentional production of false or grossly exaggerated physical or psychological symptoms, motivated by external incentives such as avoiding military duty, avoiding work, obtaining financial compensation, evading criminal prosecution, or obtaining drugs. Malingering should be strongly suspected if any combination of the following is noted:

1 Medicolegal context of presentation (e.g., the person is referred by an attorney to the clinician for examination)
2 Marked discrepancy between the person's claimed stress or disability and the objective findings
3 Lack of cooperation during the diagnostic evaluation and in complying with the prescribed treatment regimen
4 The presence of antisocial personality disorder.

From American Psychiatric Association (2000) Diagnostic and Statistical Manual of Mental Disorders, 4th Edition, Text Revision, Washington, D.C., American Psychiatric Association.

attention." The label is predicated on the intentional production of a false or grossly exaggerated physical or psychology symptom(s) for the purpose of secondary gain (see Box 18.5).

Malingering has been described by many, including the Bible (Samuel), Shakespeare, Galen, Zacchias, and Beck. The medical literature contains many case reports of elaborate schemes and personality profiles "consistent with" malingering. Antisocial personality has often been linked with deception and malingering.

Definitive research in the area has been difficult for a number of reasons. First, it is difficult to confirm malingering. Second, it is difficult to enroll people focused on deception in a study. Third, it is very difficult to obtain enough subjects to conduct a study. Fourth, design of a control group is particularly problematic. Fifth, there are several potential designs which avoid these problems, but they each have their own unique set of problems. In one of the more popular designs, individuals are offered small incentives to fake illness. The challenge then becomes developing "normal non-faking" controls. Later, the question arises whether any differences are in fact real, since neither group were true fakers. Unfortunately, the aforementioned problems have made design and implementation of definitive research virtually impossible.

In the forensic setting, the drives for avoidance of criminal responsibility and monetary compensation for damages have facilitated the utilization of preexisting neuropsychological subtests and the development of several tests to assist in evaluating possible malingering in certain types of cases. Widespread agreement regarding any definitive testing approach does not appear imminent.

Malingering can be assigned when the individual intentionally provides medical information that is proven false and a linkage can be established to a secondary gain. This is rarely, particularly without admission by the patient, an easy task. Most individuals are aware that proving intent (state of mind) and, more precisely, intent to deceive, is problematic for a multitude of reasons. In doctor-patient interactions, the patient usually has a heavy investment in not being discovered, because, among other reasons, it means complete loss of credibility with the physician. As most physicians realize, obtaining a diagnosis for certain illnesses can be challenging enough, but proving the negative in certain cases can be virtually impossible. Diagnoses of somatization disorder, pain disorder, conversion disorder, and factitious disorder can further complicate the situation, particularly for physicians not familiar with these illnesses. Linkage with a secondary medical gain may appear obvious on the face of the situation, but physicians should recognize that by giving the label of malingering they are formally proffering the opinion that there is a secondary gain with an intentional connection to the medical information. Proving the connection may be very difficult. Non-medical secondary gains may require outside investigation which may not be possible (or advisable) by the medical provider.

The potential impact of assigning a label of malingering by the medical provider can be substantial. Physicians have a bias toward believing what patients tell them unless there is substantial reason (and it is in the patients' best interest) to believe otherwise. When clinicians apply this label, they should be aware that it has very significant long-term ramifications for the patient. It may irreparably harm the current physician-patient relationship. Any physician who subsequently obtains the patient's records will probably consider this history when reviewing any medical data provided by the patient. At a minimum, the patient may lose the benefit of the doubt but, at a maximum, the patient may lose the physician's bias toward believing the patient, which makes caring for the patient very difficult. In particular, patients cannot prove their symptoms. Insurance companies may refuse to cover the individual, suspecting fraud and/or deception. In the forensic arena, the label is offered with some regularity, usually based on a substantial amount of evidence. The label itself in a legal proceeding is not as potentially damaging as a legal finding by a judge or jury that the malingering opinion is in fact legally true. This may also mean it is the opinion of the court that the patient/litigant is not only trying to fool the doctor, but also the court. While fair hearing may render the finding of malingering legally defensible, the individual's credibility is completely destroyed.

In summary, malingering is a well-appreciated phenomenon that has been described for centuries. Modern scientific research methods have not produced a reliable interview technique or test that definitively identifies malingering. The label has significant ramifications for patients, physicians, medicine, and the legal system. Finally, malingering may be most appropriately applied when the patient clearly admits the deception and/or evidence is substantial.

Malingering

PEARLS & PERILS

- Production of false symptoms is difficult to prove.
- Presentation is likely to be unique to each individual, making generalization difficult.
- Association between false symptoms and some advantage to the patient is expected but not sufficient.
- Application of the label poses problems for the administration of care.
- Useful data are lacking and, given the ethical and moral dilemmas posed by good scientific design, are likely to remain sparse.

Conclusion

Dissociative and factitious disorders are alike in that they are allegedly motivated by unconscious factors. Relatively little empirical information is available about either disorder. Neither has been empirically validated as a medical diagnosis, but both continue to play a role in clinical practice. Dissociative identity disorder is perhaps the most controversial of all psychiatric disorders and has divided the mental health field. Many professionals do not believe the disorder exists. The identification and treatment of dissociation has been widely promulgated in mental health and popular arenas without adequate scientific investigation. Physicians who are confronted with one of these patients are advised to consider diagnostic comorbidity and other psychiatric conditions for which effective treatment protocols have been established.

More work on factitious disorder is needed to help physicians manage it effectively, but previous experience indicates that direct confrontation with the patient, although seemingly desirable, may result in abrupt termination of treatment. Malingering is difficult to prove but may be worthy of consideration when there is some combination of poor cooperation with diagnosed treatment, a marked discrepancy between reported disability and objective findings, medical-legal issues that are part of treatment and comorbid antisocial personality.

Annotated bibliography

Aldridge-Morris, R (1989) *Multiple Personality: An Exercise in Deception*, London, Erlbaum.
This British monograph about multiple personality disorder is written from a skeptical point of view. It reviews the existing literature on the disorder, with well-placed dry humor in pointing out the ridiculous nature of the disorder's flamboyant presentation.

Fay, TA (1988) The diagnosis of multiple personality disorder: a critical review, *Br J Psychiatry* 153:597–606.
This article examines the phenomenology of the epidemic of MPD and reviews the relevant literature. The author is critical of recent literature for its lack of methodological attention to the reliability of diagnosis, prevalence, and the role of selection bias. He contends that MPD has not been shown to represent a distinct psychiatric disorder and instead classifies it as a hysterical symptom.

North, CS et al. (1993) *Multiple Personalities, Multiple Disorders: Psychiatric Classification and Media Influence*, New York, Oxford University Press.
This monograph examines MPD from an empirical viewpoint using the Washington University model of psychiatric nosology. It describes the research that has been done on the disorders and provides an in-depth analysis of how MPD has developed over the years in relation to the media. Existing data on MPD are critiqued, and the current state of knowledge on the disorder is reviewed in terms of clinical description of the disorder, delineation from other disorders, family history studies, follow-up studies, and laboratory documentation. This critical and balanced approach provides a valuable guide to physicians who are trying to make sense out of this confusing and controversial disorder.

Piper, A (1994) Multiple personality disorder, *Br J Psychiatry* 164:600–612.
This article critically examines five aspects of the diagnosis and treatment of MPD. It criticizes the current diagnostic criteria as being vague and overinclusive, identifies the epidemic as being artefactually produced, examines the question of personal responsibility of patients with this disorder, examines the evidence for childhood trauma as being the hypothesized cause of the disorder, and criticizes the techniques for diagnosing and treating the disorder as reinforcing its symptoms.

CHAPTER 19

Personality Disorders

C. Robert Cloninger, MD and Dragan M. Svrakic, MD, PhD

OUTLINE

Introduction

The way that people learn from experience and adapt their feelings, thoughts, and actions is what characterizes their personality. More formally, personality can be defined as the dynamic organization within the individual of the psychobiological systems that modulate adaptation to a changing environment. This includes systems regulating cognition, emotionality, and intelligence. Personality traits are stable, enduring patterns of perceiving, relating to, and thinking about oneself, other people, and the world as a whole.

The diagnosis of a personality disorder requires that patients have chronic and pervasive impairments in their ability to work and to cooperate with others. These impairments include, for example, excessive dependency, perfectionism, rigidity, social detachment or inhibition, self-centeredness, or lack of empathy. In addition, most patients with personality disorders consistently have low self-esteem and handle stress poorly. The resulting subjective distress often leads them to complain about anxiety, depression, and worries about physical health. Lastly, these patients have difficulty in maintaining healthy lifestyle choices regarding their diet and personal activities, such as drinking, smoking, and exercise. Consequently, personality and its disorders influence both objective and subjective aspects of physical health.

Individuals with personality disorders typically blame other people or external circumstances for their own physical, psychological, or social problems. This externalizing of responsibility is a result of two characteristics to which all clinicians must be alert. First, these patients do not perceive their own psychopathology and social deviance as abnormal (i.e., their symptoms are "ego-syntonic"). Second, they try to change others, instead of changing themselves; their attitude is thus described as "alloplastic." Both

these features reflect an effort to reduce subjective distress and improve perceived quality of life.

Systematic assessment of personality disorders is especially important because they are common and usually life-long disorders with extensive psychosocial disability. When antisocial personality disorder was the only personality disorder with reliable diagnostic criteria, the overall prevalence and importance of personality disorders were greatly underestimated. Now it is recognized that personality disorders are the primary psychiatric disorders in most patients with psychosocial impairment, particularly young adults. They are present in approximately one-sixth of the general population, half of psychiatric outpatients, and two-thirds of psychiatric inpatients and people who attempt suicide. Accordingly, diagnosis and treatment of any patient with psychosocial problems is incomplete without a systematic approach to assessing and classifying personality. For example, there is extensive heterogeneity in responses to antidepressant medications that cannot be predicted on the basis of depressive symptoms, comorbid psychiatric syndromes, or subtypes defined by any other known characteristic. Nevertheless, recent independent studies have confirmed that personality traits explain most of the variability in treatment response and help to select the most effective antidepressant for each individual patient. Furthermore, once the essential features of personality disorders are learned so that they can be recognized and understood, diagnosis can be made accurately with little time or expense.

Clinical features of personality disorder

Qualitative (categorical) diagnosis

Descriptive diagnostic criteria for personality disorders have been developed by the American Psychiatric Association and are summarized in Box 19.1 and Table 19.1. As shown in Table 19.1, the maladaptive behavior patterns must be "stable and enduring," that is, they must be long-term if not lifelong characteristics. The DSM-IV criteria require that the maladaptive pattern be "of long duration and its onset can be traced back at least to adolescence or early adulthood." In practice it can be difficult to distinguish long-term maladaptation pathognomonic of personality disorders and chronic personality changes caused by other factors (e.g., other mental disorders such as chronic depression) or long-term situational factors (e.g., financial dependency on one's spouse). Second, the maladaptive pattern must be inflexible and pervasive, that is, manifest in a wide range of personal and social contexts (i.e., at home, at work, with family, and friends), not only in isolated aspects of the person's life. Finally, there must be substantial evidence of subjective distress, impaired social and occupational function, or both. Subjective distress refers to low self-esteem and limited problem-solving skills, which often lead to anxiety, depression, and hypochondriasis. Social and occupational impair-

DIAGNOSIS

Table 19.1 Qualitative description of personality disorders

Discriminating features

1 A maladaptive pattern of responses to personal and social stress that is stable and enduring since the teenage years, inflexible and pervasive, and causes subjective distress and/or impaired work and/or impaired social relations.

Consistent features

1 Strong emotional reactions elicited from others (such as anger or urge to rescue).

Variable features

1 Odd or eccentric behavior.
2 Erratic or impulsive behavior.
3 Anxious or fearful attitude.

ment in people with personality disorders result from lack of self-awareness and lack of mature goals and values.

In addition to these consistent features of all personality disorders, there is a wide range of variation in specific styles of thinking, feeling, and relating. Although the *Diagnostic and Statistical Manual of Mental Disorders* (DSM) distinguishes three clusters of personality disorders (odd, erratic, and anxious), features of more than one cluster often occur in the same patient. Furthermore, although DSM-IV subdivides each cluster into discrete subtypes of personality disorder (see Table 19.2), most patients with a personality disorder have features of more than one subtype (e.g., narcissistic, histrionic, and antisocial symptoms usually occur together).

DIAGNOSTIC CRITERIA

Box 19.1 General diagnostic criteria for a personality disorder

A. An enduring pattern of inner experience and behavior that deviates markedly from the expectations of the individual's culture. This pattern is manifested in two (or more) of the following areas:
   - cognition (i.e., ways of perceiving and interpreting self, other people, and events)
   - affectivity (i.e., the range, intensity, lability, and appropriateness of emotional response)
   - interpersonal functioning
   - impulse control.

B. The enduring pattern is inflexible and pervasive across a broad range of personal and social situations.

C. The enduring pattern leads to clinically significant distress or impairment in social, occupational, or other important areas of functioning.

D. The pattern is stable and of long duration, and its onset can be traced back at least to adolescence or early adulthood.

E. The enduring pattern is not better accounted for as a manifestation or consequence of another mental disorder.

F. The enduring pattern is not due to the direct physiological effects of a substance (e.g., a drug of abuse, a medication) or a general medical condition (e.g., head trauma).

From American Psychiatric Association (2000) Diagnostic and Statistical Manual of Mental Disorders, 4th Edition, Text Revision, Washington D.C., American Psychiatric Association.

TABLE 19.2 Qualitative clusters and subtypes of personality disorders according to the American Psychiatric Association (DSM-IV-TR)

Cluster	Subtype	Discriminating features
Odd/Eccentric	Schizoid	Socially indifferent
	Paranoid	Suspicious
	Schizotypal	Eccentric
Erratic/Impulsive	Antisocial	Disagreeable
	Borderline	Unstable
	Histrionic	Attention-seeking
	Narcissistic	Self-centered
Anxious/Fearful	Avoidant	Inhibited
	Dependent	Submissive
	Obsessive	Perfectionistic
Not otherwise specified	Passive-aggressive	Negativistic
	Depressive	Pessimistic

In summary, categorical classification systems, including DSM-IV, have failed to help clinicians deal with personality disorders efficiently. The most prominent practical problem is that categorical systems do not establish a prescriptive relationship between diagnosis and treatment. In many other medical and psychiatric fields, clinical diagnosis directly indicates optimal treatment. In the field of personality disorders, however, this fundamental goal has not been achieved. The DSM categorical system usually yields multiple personality diagnoses for individual patients. In such cases, treatment priorities are easily confused. Typically, the most prominent clinical symptoms, which are not necessarily the most urgent ones to treat, are likely to be treated most vigorously. For example, people with narcissistic personality disorder are likely to be treated for their self-centered behaviors, even though their chronically fragile self-esteem generates most of the narcissistic symptoms. Furthermore, DSM-IV categories of personality disorders are symptomatically similar to some Axis I disorders (e.g., paranoid personality disorder and delusional disorder, schizotypal personality disorder and schizophrenia, avoidant personality disorder and social phobia). In fact, most Axis II personality syndromes are treated with interventions proven effective for the corresponding Axis I disorders (e.g., antipsychotics for schizotypal personality disorder). Such symptomatic treatments are generally inferior to those derived from understanding the underlying causative mechanisms. On the positive side, categorical models convey vivid, clinically useful information about rare prototypical cases, i.e., cases that perfectly fit their corresponding "pigeon-hole" in the classification.

Detailed checklists of diagnostic features are available for each of the personality disorder subtypes listed in Table 19.2. Reliable structured interviews are available to make such diagnoses, but the interviews take 90 minutes or more to complete and, as noted above, usually produce multiple diagnoses. Consequently, other approaches are needed in practical clinical work.

Quantitative (dimensional) diagnosis

The seven-factor model of temperament and character

Qualitative terms like "inflexible" and "enduring" necessitate subjective judgments and produce little precision in the diagnosis of personality disorders. When efforts were made in the past to diagnose personality disorders using such general qualitative terms, the reliability of diagnosis was low. In contrast, criteria for more specific subtypes increased reliability, but produced many overlapping diagnoses. Fortunately, quantifiable components of personality have been identified that reliably distinguish patients with personality disorders from people with other or no psychopathology. These basic features of all personality disorders are derived from the concept of "character," which involves an individual's self-awareness of his or her goals and values.

Three dimensions of character have been distinguished: self-directedness, cooperativeness, and self-transcendence. Self-directedness quantifies the extent to which an individual accepts responsibility for control of his or her goals and habits, rather than blaming other people and circumstances for his or her behavior; self-directed people are responsible, purposeful, resourceful, self-accepting, and dutiful. Cooperativeness quantifies the extent to which a person identifies with other people and feels like an integral part of society; cooperative people are tolerant, empathic, helpful, compassionate, and principled. Self-transcendence quantifies the extent to which a person feels like an integral part of the universe as a whole; self-transcendent people are intuitive, idealistic, contemplative, faithful, and spiritual. Highly creative individuals are high in all three of the character dimensions, but many well-organized (i.e., mature) people are low in self-transcendence. For highly mature and creative people, life is full of challenging opportunities, people are generally trustworthy and nice, and most things will ultimately work out right, even if difficult at the moment.

It has been repeatedly demonstrated that poorly developed character traits, especially self-directedness, increase the risk for personality disorder substantially (Table 19.3). Indeed, most individuals with personality disorder have difficulty accepting responsibility, setting long-term goals, accepting their own limitations, and/or overcoming obstacles they encounter in life. Usually, but not always, they are also uncooperative, i.e., they tend to be intolerant of others, insensitive to others' feelings, selfish, and have difficulty trusting and confiding in other people. They are often hostile

---

DIAGNOSIS

Table 19.3 Quantifiable (dimensional) features of personality disorder

Consistent features

1 Low self-directedness:
- irresponsible, blaming
- no mature goals
- resourceless, helpless
- poor self-esteem
- undisciplined.
2 Low cooperativeness:
- intolerant of others
- lack of empathy
- unhelpful
- revengeful
- unprincipled.

Variable features

1 Low persistence.
2 Low reward dependence (odd cluster only).
3 High novelty seeking (erratic cluster only).
4 High harm avoidance (anxious cluster only).
Cloninger et al., 1993; Svrakic et al., 1993.

and revengeful when others disappoint them, but are quick to take advantage of others in an unprincipled manner when the opportunity arises.

High self-directedness is not always protective against personality disorders. Some narcissistic and antisocial people may be highly self-directed, i.e., quite resourceful and purposeful and thus successful in pursuing their narcissistic or antisocial goals. Their very low cooperativeness (e.g., intolerance of others, low empathy) may so interfere with social relations that they have a personality disorder. The degree of self-directedness is indicated by an individual's responses to questions regarding goals in life, self-esteem, and ability to overcome obstacles. In a busy medical setting, this information may be most often elicited in discussions about lifestyle choices that are important for long-term health and prevention of disease, such as weight control, dietary balance, exercise, smoking, drinking, and ways of relaxing and coping with stress. The more mature individuals are, the more clear their goals and the disciplined sequence of steps they are taking to accomplish their goals despite obstacles and initial failures. Immature people (that is, individuals with personality disorders) are unsure about their goals and are unable to accept criticism and acknowledge their limitations. Consequently, when immature people are successful, they exhibit vanity; when they have problems, they blame other people and circumstances in order to avoid feelings of shame. They wish things were better but are not self-confident or determined enough to do whatever it takes to fulfill their wishes. As noted above, patients with personality disorders are also usually low in cooperativeness. The components of cooperativeness (i.e., social tolerance, empathy, helpfulness, compassion, and ethical principles) are self-explanatory and can be easily examined in a primary medical care setting. (See *Key clinical questions and what they unlock*.)

While low character traits represent core features determining the presence or absence of personality disorders, other quantifiable traits are used for differential diagnosis of the DSM clusters (odd/eccentric, erratic/impulsive, anxious/fearful) and discrete subtypes of personality disorders. These clusters are distinguished by basic emotional responses such as anger, fear, and disgust. Such basic emotions are regulated by components of personality called temperament, which develop in infancy and persist stably throughout life.

Four dimensions of temperament have been identified and have been labeled novelty seeking, harm avoidance, reward dependence, and persistence. Individuals high in novelty seeking are impulsive, quick-tempered, extravagant, and dislike rules; high novelty seeking is characteristic of individuals with antisocial, histrionic and other erratic personality disorders. Individuals high in harm avoidance are anxious, fearful, shy, and fatigable; high harm avoidance is characteristic of avoidant and other anxious personality disorders. Individuals low in reward dependence are socially indifferent, aloof, cold, and independent; such low reward

KEY CLINICAL QUESTIONS AND WHAT THEY UNLOCK

- *Do you feel responsible for what happens to you? Are you often the victim of other people and circumstances?*
  These two questions indicate how well developed a person's sense of agency (responsible, in control, not victimized) is. Responsibility is a key aspect of self-directedness, whereas feeling controlled or victimized suggests personality disorder.

- *Do you feel that your life has purpose and meaning? Do you know what you want to do in life?*
  These two questions indicate how well developed a person's sense of self-efficacy (purposeful, goal-directed, not aimless) is. Purposefulness is a key component of self-directedness in everyday activities, whereas aimlessness and lack of meaning suggest personality disorder.

- *What do you do to find a solution when problems occur?*
  This question may reveal the extent to which a person is resourceful and inventive. Resourcefulness is a key component of self-directedness.

- *What do you do to calm down when you get upset? What do you like to do to have fun?*
  These two questions may reveal what a person enjoys and how he or she deals with negative emotions and stress. Individuals with personality disorder often have poor skills in modulating negative emotions and facilitating positive emotions.

- *Tell me about your relationships with your parents and your best relationship with someone outside your family.*
  These usually reveal much about a person's capacity for trust and intimacy in social relationships. Cooperative relationships indicate maturity and capacity for a therapeutic alliance, whereas the absence of healthy relationships in the past suggests psychotherapy will proceed slowly.

dependence is characteristic of schizoid and other odd personality disorders. Individuals who are high in persistence, such as some mature and some obsessional patients, are industrious and persevering, whereas those who are low in persistence are easily discouraged.

Factor analyses have repeatedly supported the validity of these three DSM clusters of personality disorders (i.e., odd/eccentric, erratic/impulsive, anxious/fearful) except that symptoms for compulsive personality disorder tend to load separately from other personality disorders thus forming a fourth cluster. The fourth temperament dimension, persistence, has been shown to correlate with symptoms of obsessive-compulsive personality disorder.

Temperament traits regulate the primary emotions of fear (harm avoidance), anger (novelty seeking), and attachment/disgust (reward dependence). Often people with personality disorders impress others as irrational and/or excessively emotional because their behavior and interactions are dominated by extreme temperament traits that are only weakly modulated by character traits. These people have a rather limited spectrum of the three elementary emotions with which to respond to everything going on inside and around them. In contrast, mature people have a more complex emotional life, including a broad spectrum of so-called secondary emotions, such as pride, humility, compassion, empathy, equanimity, and patience. The likelihood of a well-adapted temperament and mature character is high when these complex emotions are prominent.

Each of the character and temperament dimensions is a quantitative trait with a roughly bell-shaped distribution. These traits vary independently of each other, so varied combinations of values derived from each dimension occur. The presence or absence of any personality disorder can be defined as the usual absence of self-awareness, which is associated with inadequate character development. Inadequate character development is indicated by low self-directedness and/or low cooperativeness. Furthermore, different personality subtypes can each be distinguished by a unique combination of values on the temperament dimensions. For example, histrionic personality disorder is characterized by high novelty seeking, low harm avoidance, and high reward dependence. Antisocial personality disorder has the same temperament profile except that reward dependence is low.

The seven-factor model of temperament and character provides simple and practical guidelines for integration of the categorical and dimensional models of personality disorders. As described above, poorly developed character traits represent consistent features typical of all clinical subtypes of personality disorders, whereas individual variation in the temperament dimensions (i.e., the specific temperament profile) is useful for differential diagnosis of the subtypes. It is easy to remember the discriminating features of most personality disorders as the extremes of a cube with the three dimensions defined by novelty seeking, harm avoidance, and reward dependence (see Fig. 19.1).

In general, for efficiency of assessment and for analysis of etiology and pathophysiology, it is helpful to be aware that the underlying clinical variation in personality disorders involves a small number of quantitative dimensions rather than a set of discrete diseases. Several reliable self-report questionnaires are available to allow quantitative ratings of personality dimensions for differential diagnosis of personality disorders. Different models that distinguish normal and abnormal personality have been discussed in detail by Strack and Lorr (see the *Annotated bibliography*). The most commonly used scales are the Minnesota Multiphasic Personality Inventory (MMPI), the Neuroticism-Extraversion-Openness Inventory (NEO), the Millon Clinical Multiaxial Inventory, and the Temperament and Character Inventory (TCI). The Millon inventory is designed for use only with clinical psychiatric patients and is not appropriate for general medical patients. Comparisons of the TCI, NEO, and MMPI show that the TCI is more comprehensive and better discriminating than the other two for differential diagnosis of personality disorders.

The seven-factor dimensional model of temperament and

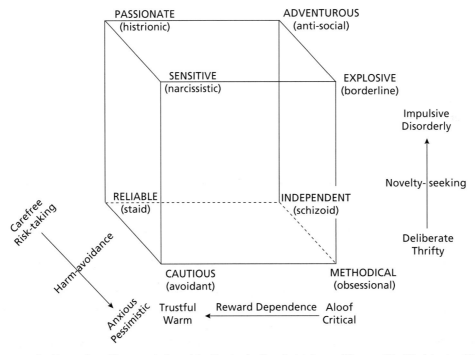

Fig. 19.1 Temperament cube. Reproduced by permission of the Center for Psychobiology of Personality, Washington University, St Louis, Missouri.

TABLE 19.4 Demographic features of personality disorder in a sample of 800 individuals representative of the general adult population of metropolitan St Louis (1994 St Louis Health Survey)

| | Personality disorder | | No personality disorder | |
| | Severe (N = 141) | Mild (N = 131) | Average (N = 276) | Mature (N = 252) |
Feature	%	%	%	%
Male	59	47	40	36
Not white	19	24	17	15
Never married	23	13	8	9
Unemployed	6	8	4	3
Did not graduate high school	17	15	13	7
Rarely go to church	56	38	27	19

character described here is the most comprehensive model of personality currently available and has been validated both in the general population and in psychiatric patients for the diagnosis of personality disorders. All of the personality dimensions are assessed by the Temperament and Character Inventory (TCI), which consists of 240 true-false questions, or the revised TCI, which uses a five-point scale so people can indicate whether an item is definitely or probably true, uncertain, or definitely or probably false. The TCI can be self-administered in about 35 minutes at home or in the office. Copies of the test and services for scoring and interpretation are available from the authors.

Epidemiology and presentation in primary medical care

About 11–23% of individuals in the general population are diagnosed as having a personality disorder using the categorical criteria in Table 19.1. However, there is no natural subdivision between more mature and less mature people when quantitative ratings are made by people themselves or knowledgeable informants. Using the sum of self-directedness and cooperativeness scores as the measure of maturity, one in every three individuals in the general population is noticeably less mature than others to those who know them. Accordingly, for descriptive purposes here, we distinguish the least mature sixth of the population (i.e., bottom 17%) as "severe" or "definite" cases and the next sixth as "mild" or "possible" cases.

It widely believed that patients with personality disorders are more often less educated, have more marital difficulties, and are more often unemployed. Our data concerning the demographic features of personality disorders in the general population are summarized in Table 19.4. Patients with personality disorders are more likely to be male, not white, never married, unemployed, high school dropouts, and rarely attend religious services. In addition, they are usually young adults because personality disorders are likely to remit with increasing age, as described later. Except for age and church attendance, however, these demographic differences are small, and no demographic group is immune to personality disorders.

Regarding general health, patients with personality disorders are less likely to report that their health is "excellent" and more likely only "fair," presumably because somatic anxiety is weakly correlated with low self-directedness ($r = .35, P < .01$). However, many report their health as "good" to "very good." Likewise, 27% of patients with personality disorders report that their health impairs their ability to work compared with 19% of those without personality disorders. Most patients with personality disorders complain of significant bodily pain during the previous month, but this is only slightly more common than in other people (51% vs 40%) and seldom severe (6%). Overall, the excess of physical health complaints in patients with personality disorders is consistent but small. This suggests that the physical health of patients with personality disorders is usually not impaired much more than is attributable to hypochondriasis and other aspects of mental health.

In contrast, patients with personality disorders differ substantially from others in their history of past psychiatric problems (Table 19.5). Use of psychotropic medications and mental health counseling are only weakly associated with personality disorders. However, psychiatric hospitalization occurs in 8–14% of patients with personality disorders and in only 4% of the population without personality disorders. Among the 6% of the general population with a history of psychiatric hospitalization, 39% have severe personality disorders and another 22% have mild personality disorders. Likewise about 7% of the general population report a past suicide attempt; 46% of these have a severe personality disorder and another 21% have a mild personality disorder. Accordingly, the possibility of personality disorders should be carefully evaluated in any patient with a past history of psychiatric hospitalization or suicide attempt.

The detection of personality disorders is helpful in treatment because it alerts the physician to the common subjective distress and psychosocial disability of these patients. At any given time, many patients with personality disorders are nervous or sad much of the time, whereas others are rarely so

TABLE 19.5

Lifetime history of past psychiatric treatment in the general population (1994 St Louis Health Survey)

| | Personality disorder | | No personality disorder | |
| | Severe (N = 141) | Mild (N = 131) | Average (N = 276) | Mature (N = 252) |
Psychiatric history	%	%	%	%
Medication	32	35	27	23
Counseling	32	23	19	18
Hospitalized	14	8	4	4
Suicide attempt	17	8	4	2

TABLE 19.6

Nervousness and mood in the past month in the general adult population (1994 St Louis Health Survey)

| | Personality disorder | | No personality disorder | |
| | Severe (N = 141) | Mild (N = 131) | Average (N = 276) | Mature (N = 252) |
Psychiatric history	%	%	%	%
In the past month, much of the time are you . . . ?				
Nervous?	25	13	7	2
Downcast?	27	24	8	1
Unable to cheer up?	13	8	4	1

TABLE 19.7

Prevalence of personality disorder by age in the 1994 St Louis Health Survey

| | Age group | | | |
| | 18–24 (N = 85) | 25–39 (N = 286) | 40–59 (N = 241) | 60+ (N = 191) |
Personality status	%	%	%	%
Personality disorder				
Severe	34	17	17	11
Mild	22	16	14	17
No personality disorder				
Average	32	33	33	39
Mature	12	34	36	33
Total column %	100	100	100	100

(Table 19.6). For example, patients with severe personality disorders are thirteen times more likely than mature people to report that they were unable to cheer up much of the past week (13% vs 1%). Accordingly, reports of anxiety and depression have different diagnostic and treatment implications depending on the presence or absence of personality disorders, as discussed below.

Natural history

The requirement of early onset and enduring impairment assures extensive chronicity for personality disorders. However, in a general population sample of varying age, people with personality disorders are more likely to be younger than more mature individuals; for example, in the St Louis Health Survey, average age varied from 40 years in severe personality disorders to 46 years in mature individuals. The proportions of individuals with severe and mild personality disorders are shown by age in Table 19.7.

The association of personality disorders with younger age indicates maturation (i.e., remission of personality disorders) with increasing age in some cases. In particular, three dimensions of personality change substantially with age according to both longitudinal comparisons of the same people at different ages and correlations of age and personality in cross-sectional studies of the general population. Novelty seeking decreases with age by approximately 18%, so that older individuals become less impulsive (more reflective), less rule-breaking (more orderly), and less quick-tempered (more stoical). Cooperativeness increases markedly in most children during school age and then increases by 12% on average after age 18. Self-directedness increases markedly in most people during adolescence and young adulthood, increasing by 9% on average after age 18.

The decreasing prevalence of personality disorders with age is attributable to the increased development of both self-directedness and cooperativeness with age. The additional tendency for novelty seeking to decrease with age explains the finding that patients with impulsive personality disorders, such as antisocial and borderline personality disorders, show even more improvement than patients with anxious or eccentric personality disorders over time. The best documented finding about change in personality disorders is the remission of criminal behavior in individuals with antisocial personality disorder. In a prospective 30-year follow-up study of children, Lee Robins found that 39% of 82 patients with antisocial personality disorder settled down and matured; that is, they became more responsible and conscientious, and they reduced criminal activities and substance abuse. In Robins' study, 12% were rated in remission and 27% much improved. Maturation most often occurred in the fourth decade (age 31–40), but there was no age at which improvement was not possible. Of those who improved, 20% did so by age 30 years, 50% from 31–40, and 30% after age 40 years. Regardless of age, they nearly always remained impulsive (high novelty seeking), risk-taking (low harm avoidance), and aloof (low reward dependence), but they became mature enough to maintain work and family life in a stable manner.

When asked to explain how the transition to maturity was achieved, patients with personality disorders usually point to meaningful emotional experiences and valued life opportunities. These include events like marriage to a caring and responsible spouse; obtaining a job that permits the development of skills, self-respect, and hope about opportunities for advancement; or a religious conversion. Often the emergent changes are sudden and associated with a new perspective on life, which cannot be achieved by logic, medication, or advice alone. Such emotional experiences and emergent insights lead to new goals and values, as confirmed by multiple randomized controlled trials of the benefits of trusted therapeutic alliances. The basic temperament traits stay nearly the same but can be satisfied by mature goals and values.

Differential diagnosis and comorbidity

Transient mood states, such as a depressive episode, may alter personality function temporarily. Increases in anxiety or depressive symptoms lead to moderate increases in harm avoidance, but do not alter other aspects of temperament. Self-directedness and cooperativeness may also be transiently reduced during depressive episodes. Consequently, a person with no enduring personality disorder may act immaturely when depressed or under stress. The diagnosis of a personality disorder should be based on enduring patterns of behavior and not limited to episodes of anxiety or depression.

Adolescent onset of alcohol or drug use usually leads to arrested character development. Mature problem-solving skills, goals, and values do not develop when a person relies on drug abuse for thrills or relief of worries. Once abstinence is achieved, character development may proceed. Meanwhile, the diagnosis of a personality disorder is justified on the basis of patients' inner experience (way of thinking and feeling) and behavior (impulse control and social relations) regardless of explanations, such as drug abuse or social deprivation.

Most patients with psychoses have comorbid personality disorders. In fact, it has been suggested that personality disorder increases vulnerability to psychosis, particularly when self-transcendence is high because such individuals are prone to magical ideation and perceptual aberrations. Alternatively, a personality disorder may represent an early manifestation of psychotic illness. Further prospective studies are needed to evaluate whether clinical features of patients with personality disorders or external influences, such as drug abuse or stress, can distinguish patients with personality disorders that eventually deteriorate with a psychosis from other patients with personality disorders. In most cases, psychoses in patients with personality disorders are brief and reactive, but sometimes psychosis may become chronic. In patients with chronic psychotic illnesses, personality disorders should be diagnosed, when indicated, because it can add useful information about the patient's behavior and treatment.

Patients with personality disorders commonly have comorbid psychiatric syndromes related to anxiety, depression, and substance abuse. The risk and severity of these comorbid syndromes varies quantitatively with the degree of immaturity. For example, the severity of depression in the previous week has been measured in the general population using a scale developed by the NIMH Center for Epidemiological Studies (CES) (Table 19.8). The CES depression scale indicates a high probability of major depression when there are many depressive symptoms (scores of 21 or more) and high probability of minor depression or dysthymia with moderate depressive complaints (scores of 16 to 20). Using these reports, the risk of major depression varied from 2% in mature individuals to 42% in severe personality disorders, and minor depression varied from 2% to 16%. Alcoholism, indicated by lifetime reports of three or more problems on the Michigan Alcoholism Screening Test, varied from 16% in mature individuals to 37% in severe personality disorders.

TABLE 19.8 Psychiatric syndromes comorbid with personality disorder in the general adult population (1994 St Louis Health Survey)

Comorbid psychiatric syndromes	Personality disorder		No personality disorder	
	Severe (N = 141) %	Mild (N = 131) %	Average (N = 276) %	Mature (N = 252) %
Depression				
Major	42	30	11	2
Minor	16	13	13	2
Alcoholism				
Definite	28	7	12	8
Possible	12	18	16	10
Cigarette smoking				
Ever	77	72	68	56
Pack/day	54	48	41	31
Current	45	40	34	23
Eating disorder				
Binging	31	25	15	9
Purging	6	6	4	4
Panic attacks	20	7	11	6
Phobias				
Specific	37	36	25	22
Social	42	37	20	14

Depression based on the Center for Epidemiological Studies—Depressed Scale (CES-D) (16–20, minor; 21+, major).
Alcoholism based on the Short Michigan Alcoholism Screening Test (SMAST).

Extent of cigarette smoking and symptoms of eating and anxiety disorders are inversely correlated with degree of maturity. Accordingly, subjective distress and difficulty handling stress are prominent features of all personality disorders (see *Pearls & Perils*).

Genetics and family history

Genetic and environmental factors interact in complex ways to influence the risk of developing a personality disorder. Robust findings from many family studies demonstrate that relatives of individuals with personality disorders often have incomplete forms of the same disorder with mild or partial features. Likewise parents with no personality disorder may produce one or several children with severe personality disorders.

Family studies, including studies of adopted-away children of biological parents with personality disorders, indicate that the risk of personality disorders in children increases in proportion to the number of disorders and their severity in their biological parents. Studies of adoptive parents and family environments also show that the risk of personality disorders depends on the severity of the psychosocial disorganization of the family of rearing. All these observations are explained by the hypothesis that there is quantitative inheritance of individual personality dimensions that influence the risk of personality disorders, rather than separate inheritance of a particular personality disorder.

More specifically, each of the seven dimensions of personality is moderately heritable. The genetic heritabilities of each dimension is about 50% according to twin studies and about 25% according to adoption studies. Each personality dimension has unique genetic determinants, although there is some overlap. Surprisingly, effects of social learning that are shared by children reared together have little influence on personality development. Instead, variables that are unique to each individual are most important in influencing personality development. Parents should be educated and supported in their efforts to provide a character-building milieu tailored to the unique personality of each child. Mature character development is most likely to occur in homes that provide security and definite limits on behavior in a compassionate manner tailored to the particular needs of each child, as well as encouragement for self-directed choice and the value of respect for other people.

Recognizing personality disorder

- Personality disorder is the primary disorder in most patients with psychosocial impairment, especially young adults.
- No demographic group is protected from personality disorders.
- Individuals with personality disorders impress others as irrational or excessively emotional because their behavior and interactions are dominated by unregulated, basic emotions (fear, anger, disgust) without integration with mature goals and values.
- Strong emotional reactions, such as anger or an urge to rescue, to a patient suggest the possibility of personality disorder in the patient, inappropriate expectations by the physician, or both. ("I often get under the skin of other people." "I don't know why people are always trying to protect me or tell me what to do when I don't want their help.")
- When there is a past history of a suicide attempt or psychiatric hospitalization, further review of school, work, and social behavior usually confirms the presence of personality disorder. (A characteristic statement is: "I don't like or trust many people.")
- A pattern of consistently blaming other people and external circumstances for one's problems in a wide range of personal and social contexts is the essential diagnostic feature of personality disorder. ("I often feel used, manipulated, or betrayed by others.")
- Transient immature behavior can occur under unusual stress and should be distinguished from the enduring and pervasive maladaptation typical of personality disorders or personality changes caused by other chronic mental and physical disorders.
- Patients with personality disorder handle stress poorly and are often mildly depressed, anxious, or hypochondriacal. ("Many things upset, bother, or frustrate me." "Nothing ever goes easy for me.")
- Severe pain and prolonged inability to work are seldom attributable to personality disorder alone. ("My health is just fair—not so bad that I cannot work, but not excellent.")
- When personality disorder is suspected, quantitative personality tests are unbiased, reliable, efficient, and inexpensive diagnostic tools that do not require referral.

Pathophysiology

Personality disorders can be understood in terms of the dynamic interactions among the components of a complex adaptive system. Temperament dimensions are inherited biases in adaptive responses to environmental stimuli. These biased adaptive response patterns, in turn, constrain the way character matures—that is, modify the way we view ourselves, others, and the world at large. Below, a few illustrative findings are summarized about temperament.

The four temperament dimensions influence differences among individuals in their responses to associative conditioning. For example, levels of harm avoidance predict the formation of conditioned signals of punishment, but not reward. In other words, individuals high in harm avoidance are more prone to worry because they acquire warning signals about danger more readily than others. Individual differences in harm avoidance are correlated with low activity in genes that promote expression of the serotonin transporter and the catabolism of dopamine. Noradrenergic mechanisms also appear to be involved in harm avoidance because Joyce and colleagues showed that high harm avoidance in women predicts response to the noradrenergic antidepressant desipramine in major depression. Genetic vulnerability to depression is expressed when individuals with low activity of the serotonin transporter promoter are exposed to stressful life events.

Likewise, levels of reward dependence predict the formation of conditioned signals of reward, but not punishment. In other words, individuals high in reward dependence are more sensitive to the exchange of signs of appreciation and approval. High reward dependence levels predict high morning cortisol levels in major depression and also antidepressant responses to serotonergic drugs like chlorimipramine and nefazadone.

Novelty seeking levels predict quick reaction times and sensitivity to incentive activation of behavior by novelty and conditioned signals of reward. Novelty seeking is modulated by dopaminergic mechanisms; high novelty seeking depends on increased excitability of prefrontal neurons resulting from low postsynaptic sensitivity to dopamine, which inhibits neuronal firing. The gene locus encoding the dopamine D4 receptor (DRD4) contributes to individual differences in novelty-seeking levels in interaction with other genetic and environmental factors that affect dopamine catabolism and reuptake. For example, novelty seeking is increased when individuals with susceptible DRD4 genotypes are reared in a hostile childhood environment.

Given these individual differences in temperament, it is possible to predict the course of character development. For example, personality disorders (i.e., low self-directedness and cooperativeness) are most likely to occur when the temperament profile combines high harm avoidance, low reward dependence, and high novelty seeking. Mature character is most likely when the temperament profile combines low novelty seeking, low harm avoidance, and high reward dependence. The remission of personality disorder involves growth in self-awareness, which depends on complex interactions among many biological, psychological, and social variables.

Treatment

Individuals with personality disorders do not perceive their behaviors and feelings as aberrant (these are ego-syntonic disorders) and seldom seek help, except when others (usually a spouse or parents) are insistent. This usually happens when maladaptive behaviors create marital, family, and career problems, or when other mental symptoms (e.g., anxiety, depression, substance abuse) or somatic symptoms (e.g., obesity) complicate the clinical picture. In general, patients with personality disorders require a multifaceted treatment plan that often combines psychotherapy and pharmacotherapy.

There are two major barriers to effective treatment of personality disorders. (Fortunately, both are within the control of the health care provider.) The first is the common loss of professional objectivity, signaled by the development of strong emotions (positive or negative) and called positive or negative counter-transference. This inappropriate personal involvement is a red flag to reassess diagnosis and treatment, and it often suggests the need for referral to a psychiatrist. Frequent discussions and counseling with colleagues are useful because even strong counter-transference feelings sometimes persist unrecognized. The second preventable error in personality disorder management is to give the patient direct advice on personal and social problems. This is counterproductive in patients with personality disorders because they usually become dependent, non-compliant, or resentful. Occasionally, direct advice may be offered to some antisocial, narcissistic, and schizoid patients who are at low risk of developing dependency and, at least initially, need precise structure and direction. However, it is most beneficial to provide guidance and support without giving direct advice. All that is usually required in supportive therapy is compassionate attention, respect for the dignity of other human beings despite their flaws, and reinforcement of patients' existing adaptive coping mechanisms.

When tempted to give direct advice to patients, physicians should remember that change in personality requires more than common sense and logic. People change when they become self-aware, usually from personal recognition of dissatisfaction with themselves and their relationships. Personal growth thus arises from new insights about oneself and the environment. Direct advice robs the patient of the opportunity to develop new insights and to learn from his or her mistakes. In summary, supporting these patients involves joint evaluation of options and encouragement to practice skills in solving problems. If the physician is unable to refrain from frequent advice giving, then referral to a psychiatrist or psychologist may be indicated.

Substantial personality change, which is invariably needed by people with personality disorders, involves an extensive reorganization of internalized concepts and coping mechanisms. Thus, it requires precise diagnostic analyses, specific treatment strategies, and, above all, expert training of the clinician. This expert treatment may include any of several available psychotherapeutic approaches, usually combined with pharmacotherapy. The major points relevant to psychotherapy and pharmacotherapy of personality disorders are summarized below.

Psychotherapy

As described earlier, individuals with personality disorders have a peculiar capacity to elicit strong emotions from other people. They are often described as aggravating, unlikable, difficult, or "bad." Alternatively, they may be seductive or dependent, and they may elicit inappropriate emotions or actions, such as sexual interest or the urge to rescue. Even professionals may have difficulty treating them with respectful objectivity because of a blurring of personal boundaries. Such loss of objectivity occurs because the patient's deeply felt assumptions about other people may often elicit interpersonal responses that are appropriate to the patient's assumptions. People's assumptions about themselves and others often become self-fulfilling prophecies because of automatic mechanisms of affect transfer. If someone smiles at a person, communicating appreciation, it is natural to experience feelings of social attachment and to smile back automatically. Likewise, if someone frowns, communicating anger, it is natural to feel defensive in preparation for his or her angry attack. For example, many patients with personality disorders are suspicious and hostile about others' motives. This distrustful attitude is communicated in many verbal and non-verbal ways and often elicits disagreement or frank hostility from others. These uncooperative responses reinforce the original negative assumptions of the patient, which in turn leads to further alienation.

CONSIDER CONSULTATION WHEN...

- The patient elicits strong emotions that the physician does not understand and control well (so-called 'counter-transference' problems). These can be either negative (e.g., anger or anxiety) or positive (e.g., sexual attraction or urge to rescue). Such feelings are professionally inappropriate and harmful.
- The relationship with the patient depends on giving advice on how to cope with problems. Patients cannot develop self-reliance when they are dependent on advice from others.
- The patient is so unstable that he or she requires excessive time, expresses frequent or serious suicidal ideation, or makes recurrent suicide attempts. Involvement of a psychiatrist or psychologist may help stabilize the patient and help the primary care provider by sharing responsibility with another professional colleague.
- The patient is not making progress. Consultation may uncover obstacles to progress or suggest new approaches to treatment.

This vicious cycle of affect transfer can only be interrupted by professional objectivity combined with patience and compassionate respect for the patient's disability. Such objectivity arises from recognizing the overall meaning and implications of the pattern of interpersonal signals, so that verbal and non-verbal communication takes on diagnostic and therapeutic, rather than personal, significance. In optimal therapeutic relationships, "patients" should be patiently hopeful and physicians should be compassionately realistic. Whenever professionals become aware of strong positive or negative emotions toward a patient (so-called "counter-transference" reactions), this should help to alert them to the possibility that the patient has a personality disorder (see *Pearls & Perils—Recognizing personality disorder*).

Because many patients with personality disorders do not recognize or admit their psychopathology, they resist and resent psychiatric diagnoses and any form of mental health treatment. Accordingly, it is prudent to let the patient define his/her treatment goals and then jointly evaluate the likelihood of a successful outcome. Initially, these goals should be as simple and concrete as possible (e.g., to develop social skills, or to reduce alcohol use, etc.). In many, but not all cases, successful completion of this initial phase will motivate the patient to define other, more complex treatment goals and to continue treatment.

An alternative approach in a busy medical practice is to focus primarily on issues that are related to general health but offer an adequate basis for the diagnosis and treatment of personality disorders. For example, a systematic focus on healthy lifestyle choices provides a non-threatening basis for evaluation of a patient's goals, values, habits, and skills (that is, their personality). Choices about diet, weight control, exercise, smoking, drinking, and ways of relaxing and managing stress are appropriate for discussion and do not threaten or stigmatize the patient. Discussion of these choices with a patient can provide a guiding stimulus for developing more self-direction and constructive planning about life. Discipline in working towards chosen goals is an indicator of maturity. Lack of success stimulates learning about goal-setting and personal growth by, for example, breaking a problem into smaller steps to be taken one at a time. In this process, patients have the opportunity to learn from experience (the type of learning invariably damaged in personality disorder patients), and in many cases this leads to the acceptance of strengths and limitations. Self-acceptance and acceptance of others usually progress hand in hand. Such patient guidance is a simplified and non-threatening form of what is usually called cognitive-behavioral therapy and can be safely practiced in a busy primary care office.

As a rule of thumb when treating patients with personality disorders with psychotherapy, it is optimal to use combinations of theoretical orientations (psychodynamic, cognitive, behavioral) and formats (individual, group, marital), whether these are carried out by an individual therapist or by a multidisciplinary team. An increasing number of professionals ignore ideological barriers dividing schools of psychotherapy and attempt both technical synthesis (eclecticism) and theoretical synthesis (integration) of various orientations. Different approaches to psychotherapy are complementary, and each can contribute to the overall efficacy of treatment of personality disorders.

Dynamic schools have been traditionally regarded as helping patients understand conflicting internal motivations, behavioral schools as assisting patients in changing the most disruptive behaviors, and humanistic approaches as assisting patients in achieving what might be called "co-operative self-assertiveness" or "altruistic individualism." No one approach is invariably superior to the others. The only exception to this is that supportive therapy, which is traditionally aimed at strengthening coping mechanisms, is not used in the treatment of personality disorders because these patients' coping mechanisms are already maladaptive. Occasionally, supportive treatment of subjective distress (achieved through compassionate listening, respectful validation, and reassurance) is aimed at developing new coping mechanisms, primarily deriving from the patient's positive experience of trust and understanding in the treatment setting.

Dynamic (insight oriented) therapies may be usefully complemented by humanistic and behavioral (action oriented) therapies because personality change only occurs when apparent growth in insight is actually confirmed by its integration into everyday behavior and social interactions. Whenever possible, individual sessions are combined with group sessions and the former elaborate relevant group experiences, i.e., those reflecting the most disruptive maladaptive behaviors. Group interactions are considered useful for patients with personality disorders to acquire social skills. However, some schizoid, borderline, or avoidant patients may resist this format because it is difficult for them to share their intimate experiences with a large group of people, to be exposed, and to tolerate the confrontations that are likely to occur in group therapy.

Simple cognitive-behavioral interventions that are not psychologically threatening (such as stimulating greater awareness of the sources and consequences of a person's attitudes, discussion of adaptive behavioral options, and education about lifestyle choices) may have many benefits beyond support. These additional benefits include reduced interpersonal conflict, increased compliance with treatment, and increased emotional satisfaction for the patient, the patient's family and friends, and the physician.

Pharmacotherapy

Psychotropic medications may be beneficial to facilitate personality change, but they are inadequate without guidance and interpretation about experience, as can be provided in

Treating personality disorder

- Patients with personality disorders usually require a multifaceted treatment plan that combines psychotherapy and pharmacotherapy.
- Effective treatment requires much work, patience, and empathy.
- Compassionate support and reassurance can be safely provided without giving direct advice.
- Creativity in inventing new "techniques," "strategies," or methods is encouraged in order to deal efficiently with frequent and frustrating no-way-out situations.
- Direct advice on personal and social problems is generally counterproductive in patients with personality disorder because they become dependent, non-compliant, or resentful.
- Personality change is based on emotional experiences that alter basic assumptions and views about oneself, others, and the world.
- Prognosis is especially poor in patients who have never had a meaningful relationship with at least one person.
- The patient should be asked to define his/her treatment goals with subsequent realistic evaluation of the likelihood of success, which is central to patient selection. Initially, these goals should be as simple and concrete as possible (e.g., "to develop certain social skills," "to reduce alcohol use," etc.). In many cases, successful completion of this initial phase will motivate the patient to define other, more complex treatment goals and to continue treatment.
- Focus on healthy lifestyle choices, like diet, exercise, and stress management, is a beneficial approach to personality disorders in primary medical care settings.
- Personality disorder can complicate medical treatment and herald onset of severe mental disorders.
- Psychotropic medications may be beneficial to facilitate personality change, but are inadequate without guidance and interpretation about experience, as can be provided in expert psychotherapy.
- Non-compliance with medical treatment or emergence of marked emotional instability warrants further evaluation by psychological testing, or, if acceptable to the patient, referral to specialists for an expert opinion about diagnosis and treatment.
- Relapses and recovery are expected features of treatment with chronic disorders like personality disorders. Consultation with colleagues helps to avoid giving up or developing inappropriate attitudes.

psychotherapy. In general, there are two approaches to the pharmacotherapy of personality disorders: (1) causal therapy, which is aimed at correcting neurochemical disturbances underlying deviant behavior traits, and (2) symptomatic therapy, which is aimed at correcting target symptoms of personality disorders. These two approaches will be described briefly.

Causal pharmacotherapy of personality disorders is still in its infancy. It is based on the hypothesis that enduring behavior changes may emerge from drug-induced modification of neurobiological dispositions to specific personality traits. As described earlier in this chapter, our psychobiological model of temperament and character provides testable hypotheses about underlying mechanisms of extreme behavior variants, i.e., it postulates that more or less distinct brain neurotransmitter networks underlie observable personality traits. Specifically, temperament traits are conceptualized as stable neurobiological dispositions that are difficult to change either by voluntary effort or by psychotherapy alone. Personality disorders are postulated to reflect extreme variants in temperament traits coupled with immature character, which ultimately lead to maladaptive behaviors. Our concept of personality disorders has numerous ramifications for both research and clinical practice.

Clinically we suggest that enduring personality changes may emerge from pharmacological modification of neurobiological dispositions to behavior traits. For example, preliminary evidence suggests that the response to antidepressants by different patients with major depressive disorder can be predicted to a substantial degree by their temperament, and not by the number, type, severity, or course of their depressive symptoms. Similarly, patients who are highly sensitive to social approval (i.e., who are high in reward dependence) are most likely to improve on selective serotonin uptake inhibitors like fluoxetine or nefazadone. In contrast, those who are highly fearful but not socially dependent are most likely to improve on noradrenergic uptake inhibitors, like desipramine. If further work confirms and refines the nature of the relationship between temperament and therapeutic response, improved treatment outcomes can be expected.

Patients with personality disorders are often treated with drugs used for schizophrenic and mood disorders based on the fact that some personality disorder subtypes have symptoms similar to some Axis I disorders (e.g., borderline personality and cyclothymia). This approach is called symptomatic treatment. Of note, pharmacotherapy cannot be systematically organized around individual subtypes of personality disorder because the target symptoms likely to respond to a particular drug are not unique to any specific subtype of personality disorder but are shared by a number of other subtypes. Target symptoms for pharmacological treatment of personality disorders are: (1) aggression and behavioral dyscontrol, (2) mood and anxiety dysregulation, and (3) psychotic symptoms and cognitive distortions. Note that these three target symptoms roughly correspond to the three temperament dimensions described by the TCI and also to the three DSM-IV clusters of personality disorders (that is, this symptomatic pharmacological treatment of personality disorders is largely dimensionalized).

Aggression

It is useful, though sometimes difficult, to distinguish different types of aggression. The most common form of aggression occurs when a quick-tempered person is provoked by frustration or threats. This is often called "affective aggression" and is common in impulsive-aggressive individuals (that is, those high in novelty seeking and low in harm avoidance). Aggression that appears to be unprovoked sometimes occurs in patients with seizure-like cerebral instability documented by an abnormal EEG and is called "ictal aggression," regardless of any associated personality traits. Predatory aggression or "cruelty" involves hostile revengefulness and taking pleasure in victimizing others, often with intact impulse control; such predatory aggression is most common in individuals who are very low in cooperativeness, such as antisocial and borderline personality disorders. Lastly, frontal lobe lesions are often characterized by "organic" aggression, poor social judgment, disinhibition, distractibility, inattention, and emotional lability.

Multiple trials have shown efficacy of lithium carbonate in the treatment of affective "hot-temper" aggression. It helps impulsive-aggressive individuals be more reflective, that is, think about consequences before acting on impulse. To a lesser extent, it may be helpful in reducing cruelty and lack of cooperativeness, but this may be an indirect result of reducing impulsivity, which often is a predisposing influence in the development of hostility and revengefulness.

Antidepressants (particularly selective serotonin reuptake inhibitors—SSRIs) are considered by many to be beneficial for impulsive subtypes of personality disorders (e.g., borderline, histrionic, antisocial). Occasionally, monoamine oxidase inhibitors (MAOIs) are effective in some dysphoric states with somatic anxiety and hostility.

Atypical neuroleptics may be useful in reducing affective or predatory aggression. A number of these new medications have been recently approved for non-psychotic manic episodes, which will certainly encourage trials for other non-psychotic symptoms, including mood instability, aggression, and behavior dyscontrol in patients with personality disorders. Certainly, decisions to use neuroleptics long-term should involve a consideration of the potential side effects such as weight gain, diabetes, and tardive dyskinesia (see Chapter 22) and should be made with the informed consent of the patient.

Anticonvulsants, such as valproate, lamotrigine, carbamazepine, and oxcarbazepine, reduce both the intensity and the frequency of unprovoked angry outbursts in many patients, regardless of normality of their EEG. "Ictal aggres-

sion" is treated with anticonvulsants and occasionally long-acting benzodiazepines, such as clonazepam.

Double-blind trials have shown that psychostimulants and catecholamine agonists, such as methylphenidate, can be beneficial in the treatment of inattentive and hyperactive adults who are impulsive and aggressive (frontal lobe aggression), especially when symptoms began in early childhood. In other cases, anticonvulsants and SSRIs may be helpful.

Lithium should not be given to antisocial people without aggression and impulsivity; it does not diminish non-aggressive antisocial behaviors (such as lying, cheating, and stealing) and is poorly tolerated by anxious schizoid individuals. Likewise, benzodiazepines and alcohol have disinhibiting effects on violence, reduce conditioned avoidance behavior ("loosen inhibitions"), and further impair passive avoidance learning in impulsive antisocial people. In general, the use of benzodiazepines for patients with personality disorders seems appropriate only in non-aggressive subtypes from the anxious/fearful cluster (avoidant, dependent, or obsessive) and some subtypes from the odd/eccentric cluster (schizoid personality disorder).

Mood dysregulation

Mood dysregulation includes chronic anxiety, emotional lability, emotional detachment, and atypical depressive symptoms or dysphoria. Atypical depressive symptoms, for example, may include mood reactivity, increased sleep or appetite, and extreme responses to interpersonal rejection.

Patients with personality disorders often present with both cognitive anxiety (anticipatory worry) and somatic anxiety (concerns about bodily pains and psychophysiological reactions). Cognitive anxiety is most responsive to SSRIs, benzodiazepines and certain anticonvulsants (valproates, gabapentin, lamotrigine). Somatic anxiety is more responsive to MAOIs, SSRIs, and buspirone. Benzodiazepines are rarely used in these patients because treatment is chronic, which increases the likelihood of addiction. Avoidant traits can also be effectively treated with either SSRIs or MAOIs. Some components of somatic anxiety, such as sweating, palpitations, diarrhea, and tremor, can be treated with beta-blockers. Severe, psychotic-like anxiety responds to low-dose neuroleptics, especially drugs with relatively low D2 affinity (e.g., quetiapine). Despite relative safety of novel antipsychotic agents, caution about prolonged use is necessary.

Emotional instability (manifested as severe mood swings) is usually responsive to lithium (for those with frequent episodes of euphoria) or lamotrigine (for those with more frequent depressive episodes) or both (for patients with both euphoric and depressive episodes). Occasionally, atypical psychotropics are used as well. Tricyclic antidepresssants (TCAs) like imipramine tend to increase impulsivity and anger in emotionally unstable patients (e.g., borderline, narcissistic, histrionic, dependent). As TCAs are also extremely dangerous if a patient were to overdose, these drugs ought to be used with caution in patients with personality disorders.

Emotional detachment, cold and aloof emotions, and disinterest in social relations ("chronic asociality") is observed in schizoid and schizotypal people, and, to a lesser extent, antisocial, paranoid, and some narcissistic personalities. In cases where these symptoms reflect an underlying depression, antidepressants (SSRIs or MAOIs) often help. One should be cautious with TCAs in schizotypal personality disorder, for they may worsen or trigger psychosis. In many cases, emotional detachment responds to atypical neuroleptics like aripiprazole, olanzapine, or risperidone, which may reduce social withdrawal and other features of eccentric personality disorders with less risk of extrapyramidal symptoms than with typical neuroleptics. However, dose adjustment is crucial to maintain compliance because patients with personality disorders often have little tolerance for side effects.

Atypical depressive symptoms and dysphoria accompanying personality disorder are rarely responsive to TCAs. (In fact, at least half of the subjects with personality disorders suffering from atypical depressive symptoms worsen on TCAs.) SSRIs, MAOIs, or possibly atypical neuroleptics (aripiprazole is especially promising) are better choices. Again, antipsychotics should only be used after careful consideration of the risk-benefit ratio. In contrast, classic major depressive episodes, which often complicate personality disorder, are treated with antidepressants, including heterocyclics, in doses suggested for the treatment of primary major depression.

Psychotic symptoms and cognitive distortion
Acute, brief reactive psychoses may complicate most subtypes of personality disorders. These are treated symptomatically, according to accepted pharmacological practices. In general, psychotic patients with personality disorders are likely to respond to and comply with either low doses of powerful neuroleptics or atypical neuroleptics. As a result of much better safety and tolerability, new antipsychotics are now the first-choice treatments for these symptoms. Acute psychotic symptoms requiring medication may subside when environmental stressors are brought under control; thus one should be ready to lower the dose or discontinue the medication.

Some patients with personality disorder manifest chronic, low-level psychotic-like symptoms, such as peculiar thought content (ideas of reference, magical thinking, odd fantasies, suspiciousness), unusual perceptual experiences (illusions), and eccentric speech (sometimes called "nonpsychotic formal thought disorder"). These chronic, low-level, psychotic-like symptoms may respond to low-dose powerful neuroleptics like haloperidol. There are no data on atypical neuroleptics for these symptoms, although it seems reasonable to expect them to be efficacious. Some chronic cognitive disturbances, such as mild ideas of reference or suspiciousness, tend to subside when the background emotional tension is reduced. For example, alprazolam has been found to be beneficial in patients with borderline personality, particularly those with a history of drug abuse and suspiciousness. Again, long-term use of benzodiazepines is associated with high risk of drug dependence, particularly in patients with personality disorders, so these drugs should be prescribed only after careful consideration of the risk-benefit ratio. Their use should be carefully monitored for evidence of abuse or dependence.

Table 19.9 summarizes possible drug choices for various target symptoms of personality disorders. It should be emphasized that advanced psychotherapy or use of psychotropic medications for treatment of PD requires expert training or close supervision by a psychiatrist. This is a rapidly advancing area of psychiatry and decisions about the use of drugs with the potential for serious side effects or dependence should be made thoughtfully.

Summary

Personality disorders are the primary psychiatric illnesses observed in most patients with psychosocial complaints, particularly young adults. They are present in one-sixth of people in the general population, half of all psychiatric outpatients, and two-thirds of patients with a history of psychiatric hospitalization or suicide attempt. Reliable diagnosis of personality disorder can be made in routine clinical practice by brief assessment of two essential features—low self-directedness and low cooperativeness—that indicate reduced ability to work and to get along with other people.

Personality disorders are usually lifelong disorders but can mature (remit) spontaneously or with treatment. The temperament and character components of personality disorders are all moderately heritable. Neurobiological findings about personality explain the benefit of differential pharmacotherapy for different subtypes of personality disorders. Supportive and cognitive-behavioral treatment of personality disorders within primary medical care is feasible and often benefits compliance with other aspects of medical treatment. Pharmacotherapy of personality disorders usually requires psychiatric consultation.

TABLE 19.9

Choice of drugs according to target symptoms of personality disorders

Target symptom	Drug of choice	Not recommended
I Behavior dyscontrol		
*Aggression/impulsivity**		
Affective aggression	LITHIUM	
("hot temper" with normal EEG)	SSRIs	
	ANTICONVULSANTS	
	atypical neuroleptics	
Predatory aggression	ATYPICAL NEUROLEPTICS	Benzodiazepines
(hostility/cruelty)	lithium	
Organic-like aggression	catecholamine agonists	
	anticonvulsants	
	SSRIs	
Ictal aggression (abnormal EEG)	ANTICONVULSANTS	Low-potency "old"
	benzodiazepines	neuroleptics
II Mood dysregulation		
Emotional lability	LITHIUM	
	LAMOTRIGINE	
	atypical neuroleptics	TCAs
Depression		
Atypical depression/dysphoria	MAOIs	
	SEROTONERGIC DRUGS	
	atypical neuroleptics	
Classical depression	ANTIDEPRESSANTS	
Anxiety		
Chronic cognitive	SEROTONERGIC DRUGS	
	ANTICONVULSANTS	
	Benzodiazepines	
Chronic somatic	MAOIs, SSRIs	Benzodiazepines
	buspirone	
	beta blockers	
Acute and severe	atypical neuroleptics	
	(e.g. quetiapine)	
Emotional detachment	ATYPICAL NEUROLEPTICS	
	(e.g., aripiprazole)	
III Psychotic symptoms		
Acute & brief psychotic	ATYPICAL NEUROLEPTICS	
episodes	low-dose typical neuroleptics	
Chronic & low-level	ATYPICAL NEUROLEPTICS	
psychotic-like symptoms	low-dose typical neuroleptics	
	anxiolytics	

Capital letters indicate drug of choice.

Annotated bibliography

Beck, AT, Freeman A, and Associates (1990) *Cognitive Therapy of Personality Disorders*, New York, Guilford Press.
This book describes the application of cognitive-behavioral therapy to each of the individual subtypes of personality disorder classified according to criteria of the American Psychiatric Association.

Cloninger, CR (2004) *Feeling Good: The Science of Well-Being.* Oxford University Press.
This book provides a comprehensive description of the biopsychosocial foundations needed to understand personality and to treat psychopathology. It includes an extensive bibliography of recent research and methods for assessing personality and self-aware consciousness.

Cloninger, CR, Przybeck, TR, Svrakic, DM, and Wetzel, RD (1994) *The Temperament and Character Inventory (TCI): A Guide to Its De-*

velopment and Use, St Louis, Washington University Center for Psychobiology of Personality.

This book provides a comprehensive description and bibliography of the seven-factor model of personality, including its psychobiological and genetic basis, psychometrics, normative data from general and diverse clinical populations, use, and interpretation. It describes the practical clinical use of the TCI and available scoring and interpretation services for clinicians in practice. It can be ordered by fax at 314–362–5594 or at http://ta.wustl.edu.

Cloninger, CR and Svrakic, DM (2000) Personality Disorders, in Sadock, BJ and Sadock, VA, (eds) *Comprehensive Textbook of Psychiatry*, New York, Lippincott Williams & Wilkins: 1723–1764.

This chapter provides a thorough description of individual personality disorders from the perspective of both DSM-IV and the dimensional approach of the biopsychosocial approach to personality assessment and treatment.

Strack, S and Lorr, M (eds) (1994) *Differentiating Normal and Abnormal Personality*, New York, Springer Publishing Co.

This book provides a comprehensive review of theories and measurement techniques for distinguishing normal and abnormal personality variants. Articles on alternative dimensional and categorical models are presented by their originators and compared critically.

Vaillant, GE (1977) *Adaptation to Life*, Boston, Little, Brown & Co.

This book describes and clearly illustrates mature and immature psychodynamic mechanisms used to cope with life stress across the lifespan.

CHAPTER 20

Trauma-Related Syndromes

Carol S. North, MD

Clinical relevance: importance and scope of the problem

Scientific advances have contributed to worldwide risks for large-scale catastrophes such as technological accidents and terrorist acts. Examples of technological disasters are transportation accidents such as airplane, subway, train, and motor vehicle collisions; the collapse of buildings and transportation structures such as stadiums and bridges; and industrial tragedies including explosions and toxic chemical spills. Terrorist and other large-scale violent acts include bombings of crowded public structures; release of noxious gas in congested subways; shooting of innocent people in busy public venues such as post offices and courthouses; and use of weapons of mass destruction such as nuclear bombs in metropolitan centers, intentional infectious epidemics, and chemical attacks. The world still endures catastrophic stresses of major wars and atrocities of genocide.

Natural calamities such as tornadoes, hurricanes, earthquakes, volcanoes, wildfires, and floods strike with unexpected yet unrelenting frequency. Disasters may contain elements of both technological and natural catastrophes, such as the Mexico City earthquake, during which devastation was magnified by inadequate antiearthquake construction of buildings, and the Great Midwest Floods of 1993, in which water-containment procedures by the Army Corps of Engineers were criticized.

Besides these dangers, ongoing levels of endemic violence and accidents traumatize members of communities on a daily basis. Drug abuse and violent crime in American cities and associated gang warfare in indigent areas make trauma related to violence a part of daily life in some places. In unsafe neighborhoods where violence is routine, the population has to cope with ongoing, repeated traumatization of extent and intensity sometimes resembling military combat. Even the most affluent neighborhoods, however, are not immune to random violence and accidental trauma, such as motor vehicle accidents, assaults, rapes, robberies, carjackings, and murders, that are sporadic and shocking. Within the assumed safety of families, reported instances of child abuse and molestation are on the rise and may be associated with serious psychological problems among those who are victimized.

With the world's accelerating vulnerability to technological accidents and terrorism, physicians and other health professionals can increasingly expect to encounter psychologically traumatized individuals in clinical practice. After community-wide disasters, physicians may find themselves in positions of leadership, helping communities cope with major disasters as well as with ongoing endemic violence within communities. With some review of posttraumatic syndromes and management techniques, physicians can deal with these syndromes effectively in community and treatment settings.

History of posttraumatic stress disorder

Although the diagnosis of posttraumatic stress disorder (PTSD) is relatively new in official psychiatric nomenclature, posttraumatic syndromes are well known throughout history and have been described in soldiers of the American Civil War, the Crimean War, and World War I as syndromes of physical and nervous exhaustion and under names such as soldier's heart and shell shock. PTSD has been studied most extensively in combat veterans, especially Vietnam veterans throughout the 1980s and 1990s. The current term PTSD first appeared in DSM-III in 1980, and the criteria have been refined in subsequent editions of the diagnostic manual.

An extensive, relatively new body of literature addresses the development of adult psychiatric syndromes in relationship to reports of childhood trauma, especially childhood sexual abuse. In particular, the literature on dissociative

Box 20.1 Posttraumatic stress disorder

A. The person has been exposed to a traumatic event in which both of the following were present:
- the person experienced, witnessed, or was confronted with an event or events that involved actual or threatened death or serious injury, or a threat to the physical integrity of self or others.
- The person's response involved intense fear, helplessness, or horror. **Note**: in children, this may be expressed instead by disorganized or agitated behavior.

B. The traumatic event is persistently reexperienced in one (or more) of the following ways:
- recurrent and intrusive distressing recollections of the event, including images, thoughts, or perceptions. **Note**: in young children, repetitive play may occur in which themes or aspects of the trauma are expressed
- recurrent distressing dreams of the event. Note: in children, there may be frightening dreams without recognizable content
- acting or feeling as if the traumatic event were recurring (includes a sense of reliving the experience, illusions, hallucinations, and dissociative flashback episodes, including those that occur on awakening or when intoxicated). **Note**: In young children, trauma-specific reenactment may occur
- intense psychological distress at exposure to internal or external cues that symbolize or resemble an aspect of the traumatic event
- physiological reactivity on exposure to internal or external cues that symbolize or resemble an aspect of the traumatic event.

C. Persistent avoidance of stimuli associated with the trauma and numbing of general responsiveness (not present before the traumatic event), as indicated by three (or more) of the following:

- efforts to avoid thoughts, feelings, or conversations associated with the trauma
- efforts to avoid activities, places, or people that arouse recollections of the trauma
- inability to recall an important aspect of the trauma
- markedly diminished interest or participation in significant activities
- feeling of detachment or estrangement from others
- restricted range of affect (e.g., unable to have loving feelings)
- sense of a foreshortened future (e.g., does not expect to have a career, marriage, children, or a normal life span).

D. Persistent symptoms of increased arousal (not present before the traumatic event), as indicated by two (or more) of the following:
- difficulty falling or staying asleep
- irritability or outbursts of anger
- difficulty concentrating
- hypervigilance
- exaggerated startle response.

E. Duration of the disturbance (symptoms in criteria B, C, and D) is more than one month.

F. The disturbance causes clinically significant distress or impairment in social, occupational, or other important areas of functioning.

Specify if:
- acute: if duration of symptoms is less than three months
- chronic: if duration of symptoms is three months or more.

Specify if:
- with delayed onset: if onset of symptoms is at least six months after the stressor.

From American Psychiatric Association (2000) Diagnostic and Statistical Manual of Mental Disorders, 4th Edition, Text Revision, Washington, D.C., American Psychiatric Association.

---

disorders indicates that the vast majority of patients with these disorders report childhood abuse (often severe and in some cases allegedly at the hands of satanic cults). These reports have provided a stimulus for theories of dissociative disorders as posttraumatic syndromes that arise from childhood abuse.

Clinical features

Diagnosis

In current psychiatric diagnostic classification, PTSD is officially classified with the anxiety disorders. DSM-IV-TR criteria for PTSD are summarized in Box 20.1. PTSD is the only major psychiatric disorder defined in relation to a stressor.

The single most important aspect of the diagnosis of PTSD is an identifiable traumatic event causing physical injury or threat to life or limb (Table 20.1). Additionally, the traumatic event must evoke a response of intense fear, helplessness, or horror.

Qualifying types of traumatic events may include violent personal assault (such as kidnapping, mugging, physical assault, rape, or torture); violent accidents (for example, motor vehicle accidents, falling from a building or a cliff, or being crushed by heavy machinery): natural and manmade disasters; military combat; being taken hostage; detainment in a concentration camp or as a prisoner of war; and being diagnosed with an acute life-threatening illness. Witnessing a violent injury or death, or unexpectedly seeing a dead body or dismembered body parts qualifies as a traumatic event, as

DIAGNOSIS

Table 20.1 Posttraumatic stress disorder

Discriminating features

1 Requires a traumatic event causing physical injury or threat to life/limb.
2 Categories of symptoms are re-experiencing, avoidance and numbing, and hyperarousal.
3 Lasts more than one month.

Consistent features

1 Symptoms are an amalgam of anxious, depressive, and dissociative symptoms that are new after the event.
2 Higher rates in women.
3 PTSD is more likely after more severe events with high numbers of fatalities or gruesome scenes (e.g., a collapse of a ten-story hospital might be more traumatic than the collapse of a two-car garage).
4 PTSD is more likely with greater exposure to event (e.g., people trapped inside a burning building have more severe exposure than onlookers).

Variable features

1 Psychiatric comorbidity, especially anxiety and depressive disorders.
2 Associated with prior psychiatric illness, especially cases with less serious trauma or less exposure.
3 Delayed onset PTSD begins more than six months after the event; chronic PTSD persists at least three months.

does learning of a sudden, unanticipated death or violent injury of a family member or close friend. Nonviolent events such as watching a scary movie, being fired from a job, or being served with divorce papers are not considered qualifying events. Related to the September 11th terrorist attacks, candidates for PTSD might include those who were caught in the World Trade Center towers after the planes struck, those who watched the horrific scenes from close by, and those whose close family members were in the World Trade Center. People whose only exposure to the disaster was viewing the event on television (even those who witnessed the live coverage or viewed repeated coverage) would not be candidates for PTSD. This is not to discount the intensity of their emotional response, but the psychological experience is not the same as for those directly in harm's way.

Posttraumatic symptoms evoked by the traumatic event are divided into the following three categories: persistent re-experience of the event (Group B symptoms), persistent avoidance of reminders and emotional numbing (Group C symptoms), and persistent arousal (Group D symptoms). Symptoms of persistent re-experience include distressing intrusive memories, vivid visual images of the event, dissociative "flashback" episodes in which the person relives the

event, and recurring or distressing dreams of the event. For example, a survivor of a mass-murder episode complained of being tormented by unrelenting visual images that she described as "snapshots" of the victims' heads being blown apart as they were shot at point-blank range by a large-bore gun. Persistent avoidance and numbing responses include active efforts to escape reminders of the event (for example, going out of one's way to avoid travel near the location of the event), "psychic numbing" or "emotional anesthesia," restricted range of emotional expression, loss of interest in previously enjoyed activities, and feelings of detachment from others. Persistent arousal responses include difficulty falling or staying asleep, exaggerated startle responses such as jumpiness in response to loud noises, and hypervigilance. For example, a woman who survived a public shooting spree described inability to sit in a room with her back to the door, and another woman complained that she now involuntarily scanned for a gun in the hands of every new person entering the room.

Re-experience symptoms qualify toward the diagnosis of PTSD only if they are specific to the event, meaning either directed toward the event or beginning only after the event. Nightmares count, for example, only if the content pertains directly to the event. Avoidance/numbing and hyperarousal symptoms qualify toward the diagnosis only if they present after the event or if pre-existing symptoms are greatly magnified after the trauma; pre-existing difficulties do not count.

Re-experience and hyperarousal symptoms are more common than avoidance/numbing symptoms, but the avoidance/numbing symptoms are more pathological. For example, about 80% of survivors of the direct bomb blast in the Oklahoma City bombing met Group B (re-experience) and Group D (hyperarousal) criteria, but only about one-third met Group C (avoidance/numbing) criteria. More than 90% of those meeting Group C criteria met full PTSD criteria, and showed many other indicators of illness. Group B and D criteria by themselves did not predict PTSD or other indicators of illness.

For a diagnosis of PTSD, the symptoms must also cause significant distress or social impairment. Symptoms of the disorder must be present for more than one month for the diagnosis to be made. Subclassification according to length of illness defines acute PTSD as lasting for fewer than three months and chronic PTSD as lasting three months or more. Delayed onset PTSD is defined by the passage of at least six months from the traumatic event to onset of the symptoms.

Both clinicians treating patients and researchers studying posttraumatic syndromes encounter traumatic responses arising during the first month before a diagnosis of PTSD technically can be made. To cover this situation, the diagnosis of acute stress disorder was introduced in DSM-IV in 1994 to describe symptoms arising after the same type of traumatic event as described for PTSD but not meeting full criteria for PTSD. Criterion symptoms of acute stress disorder include dissociative symptoms, persistent re-experiencing of the event, avoidance responses, and hyperarousal. As with PTSD, the symptoms must interfere with a person's usual functioning for diagnosis of acute stress disorder. The symptoms must last for at least two days, and they must occur within the first month after the event.

The character of PTSD symptoms has variable manifestations in different populations. The post-Vietnam War syndrome involves severe and vivid flashbacks, causing its sufferers to relive the war experience with immediate intensity. Compared to survivors of civilian traumas, combat veterans more commonly report emotional numbing, amnesia, social isolation, and survivor guilt. Survivor guilt has been dropped from the PTSD criteria because of its uncommon appearance in other traumatized populations. Combat veterans in general are a special population characterized by male predominance, combat-readiness training, expectation of military combat experience, and exposure to trauma (combat) that may be longlasting and repetitive. Vietnam veterans also faced the distinctive stress of the politically charged anti-war atmosphere on their return to American society, an added psychosocial burden. War veterans would be expected to show different responses to combat traumas than other populations subjected to different traumas, such as community-wide catastrophes or random and singular acts of violence in the community. Therefore, not only do members of other populations experience different types of traumatic agents, but they may also have different vulnerabilities to traumatic experiences and varied coping abilities. Finally, the symptoms characteristic of dissociative disorders following violent adult trauma are quite different from symptoms described by patients reporting traumatic childhood events (see Chapter 18).

An important clinical aspect of posttraumatic experience is the recognition that although most people briefly develop at least some psychological symptoms after catastrophic traumas, most individuals do not become psychiatrically ill. The ability for most individuals to emerge psychologically intact from severely catastrophic events bears witness to human resilience and the capacity of the mind to process and cope with extremes of traumatic experience.

Natural history

Symptoms of PTSD may begin within hours, and they usually begin within a few days, of the event. Delayed onset (by definition, longer than six months after the trauma) of PTSD is uncommon, but cases beginning as much as several years after the event have been described by Helzer and colleagues in 16% of PTSD cases in Vietnam veterans sampled from the general population. In studies conducted by Archibald and Tuddenham, World War II veterans showed no evidence of delayed PTSD. A 14-year follow-up study of survivors of the

Buffalo Creek dam break and flood found that 20% of all identified PTSD cases were delayed cases (that is, they met PTSD criteria at the time of the follow-up study but not at the time of the index)—but the fact that this was a litigant sample may have affected the natural course of the symptoms. A series of studies of more than 2,000 survivors of major disasters by the Washington University disaster research team found virtually no delayed-onset PTSD.

PTSD symptoms typically start to fade within weeks of the event, but their character and intensity can vary over time. Helzer and colleagues found that approximately half of the cases in the general population resolve within six months. A resurgence of symptoms at the one-year anniversary of the event is characteristic and may become an annual phenomenon with diminishing intensity in subsequent years. Such anniversary reactions are thought to be further stimulated by media attention reminding people of the event.

Chronic PTSD with symptoms persisting for many years has also been described. More than one-half of PTSD cases in a community study were found to persist for more than one year. In a study by Helzer and colleagues, one-third of PTSD cases persisted for at least three years. Chronicity has been predicted by the presence of preexisting psychiatric disorders, neuroticism, a history of early separation from parents in childhood, and a family history of anxiety or antisocial behavior. Among disaster survivors, litigation is thought to keep symptoms alive, slowing the recovery process, which apparently rebounds relatively quickly once the litigation is completed. Prisoners of war appear to have the greatest chronicity. After 40 years, 58–90% of World War II prisoners of war with PTSD were found to still meet criteria for active PTSD.

Differential diagnosis (comorbidity)

PTSD is differentiated from acute stress disorder by the persistence of symptoms for at least one month, as well as a greater number of symptoms in discrete groups. The diagnosis of acute stress disorder, unlike PTSD, requires an onset of symptoms within one month of the traumatic event and lasts for less than a month. If an individual with acute stress disorder subsequently fulfills criteria for PTSD, the diagnosis is changed from acute stress disorder to PTSD.

PTSD is differentiated from adjustment disorder by the extreme nature of the stressor (physically injurious or life-threatening) required for PTSD, compared with the stressor in adjustment disorder, which can be of any type or severity. After traumatic events, symptoms that do not meet criteria for PTSD, acute stress disorder, or another psychiatric disorder might be diagnosed as adjustment disorder. This diagnosis might also be made for posttraumatic symptoms occurring in response to a nonqualifying type of stressor.

Other psychiatric disorders with symptoms that can be confused with PTSD include obsessive-compulsive disorder

(OCD), which has obsessions and compulsions that are recognized by the individual as inappropriate and which do not occur in response to a traumatic event, and psychotic disorders, which have hallucinations and other perceptual disturbances that must be differentiated from the characteristic flashbacks of PTSD. PTSD should be differentiated from malingering in situations in which an individual stands to gain financially or personally (for example, eligibility for disability benefits or forensic determination of criminal responsibility).

According to DSM-IV-TR, comorbid psychiatric disorders associated with PTSD may include panic disorder, agoraphobia, social or other phobias, OCD, major depressive disorder (MDD), somatization disorder, and substance use disorders. The manual further states that no information is available on the extent to which these comorbid disorders may precede or follow the onset of PTSD—meaning that they may occur as additional psychopathological conditions along with PTSD after a traumatic event or that they may be predisposing conditions. Further research is needed to determine these relationships. Virtually all of the highly prevalent alcohol abuse and dependence found in firefighters rescue and recovery workers after the Oklahoma City bombing was found to be pre-existent.

The disaster literature has examined psychiatric comorbidity with PTSD in some detail. Rates of psychiatric comorbidity with PTSD found after disasters range from approximately 20% in studies of survivors of a volcano eruption and of a plane crash into a hotel to 89% in survivors of a multiple-agent disaster setting. MDD appears to be the most common comorbid disorder. General population studies find that other psychiatric disorders are twice as prevalent in people who suffer from PTSD than in the rest of the population. Approximately 80% of people with PTSD are found to meet criteria for an additional diagnosis. Disorders most closely associated with PTSD in the general population are OCD, mood disorders, and substance abuse. Three-fourths of people with PTSD have a preexisting personal or family history of anxiety disorder.

Further work on psychiatric comorbidity with PTSD has been carried out in military combat populations. Veterans with PTSD have been found to have comorbidity rates of up to 80%. The most commonly associated psychiatric disorders in veterans with PTSD are MDD, anxiety disorders, substance abuse, and antisocial personality disorder. Prisoners of war appear to have the highest rates of comorbidity with PTSD, with more than 90% meeting criteria for a second diagnosis.

Comorbidity of personality disorders with PTSD has received insufficient attention. This has been perhaps best studied in military populations. More than two-thirds of Vietnam veterans with PTSD have been found to meet criteria for a personality disorder diagnosis. It is not clear whether associated personality findings represent enduring

changes in personality function as a result of psychological trauma, or preexisting psychopathological conditions with known risk for exposure to traumatic events and posttraumatic difficulties. In clinical settings, personal difficulties in relation to traumatic events and posttraumatic syndromes are frequently seen in association with prominent borderline (and other Cluster B) personality features and somatoform symptoms, which are further associated with dissociative syndromes and potential for substance abuse. Failure to recognize these comorbidities or to discount their significance by attributing them to the traumatic exposure may lead to serious difficulties in management of these patients.

PTSD symptoms overlap considerably with symptoms of other psychiatric disorders. Sleep disturbance, one of the most common PTSD symptoms, is also one of the criterion symptoms of MDD. Loss of interest in usual activities and difficulties concentrating, which are criteria for PTSD, are also criterion symptoms of MDD. The hypervigilance of PTSD is also seen in other anxiety disorders. Amnesia and feelings of numbness and detachment described in PTSD are hallmark symptoms of dissociative disorders.

Because of the great degree of symptom overlap, the validity of PTSD as a separate clinical entity has been questioned. In essence, the diagnostic criteria for PTSD are an assimilation of symptoms from the following three recognized psychiatric categories: MDD, generalized anxiety disorder (GAD), and dissociative disorders. The documented overlap of PTSD with other disorders in traumatized populations may be at least in part a function of this overlap in symptom criteria. Controversy persists as to whether PTSD belongs with the anxiety disorders or whether it is more appropriately grouped with the dissociative disorders. Even more fundamentally, however, standard procedures for validation of PTSD as a distinct diagnosis have yet to be completed.

Genetics and family history

The genetics of PTSD are unknown. A family history study of 36 military veterans with chronic PTSD found evidence of psychiatric illness in two-thirds (66%) of the families. Substance abuse (60%), anxiety disorders (22%), and MDD (20%) were the most prevalent disorders in families. Only 6% of families had one or more members with PTSD. The familial association of PTSD with a variety of other disorders and not with PTSD argues against the assumption that PTSD as currently defined describes a unified syndrome.

Epidemiology

Between 1% and 14% of the general population have been found to meet lifetime criteria for an episode of PTSD. Experiences of violent trauma are far more prevalent than PTSD. Most people who have such an experience do not develop PTSD. The population study by Breslau's group found that

39% of the population had experienced a violent traumatic event. The most common violent trauma was a violent accident or injury (9%), followed by physical assault (8%). A study by Norris of a community sample of 1000 adults found that a higher proportion (69%) had experienced a traumatic event, including 21% who had experienced a traumatic event in the previous year alone. Robberies (25%) and motor vehicle accidents (23%) were the most common traumatic events in this study. Men were significantly more likely than women to report a traumatic event, with 74% indicating such a history.

In the Breslau study, nearly one-fourth (24%) of people who had experienced a traumatic event developed PTSD in relation to it. Overall, 9% of the population was found to have experienced an episode of PTSD. The type of event most likely followed by PTSD was rape among women, resulting in PTSD in 80% of the cases. A general population study by Helzer's group found lower rates of PTSD—0.5% in men and 1.3% in women. In the Norris study, the lifetime rate of PTSD was 5%.

Studies conducted in psychiatric treatment settings find high rates of PTSD and reported traumatization. The majority of psychiatric outpatients (68%) and inpatients (81%) report a history of physical or sexual victimization. Drug-abusing women in treatment almost universally (99%) report a history of violent trauma, and 59% of those with a history of trauma qualify for a diagnosis of PTSD.

The prevalence of PTSD after disasters varies widely according to the type of disaster and the population affected. Studies of tornadoes, volcanoes, mudslides, floods, and dioxin contamination have yielded rates of PTSD from 2% to 8%. Higher rates of PTSD were found among survivors of a plane crash into a hotel (22%), among victims of a shooting massacre in a Texas cafeteria (29%), and in survivors of the Oklahoma City bombing (34%). Even higher rates of PTSD (44% to 54%) have been recorded in studies of survivors of a dam break and flood, bushfires, and an airplane crash-landing.

Studies of Vietnam combat veterans have identified rates of PTSD in the range of 15% to 31%, but only 9% of Desert Storm soldiers were diagnosed with PTSD 6 months after their return from the Persian Gulf. Higher rates of PTSD have been documented in prisoners of war (50% to 78%). It can be seen that the prevalence of PTSD varies considerably and is highly dependent on the type and features of the event as well as preexisting characteristics of the population involved.

Risk factors

Specific characteristics of evocative trauma agents predict human response to them. The highest rates of psychiatric difficulties are associated with disaster agents with the most severe elements of terror (that is, threat to life or limb), horror (witness to grotesque scenes), suddenness and unexpected-

ness of occurrence (tornadoes and plane crashes), long duration (floods continuing for months), repetitive occurrence (repeated crests of floods in a single season), intensity (sheer numbers of lives lost and catastrophic financial damages to communities), degree of personal damages (physical injury, total destruction of a home), and grief over loss of loved ones. Disasters with the additional element of causation by human factors, particularly willful acts of terrorism (for example, bombings and shooting massacres) even more than accidents caused by human error, are thought to evoke more pathological human responses.

The personal attributes of individuals exposed to traumatic events predict both exposure to traumatic events and psychiatric response. Individual vulnerability to exposure to traumatic events varies among populations and individuals. Whereas certain freak accidents, such as plane crashes into buildings, and unprecedented terrorism, such as bombings of public buildings, are virtually equal-opportunity events, many traumatic stressors target individuals with attributes that increased their likelihood of exposure. Demographic and personal characteristics found to predict exposure to violent trauma in the community include lack of education, male gender, early conduct problems, and extroverted personality style. Psychiatric disorders—especially illicit drug use disorders, alcoholism, and antisocial personality disorder—put people at risk for exposure to violent trauma in excess of that in the rest of the population.

Among military populations, pre-service variables predict likelihood of combat exposure. These predictors include youthfulness, lack of education, history of juvenile conduct problems, and preexisting psychopathology. Therefore, those least likely to tolerate the horrors of combat may be those most likely to be placed in combat.

People of any age, either gender, and any race may develop PTSD. Somewhat different factors are found to predict psychiatric illness after a traumatic event than those that predict the likelihood of exposure to the event. Among populations exposed to traumatic events, the demographic characteristics of survivors can further predispose them to a psychiatric disorder after the event. After disasters, women tend to have higher rates of PTSD than men. Lower socioeconomic and educational status may predict a greater degree of postdisaster psychopathology. Although one study found that older people are at increased risk for psychiatric problems after disasters, a number of other studies have determined that age is a weak predictor or nonpredictor of postdisaster adjustment. Personal support networks, or at least a perception of them, are associated with improved outcome after disasters; women have been found to experience spousal and social relationships as more burdensome than supportive after highly stressful events. Female gender, youth, less education, and ethnic minority group membership have been found to predict vulnerability to developing PTSD after violent trauma in communities. Combat-related

PTSD has also been found to be associated with lower educational achievement.

In all trauma-exposed populations, preexisting psychopathology has repeatedly been found to be the greatest predictor of trauma-associated psychopathology. In survivors of major disasters, predisaster psychiatric illness strongly predicts the postdisaster psychopathological state, especially after low-impact disasters and among less exposed individuals. With increasing disaster intensity and greater individual exposure to the disaster agent, personal vulnerability becomes less predictive; more people with no history of psychiatric problems succumb to the psychological impact of traumas of a catastrophic magnitude that would theoretically overwhelm even the most resilient person.

Among combat veterans, the pre-service psychopathological state is similarly predictive of postwar psychiatric adjustment. Even when controlling for the degree of combat exposure, combat-related PTSD and PTSD symptoms are predicted by pre-service Minnesota Multiphasic Personality Inventory (MMPI) ratings of hypochondriasis, paranoia, depression, hypomania, psychopathic deviation, social introversion, and diminished masculinity. A history of juvenile behaviors consistent with conduct disorder symptoms was found to predict PTSD symptoms in combat veterans in a general population sample. Antisocial personality disorder in combat veterans predicted drug and alcohol abuse but not PTSD. Postwar factors have also been found to predict the psychiatric outcome of combat veterans. Psychiatric difficulties have been found in association with other negative life events and lack of social support networks after returning home.

In community survivors of violent trauma, preexisting psychiatric disorders also predict PTSD. PTSD is associated with a history of childhood behavior problems and with preexisting neuroticism, drug abuse (particularly cocaine and opiate abuse), anxiety, and depression.

Pathophysiology

The hypothalamic-pituitary-adrenal axis is one of the main hormonal systems mediating the physiological stress response and is considered pivotal in the generation of PTSD symptoms. Under stress, the adrenals release glucocorticoids, including cortisol. Relative to healthy controls, patients with PTSD excrete more urinary epinephrine and norepinephrine and less cortisol, and have elevated plasma adrenocorticotropic hormone levels. Central nervous system lymphocyte glucocorticoid receptors may be upregulated in PTSD, suggesting mechanisms of hypersensitivity of feedback inhibition of corticosteroids in the hypothalamic-pituitary-adrenal axis system in the generation of PTSD symptoms.

It has been hypothesized that neurotoxic effects of chronic stress hormone exposure may damage the hippocampus. Supporting evidence of this has been suggested by magnetic resonance imaging (MRI) studies indicating smaller hippocampal volumes in PTSD patients, correlating with 24-hour urinary cortisol, compared with matched controls. Ongoing stress with its resultant chronic corticosteroid stimulation in PTSD is hypothesized to exert a neurotoxic effect on hippocampal structures, which could be related to the memory impairment associated with PTSD in some studies. Recent studies involving serial examination of trauma victims prospectively over time, however, have not observed loss of hippocampal volume, deflating theories of hippocampal damage as the mechanism of PTSD development.

Combat veterans with PTSD demonstrate heightened autonomic responses, including elevated heart rate, blood pressure, and electrodermal responses. Those suffering from PTSD are hypothesized to experience continuous and repeated autonomic arousal through conditioning of a persistent startle reaction as well as internally generated imagery in the form of flashbacks and intrusive recollections of the traumatic event. Persistence or nonhabituation of the autonomic response to repetitive tone stimuli has been observed in Israeli combat veterans relative to controls and is thought to support a chronic autonomic arousal model of PTSD. Chronic autonomic arousal in PTSD may overstimulate the hypothalamic-pituitary-adrenal-axis and lead to exhaustion of adrenal cortical function. Suppression of affective arousal described in PTSD (emotional numbing) theoretically reflects this adrenal exhaustion. It is not clear whether such nonhabituation might reflect antecedent constitutional risk or an acquired abnormality resulting from traumatic experience.

Military veterans with combat-related PTSD demonstrate increased latency and decreased amount of rapid eye movement (REM) sleep, reduced Stage IV sleep, and lowered sleep efficiency. Nightmares related to PTSD occur in various stages of non-REM sleep, further supporting the theory that PTSD is a disorder of general hyperarousal.

Treatment

Fundamental to management of posttraumatic syndromes is completion of a full diagnostic evaluation. Prominent avoidance and numbing symptoms are strongly suggestive of PTSD, and their presence should stimulate the clinician to pursue a focused examination for PTSD. Additionally, one or more important comorbid conditions often accompany the presentation of PTSD. The greatest potential error in this process is to abandon the diagnostic investigation once PTSD has been identified. Treating PTSD without careful consideration of comorbid disorders invites difficulties in care of these patients. The comorbid conditions, most often mood and anxiety disorders, substance abuse, and personality disorders, can confuse and confound treatment if not recognized and managed. Treatment of these comorbid disorders in the usual manner is recommended along with attention to PTSD. These other disorders may overshadow PTSD in clinical relevance, have implications for management, and contribute to outcome.

Psychotropic management of posttraumatic syndromes can be approached in two ways, symptomatically and diagnostically. The symptomatic approach utilizes short-term sedation usually with a benzodiazepine for relief of early posttraumatic anxiety, agitation, and insomnia. This approach is often utilized in the early posttraumatic period, particularly during the first 2–4 weeks before major depression and PTSD can be diagnosed. Benzodiazepines have the potential to induce amnesia, block restorative cognitive processes, and disinhibit predisposed individuals. Long-term use of potentially habit-forming medications has not been demonstrated to be effective treatment of PTSD and generates the potential for tolerance and dependence. Behavioral disinhibition and potential for sedative abuse are of particular importance in clinical settings where comorbidities often involve personality, somatoform, and substance use disorders—a sound reminder of the importance of solid diagnostic assessment.

The diagnostic approach to pharmacologic management of PTSD involves longer term pharmacotherapy for patients who fulfill criteria for PTSD. Two SSRI agents, sertraline and paroxetine, have received indications for treatment of PTSD by the FDA. A more extensive literature also suggests utility for other antidepressant agents, including tricyclic antidepressant agents (TCAs), monoamine oxidase inhibitors (MAOIs, for example, phenelzine), other SSRIs and possibly other antidepressants, in effective treatment of PTSD. Because major depression and other anxiety disorders are frequent concomitants of PTSD, use of antidepressant medications is a parsimonious choice. However, the posttraumatic effect is independent of antidepressant properties, and therapeutic response is seen in all three groups of PTSD symptoms (intrusive recall, avoidance/numbing, and hyperarousal). Pharmacotherapy of PTSD with antidepressants follows principles of use of these agents in treatment of other anxiety disorders and major depression. Other agents that have been tried with limited and anecdotal success include propranolol, lithium, clonidine, prazosin, antihistamines, anticonvulsants, and antipsychotics.

In the absence of an extensive therapeutic trial literature on medications for PTSD, theories involving physiological mechanisms and hypothesized pharmacologic action have provided direction for choosing therapeutic agents. Benzodiazepines and anticonvulsants have been suggested to reduce "kindling" in the genesis of PTSD. Serotonergic synergism and anti-panic mechanisms of TCAs are considered likely to dampen posttraumatic hyperarousal. Alpha$_2$ agonists have been hypothesized to down-regulate activation of sympathetic outflow from the locus ceruleus.

Psychotherapy is an important management tool in posttraumatic settings, but the relevant research literature is in-complete and controversial. Cognitive behavioral and exposure therapies have been demonstated to be effective in the treatment of PTSD.

Normal processes of emotional healing after psychologically traumatic events typically involve sharing the experience with others, serving to facilitate cognitive processing and healthy habituation and assimilation of memories of horrifying experiences that are not supposed to be a part of life. Therefore, clinical management of PTSD and other posttraumatic syndromes begins with taking a history that allows the patient to share the experience, which is in itself a comforting and self-validating process. Recounting the event also serves to bond the storyteller to the listener. Available data are not sufficient to determine when and under what circumstances a person should be encouraged to talk about the experience or to avoid thinking or talking about it. Traumatized individuals relying on denial and avoidance as their main coping method may find direct confrontation with the memory of the event overwhelming and retraumatizing. Therefore, proceeding cautiously and not pushing against resistance in pursuit of discussion of the event are recommended, especially in the early posttraumatic stages.

The psychotherapeutic tools for symptom management of PTSD symptoms differ for symptom groups. Management of intrusive memories and hyperarousal involves relaxation procedures and peaceful imagery, strengthening and substituting pleasant old associations for traumatic reminders of the event, graded re-exposure to reminders of the event, cognitive restructuring to identify and replace maladaptive cognitions with rational ideas, thought-stopping techniques, and application of sleep hygiene. Management of avoidance and numbing symptoms involves establishment of positive, tolerable memories and associations to replace disaster reminders, cultivation of gratifying emotional states and social experiences, and graded resumption of pleasurable activities and social relationships.

Survivors of traumatic events who do not develop PTSD have needs that differ from those for individuals with the disorder. Fundamental processes of management for these more resilient individuals are reassurance and education, with continued monitoring for development of PTSD or other disorders. Reassurance and educational procedures include validation and normalization of disturbing feelings and thoughts that people often have after extremely upsetting events, providing coping skills, and boosting social support. The experience must be assimilated into the unique personal context of each individual's private system of meaning and organization of life and existence. This process may include philosophical and spiritual dimensions that lie within the individual's personal and cultural framework.

Group sharing of experiences after community-wide disasters can be a useful avenue for communities to respond to the catastrophe. Mitchell's method for critical incident stress management provides one or two group debriefing sessions involving systematic sharing and cognitive processing of the experience in a socially supportive setting, education to legitimize and normalize members' distressing experiences and provide coping and problem-solving strategies, and identification of individuals at risk for serious psychiatric problems. Over the last several years, group debriefing procedures have been promoted around the world for coping with international catastrophes, without empirical testing. Recently, research has found that group debriefing not only does not prevent PTSD, but it may be harmful to some people. A more appropriate goal for debriefing is to help basically healthy people accommodate to their experience. Highly traumatized individuals with prominent avoidance and numbing profiles may be retraumatized by confrontation of the experience in debriefing groups, and should be triaged to formal treatment.

PEARLS & PERILS

- A pivotal aspect of the diagnosis of PTSD is identification of sufficient exposure to an appropriate traumatic agent, that is, one causing physical injury or threat to life or limb to the individual (or witnessing a violent event or learning that a close family member experienced an acute life-threatening trauma). Nonviolent stressors such as being fired from a job and divorce do not qualify.
- Symptoms of PTSD must be specifically related to the event or new after the event to qualify; pre-existing symptoms do not count toward the diagnosis.
- The best predictors of psychiatric illness after disasters are preexisting psychopathology (especially after milder events) and female gender. With increasing intensity of the event and exposure to it, more individuals with no past psychiatric history may develop postdisaster difficulties.
- When PTSD is present, comorbid psychiatric diagnoses are common and should not be overlooked. They may be important in shaping treatment strategies.
- An important clinical aspect of posttraumatic experience is the recognition that although most people briefly develop at least some psychological symptoms after catastrophic traumas, most do not become psychiatrically ill. This information is helpful to reassure people after traumatic events and to normalize their experience as a legitimate response to an extreme event.
- SSRI agents are the treatment of choice for PTSD (sertraline and paroxetine having FDA approval), but other types of agents have also been tried.
- Social support and psychotherapy help patients cognitively process and assimilate the traumatic experience. People with PTSD and prominent avoidance and numbing profiles may be retraumatized by confrontation with the experience they are unable to face, and for them, more gradual and indirect approaches to psychotherapy are indicated.

KEY CLINICAL QUESTIONS AND WHAT THEY UNLOCK

- *Inquire specifically about the presence of avoidance and numbing symptoms.*
  These symptoms are the most predictive of the full spectrum of PTSD.
- *Inquire about a prior history of psychopathology.*
  Such a history may predispose patients to PTSD as well as comorbid psychiatric disorders.
- *How does diagnostic assessment direct decisions about intervention?*
  Treat both PTSD and comorbid disorders with standard management. If PTSD is not present, other approaches for post traumatic distress (education, reassurance, social support) are indicated.

Special issues

Social and political forces in the mental health field during the 1980s increased public attention to matters of child abuse and its potential long-term effects. These forces have helped mold popular conceptualizations of posttraumatic syndromes. In this climate, popular books such as Bass and Davis' *The Courage to Heal* have identified a host of psychopathological syndromes as adult sequelae of child abuse. These materials urge therapists and patients to work together to uncover memories of childhood abuse and resolve the traumatic experience as necessary to achieving mental health. A parallel, rapidly expanding professional literature identifies chronic adult posttraumatic syndromes as a consequence of childhood abuse. Dissociative disorders have rapidly grown to epidemic proportions in the last three decades and are considered by many to represent adult syndromes arising from childhood abuse, although empirical validation of these notions are lacking. The reader is directed to more extensive discussion of dissociative disorders in Chapter 18.

Mullen and colleagues examined the relationship of childhood sexual abuse and adult mental health in women in a community sample. Although reported childhood abuse was most prevalent among women from disrupted and dysfunctional homes and predicted several types of adult psychopathological conditions, the authors made several cautionary statements. They indicated that rather than abuse being the direct causal factor, other explanations might account for the association, including sexual abuse as a possible marker for other variables that might be the operative causal factors in adult psychopathological conditions or at least part of a broader etiological scenario.

Further analysis of the data from Mullen and colleagues showed that although a report of sexual abuse predicted adult psychopathological disorders beyond what other predictive factors contributed, other problems in the childhood home life were important predictors of the sexual abuse as well as of the psychopathological state independent of the sexual abuse. This study illustrates the importance of examining all the factors together rather than restricting the focus to childhood sexual abuse as a predictor of adult psychopathological conditions in a social and environmental vacuum. Lack of attention to these principles leads to unwarranted and unsupported conclusions about dissociation and other disorders as posttraumatic syndromes with etiological roots in childhood trauma and abuse. To reiterate an earlier statement, the only psychiatric disorder whose definition is etiologically based on traumatic experience is PTSD.

Conclusion

Although PTSD is a relatively new entity in official psychiatric criteria, trauma-related syndromes have been recognized for ages. Considerable work is needed to further define PTSD, delineate it from other psychiatric syndromes, determine underlying pathophysiology, and develop effective treatments.

In managing posttraumatic syndromes, the physician is advised to search for comorbid psychiatric disorders that are often present and to treat them in the usual manner, applying diagnosis-specific pharmacologic agents and using antianxiety and sedative agents when necessary for brief symptomatic relief. The general mainstay of psychotherapy is the provision of a supportive psychotherapeutic environment for emotionally traumatized individuals to ventilate feelings; validation and reassurance of the normalcy of their feelings after extreme events; and assistance with processing, coping with, and assimilating the trauma experience. Time heals posttraumatic distress, and the physician functions to facilitate that healing.

CONSIDER CONSULTATION WHEN...

- A patient has experienced an extreme traumatic event with threat to life or limb (e.g., being run over by a train, kidnapped at gunpoint and raped, or assaulted with intent to kill), and prominent avoidance and numbing features are present.
- Factors predicting a difficult course are present, such as a history of previous psychiatric problems; comorbid psychiatric disorder such as substance abuse, major depression, or anxiety disorder; prominent dissociative features; inadequate social support or significant other life problems; and inability to function or severe subjective emotional distress.

Annotated bibliography

Journal of Traumatic Stress, New York, Plenum Press.
 This journal, published by the International Society for Traumatic Stress Studies, provides an interdisciplinary forum for the publication of peer-reviewed original academic papers on the biopsychosocial aspects of trauma. Issues addressing theory, research, treatment, prevention, education/training, and legal and policy concerns are included. Its topics include war, disaster, accident, violence or abuse, hostage-taking, and life-threatening illness. Published quarterly, this journal is aimed as a primary reference for professionals who study and treat people exposed to extreme human trauma.

Lystad, M (ed.) (1988) *Mental Health Response to Mass Emergencies: Theory and Practice*, New York, Brunner/Mazel.
 This text is a volume of a "refereed" book series ensuring the highest academic quality of its content. An internationally respected field of researchers has provided contributions to this very readable text that covers individual and community responses to disaster, social and clinical intervention programs, and public/education/planning programs with practical material that can be directly implemented in communities.

Ursano, RJ, McCaughey, BG, and Fullerton, CS (eds) (1994) *Individual and Community Responses to Trauma and Disaster: The Structure of Human Chaos*, Cambridge, Cambridge University Press.
 This comprehensive and scholarly volume, written by an international collection of leading researchers in the field, covers the entire range of extreme traumas and disasters: technological, natural, and manmade. Empirical studies and observational reports, as well as practical clinical methods of debriefing victims and helpers and providing psychological relief, are presented.

Wilson, JP and Raphael, B (eds) (1993) *International Handbook of Traumatic Stress Syndromes*, New York, Plenum.
 This tome of more than 1,000 pages is the ultimate information source on trauma-related syndromes, as well as an extremely useful handbook for clinicians and researchers. Written by the top authorities on the subject in the world, this book covers a wide range of topics, including theoretical and research methodology strategies; war trauma and civil violence; trauma from torture, detention, and internment; disaster-related syndromes; trauma syndromes in children and adolescents including violence, incest, and transgenerational syndromes; dissociative disorders; intervention strategies; and social policy.

SECTION 3

Important Topics in Clinical Medicine

Barry A. Hong, PhD

CHAPTER 21

Psychotherapy

Richard D. Wetzel, PhD and Barry A. Hong, PhD

Introduction

What is psychotherapy? Is it properly the province of only the psychiatrist and the other mental health professionals? Our answer is No! If one considers psychotherapy as planned changes in emotions, thinking, and behavior, then every medical specialist practices psychotherapy and/or psychotherapeutic communication.

Relating to the patient

Almost all schools of psychotherapy would recognize that the clinician-patient relationship is central both to the practice of medicine and to the practice of psychotherapy. The first task in psychotherapy is to understand, develop, and maintain a relationship with the patient. This relationship is an important basis in any physician's practice, not just in that of mental health specialists. In the psychotherapy literature, this is the development of a "therapeutic alliance" when a patient and physician work in a trusting, deliberate, and collaborative manner.

The physician, especially one with ongoing responsibility for the patient, can and ought to provide a therapeutic relationship, whether the patient's illness is cancer, stroke, arthritis, depression, panic attacks, AIDS, diabetes, tuberculosis, or epilepsy. In fact, any patient confronting an illness associated with chronic or recurrent pain, disability, or early death deserves support and therapeutic conversations. Therapeutic conversations are not formal psychotherapy sessions, but are brief exchanges with patients that give insight, boost motivation, encourage better thoughts, and recommend pleasant/positive experiences.

Psychotherapy nearly always implies important and personal communication with the patient. It is very helpful for the patient to believe that the physician or therapist cares about him/her and is genuinely interested in helping the pa-
tient understand their medical condition (when there is one) and their overall life situation. The patient must develop confidence that the physician/therapist respects the patient and sympathizes and empathizes with the patient's symptoms, suffering, and relevant experiences. How are patients likely to come to such conclusions? Primarily by the therapist's demeanor, action, and communication. Sometimes it is necessary to say these things directly. By one's behavior, this caring, therapeutic climate is clearly established.

Psychotherapeutic interaction with patients depends on showing sympathy, respect, patience, and interest, both verbally and in body language. The patient's concerns, worries, fears, and other difficulties must guide the interaction to a substantial degree. Psychotherapeutic communication requires careful and attentive listening. In general, the patient should be doing most (but not all) of the talking if the exchange is to be maximally useful and therapeutic. The patient must be encouraged to talk more, steadily providing more information. "Tell me more," "And then what happened?", "How did you feel?", and "What did you do or say?" show that the interviewer really is interested in what the patient has to report or say. This behavior dispels the notion that the clinician is ready to rush off to the next patient. These responses elicit more information and indicate to the patient that the clinician welcomes significant involvement from the patient.

In addition to encouraging questions, the therapist may offer comments which reflect how a person feels such as "You were upset," "You sound angry even now," "You sound hurt," "I wonder if you showed that you were upset (angry, hurt)," and "I wonder how much it still troubles you." Such comments make it clear to the patient that it is proper to consider their feelings and to try to describe them as well as the facts of the situation. Patient responses can then be moved along by returning to basic requests for additional information. Asking for additional information gives the patient the idea that you are truly interested in them.

Some patients may have difficulty in responding. When this is the case, it should be recognized openly. The patient may be told that "You seem to find it hard to talk about such things" or "Are you aware that it is not easy for you to talk about these feelings?" The specific words or phrases are not important. Reassuring the patient is essential. It is important that the patient not be allowed to become discouraged by thinking he or she is doing poorly. It is equally important because it identifies what the patient is expected to do in the session. Asking simple, straightforward questions or pointing out fairly obvious observations or making relatively obvious inferences are what will help the patient continue talking and thinking about his or her experiences. (Brilliant leaps of insight are best displayed at cocktail parties to one's friends and colleagues who can appreciate them. Even if the clinician is correct, quick interpretations can be frightening to the patient.) If the patient can be encouraged to talk about feelings, troubles, worries, or fears, progress is being made. Asking "why" questions in contrast is not helpful, "Why do you feel this way?" Sometimes people don't understand why they feel a particular way.

As the patient talks more openly and freely, the physician or therapist can try to tie together what the patient says with the patient's presenting problem. Restating the patient's presenting problem is useful for both the patient and the physician. If the patient offers some relevant observations, the physician can reinforce the usefulness of such thinking. Again, the goal is to encourage the patient to talk about feelings, experiences, and circumstances that are relevant to the clinical problem and to the patient's ways of coping with the disorder and its associated difficulties.

The exact language is not important. In fact, psychological jargon can be off-putting or offensive. The aim is to make clear that the physician is interested in the patient's concerns and circumstances and wants to be helpful. All patients appreciate such interest. Patients interpret the physician's interest as evidence that the physician cares and recognizes the human being involved in the illness. Even patients who are not certain that such discussions make sense usually respond favorably to the physician's interest if an adequate relationship has been established. In either case, increased trust, confidence, and hope are often the result of such physician strategies. Expression of interest in and concern for the patient can never be delegated successfully to another person or physician extender. This is also a helpful stance even with physical symptoms, disease progression or partially successful treatments.

The psychotherapeutic relationship permits the physician/therapist to make observations and suggestions that may be uncomfortable or even unwanted by the patient at times. Usually, patients can tolerate and accept such communications when the relationship is properly established.

Furthermore, the proper psychotherapeutic relationship permits the patient to disagree with the physician/therapist in a way that fosters further exploration and greater mutual understanding. For that reason, psychotherapy is not like conversation among friends. It has a different goal. Sometimes you must say things people don't like hearing or seem rude in a different social situation. Patients who disagree with their doctor are not stupid; they frequently provide useful information not previously considered. The goal is always to help the patient to understand as much as possible about the illness or other problems and about the patient's ways of interpreting and dealing with these.

The process of psychotherapy

Because the physician is uniquely qualified to understand the disease processes in his/her area of specialization, the treatments involved, and the usual reactions of patients to the illness and its treatment, frequently the physician is the best qualified health care provider to help patients understand and deal with these problems. When this therapeutic relationship is adequately developed and working well, the focus will usually turn naturally to educating the patient and clarifying the patient's understanding of the illness or related problems. The patient's temperament and personality help frame the patient's reaction to the illness and affect how the patient regards his/her treatments. The discussion generally will deal with the patient's attitudes, coping style, important relationships, and life circumstances, as these interact with the patient's illness and course. Adherence behaviors are good examples of these effects.

Psychotherapy or at least therapeutic conversations can and should be part of each physician's treatment plan in patients whose clinical problems warrant the time and effort. In the presence of a warm, supportive, and nurturing relationship, the clinician and the patient define the problem, agree on a preferred and acceptable outcome, and identify the steps to be taken to reach that goal. This is an iterative process in which the patient hopefully develops more insightful, more nuanced and complex understanding of the problem, the goal, and the decisions, skills, and actions needed to reach the goal. Frequently the goals will be modified or expanded over time. Generally, experienced clinicians begin with a simpler problem as a first step that the patient can solve rather easily in order to build the patient's confidence in the process and in themselves.

In some sense the patient's and the clinician's understanding of the problem is like a parable or a myth in the literary or religious sense of the word. Some feel that psychotherapy replaces one myth with a more functional and useful myth. Different schools of psychotherapy teach the patient to attend to slightly different aspects of their feelings and behavior. Most psychotherapies help patients. Absolute scientific and historical precision is not required to be helpful. The understanding only needs to be sufficient to tell the clinician and the patient what to do.

A common issue relevant to psychotherapy is "the meaning of illness." Some individuals are predisposed to search for and often find "meaning" in all important life experiences, including illnesses. Typically, efforts to give "meaning" to illness or other suffering involve plausible stories that may be independent of scientific validity. These stories or interpretations during psychotherapy frequently may seem to be helpful to the patient. It should be recognized clearly, however, that such meaning is quite different from what physicians have always understood by etiology or causation. It is important to realize that "meanings" can change over time and not be a misperception or distortion. For example, your graduation day from high school will have different meanings to you over the course of your life.

In some cases, referring to an illness as "a chemical imbalance" may be enough to motivate the patient to take helpful medicines without specifying the exact neurotransmitter, the exact brain site, the genetic allele(s) involved, and the time when the gene switched on or off. In others, "your blood pressure is too high" may be adequate to motivate changes in diet and exercise patterns and to accept appropriate medication. In other cases, the obstacles to change by the patient may require a more intensive, prolonged and affective-laden process. It is not unusual for this intensity to vary during the course of clinical management.

This model of the psychotherapeutic process applies well to most problems in medicine, psychiatry, and psychology. It allows both the clinician and the patient to tell whether or not they are working in a helpful manner or spinning their wheels.

Types of goals of psychotherapy

In medicine, treatment can be aimed at ameliorating, curing, or ending a disease process. Alternatively, it can be aimed at preventing or reducing the complications of a disease process. Finally, it can be used to reduce the burdens of life (psychological, social or medical) that will make management of the disease easier.

Affecting the disease process

In general, the pathophysiology of psychiatric disorders is not well enough understood to allow one to assess scientifically whether the underlying process has been affected. Clinically, there is dispute. The closest, in our opinion, to definitive evidence is the observation that naloxone administered one-half hour prior to behavior desensitization for phobias blocks the effect of the treatment. Unfortunately, blocking the opiate receptor does not tell one about the physiological cause (mechanism) for phobias any more than

the use of electroconvulsive therapy informs one about the pathophysiology of depression.

In our personal experience with treating depressed patients with cognitive-behavioral therapy, it seems clear that some patients learn that distraction from distressing thoughts helps. Others learn that antidepressant behaviors (do something) improve their mood. Only some seem to learn to identify cognitive distortions and the underlying attitudes they serve. Until the pathophysiology is understood and ascertainable, no one can say whether each of these different learnings use the same mechanisms in the brain.

Interestingly, this lack of knowledge about the pathophysiology of psychiatric diseases has led to the burgeoning of psychotherapy research on patients with medical disease because the effects of treatment on disease process can be evaluated. As examples, cognitive therapy in diabetes can be evaluated by examining glycosated hemoglobin levels and the outcome of treating depression can be assessed by measuring cardiac events.

Preventing and reducing complications

There is no doubt that psychotherapy can be used to educate the patient and to help them avoid some of the more serious complications of a specific syndrome, particularly if the complication is affected by patient behavior.

The burdens of life

Patients have problems beyond their illnesses and beyond problems with their clinical providers. Work, financial, marital, family, school, and other life problems can absorb their time and energy. It is well accepted that stress can exacerbate (but not usually cause) an existing medical or psychiatric problem. The caring physician, sensitive to the additional life burden imposed by such problems, can offer simple counsel or referral to appropriate sources of help for these non-medical problems. When patients do better, their illnesses frequently do better as well. When the physician offers wise counsel, the patient obtains relief from the problem and the relationship between clinician and patient is strengthened. However, this is a situation in which referral to non-medically trained counselors and professionals is most likely to be helpful to the patient and the physician simply because of the time and effort involved.

Two models of psychotherapy

Psychotherapy as rehabilitation

This concept of psychotherapy championed by our mentor and colleague, Samuel B. Guze, and others has been termed "rehabilitative psychotherapy" because it is based on certain fundamental principles in rehabilitation medicine. As in much of rehabilitation medicine, the focus is less on etiology and more on disability. In most treatment programs in rehabilitation medicine, the emphasis is not on how the injury or disability was caused, but on the nature and severity of the disability and on the individual's personality and temperament as these may affect the patient's energy, motivation, flexibility, and cooperation. Clearly, the approach to psychotherapy advocated here is similar. It is not primarily focused on etiology, which is still largely unknown in psychiatry and psychology, but is focused on helping the patient cope with disability, increasing self-confidence, and developing skill in achieving optimal solutions to clinical and life problems.

Psychotherapy as an investigative tool in psychiatry

Others in the field have different beliefs about psychotherapy and what it can tell us. Our colleague, Saul Rosenzweig, has pointed out cogently that some are interested in discovering the commonalities in psychiatric disorder; he called this the nomothetic approach. Others have been interested in discovering the unique aspects, internal logic and rules of each individual, regardless of their universality; he termed this the idiographic approach. This difference in interest explains to some degree much of the controversy in psychology and psychiatry about psychotherapy.

Freud believed and taught that the analytic method was a procedure capable of advancing the scientific understanding of personality and psychiatric disorder. With some modifications, many psychiatrists and psychologists believe this today. Since Freud and the advent of psychoanalysis, practitioners of psychotherapy in the "psychodynamic" tradition have been guided by the conviction that "dynamic" psychotherapy deals with unconscious psychological forces crystallized during early development. These are thought to be centrally responsible for much or for all psychopathology, which, according to this model, represents an adjustment or compromise between instinctive drives, personality needs, defenses, and the environment. Many would add the family genetic background to this mix. In other words, psychodynamic psychotherapy has been understood to be directed at identifying and correcting what are believed to be the mechanisms formed by the original etiological factors and leading to or maintaining the current psychiatric or psychological problems.

Thus, psychodynamic psychotherapy, in its varied permutations, reflects a set of related beliefs concerning the central causes of psychopathology. Crucial to these beliefs is the concept of defenses, particularly repression, emphasized by Freud. Repression in this context refers to the hypothesis of motivated unconscious forgetting. The presumption is that a fundamental psychological process exists in at least some humans for forgetting painful and frightening memories. It is argued that this unconscious process is called into action in order to protect the individual from the associated fear, guilt, other unacceptable emotion, or unwanted social consequences of fully experienced emotion. While the repression may leave the individual without any memory of the repressed experience, very often the repression is not entirely complete and the individual experiences a variety of psychopathological disturbances.

It must be understood, however, that very little evidence exists from systematic controlled studies to support the concept of repression except from the clinical reports of psychotherapists who accept the idea to begin with. The absence of credible scientific evidence for the existence of repression is not hard to understand. Currently, there is no way to determine the presence or absence of a memory, repressed or not. In addition, borrowing an analogy from the computer field, if one were able to detect that a memory existed, one would also have to be able to determine when the memory was first filed and whether or not it had been edited or censored.

The absence of satisfactory evidence in favor of the existence of dynamic repression does not prove that the hypothesis is invalid, but it does mean that a reasonable level of skepticism is called for in approaching the subject. The widespread epidemic in the United States of the often correlated phenomena of recovered memories of childhood sexual abuse, reports of satanic ritual abuse, multiple personality, and other so-called dissociative phenomena, all of which depend upon dynamic repression or dissociation as the central explanation, may attest to the consequences of uncritical acceptance of what remains an unproved and probably unprovable concept. Unfortunately, mental health always has popular and fad-like concepts, though many areas lack scientific support or verification.

Psychotherapy based on the belief that the causes of psychiatric disorders are to be found in the unconscious psychological residues of early development and experience can be characterized as etiology-directed. Such psychotherapy assumes that these psychological processes are to be recognized and confirmed by exploring free associations, dreams, symptoms, projective tests, and transference phenomena (the belief that the patient's reactions to the physician/therapist reflect unconscious tendencies to transfer repressed feelings and attitudes from childhood to a substitute for the patient's parents or other close relatives). Some modifications of traditional psychodynamic psychotherapy reflect efforts to shorten the process. These modifications (modern-day) focus on the assets or strengths the patient brings to the situation and try to increase coping ability, frustration tolerance, and the like. We would like to claim such modifications are closer to the rehabilitation model we espouse.

Assumptions that the causes of psychiatric disorder are well known and adequately understood are not confined to psychoanalytically oriented psychotherapists. One can easily find such over-confidence in some cognitive therapists, rational emotive therapists, and in biomedically oriented psychiatrists.

We believe it is crucial to recognize what we know and do not know. Non-etiologically based, "rehabilitation" psychotherapy is predicated on the belief that patients often can benefit from frank discussions with the physician/therapist about anything of importance to the patient. Many of us prefer the belief that the etiology of most psychiatric disorders is unknown or very imperfectly understood. We believe or hope that extensive genetic, epidemiologic, and neurobiologic research is beginning to point to potential causal factors.

Despite our lack of knowledge about the cause of psychiatric disorder, we believe that some psychotherapeutic strategies can be and often are helpful in treating a wide range of clinical problems. A number of psychotherapeutic approaches have been suggested and implemented that do not depend upon any as yet unproven theories of etiology. These approaches are based upon the goal of helping patients understand their disorders better and improve their abilities to cope more effectively with the consequences of their conditions and associated disability. Many psychotherapies based on inadequately proven causal theories also benefit patients. Fortunately, there are many problems which can be helped with proven effectiveness, even though the specific causes for the problem are not fully understood.

Psychotherapy need not be based upon any specific causal hypothesis to recognize and work with certain widely accepted assumptions about people in pain, in distress, fearful about their futures, or contemplating serious disability or early death. Nearly all such people can benefit from the opportunity to review, consider, and discuss what is happening to them with an individual whom they trust and in whom they place confidence. Such discussions should be meant to clarify patients' understanding of their conditions and situations, acknowledge and express their emotions and feelings, and explore various ways of coping better. Such discussions, properly carried out, often provide important emotional support, stimulate greater confidence in one's ability to manage optimally, and convey a sense that one is not entirely alone in dealing with the particular problems one is confronting.

Ideally, psychotherapy should be an integral part of the strategy for treating all such patients. In fact, all interaction with patients in all specialties should be carried out within a psychotherapeutic framework. Eliciting the initial history, continued elaboration of the history, repeated and ongoing evaluations of the patient's mental status, explaining the illness and the elements of the treatment, discussing possible complications and prognosis all offer rich opportunities for helpful psychotherapeutic intervention.

- The first task in a clinical undertaking is to understand, develop, and maintain a relationship with the patient. This is also true of psychotherapy.
- Good clinical care involves a lot of careful and attentive listening. This is also true of psychotherapy.
- The goal of clinical management is to help the patient understand as much as possible about the illness or other problems and about his way of interpreting and dealing with these problems. This is also true of psychotherapy.
- Psychotherapy can focus on the disability associated with an illness and other life problems. Helping the patient cope with disability, increase self-confidence, and develop skills in obtaining optimal solutions is central.
- Psychotherapy is frequently quite successful. Different therapists and different schools of therapy give the patients different models of the illness, its cause, and its cure. Although these models remain speculative, many share common elements and can be effective, however. There may be more commonalities between psychotherapies than actual differences.

Problematic practices related to psychotherapy

The widespread practice in some managed care systems of assigning responsibility for psychotherapy to another mental health professional, most frequently a social worker or counselor, appears to be derived from a number of assumptions, erroneous in our opinion, about psychotherapy. Instead of understanding psychotherapy as an integral part in treatment to be interwoven with the other elements of care, it is conceptualized as a separate and distinct therapeutic effort. This practice appears to be illogical. It separates the care of the patient into different realms: one for the consideration of physical phenomena and the other for psychological phenomena. Hardly any knowledgeable person considers such a division desirable or truly defensible.

In an optimally organized arrangement, many patients might require only a brief consultation with a physician and then be referred to a psychiatrist, psychologist, social worker, nurse, or other professional. Such patients might include those with marital problems, dissatisfaction at work, problems coping with parents, interpersonal conflicts, etc. In each case, the physician's initial responsibility would include ascertaining whether or not such problems were associated with recognizable psychiatric disorders. If the diagnosis was in doubt, consultation with a psychiatrist would certainly be justified. If such an association existed, the physician would consider the appropriateness of a psychiatrist following the patient personally rather than referring the patient to a non-psychiatric colleague.

Sometimes, even in the presence of a diagnosable psychiatric disorder, referral to a non-psychiatric colleague might be appropriate, especially if the psychiatrist concludes that medication is not indicated for that patient. In all cases, however, the physician should continue to monitor the patient's course and response to treatment. This might sometimes warrant another face-to-face encounter with the patient and even the patient's family.

Many people, including a large percentage of psychotherapists, think of psychotherapy as a specific form of treatment, akin to surgery or medication, to be administered by experts trained to carry out the arcane procedures. Psychotherapy is not recognized as appropriate and helpful primarily as part of a comprehensive and integrated approach to the care of certain patients. This is truly unfortunate. Recognizing and appreciating the need for an integrated approach to care at the level of the individual patient with a particular set of clinical problems is the key to effective psychotherapy.

Psychotherapy for patients with significant psychiatric illness should be part of an integrated clinical approach with a psychiatrist responsible for oversight of the entire intervention. Where a primary care physician has had appropriate training, the oversight might be that of the primary physician.

Summary

In 1992, SB Guze wrote:

> Psychotherapy can provide much needed emotional support, the chance to discuss and understand one's self better, an opportunity to consider the meaning of one's illness and related experiences, a safe and protected situation in which to explore various options and possibilities that take into consideration one's personal attributes and circumstances, and a special environment in which frustrations and anger may be freely expressed. The psychotherapeutic process can also lead to hypotheses about etiology, but it does not allow for the critical testing of such hypotheses. Psychotherapy offers no way to control for the preexisting assumptions of the therapist or the patient, nor for the effect on the patient's communications of the therapist's interpretations and suggestions. And, significantly, the psychotherapeutic process does not allow one to determine the causal relationships between phenomena of interest considered during psychotherapy and the patient's clinical problems. Nevertheless, psychotherapy, especially when based upon a rehabilitation strategy, is fully compatible with the medical model. Only those who believe that psychotherapy is the best path to identifying etiology are likely to object seriously to the basic arguments presented here.

Annotated bibliography

Guze, SB (1988) Psychotherapy and the etiology of psychiatric disorders, *Psychiatric Developments* 3:183–193.

Guze, SB and Murphy, GE (1963) An empirical approach to psychotherapy: the agnostic position, *American Journal of Psychiatry* 120:53–57.
The two articles listed above present a fuller consideration of the basis for considering psychotherapy a rehabilitative process.

Luborsky, L, Singer B, and Luborsky, L (1975) Comparative studies of psychotherapies. Is it true that "every one has won and all must have prizes"?, *Archives of General Psychiatry* 32: 995–1008.
When you look to the literature, there is evidence for every form of psychotherapy. Few studies are randomized trials and meta-analysis of this field can be misleading. Thus, "everyone" is a winner.

Spence, DP (1982) *Narrative Truth and Historical Truth*, New York, WW Norton & Company.
This is a clear discussion of the problems inherent in all psychotherapeutic interpretation.

CHAPTER 22

Pharmacotherapy

John G. Csernansky, MD

Introduction

Most of the major classes of psychotropic drugs used today were discovered through serendipity in the 1950s and 1960s. For example, the monoamine oxidase inhibitor antidepressants (MAOIs) were discovered when the "activating" effects of iproniazid, a prototype MAOI, were noticed in patients being treated for tuberculosis. Until recently, new members of each major psychotropic drug class were highly similar (that is, "me-too drugs"), developed by making slight modifications to the chemical structures of the original drugs. Too little was known about the underlying neurobiology of severe mental disorders to permit more innovative approaches to drug development.

Psychotropic drug development is now surging forward because of two new innovations. First, new drugs are being designed by targeting particular neurotransmitter receptors or other proteins (for example, monoamine transporters) that have been experimentally linked to the neurobiology of severe mental disorders. Second, an increasing number of neurotransmitter receptors and other proteins have been discovered by molecular biologists using cloning techniques, thereby providing new targets for drug action. In addition to these new approaches, psychotropic drugs continue to be discovered by empirical observation—for example, anticonvulsants for the treatment of patients with bipolar disorder. Thus, a variety of new drugs have become available for the treatment of patients with psychotic, affective, and anxiety disorders that are substantially different from the classic drugs developed in the 1950s and 1960s. These drugs include second-generation antipsychotic drugs (i.e., risperidone, olanzapine, quetiapine, ziprasidone, aripiprazole) for the treatment of schizophrenia; carbamazepine, sodium valproate, and other anticonvulsants for the treatment of bipolar disorder; fluoxetine, sertraline, paroxetine, and other second-generation antidepressants for the treatment of depression; and clomipramine and fluvoxamine for the treatment of obsessive-compulsive disorder (OCD). For the first time since the discovery of the original psychotropic drugs, physicians must choose from among drugs with substantive differences in efficacy and side effects to treat their patients.

In this chapter, the clinical characteristics of the major classes of psychotherapeutic drugs are reviewed and guidelines for drug use and for evaluating the scientific literature in this area are provided. Detailed discussions of the pharmacokinetics and pharmacodynamics of psychotherapeutic drugs can be found in other texts.

Major classes of psychotherapeutic drugs

Antidepressants

Contrary to some popular beliefs, antidepressant drugs are not stimulants. They only relieve symptoms of depression, that is, produce a mood-elevating effect, in patients with a mood disorder. In other individuals, they have no perceptible effects other than their side effects (such as sedation).

The efficacy of antidepressant drugs has been best demonstrated for individuals with major depressive disorder (MDD). The symptoms of MDD have been summarized in Chapter 8 and include low mood, hopelessness, guilt, suicidal thoughts, sleep changes, appetite and weight changes, and loss of sex drive. These symptoms usually remit during treatment; however, a delay of several weeks before symptom remission is expected. Among patients with MDD, approximately two-thirds respond to antidepressant drugs. MDD can be successfully treated with antidepressant drugs whether it occurs in patients with unipolar or bipolar mood disorder. Attempts have been made to treat other mood disorders with antidepressant drugs, but in these cases the efficacy of treatment is much less certain. These other disorders

325

TABLE 22.1

Antidepressant drugs

Drug (generic name)	Representative doses (mg/day)*	Half-life (hours)
Tricyclic antidepressants		
Amitriptyline (AMI)	75–200	30–46
Clomipramine	150–300	22–80
Desipramine (DMI)	75–200	14–40
Doxepin	75–300	8–24
Imipramine (IMI)	75–200	8–24
Nortriptyline (NTP)	75–150	18–80
Protriptyline	20–40	50–140
Serotonin reuptake inhibitors		
Citalopram	20–40	30–35
Fluoxetine	10–60	24–100
Fluvoxamine	100–300	12–18
Paroxetine	20–40	18–24
Sertraline	50–150	20–26
Venlafaxine**	75–375	8–12
Monoamine oxidase inhibitors		
Phenelzine	45–90	
Tranylcypromine	10–30	
Unusual structure or mechanism		
Bupropion	75–300	10–16
Mirtazapine	15–45	8–12
Nefazodone	300–600	2–4
Trazodone	150–600	4–8

* Specific information regarding medication titration, interactions, and use of plasma levels is available in pharmacology texts or in the manufacturers' information for physicians.

** Venlafaxine blocks both serotonin and norepinephrine uptake.

include minor depressive disorder, cyclothymia, and dysphoria associated with some personality disorders.

One can identify four major classes of antidepressant drugs (Table 22.1). Three of these classes include tricyclic antidepressants (TCAs) (including imipramine, amitriptyline, desipramine, and nortriptyline), MAOIs (phenelzine and tranylcypromine), and serotonin-selective reuptake inhibitors (SSRIs) (including fluoxetine, sertraline, paroxetine, and citalopram). Additionally, some individual drugs (trazodone, nefazodone, bupropion, and mirtazapine) remain difficult to classify into one of these three because they have unusual chemical structures and/or pharmacological mechanisms of action, and so may constitute a fourth class.

All four classes of drugs appear of equivalent efficacy, but are distinguishable by their side effects. The side effects of TCAs derive from the following three major mechanisms: (1)

muscarinic cholinergic receptor blockade, (2) $\alpha_1$adrenergic receptor blockade, and (3) quinidine-like effects on cardiac conduction. In the case of the anticholinergic effects of the TCAs, dry mouth, blurry vision, constipation, urinary hesitancy, and sedation are common and occur in a dose-dependent fashion. Blockage of α_1-adrenergic receptors can cause problematic hypotension, which can lead to fainting and falls. Finally, TCAs can slow conduction through the AV node and ventricles, increasing the possibility of ventricular (but rarely fatal) arrhythmias. MAOIs also commonly cause hypotension. However, when foods or other drugs containing tyramine or adrenergic agonists are consumed along with an MAOI, sudden and severe hypertension can occur (that is, hypertensive crisis).

People taking MAOIs also need to avoid agents that enhance the serotonergic system in order to prevent the development of a "serotonin syndrome." This syndrome can include restlessness, hyperreflexia, decreased coordination, shivering, and cardiovascular instability. Thus, there are many dietary and pharmacologic restrictions when MAOIs are used. The classic MAOIs are irreversible and nonselective with respect to the isoenzyme of monoamine oxidase inhibited. Interestingly, more recently developed MAOI drugs are either selective (for the monoamine-oxidase A isozyme) or fully reversible inhibitors of monoamine oxidase. At the time of this writing, however, such agents are not available in the United States. These selective MAOIs appear to have fewer and less severe side effects. The SSRIs are the best tolerated of all antidepressants, and they are surprisingly safe even in overdose. Their side effects include nausea, headache, insomnia, agitation, and sexual dysfunction (for example, delayed orgasm), attributable in all likelihood to their serotonin-enhancing actions.

Because of the highly favorable safety profile of SSRIs, they are usually the initial choice for the treatment of a patient with MDD and other mood disorders. However, when this class of drugs fails, drugs in the other three classes can and should be tried. There is no simple explanation for the approximate one-third of patients who do not respond to antidepressant drugs. In some cases, the dose of drug and duration of treatment have been inadequate. However, when this is not the explanation, there is usually no other that can be proven. The efficacy of antidepressant drugs has been variously enhanced by adding lithium or thyroid hormone. Finally, when trials of 2–3 different antidepressant drugs in more than one class have failed, electroconvulsive therapy (ECT) remains an invaluable option and should be considered (see Chapter 23).

The approach to drug development for the treatment of depression has thus far been focused on presynaptic mechanisms. That is, TCAs and SSRIs block the reuptake of biogenic amines (such as serotonin and norepinephrine) into the presynaptic terminals where they are ordinarily destroyed. In the case of the MAOIs, monoamine reuptake is not blocked, but metabolism of the amine by monoamine oxidase after reuptake into the presynaptic terminal is prevented, thus spilling the monoamine back out into the synaptic cleft. Additionally, chronic treatment with many of these drugs decreases the functioning of inhibitory presynaptic autoreceptors, which variously slow monoamine synthesis and release, as well as the firing rate of the cell. In all cases, the net effect of treatment appears to be an increase in the rate of monoamine transmission, and among the monoamines, changes in serotonin transmission appear to be most essential.

More recent antidepressant drugs target postsynaptic mechanisms. For example, some drugs (such as trazodone and nefazodone) are antagonists at postsynaptic serotonin $5HT_{2a}$ receptors. Mirtazapine is an agent that influences both presynaptic and postsynaptic mechanisms.

Anxiolytics

Benzodiazepines are the most commonly prescribed anxiolytic drugs in the United States (Table 22.2). They are far safer and less likely to cause physical tolerance than the barbiturates and meprobamate, which they have replaced. Benzodiazepines act by binding to specific sites on the γ-aminobutyric acid (GABA) receptor–chloride channel macromolecular complex and thereby enhance the actions of that inhibitory transmitter. These drugs have a variety of effects in addition to anxiolysis, including sedation, muscle relaxation, and seizure inhibition. From the point of view

of this chapter, these other actions may be considered side effects; however, benzodiazepines are used as hypnotics, muscle relaxants, and anticonvulsants in other settings.

Recently, drugs such as zolpidem and zaleplon have been developed. Although these agents are not structurally benzodiazepines, they bind to a specific subtype of the benzodiazepine-GABA receptor-chloride channel macromolecular complex. These agents have hypnotic properties but are not anxiolytics. Buspirone is an anxiolytic, but it is not a benzodiazepine. It does not influence the GABA system—rather it is a partial serotonin ($5HT_{1a}$) agonist. In distinction to the benzodiazepines that have acute effects, the anxiolytic effects of buspirone require several weeks of treatment.

Anxiety is experienced by all people. In some individuals, anxiety is transient, but it is of such severe intensity that treatment with a drug is indicated. In others, anxiety along with other symptoms becomes a chronic problem and necessitates treatment. DSM-IV lists a variety of such anxiety disorders, including generalized anxiety disorder (GAD) and panic disorder. However, anxiolytics are prescribed much more often for anxiety as a single symptom than for one of these DSM-IV anxiety disorders.

As mentioned earlier, sedation is a common side effect of the benzodiazepines. The fact that the degree of sedation varies among different anxiolytics has been exploited to promote the use of some drugs in this category as anxiolytics (drugs with little sedation) and some as hypnotics (drugs with more sedation). A serious drawback to the use of benzodiazepines is that physical tolerance can develop within even several days of regular use. Withdrawal syndromes have also been described, although they are usually mild and difficult to distinguish from the reemergence of the original symptoms of anxiety for which treatment was given. Tolerance and withdrawal phenomena have been more commonly described for drugs with half-lives of 8–12 hours (such as alprazolam and lorazepam) than for drugs with either shorter or longer half-lives. In rare cases, seizures and even delirium tremens have been described after stopping chronic benzodiazepine use. The possibility of tolerance and dependence should be considered when determining how long a patient should be prescribed these agents. In cases where the symptoms of a chronic anxiety disorder warrant long-term drug treatment, the use of buspirone (for GAD) or an antidepressant may be preferable.

Many people with situational anxiety (not necessarily associated with an anxiety disorder) may experience, even acutely, the anxiolytic effects of benzodiazepines. However, the response of patients with GAD, panic disorder, or obsessive-compulsive disorder (OCD) to drug therapy is less predictable. The reasons for lack of response in such patients are unknown.

Serotonergic mechanisms appear to play a role in the pathophysiology of anxiety and anxiety disorders. Therefore, research has been directed toward identifying new

TABLE 22.2 — Anxiolytic drugs

Drug (generic name)	Representative dose (mg/day)*	Half-life (hours)
Benzodiazepines		
Alprazolam	0.5–2.0	6–20
Chlordiazepoxide	10–75	10–30
Clonazepam	1–10	20–40
Clorazepate	15–60	50–80
Diazepam	2–20	15–60
Lorazepam	2–6	8–20
Oxazepam	20–60	6–20
Beta-blockers		
Atenolol	50–100	6–8
Metoprolol	100–200	2–4
Nadolol	40–80	15–20
Propranolol	40–80	2–6
Other		
Buspirone	20–60	2–4

* Specific information regarding medication titration and interactions is available in pharmacology texts or in the manufacturers' information for physicians.

drugs that act through serotoninergic mechanisms to relieve anxiety. Buspirone is a prototype drug in this class. Because of decreased concerns regarding tolerance and sedation, it may offer some advantages for the long-term treatment of anxiety disorders. The SSRIs, particularly fluoxetine, paroxetine, and fluvoxamine, are also being used for the treatment of panic disorder and OCD.

Finally, a word should be mentioned about the use of β-blockers in patients with anxiety disorders. These drugs are very effective in blocking the peripheral manifestations of anxiety, such as trembling, sweating, and tachycardia; however, they have no effects on more central symptoms, such as worry or dread. Thus, they can be useful for common forms of stage fright or social phobia, in which the person being treated is primarily concerned about others noticing their physical tension.

Antipsychotics

Until the discovery of antipsychotic drugs in the early 1950s, there were few effective treatments for psychotic illnesses. The one exception to this rule was ECT (see Chapter 23). During the 1960s and 1970s, a multitude of antipsychotic drugs were developed and marketed, all of which shared a common pharmacological action in that they blocked dopamine (D_2) receptors. Over the last several years, a second generation of antipsychotic drugs (including risperidone, olanzapine, quetiapine, ziprasidone, and aripiprazole) have been developed that have atypical mechanisms of action. These mechanisms of action include blockade of both serotonin and dopamine receptors or partial agonism at dopamine receptors.

Clozapine, which is a member of the new class of antipsychotic drugs, has been shown to be helpful in many patients who are treatment-resistant to first-generation antipsychotics. Its use is limited by significant side effects, including potentially severe leukopenia and occasional agranulocytosis. Regular monitoring of a patient's white cell count is required. Movement disorder side effects are uncommon with this agent, and its mechanism of action remains to be fully elucidated.

The second-generation antipsychotic drugs were originally referred to as atypical, because of their unusual mechanisms of action and the fact that they offered antipsychotic efficacy without extrapyramidal side effects (see below). However, because of their increased tolerability and efficacy, the use of these drugs has grown rapidly, and they now account for the large majority (>70%) of drug prescriptions in patients with psychotic disorders. Thus, it seems peculiar to still call them atypical. In fact, their use is typical, and so it seems more appropriate to refer to this class of drugs as second generation.

Antipsychotic drugs are used for the treatment of psychotic symptoms occurring in a variety of psychiatric dis-

TABLE 22.3

Antipsychotic drugs

Drugs (generic name)	Representative dose (mg/day)*	Half-life (hours)
Examples of first-generation agents		
Chlorpromazine	100–1000	20–40
Fluphenazine	2–20	20–40
Haloperidol	2–20	12–30
Perphenazine	8–64	20–40
Pimozide	2–6	50–80
Thiothixene	6–60	20–40
Trifluoperazine	4–20	20–40
Second-generation agents		
Aripiprazole**	10–30	48–96
Clozapine	300–900	6–30
Olanzapine	10–20	20–50
Quetiapine	300–800	5–10
Risperidone	2–8	2–8
Ziprasidone	40–160	5–10

* Specific information regarding medication titration, interactions, and use of plasma levels is available in pharmacology texts or in the manufacturers' information for physicians.

** Among second-generation drugs, aripiprazole has an unusual mechanism of action; that is, partial agonism at the dopamine D_2 receptor, antagonism at the $5HT_{2a}$ receptor and partial agonism at the $5HT_{1a}$ receptor.

orders (Table 22.3). The most common illness in this category is schizophrenia, and antipsychotic drugs are the mainstay of treatment for this often disabling condition (see Chapter 13). Some individuals develop complex delusions in the absence of other symptoms of schizophrenia; these individuals are classified as having delusional disorder. Patients with bipolar disorder often require the combination of both an antipsychotic drug and a mood stabilizer, especially when psychotic symptoms complicate the presentation of their illness (see Chapter 8). Patients with unipolar depression may also develop hallucinations and delusions that require the use of antipsychotic medications. Psychotic symptoms can occur after the use of hallucinogens or stimulants, and antipsychotic drugs are also useful in mitigating these temporary conditions. Examples of other illnesses in which antipsychotics may be considered include psychosis or severe agitation associated with delirium or certain dementias.

The side effects of the first-generation antipsychotic drugs can be divided into categories. First, neurological side effects typically occur as a result of dopamine D_2 receptor blockade in the nigrostriatal pathway and can include pseudoparkinsonism and dystonia. Akathisia, neuroleptic malignant syndrome, and tardive dyskinesia have also been linked to such unwanted dopamine receptor blockade. Second, a variety of side effects can occur as a result of the blockade of receptors for other neurotransmitters, such as acetylcholine (resulting in blurred vision, urinary hesitancy, constipation, and confusion), norepinephrine (orthostatic hypotension and sedation), and histamine (sedation, weight gain). First-generation antipsychotic drugs with high potency and relative selectivity for the D_2 receptor in relationship to other neurotransmitters (such as haloperidol, fluphenazine, and thiothixene) are available that have lower incidence of the second category of side effects. However, these drugs still cause neurological side effects in the majority of patients, so these drugs are only used when second-generation antipsychotic drugs have failed. Lower potency, first-generation antipsychotic drugs (for example, chlorpromazine and thioridazine) cause both neurological side effects and other side effects, such as sedation and orthostasis, calling into question the continuing use of such drugs.

Unfortunately, second-generation antipsychotic drugs still have unwanted side effects, although the neurologic side effects noted above are much less common. In fact, because of the propensity of these drugs to block neurotransmitter receptors other than the dopamine D_2 receptor, metabolic side effects are common. Blockade of $5HT_{2c}$ receptors and histamine H_1 receptors has been linked to weight gain and illnesses, such as heart disease and diabetes, that are commonly associated with weight gain. The influence of some of these agents on weight gain and glucose homeostasis can be substantial, and patient monitoring is appropriate. Blockade of noradrenergic α_1 receptors can still occur with these drugs and has been linked to falls. Finally, although blockade of $5HT_{2a}$ receptors appears to mitigate the neurological side effects of the second-generation antipsychotic drugs, this action does not mitigate the ability of some of these drugs to block dopamine D_2 receptors in the tubero-infundibular pathway and increase serum prolactin concentrations. Recently, increasing concern has developed about prolactin elevation induced by antipsychotic drugs, because of the link between this effect and loss of sexual interest. Aripiprazole is unusual among the second-generation antipsychotic drugs because it is a partial agonist at the dopamine D_2 receptor as well as an antagonist at the $5HT_{2a}$ receptor. Evidence from clinical trials suggests that this drug retains sufficient ability to block excess dopamine transmission so that it is an effective antipsychotic drug, but does not cause the complete D_2 receptor blockade linked to increases in prolactin levels. Further, because this drug is devoid of $5HT_{2c}$ and H_1 blockade, weight gain appears to be minimal.

Today, 30–40% of patients with chronic schizophrenia still do not respond adequately to antipsychotic drug treatment. This rate of nonresponse may be lower (approximately 20%) among schizophrenic patients in their first episode. There is no clear explanation as to why patients with apparently similar clinical presentations respond differently; differences in neurobiological parameters are presumed but unproven. Of the patients with schizophrenia who are refractory to antipsychotic drugs, 30–50% respond to the atypical drug clozapine. Although the more widespread use of clozapine is limited by its propensity to cause leukopenia, the availability of this drug is critical for this minority of patients.

Many patients with schizophrenia fail to take their antipsychotic drugs as prescribed, sometimes because of drug side effects, but often because they lack insight into their illness and the need for treatment. For these patients, long-acting, injectable formulations of antipsychotic drugs can be very helpful. Such formulations of the first-generation drugs haloperidol and fluphenazine were produced by linking the drug to a long chain fatty acid (decanoic acid) through an ester bond. Such decanoate preparations are administered by intramuscular injection (where endogenous esterase enzymes gradually release the drug) and have durations of action of 2–4 weeks. Risperidone also is now available in a long-acting, injectable formulation, although in this case the drug will be suspended in a synthetic polymer, which is slowly degraded by the body after injection. Risperidone in this formulation has a duration of action of two weeks.

Efforts at further antipsychotic drug development are being focused on developing drugs with yet other mechanisms of action. A variety of hypothetical mechanisms of action are being investigated, such as blockade of dopamine receptors other than D_2 (i.e., D_3 and D_4), blockade of serotonin receptors other than $5HT_{2a}$ (i.e., $5HT_6$ and $5HT_7$), stimulation of muscarinic M_1 receptors, and blockade of peptide receptors, such as receptors for neurotensin and neurokinin. The goal of such research is the successful treatment of a higher proportion of patients with schizophrenia and other psychotic disorders. However, the realization of this goal may occur only when there is a thorough understanding of the pathophysiology of schizophrenia and the particular neural circuits involved, as well as their component neurotransmitter receptor targets.

Mood stabilizers

The first mood stabilizer was hardly a drug at all but an ion. Lithium's antimanic effect was discovered in 1949 by John Cade, an Australian psychiatrist. Cade, studying toxic substances in the urine of patients with bipolar disorder, administered combinations of urea and uric acid (the latter substance was thought to be protective) to rodents and noticed a calming action of the uric acid. This was in all likelihood a result of the fact that he had given the uric acid as its most soluble salt, lithium urate. This observation led Cade to discover the calming effects of lithium carbonate (which was less toxic than lithium urate). He subsequently administered lithium to patients with bipolar illness. His choice of dose (600 mg, three times per day) was highly fortuitous; all ten of his first patients improved dramatically.

TABLE 22.4

Mood-stabilizing drugs

Drug (generic name)	Representative doses (mg/day)*	Recommended blood level (as noted)	Half-life (hours)
Lithium preparations			
Lithium carbonate	900–1800	0.6–1.2 mEq/L	20–24
Lithium citrate	900–1800	0.6–1.2 mEq/L	20–24
Anticonvulsants			
Carbamazepine	600–1200	6–12 µg/ml	30–36
Clonazepam	2–5		20–40
Lamotrigine	100–200		15–60
Sodium valproate	1000–2000	30–100 µg/ml	10–20

* Specific information regarding medication titration, interactions, and use of plasma levels is available in pharmacology texts or in the manufacturers' information for physicians.

Lithium salts and anticonvulsants are two classes of mood stabilizers (Table 22.4). Lithium carbonate can be administered in a slow-release preparation administered twice daily (lithobid) or in several regular preparations. Lithium citrate is available as a liquid, and it can be used when compliance with lithium carbonate capsules is in question. At least three anticonvulsants are now known to have mood-stabilizing properties. The first discovered was carbamazepine, and clinical trials have demonstrated the efficacy of this compound in acute mania and depression, as well as in prophylaxis against episodes of bipolar disorder. Evidence is now available to show that sodium valproate is similarly effective. More recently, lamotrigine has been shown to have mood-stabilizing properties.

The dosing of lithium carbonate and lithium citrate must be carefully guided by monitoring blood levels. Serum concentrations of 0.6 to 1.2 mEq/L are usually optimal. Blood levels are also readily obtainable for both carbamazepine and sodium valproate and can be used to guide dosing. However, there is no evidence that optimal efficacy is achieved for the treatment of bipolar disorder using blood level ranges developed for the treatment of seizures. Blood level monitoring is useful for avoiding toxicity and monitoring compliance.

As alluded to earlier, mood-stabilizing drugs are useful for the treatment of manic episodes and may be useful for reducing the risks of future episodes of mania. Lithium may be helpful in lowering the long-term risk of suicide. Mood-stabilizing drugs are also effective, although somewhat less so than antidepressants, in treating episodes of bipolar depression. However, when used for the treatment of bipolar depression, they are not likely to precipitate a "switch" of the patient from depression to mania. Characteristics that may identify those patients with bipolar disorder who are most effectively treated with anticonvulsants rather than lithium include rapid cycling and a negative family history for bipolar disorder.

Another class of agents that may be helpful in treating manic or mixed episodes is the second-generation antipsychotic drugs. The hypothetical mechanism of action for these drugs is that blockade of dopamine D_2 receptors would be beneficial for reducing manic symptoms, while blockade of $5HT_{2a}$ receptors would be beneficial for reducing (or preventing the development of) depressive symptoms. However, long-term studies clearly demonstrating the prophylactic properties of monotherapy with second-generation antipsychotic drugs are still needed before clinicians can consider such treatment as a substitute for more classic mood stabilizers, such as lithium and the anticonvulsants. Also, risks of long-term treatment with the various categories of agents need to be considered.

Mood-stabilizing drugs have also been proposed as treatments for other psychiatric disorders that have a cyclical or oscillating character, such as cyclothymic disorder and intermittent explosive disorder. However, firm evidence from controlled clinical trials demonstrating efficacy in these situations is lacking. Mood-stabilizing drugs have also been suggested as adjunctive treatments to antipsychotic drugs for the treatment of refractory cases of psychoses, such as schizophrenia disorder. However, evidence from controlled trials remains inconclusive in this situation, also.

The common side effects of lithium include nausea, diarrhea, tremor, lethargy, polyuria, and weight gain. Reversing initial concerns, the drug is now known to be relatively free of cardiovascular side effects. T-wave flattening or inversion is a common, but usually benign, side effect. Lithium should not be given to patients with sick sinus syndrome, because it can aggravate the bradycardia associated with this syndrome and occasionally precipitate cardiac arrest. Since lithium inhibits the release of thyroid hormone (T_4), it may cause hypothyroidism and goiter. However, such side effects do not always require that treatment with lithium be stopped. Rather, thyroid hormone can be given. There remains concern regarding the chronic effects of lithium on renal function, in particular the development of interstitial nephritis, which might lead to irreversible decreases in creatinine clearance. Although this side effect appears to be much rarer than originally thought, renal function should still be monitored. Lithium is also known to cause severe fetal cardiovascular abnormalities, particularly when given during the first trimester of pregnancy.

In overdose, lithium can be lethal. Delirium, followed by coma, cardiovascular collapse, and death is the usual progression. Monitoring lithium serum concentrations as the sole guide to treatment during overdose can be dangerous, since the serum concentrations may change rapidly and unpredictably and may not always faithfully reflect tissue levels of the drug. Clinical judgment and careful examination are an essential accompaniment to blood level monitoring. Lithium overdose can be rapidly reversed with renal dialysis.

The common side effects of anticonvulsants include sedation, nausea, weakness, ataxia, diplopia, and nystagmus. These side effects are dose-dependent and can be mitigated by dose reduction. Carbamazepine is also well known to cause leukopenia. Although this rarely leads to agranulocytosis, blood counts should be monitored during carbamazepine treatment, particularly during the first six weeks. Sodium valproate lacks many of the side effects of carbamazepine. However, sedation and increases in liver enzymes are common. Certain anticonvulsants, including carbamazepine and sodium valproate, can cause cranial-facial birth defects and therefore should be avoided in pregnant patients. Lamotrigine has been associated with the Stevens-Johnson syndrome, which can be fatal. Guidelines suggest starting this agent at a low dose and increasing the dose only gradually.

Lithium is effective in treating approximately 70% of manic episodes but only 50–60% of depressive episodes in patients with bipolar disorder. Lithium's efficacy as a prophylactic treatment in patients with bipolar disorder lies approximately midway between these two estimates. The rates of success for treating the various aspects of bipolar disorder with anticonvulsants are less well defined, but they appear to be approximately the same as for lithium. When one mood-stabilizing drug has failed in treating a patient with bipolar disorder, others should be tried. Additionally, lithium and an anticonvulsant can be used together, and in some cases this combination has resulted in increased efficacy. For patients with bipolar disorder who are refractory to these mood-stabilizing drugs, ECT is also indicated (see Chapter 23).

A larger arsenal of mood-stabilizing drugs would be desirable. When lithium was first discovered to be effective as a mood-stabilizing drug, other ions were explored also, but were not found to be effective. Current efforts in drug development have focused on testing the efficacy of newly developed anticonvulsant drugs. However, these efforts have not been uniformly successful (i.e., not all anticonvulsant drugs have mood-stabilizing properties), perhaps because they have not been based on a clear understanding of the pathophysiology of bipolar disorder, or in some cases, the mechanism of action of the anticonvulsant drug.

Phases of treatment

Most psychiatric illnesses are lifelong, and none of the drugs available to treat them is curative. Whereas past efforts to treat psychiatric disorders have emphasized the treatment of acute episodes, current efforts are directed more toward preventing episodes of illness.

There are two important rationales for this change in emphasis. First, if the acute episodes of illness can be prevented, the costs of inpatient hospitalization needed to treat those episodes can be avoided. Second, evidence is accumulating that episodes of certain illnesses, such as schizophrenia, may unleash "toxic" processes that worsen the prognosis and undermine the capacity for subsequent treatment response.

Treatment of acute episodes of illness

Most patients begin treatment for psychiatric illness in the midst of an acute episode. In this situation, there is almost always a sense of urgency among the patient's family and friends. Initial treatment for an acute episode of psychosis, mania, or depression is often undertaken in an emergency room or hospital. Rapid initiation of treatment is necessary because of the patient's agitation, the family's concern, and institutional pressures to reduce the duration of hospitalization. Unfortunately, most drug treatments for psychiatric illness do not have immediate effects.

Antipsychotic drugs are effective within a few days for some patients, but in the majority, clinical response develops gradually over 2–4 weeks. Increasing the dose of antipsychotic drug has not been shown to speed up this process, suggesting that the clinical response to antipsychotic drugs depends on intrinsic brain mechanisms with fixed latencies. The clinical response to antidepressant drugs also develops gradually, usually within 2–3 weeks. In some patients, even longer periods are required. Therefore, the physician should not conclude that a depressed patient cannot respond to an antidepressant until treatment has been under way for at least six weeks at therapeutic doses. In the case of mood stabilizers, including lithium and mood-stabilizing anticonvulsants, there are also latencies in response, usually on the order of 1–2 weeks. A drug group for which there is no latency before a clinical response is the group of benzodiazepine anxiolytics. In this case the response is immediate. It is useful to teach patients and caregivers about latencies of response.

The fact that most patients respond to psychotropic drugs

after a latency period is at odds with the need most physicians feel to treat acute episodes of psychiatric illness quickly. As mentioned above, increasing the dose of a drug does not shorten the latency. The dose ranges for most psychotropic drugs are listed in Tables 22.1 through 22.4. Additionally for certain drugs, obtaining serum or plasma levels can assist in achieving an optimal dose. Lithium offers the best example for this practice because its therapeutic serum level range has been clearly established (see Table 22.4). Among antipsychotic drugs, haloperidol blood levels are most interpretable because they have been well studied and haloperidol has few active metabolites, which can render blood level monitoring of the parent drug meaningless. Among antidepressant drugs, monitoring blood levels of nortriptyline has been best validated. Research to determine valid blood level ranges for other psychotropic drugs continues.

Using higher-than-optimal drug doses during the treatment of acute episodes of psychiatric illness is inadvisable for several reasons. First, unnecessary side effects that complicate treatment can occur. Second, the patient may be less likely to comply with long-term treatment with any drug given in excess. Third, the costs of newer drugs (for example, SSRIs and second-generation antipsychotic drugs) can be substantial and excess dosing can be a financial burden to the patient, the caregiver, and the system of care. In some cases of depression, mania, and particular types of schizophrenic psychosis (that is, catatonic schizophrenia), ECT may work more quickly than treatment with a psychotropic drug. However, the use of ECT as a first therapy in such cases is still considered unusual.

Continuation treatment

Continuation treatment is defined as drug treatment after the acute response to treatment has occurred but before the underlying episode has concluded. The period of continuation treatment may vary, but it almost always consists of weeks to months. Despite the fact that changes in symptoms may be few during continuation treatment, it is almost always necessary to sustain the initial efficacy of drug treatment.

Continuation treatment should not be confused with maintenance treatment (see the following section). An indicator of interrupting continuation treatment (that is, before the underlying episode of illness is over) is immediate relapse. In contrast, relapse during the maintenance phase of treatment often occurs weeks to months after drug treatment has stopped. As drug treatments for psychiatric illness have become less troubled by side effects, there is little reason for interrupting treatment during the continuation phase. Such interruptions are most often done by patients themselves and usually lead to relapse and rehospitalization.

Maintenance treatment

Increasing emphasis is being placed on maintenance treatment of psychiatric illness. Although it is simple to undertake, patients and sometimes their families may not understand the critical need for it. It is essential that patients with unipolar and bipolar mood disorders, schizophrenia, and other serious mental disorders understand that the illness is not resolved with conclusion of the first acute episode. These illnesses may be lifelong, with episodes of illness interspersed with periods of wellness. As noted, many patients do not regain their original "baseline" after an acute episode of psychiatric illness. Therefore, the prevention of such episodes should be a major goal for the management of psychiatric disorders.

In almost all cases, the same drug is used for acute and maintenance treatment. As described above, acute treatment and maintenance treatment are bridged by the continuation phase. Clinical experts, at one time, recommended that lower drug doses be used during the maintenance phases of treatment of depression and psychosis. However, this advice has become obsolete for two principal reasons. First, it is often possible to achieve optimal doses of psychotropic drugs during acute treatment through the use of blood-level monitoring and structured treatment protocols. Second, more recently developed psychotropic drugs tend to have fewer side effects and are better tolerated without the need for repeated dose adjustments. Today, maintenance treatment of depression, mania, and psychosis should be performed with the same drug at the same dose that was used to successfully treat the acute episode. However, when several categories of drugs are used to help during the earlier phases of treatment, it may be possible to eventually simplify the treatment regimen.

Often, maintenance treatment is continued for an indefinite time. In patients with schizophrenia or bipolar disorder, this is usually the rule. In patients with unipolar depression, indefinite treatment with antidepressant drugs is becoming more common.

General guidelines for use of psychotropic drugs

The ideal psychotropic drug has the following characteristics: (1) it acts directly and specifically on pathogenic mechanisms; (2) it benefits all patients with the indicated disorder; (3) it acts immediately; (4) it does not cause tolerance or dependence; (5) it is not toxic at therapeutic doses or after overdose; and (6) it has no side effects. Of course, no current drug meets these criteria, and for that reason, using clinical judgment to choose among a number of imperfect drug options remains an essential ingredient of practice. To optimally use the psychotropic drugs available today, the following guidelines are suggested (see *Pearls & Perils*).

Guidelines for drug therapy

- Before prescribing a psychotropic drug, the physician should establish the patient's diagnosis with certainty.
- The physician should develop a sequence of treatment options in decreasing order of predicted value.
- One psychotropic drug variable should be changed at a time.
- The physician should allow for time-dependent clinical effects.
- The minimum effective dose of the psychotropic drug should be given.
- The physician should rely on the results of controlled clinical trials to guide practice.

Example of a drug treatment algorithm

1 Diagnosis of an outpatient with major depression. No prior history of treatment.
2 Treatment with an SSRI for four weeks (e.g. paroxetine, 20 mg/day).
3 If the patient has no response and no intolerable side effects, increased dose for four additional weeks (paroxetine, 40 mg/day).
4 If no response, consideration of alternate drug or augmentation of the initial drug (for example with lithium). Continued treatment for an additional four weeks.
5 If no response, consider cessation of drug treatment, and initiation of ECT.

Special note: options for drug treatment should be discussed in an open interchange with the patient, and if appropriate, their family. When choosing among some options (see step 4), there may not be clearly superior alternatives. In such cases, it is often wise to follow the patient's wishes. In this way, compliance later in treatment can be enhanced. Also, ECT may become the best treatment option at any point in treatment if symptoms become acutely severe or if suicidal ideation becomes intense and rapid response is wanted.

First, the patient's diagnosis should be established with as much certainty as possible. In this way, the physician can relate choices among treatment options to literature findings, and the patient's chances of responding to the first drug chosen are optimized. Second, the physician should develop a sequence of treatment options (Box 22.1). None of the drug treatments available works in all patients. Therefore, a physician usually prescribes one drug after another in a trial-and-error fashion. When the physician faces this possibility from the outset of treatment, the trials can proceed more smoothly and without hesitation. Third, only one variable at a time should be changed. When searching for an optimal treatment, the physician can vary one or another drug and the dose of each drug. Although the desire to speed treatment may tempt a physician to change more than one of these parameters at a time, confusion usually follows from this practice. Additionally, even if the physician does find a regimen that works, the physician would not know which of the drugs produced the desired therapeutic effect. In this way, the patient can become committed to continuation and maintenance treatment with unnecessary drugs. Fourth, it is important to allow for time-dependent clinical effects. Keeping in mind that almost all psychotropic drugs act gradually over time, the patient and the physician must have patience and resist pressure from various sources to rush the process of therapeutic decision making. Fifth, the minimum effective dose should be used. Higher-than-optimal doses are likely to be associated with avoidable side effects, and opportunities for downward dose titration during continuation and maintenance treatment are rarely realized. Blood-level monitoring can assist in this endeavor in some cases. Sixth, the physician should rely on the results of controlled clinical trials whenever they are available. While one's own clinical experience can be invaluable, apparently compelling anecdotes can be misleading. Such anecdotes should not be the basis for routine practice; rather, they should point the way for designing future controlled trials.

Development of new psychotherapeutic drugs

Clinical anecdotes and ideas

The development of new psychotropic drugs often is a result of astute clinical observation. Such observation may occur when a drug is used in groups of patients for which it was not originally intended or when symptoms other than those originally targeted in the intended group appear to respond. Whatever the situation, the idea for a new drug treatment develops. However, single anecdotes are rarely sufficient reason to launch a clinical trial. The physician or researcher usually collects reports of similar cases to show that the new treatment is plausible and safe. The value of collecting and reporting such case series should not be underestimated. In the absence of a fundamental understanding of the pathophysiology of most psychiatric disorders, such reports can be the source of important new approaches to treatment.

Toxicity and pharmacokinetic trials

The first hurdle in the clinical development of a new drug is testing for toxicity. Although toxicity can be tested in a variety of animal species before the new drug is given to humans, only humans can report on the subjective mental effects of a drug. This phase of drug development, called phase I, is almost always carried out with volunteers who do not have psychiatric illness. Such trials are small, involving a few dozen subjects, and usually are designed to study the pharmacokinetics of the drug as well.

Preliminary clinical trials

The goals of the first clinical trials in patients, called phase II, are to evaluate efficacy and to detect unintended side effects. Patients with psychiatric disorders often are more or less sensitive to the sedation, dysphoria, or agitation caused by a psychotropic drug. Therefore, these side effects are often difficult to detect in volunteers without psychiatric illness. Early clinical trials are often either uncontrolled or placebo controlled, but not double blinded. In this way, only a preliminary estimation of the degree and type of efficacy can be made. Information about doses and latencies required for efficacy is also collected at this time, so that it can be used in the design of subsequent larger trials. Phase II trials usually involve relatively small numbers of subjects, perhaps 100 or so. Few definite conclusions about the potential for a new drug should be drawn at this stage.

Controlled clinical trials

Controlled clinical trials, called phase III trials, are the mainstay of drug development. Usually the Food and Drug Administration (FDA) requires two phase III controlled clinical trials called pivotal studies; in each one the new drug is compared with a different existing drug for the indication. Whether an additional comparison with placebo is necessary varies for each new psychotropic drug. Since an existing drug may show only minimal efficacy in a controlled trial, the degree of efficacy of the new drug may not be properly evaluated when a placebo control is omitted. However, treatment of serious psychiatric disorders with placebo, particularly for an extended time, runs counter to current treatment recommendations and may be unethical. Nonetheless, the theoretically ideal controlled trial compares the new drug with an existing drug and placebo simultaneously. In this way, both the absolute and relative efficacy of the new drug can be definitely tested. The results of such a trial are the firmest foundation for routine clinical practice.

Conclusion

It is difficult to overstate the importance of psychotropic drugs for patients with psychiatric disorders. The treatment of disorders such as schizophrenia and bipolar disorder was largely a disappointment before the discovery of such drugs. Today we have effective drugs for depression, anxiety, mania, and schizophrenia. There is hope that many patients with even the most severe disorders, such as schizophrenia and bipolar disorder, can lead relatively normal lives. The discovery of such drugs has also had a profound effect on our thinking about psychiatric illness. Before their discovery there were few clues to help physicians understand the pathophysiology of psychiatric disorders. Today, most theories about the neurobiology of psychiatric disorders have been developed at least in part by reasoning backward from the discovered pharmacological effects of effective psychotropic drugs. Hopefully, in the future, this process will be reversed and advances in our understanding of the etiology and pathogenesis of psychiatric disorders will drive new drug development.

Annotated bibliography

Davis, KL, Charney, D, Coyle, JT, and Nemeroff, C (eds) (2002) *Neuropsychopharmacology: The Fifth Generation of Progress*, New York, Raven Press.
This large reference text provides an exhaustive compilation of reviews on the neurobiology of psychiatric disorders and the molecular mechanisms of psychotropic drug actions. Additionally, the use of each of the major classes of psychotropic drugs in the acute, continuation, and maintenance settings is reviewed. There are also selected chapters on new drug design and development and methodology of controlled clinical trials.

Goodman, LS, Gilman, AG, Gilman, AG, Limbird, LE, and Hardman, JG (eds) (2001) *Goodman and Gilman's The Pharmacological Basis of Therapeutics*, 10th Edition, New York, Pergamon Press.
This book contains comprehensive information about the pharmacokinetics and pharmacodynamics of psychotropic drugs. Up-to-date guidelines regarding indications, dosing, and side effects can also be found.

Stahl, SM (ed.) (2000) *Essential Psychopharmacology*, 2nd Edition, Cambridge, Cambridge University Press.
This book is a concise, readable text that reviews the pharmacology and clinical uses of all major classes of psychotropic drugs. The illustrations are especially clear and informative. In addition, there is a CD-ROM version that features animated illustrations, which help to make the principles of synaptic function and other elements of neuropharmacology easy to understand.

CHAPTER 23

Electroconvulsive Therapy

Charles F. Zorumski, MD and Keith E. Isenberg, MD

Introduction

Psychotropic medications are the first-line treatment for most patients with mood and psychotic disorders. However, a significant minority of these individuals is either medication resistant or intolerant of medication side effects. Other patients have severe, life-threatening symptoms requiring interventions that act more rapidly than medications. These symptoms include suicidal intent, starvation, severe agitation, and exhaustion. For patients with refractory or severe symptoms, electroconvulsive therapy (ECT) can be a safe and effective alternative to psychotropic medications. This chapter will discuss the use of ECT in the management of psychiatric disorders, with emphasis on the use of ECT in patients with coexisting medical illnesses. Interest in providing treatment alternatives for patients with psychiatric symptoms unresponsive to current approaches is encouraging the development of new procedures/devices such as magnetic stimulation of the brain, briefly described at the end of the chapter.

Historical background

The use of convulsive treatments for psychiatric disorders dates to Meduna, a Hungarian psychiatrist, in the 1930s. Based on a perceived "biological antagonism" between epilepsy and schizophrenia, Meduna reasoned that induced seizures would have clinical benefit. This led him to examine the effects of camphor and pentylenetetrazole injections as ways to induce seizures in schizophrenic patients.

Meduna's initial observations suggested improvement in about half the subjects treated. There were significant problems associated with the chemoconvulsants, including discomfort and poor reliability in producing seizures. This prompted a search for more effective and better tolerated ways to induce therapeutic convulsions. In 1938, Cerletti and Bini administered the first electrically induced therapeutic seizures in humans. Their initial patient was a 39-year-old man with acute psychosis, incomprehensible speech, and periodic mutism, who had previously responded well to pentylenetetrazol seizures. The patient received a series of 11 electrical treatments and demonstrated marked clinical improvement. These observations served as proof of a concept that electrical stimulation could serve as a relatively simple, safe, and effective way to induce seizures in humans. In the early days, ECT was administered without anesthesia. This resulted in substantial discomfort and was associated with numerous complications including fractures, soft tissue injuries, and hypoxia. ECT technique has evolved greatly since that time and now routinely includes the use of general anesthetics, muscle relaxants, and brief pulse electrical stimulators. These innovations maintain the benefits of electrically induced seizures while greatly diminishing side effects. Presently, ECT is used to treat a variety of neuropsychiatric disorders and has its greatest utility in managing severe mood disorders and acute psychosis.

Indications for ECT

Major depression

Severe major depression is the most common psychiatric disorder treated with ECT. However, advances in psychopharmacology have resulted in ECT being considered a second- or third-line treatment for most patients (Fig. 23.1). Presently, ECT is most commonly used in patients with

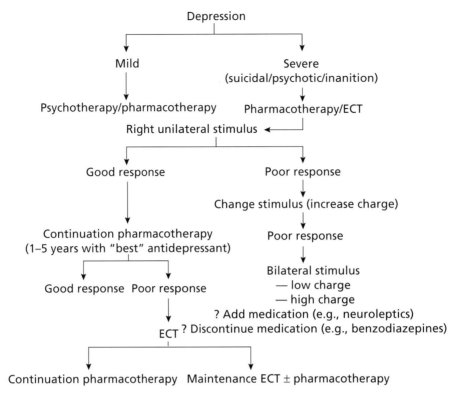

Fig. 23.1 Use of ECT in the treatment of depression. ECT is usually administered to severely depressed patients as indicated by suicidality, psychosis, or severe disability; most patients will have failed multiple trials of pharmacotherapy and psychotherapy. A non-dominant (right-hemisphere) unilateral stimulus using an electrical charge that is at least 2.5 times the seizure threshold is usually the treatment of first choice. For patients with a poor response to non-dominant hemisphere ECT, options include increasing the electrical charge or switching to low-charge (minimally suprathreshold) bilateral ECT. Failure to respond to low-charge bilateral ECT should be followed by high-charge bilateral treatments. Following a successful course of ECT, continuation therapy with an antidepressant medication diminishes the risk of relapse. Patients who subsequently relapse are candidates for maintenance ECT.

depression who have failed to respond to one or more "adequate" trials of antidepressant medications. The definition of "adequate" antidepressant medication trial varies greatly, but generally it refers to a 4–6-week trial at therapeutic doses. It is not uncommon for patients to have failed two or more trials of antidepressants before referral for ECT. This raises the question whether patients who are non-responsive to medications have diminished responses to any treatment, including ECT. Several studies have demonstrated a favorable response to ECT in medication-non-responders with significant improvement in depressive symptoms in about 50% of patients, depending on the criteria used to rate improvement. Thus, medication non-response does not necessarily predict ECT non-response, and failure to respond to one or more trials of antidepressant therapy is an indication for the primary care physician or psychotherapist to make a referral to a psychiatrist with expertise in ECT.

There are several categories of depressed patients for whom ECT could be considered a first-line treatment. These include patients with prior history of medication non-response who have previously responded to ECT. In such patients, repeated trials of medications are often unhelpful. It is not unusual for patients who have had a good response to a prior course of ECT to request this form of treatment if they relapse. A second group of depressed patients for whom ECT should be considered early are those who develop psychotic symptoms (delusions and hallucinations). Psychotic depression can be difficult to treat with psychotropic medications and usually requires combined administration of antipsychotic and antidepressant medications. Patients with psychotic depression generally have a favorable response to ECT.

An unfortunate aspect of most antidepressant medications is that therapeutic responses can be delayed for weeks. Thus, an adequate medication trial takes 4–6 weeks at appropriate doses. Because of this delay, patients with life-threatening symptoms are sometimes referred for ECT early in an episode. These include patients with severe suicidal ideation (particularly after a recent psychologically or medically serious suicide attempt) or refusal to eat and evidence of starvation. In these individuals delays in treatment response could place the patient at significant risk. Assessment by the primary care physician or therapist can help to establish the presence of severe depression in these patients as well as assist the psychiatrist with the management of concurrent medical complications that are common in severely ill individuals.

While there are no absolute predictors of patients who will have a good response to ECT, clinical experience suggests that the more "endogenous" symptoms a depressed patient has, the more likely the patient is to respond to ECT. These features include marked psychomotor retardation or agitation, sleep disturbances with early morning awakening, poor appetite with weight loss, and diurnal variation of symptoms with worsening in the morning. Such patients, particularly if they have not previously failed a trial of antidepressant medications, can have response rates of 80% or greater to ECT, making ECT one of the most effective forms of treatment available. Some patients (~10%) show a partial response to ECT, and even individuals who fail to respond to ECT may benefit from subsequent treatment with antidepressants.

There are some depressed patients for whom ECT may be less useful. These include those who develop depression in the context of somatization disorder and possibly obsessive-compulsive disorder. Additionally, patients with dysthymia, a chronic (at least two-year) form of depression in which symptoms do not meet criteria for a major depressive episode, may have a less favorable outcome with ECT. However, periodic episodes of major depression arising in the context of dysthymia may respond well to ECT. In patients with dysthymia, a major difficulty arises when judging ECT response relative to the patient's baseline mood state. Regardless of depression subtype, some patients opt to receive ECT when presented with the fact that ECT is a highly effective treatment capable of achieving rapid results.

Mania

ECT is generally considered a second- or third-line treatment for acute episodes of mania. This is based on the fact that most patients with acute mania respond well to mood-stabilizing medications (e.g. lithium, valproic acid, and lamotrigine) with or without antipsychotic medications. Nonetheless, ECT can be effective in the management of mania in patients who demonstrate a poor response to mood stabilizers or who cannot tolerate medication side effects. As in patients with major depression, patients with severe symptoms, including marked agitation, assaultiveness, and exhaustion, may be candidates for early intervention with ECT, although there is little systematic evidence that these patients respond better to ECT than to psychotropic medications. Some data suggest that about 80% of patients with acute mania respond favorably to ECT. Patients who experience multiple episodes of mania and depression in a single year, a phenomenon known as "rapid cycling," may

note a reduction in the number of episodes after a course of ECT.

Catatonia

Catatonia is a complex syndrome characterized by psychomotor retardation, mutism, and posturing. Psychiatric disorders associated with catatonia include mania, schizophrenia, and major depression. Additionally, catatonia can occur in the context of several neurological and medical illnesses. Regardless of underlying illness, catatonia generally has an excellent response to ECT with marked improvement occurring within three or four treatments. Catatonia also responds to psychotropic medications, and it is unclear whether the response to ECT is better than the response to pharmacological treatment with antipsychotic medications or benzodiazepines.

Schizophrenia

As is generally true of treatment with most antipsychotic medications, ECT has little effect on chronic symptoms of schizophrenia, including blunted affect, thought disorder, and long-standing delusions and hallucinations. However, patients with schizophrenia are most often hospitalized because of acute episodes of agitation, hallucinations, delusions, and thought disorder. Although acute exacerbations usually respond to adjustments in antipsychotic medications, ECT can also be effective, particularly in patients with severe symptoms or medication intolerance. It is estimated that about 70% of patients with schizophrenia in an acute relapse respond favorably to ECT. In contrast, only 5–10% of patients with chronic, residual symptoms of the disorder benefit from the treatment. In the past, prolonged courses of ECT (20–30 treatments or more over a several-week period, referred to as "regressive ECT") were used to treat chronic schizophrenics. The benefits of this form of treatment are unclear and do not outweigh the marked memory impairment and confusion associated with protracted ECT courses.

Other disorders

ECT has been used to treat a variety of other psychiatric disorders, including somatization disorder, personality disorders, obsessive-compulsive disorder, eating disorders, and alcohol and drug dependence. Although there are reports of benefits in some patients, it appears that ECT is not a useful treatment for these disorders. In these cases, ECT should be reserved for patients who develop major depressive episodes that are either non-responsive to pharmacological management or associated with severe symptoms.

Patients with a variety of neurological disorders may benefit transiently from ECT. There is evidence that patients with Parkinson's disease, who exhibit marked motor slowing and are subject to depressive episodes, show improvement in both the motor symptoms and mood disorder following ECT. The beneficial effects of ECT on the motor symptoms of Parkinson's disease appear to be independent of the beneficial effects on mood because some patients without a mood disorder show motor improvement with ECT. The effects of ECT on motor symptoms are typically time-limited unless maintenance treatments are given. Longer-term follow-up data on patients with Parkinson's disease treated with ECT are lacking but some evidence suggests benefits lasting several years with maintenance treatments.

Repeated generalized seizures have anticonvulsant effects. Clinically, these anticonvulsant effects are manifest as an increase in seizure threshold and a decrease in seizure duration over a course of ECT. In the past, the anticonvulsant effects of ECT were used to treat patients with refractory epilepsy. However, the anticonvulsant effects of an acute course of ECT subside over days to weeks, and there is no evidence that ECT is as effective as presently available anticonvulsant medications.

Contraindications to ECT

There are no absolute contraindications to ECT. However, some individuals may be at high risk for serious complications, and this should be considered carefully when evaluating patients for the procedure. Because ECT causes acute increases in cerebral blood flow and intracranial pressure, patients with space-occupying lesions of the central nervous system (CNS) are at risk for brain herniation and neurological decompensation. For these reasons, the presence of a space-occupying brain mass was previously considered an absolute contraindication to ECT. However, there have been reports of patients with intracranial tumors who have been successfully treated with ECT for psychiatric disorders. All patients with space-occupying lesions are at high risk for complications from ECT. Patients at greatest risk are those with focal neurological signs (particularly recent changes in the neurological examination), headaches, papilledema, or evidence of a shift in intracranial contents on brain imaging studies. Patients with small masses that are not associated with the above findings are at somewhat lower risk. Since changes in cerebral blood flow and intracranial pressure are related to changes in systemic blood pressure, it is important to manage blood pressure changes associated with ECT carefully in patients with CNS tumors. Patients with CNS tumors may also benefit from treatment with dexamethasone to limit swelling in the region of the tumor during ECT.

For several months following a myocardial infarction or cerebrovascular accident, there is increased risk of complications from general anesthesia. Additionally, the blood pressure and heart rate changes that accompany ECT compound this risk. Although ECT can be used in these patients, the relative risks versus benefits must be considered carefully. It appears that the period of greatest risk is in the first six weeks following a myocardial infarction or stroke.

Cardiovascular responses to ECT

To assess medical risks in patients undergoing ECT, it is important to understand the changes in cardiovascular function that accompany each treatment (Fig. 23.2). During and immediately following the electrical stimulus, parasympathetic tone is increased resulting in bradycardia or asystole lasting up to several seconds. This initial decrease in heart rate is prevented by pretreatment with anticholinergic medications (atropine or glycopyrrolate). During the generalized seizure, there are marked increases in heart rate (sometimes reaching rates of 120–160 beats per minute) and blood pressure (systolic blood pressures as high as 220–250 mm Hg and diastolic pressures up to 120–150 mm Hg), likely reflecting the release of catecholamines during the seizure. The hyperdynamic changes persist throughout the seizure and can last for 5–15 minutes or longer following the seizure. In some patients, the post-seizure period is marked by a rebound bradycardia that can last several minutes.

Patients with cardiovascular illnesses are at risk for myocardial ischemia and arrhythmias during ECT. Most ECT-induced arrhythmias and electrocardiographic (EKG) changes are time-limited and do not require specific treatment. However, serious arrhythmias that compromise hemodynamic function require appropriate management. Thus, it is imperative that medications and equipment for cardiac emergencies be available in the treatment room. Ventricular arrhythmias (tachycardia and fibrillation) and myocardial infarction are the most common causes of death during ECT. Despite the marked increases in blood pressure, the occurrence of a cerebrovascular bleed or a ruptured aneurysm is extremely uncommon.

Several measures can improve the safety of ECT and dampen the cardiovascular responses to the treatment. Careful pre-ECT evaluation of cardiac function is important, and appropriate treatment of underlying disorders should be initiated. One to two hours prior to an ECT treatment, routine oral cardiac medications should be administered. As described below, the judicious use of beta-blockers can also help in selected patients. Patients at high risk for myocardial ischemia can be premedicated with nitrates.

ECT technique

General management

ECT treatments are usually administered with informed patient consent. This requires a thorough discussion with the patient and, if possible, with the patient's family of the ECT indications, procedure, risks, and benefits. This also should include a discussion of the risks of not treating the

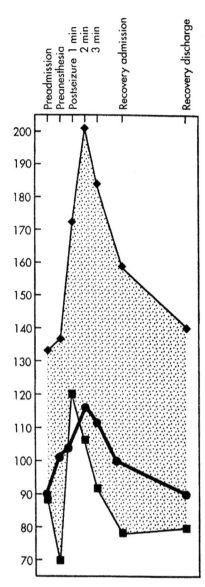

Fig. 23.2 ECT-associated cardiovascular changes. ECT seizures are associated with sympathetic (central and adrenal) discharges that result in transient elevations of heart rate (circles) and blood pressure (diamonds and squares represent systolic and diastolic blood pressures, respectively). The graph shows typical changes encountered during a single ECT treatment. The timing of the measurements is indicated at the top of the graph. Note that the ECT-induced changes reverse rapidly after the treatment; by the time the patient has recovered sufficiently from the treatment to be discharged from the ECT area (about 45 minutes after pre-admission), blood pressure and heart rate have returned to baseline.

underlying disorder. Some patients who suffer from severe psychiatric disorders may be unable or unwilling to give informed consent. Administration of ECT is subject to various legal regulations, although many jurisdictions permit involuntary treatment in severe cases after appropriate legal review. In all cases of involuntary ECT, it is important to

consider carefully the severity of the psychiatric symptoms, the response to pharmacotherapy, and the consequences of treatment.

The evaluation of patients prior to ECT requires detailed psychiatric and medical histories and a thorough physical examination. The psychiatric history should include information about psychiatric diagnosis, indications for ECT, and prior responses to psychotropic medications, psychotherapy, and ECT. The medical examination should emphasize cardiovascular, pulmonary, gastrointestinal, and neurological systems. Any prior history of surgical or anesthetic complications in the patient or patient's family should be documented, with emphasis on conditions that interfere with anesthesia (e.g. medication intolerance, pseudocholinesterase deficiency, or gastroesophageal reflux disorder).

The pre-ECT laboratory evaluation need not be extensive, but it should emphasize potential problems identified in the history and physical examination. Minimal recommended tests include serum electrolytes and EKG. Patients with histories of cardiopulmonary illnesses should have a chest x-ray prior to treatment. Spine x-rays are not required for ECT, but they should be considered in patients with a history of significant back or spine problems. Routine brain imaging studies are not necessary for most patients prior to ECT, but they should be obtained in patients with suspicious neurological histories and examinations.

Anesthesia

Prior to ECT, patients are not allowed to eat or drink for 6–8 hours. However, cardiovascular medications or medications to diminish gastric acid secretion can be administered orally under supervision 1–2 hours prior to treatment.

In general, anesthetic standards for outpatient surgery are appropriate for ECT. These include standards for anesthetic administration and postoperative care. In some centers, ECT is administered in an operating room setting, while in others ECT is given in a specialized suite. Prior to treatment, all patients are evaluated by the anesthesia provider to minimize anesthetic risk, and, in consultation with the treating psychiatrist, maximize therapeutic benefit. At the time of treatment, the patient's blood pressure, pulse, three-lead EKG, and level of oxygen saturation are monitored. A catheter is inserted into a peripheral vein and two or three medications are routinely administered at each session. For some patients, an anticholinergic medication, usually atropine (0.4–0.6 mg, i.v.) or glycopyrrolate (0.2–0.4 mg, i.v.), is administered to diminish the bradycardia that follows electrical stimulation. If oral secretions are a problem, the anticholinergic can be administered 30–60 minutes prior to treatment, intramuscularly. In many ECT centers, anticholinergics are administered to all patients. However, anticholinergics increase heart rate and could compound the tachycardia occurring during a seizure. This has led some practitioners to use these medications on a case-by-case basis, reserving anticholinergics for patients who have histories of bradyarrhythmias or who are taking medications that compound the bradycardia that occurs during ECT (e.g. beta-blockers, digoxin, and verapamil). Atropine has the added disadvantage that it is centrally acting and could increase the cognitive impairment associated with ECT.

Prior to administering the anesthetic, patients are preoxygenated with 100% oxygen by mask. Oxygen is administered throughout the procedure until the patient resumes normal respiration. This usually takes about ten minutes. The use of oxygen diminishes the risk of cardiac ischemia during ECT and may diminish cognitive side effects.

Methohexital (1 mg/kg, i.v.), a short-acting barbiturate, is the most commonly used anesthetic for ECT. Methohexital has a rapid onset, short duration of action (5–10 minutes), and is inexpensive. Potential problems with methohexital include respiratory depression at high doses and laryngospasm at low doses. In recent years, there has been increasing difficulty in obtaining methohexital, prompting the use of other anesthetics including thiopental, etomidate, ketamine, and propofol. Although most intravenous anesthetics, including the barbiturates, have anticonvulsant effects that diminish the ability to induce a seizure, this seems to be most problematic with propofol and least with ketamine. In adults, ketamine can produce significant side effects, including increased blood pressure responses during ECT and psychotic symptoms.

In the early days of ECT, fractures of vertebrae and long bones, resulting from muscle contractions during the electrical stimulus and seizure, were major complications. Routine pretreatment with muscle relaxants has eliminated this problem. Succinylcholine (1 mg/kg, i.v.), a depolarizing muscle relaxant, is the agent of choice for ECT. Advantages of succinylcholine include rapid onset, brief duration of action (5–10 min), and low cost. Because succinylcholine acts by depolarizing muscle cells and causes an acute increase in extracellular potassium, patients with neuromuscular disorders, recent trauma, or burns are at risk for developing severe hyperkalemia following succinylcholine. Patients with neuromuscular disorders are also at increased risk for developing malignant hyperthermia following succinylcholine. Other patients have genetic or drug-induced alterations in the activity of pseudocholinesterase, the enzyme that degrades succinylcholine. Deficiencies in pseudocholinesterase can cause prolonged paralysis requiring intubation and assisted ventilation. For patients at risk for complications from succinylcholine, non-depolarizing muscle relaxants such as mivacurium can be used.

Despite the routine use of muscle relaxants, direct electrical stimulation of the jaw muscles during the ECT stimulus causes clenching of the teeth. Thus, to protect the teeth and tongue, patients routinely have a bite block inserted in the mouth prior to electrical stimulation. The bite block can be removed after the electrical stimulus.

Each ECT-induced seizure is associated with increases in heart rate and blood pressure lasting several minutes. In young, medically healthy patients these cardiovascular changes are well tolerated, but could predispose patients with heart disease to serious arrhythmias or myocardial ischemia. Preoperative evaluation of patients on cardiovascular medications may show the need to adjust the medication regimen prior to instituting ECT. In selected patients, blood pressure and heart rate can be controlled during ECT by treatment with esmolol (0.2 mg/kg i.v.), a short-acting beta-blocker, or labetalol (5–20 mg, i.v.), a combined beta- and alpha-adrenergic antagonist. Esmolol may be the preferred drug because of its shorter duration of action. Because beta-blockers enhance the initial bradycardic response to ECT, patients on these medications are often pretreated with an anticholinergic medication. Alternatively, esmolol or labetalol can be administered intravenously following the electrical stimulation and the onset of generalized seizure activity. More serious sustained blood pressure changes can be blunted by premedication with calcium channel blockers such as nifedipine (10–20 mg, sublingually) or administration of nitrates 30 minutes prior to ECT. Some centers prefer nicardepine, a shorter-acting calcium channel blocker that can be administered intravenously.

The decision to use drugs to control heart rate and blood pressure is best made on a case-by-case basis, involving the anesthesia provider in the process. Importantly, ECT has been used as a treatment for more than 60 years and has had very low morbidity and mortality from cardiovascular complications. Potential problems with agents used to treat the cardiovascular changes associated with ECT include hypotension and bradyarrhythmias. These side effects can pose serious risks for elderly patients, in whom falls are a major concern. In general, conservative management is recommended for the cardiovascular changes accompanying ECT. The most appropriate pharmacological treatments for acute hemodynamic changes are those that have a short duration of action matched to the time course of ECT-related changes.

Electrical stimulation

To achieve therapeutic benefits, a generalized seizure must be produced at each ECT session. Seizures are induced by passing a brief electrical stimulus across the head from two electrodes that are positioned either bitemporally (bilateral ECT) or over the non-dominant cerebral hemisphere (unilateral ECT). A temporoparietal electrode placement is used most often for unilateral ECT (Fig. 23.3). Other placements of the stimulating electrodes are of uncertain value. For right-handed patients, electrodes are placed over the right cerebral hemisphere. Because most left-handed patients (~70%) are

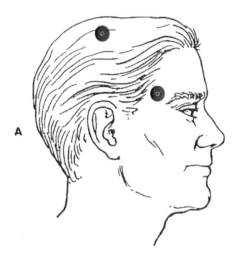
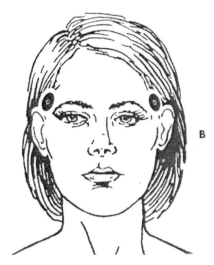

Fig. 23.3 Electrode placement for ECT. Stimulation can be administered either unilaterally (A) or bilaterally (B). Non-dominant unilateral stimuli are administered using the d'Elia placement (A), which is relatively memory-sparing, compared with bilateral electrode placements. Prior to electrode application, the placement sites are cleaned with a saline-soaked pad and an electrical conducting gel is applied to the ECT electrodes. With constant current stimulators, a low-amplitude, subconvulsive electrical stimulus is used to estimate the interelectrode impedance. Excessive impedance usually results from poor preparation of the electrode sites. To prevent electrical tissue burns, most constant current ECT stimulators have a failsafe that prohibits administering the convulsive stimulus if the interelectrode impedance exceeds certain values.

left hemisphere dominant for language, a right-sided electrode placement is also appropriate for most of these patients as well. Both unilateral and bilateral forms of treatment are effective, but bilateral ECT is associated with greater memory impairment and confusion. For this reason, nondominant unilateral ECT is often the preferred initial mode of treatment. However, unilateral stimulation results more frequently in missed or partial seizures unless the electrical dose is carefully adjusted. Additionally, some patients do not respond well to unilateral ECT, and the response to unilateral ECT can be slower to develop.

ECT-induced seizures are monitored by a two-channel electroencephalogram (EEG) and by observing convulsive motor movements. Because treatments are done with muscle relaxation, peripheral movements are monitored by occluding the flow of the muscle relaxant into a limb with an inflated blood pressure cuff or tourniquet. The isolated limb is usually ipsilateral to the side of the head that is stimulated in unilateral treatments, allowing determination of whether a generalized seizure is produced with the electrical stimulus.

Electrical stimuli that are subconvulsive or that induce focal seizures produce no clinical benefit. Similarly, treatments that terminate seizure activity shortly after electrical stimulation (e.g. lidocaine, anticonvulsants) diminish the effectiveness of the treatments. The typical duration of an ECT seizure is 30–90 seconds by EEG. Seizures lasting less than 25 seconds may be less therapeutic, but this is controversial. In patients who develop short seizures during ECT (defined as less than 25 seconds on EEG), intravenous caffeine (250–500 mg) can be used to lengthen the seizures. Alternatively, reductions in the dose of anesthetic agent or switching to a different anesthetic (e.g. etomidate or ketamine) will lengthen seizures in some patients. Prolonged seizures, defined as seizures longer than 180 seconds, are terminated by an intravenous anticonvulsant, usually methohexital or lorazepam. Status epilepticus is rare during ECT and is managed with agents typically employed for this problem in other settings. Status epilepticus is an indication for neurological consultation.

There is now reasonable evidence that the electrical dose used to induce seizures is important in determining clinical response. With bilateral ECT, stimuli that are just above seizure threshold (defined as the minimal amount of electrical charge needed to induce a seizure) produce good clinical effects. These lower charge bilateral treatments also appear to diminish the cognitive side effects of bilateral ECT. In contrast, unilateral ECT administered at minimally suprathreshold doses results in limited clinical benefit despite inducing generalized seizures of adequate duration. Furthermore, administering unilateral treatments at electrical doses that are more than 2.5 times the seizure threshold greatly improves the efficacy of unilateral ECT, while maintaining the cognitive benefits of the treatment relative to bilateral ECT. Present evidence suggests that unilateral treatments should be administered at electrical doses that are five-to-six times the seizure threshold. Patients who fail to respond at this level should receive maximal charge unilateral ECT (using presently available commercial ECT stimulators with maximal outputs of 500–600 milli-coulombs). Those failing maximal charge unilateral treatments should be switched to bilateral ECT. A patient should not be considered to have failed ECT until a trial of high-charge bilateral ECT has been administered.

During ECT, most of the administered current is shunted between the stimulating electrodes. This is because the resistivity of the scalp is much less than that of the skull (about 200 Ω/cm vs. 17,000 Ω/cm). It is estimated that less than 20% of the electrical stimulus enters the cranial cavity. Caution must be exercised in treating patients who have skull defects in the area where the electrodes are placed, because skull defects allow greater current flow into the cranium and could result in electrolytic tissue damage.

ECT stimulators generate either a constant current or constant voltage output. Constant current stimulators are used most commonly and have greater ease in quantifying the electrical dose because the amplitude of the output waveform does not depend on the impedance between the electrodes. A major consideration in selecting an ECT stimulator is the electrical waveform generated by the stimulator. Most ECT devices use either brief electrical pulses (i.e. a series of square wave pulses of specified amplitude and duration that rise and fall almost instantaneously) or sine wave outputs. Compared to sine wave generators, seizures can be induced at significantly lower charges using brief (0.5–2.0 msec) electrical pulses delivered at frequencies of 30–90 Hz for 0.5–8.0 seconds. The difference in seizure threshold arises from the fact that sine waves are highly inefficient and provide much of their current flow at subconvulsive levels during neuronal refractory periods when action potentials cannot be generated. Brief pulse stimulation is also associated with fewer cognitive side effects than sine wave stimulation. For these reasons, it is strongly recommended that only brief pulse stimulators be used for ECT. Typical seizure thresholds using brief pulse stimulation range from less than 25 millicoulombs to several hundred millicoulombs. Most ECT stimulators used clinically in the United States have maximal outputs of 500–600 millicoulombs. For comparison to cardioversion, this is equivalent to less than 100 watt-seconds (joules), assuming an interelectrode impedance of about 200 Ω.

Side effects and risks of ECT

Because ECT requires general anesthesia and electrical stimulation, is associated with marked changes in cardiovascular function, and is often used in the treatment of psychiatric disorders in patients with serious medical illnesses, it is not surprising that ECT is associated with some risk of death. It is estimated that an ECT-related death, defined as a death occurring within 24 hours of a treatment, occurs in about 2–4 of every 100,000 treatments. Importantly, this risk is not greater than the risk of general anesthesia alone. Since most centers administering ECT give fewer than 1000 treatments per year, practitioners rarely encounter an ECT death.

The cause of death is most often an adverse cardiovascular event (myocardial infarction or ventricular arrhythmia). In weighing the risk of death it is important to consider that untreated major psychiatric disorders are also associated with significant risks of morbidity and mortality from suicide and deterioration in health. About one in six individuals hospitalized for severe depression will kill themselves over their lifetime, an enormously greater risk than that associated with ECT.

Confusion and memory impairment are major side effects of ECT. It is important to emphasize that cognitive impairments are adverse effects of the treatment and play no role in the therapeutic benefits of ECT. Following an ECT treatment there is a period of postictal and postanesthetic confusion lasting minutes to hours. During this time, some patients become agitated and require treatment with benzodiazepines or antipsychotic medications. This immediate post-ECT confusion may worsen with increasing number and frequency of ECT treatments.

The memory impairment associated with ECT has both retrograde and anterograde components. In general, memory is worst for events occurring during the ECT course, although some patients report deficits in the recall of items of past personal information as well. ECT-induced memory loss tends to improve with time following the last ECT treatment, returning to baseline levels in about 6–8 weeks in most patients. Because certain psychiatric disorders, particularly depression, are associated with deficits in concentration and information processing, many patients report that their memory actually improves following a successful course of ECT, compared to a baseline when ill. Some patients report longer-lived deficits in autobiographical memories following ECT, but these are difficult to document systematically. Memory impairments worsen with increased number and frequency of treatments. Bilateral ECT produces significantly greater memory impairment than non-dominant hemisphere unilateral stimulation. It also appears that the cognitive side effects of ECT are increased by use of high electrical charges and perhaps by high doses of anesthetic medications and CNS-active anticholinergic drugs. The influence of electrical dose on memory and the role of electrical dose in ECT efficacy provide arguments for titrating seizure threshold and adjusting the administered electrical dose carefully in individual patients. Similarly, in order to spare memory to the maximum extent possible unilateral ECT should be considered for most patients. Despite advances in ECT technique, effects of ECT on memory are a significant limitation of this treatment.

Other side effects of ECT include muscle soreness, nausea, vomiting, and headaches. Muscle soreness results, at least in part, from fasciculations produced by succinylcholine, although direct muscle depolarization during the electrical stimulus and movements during the seizure contribute in some patients. Prior to the use of muscle relaxants, fractures of long bones and vertebrae were complications of ECT, but these are extremely rare in patients adequately treated with muscle relaxants. In patients with a prior history of back, joint or bone problems, careful monitoring of muscle relaxation is important. The nausea, vomiting, and headaches that some patients experience following a treatment usually respond to simple interventions. Typical agents include metoclopramide (10 mg i.v.) for nausea and ketorolac (30 mg i.v.) for headaches.

Acceptance of ECT can be difficult to achieve. In part, difficulties reflect anxiety associated with any medical procedure. Clear communication of indications, benefits, and risks to patients and their families verbally, in written form and, when available, in video form diminishes anxiety and is an important part of the informed consent process. Routine premedication for anxiety (e.g. benzodiazepines) is undesirable because of possible inhibition of seizure induction and perhaps adverse impact on ECT efficacy. Unfavorable perception by the general public, to the extent this influences use of ECT, may reflect overly dramatic media portrayals.

ECT in patients with concurrent medical illnesses

Treatment of psychiatric disorders in patients with severe medical illnesses can be difficult because many psychotropic medications have side effects that limit their use in this population. Because of its rapid effectiveness and relative safety, ECT is important to consider in treating medically ill patients with major affective or psychotic disorders. Although there are no absolute contraindications to ECT, patients with severe cardiovascular illnesses are exposed to marked hemodynamic changes during ECT. Thus, ECT can be viewed as a form of myocardial stressor producing significant changes in heart rate and blood pressure with each treatment. To diminish cardiovascular risks of ECT, nonpsychiatric physicians are often involved in the evaluation of medically ill patients prior to ECT and at times may be asked to participate in the administration of treatments.

ECT has been successfully used to treat patients who have a variety of cardiovascular illnesses. Consultation with a practitioner knowledgeable about the management of cardiovascular disorders may suggest strategies (e.g. antihypertensives) that minimize ECT-related cardiovascular stress. Most medications used to treat cardiovascular illnesses, including hypertension, present no specific problems during ECT. A possible exception is reserpine, an agent that has been associated with ECT-related deaths. Certain antiarrhythmic drugs (e.g. phenytoin, procainamide, lidocaine) increase seizure threshold and make it more difficult to induce therapeutic seizures. The presence of uncompen-

sated congestive heart failure presents significant anesthetic and ECT risks. Following appropriate medical management, patients with congestive heart failure can be treated successfully with ECT, although they are at risk for decompensation. Patients with cardiac pacemakers can be treated with ECT provided that there is adequate grounding of the electrical equipment used to administer treatments. A pacemaker magnet should be available at the time of treatment to help control heart rate if necessary. Patients with vascular aneurysms can be treated with ECT but careful attention should be paid to limiting the hemodynamic changes. Similarly, patients who have had cardiac surgery including valve replacements, coronary artery bypass grafts or cardiac transplants have been treated successfully with ECT. The valve replacement patients are typically on anticoagulant medications. These medications can be used concurrently with ECT without inordinate risk.

There are risks associated with the use of ECT in patients with pulmonary illnesses (emphysema, bronchitis, and asthma) because each treatment requires general anesthesia. However, respiratory illnesses do not preclude the use of ECT. Endotracheal intubation is not routinely used for ECT and is to be avoided because of the need for multiple treatments and hence multiple intubations over a several week period. Intubation is usually reserved for patients with severe gastroesophageal reflux, although conservative management with medications that diminish gastric acid secretion (antihistaminics or omeprazole) and cricoid pressure during ECT is the preferred mode of treatment. Theophylline is used in the treatment of some patients with respiratory disorders and has been associated with prolonged seizures and status epilepticus during ECT. For this reason, it is recommended that theophylline levels be kept as low as possible ($<20\,\mu g/ml$) or that the medication be discontinued during a course of ECT. Pretreatment of patients with reactive airway disease may facilitate management. Administration via inhaler of albuterol, a selective beta-2 adrenergic agonist, or other rapidly acting agent is usually performed immediately before treatment.

Patients with diabetes mellitus can be treated successfully with ECT. Prior to treatment, blood sugar is monitored by finger stick and should be at a level deemed non-emergent. In patients on insulin, the morning dose is usually withheld until after ECT when patients can resume oral intake. ECT is reported to have variable effects on blood sugar levels in diabetic patients, but these effects do not appear to be a clinical problem provided that patients are monitored closely through their ECT course.

Patients with coexisting neurological disorders have been treated successfully with ECT. Blood pressure and heart rate changes in patients with CNS tumors or cerebrovascular disorders should be monitored carefully and limited to the extent possible. Although spontaneous seizures following ECT have been described, patients with epilepsy are not at marked risk during ECT. In fact, there may be diminished seizure frequency during ECT because the treatment has anticonvulsant effects. Patients on anticonvulsant medications for the treatment of a seizure disorder should be maintained on these medications throughout their ECT course because there are substantial risks associated with discontinuing or diminishing the dose of these agents in epileptic patients.

Intraocular pressure increases during ECT. However, these changes are short-lived and usually do not present a clinical problem. Patients with glaucoma should be maintained on their routine medications during ECT. One potential problem concerns the use of ECT in patients treated with ecothiophate eye drops. Ecothiophate inhibits pseudocholinesterase and has been associated with prolonged paralysis following use of succinylcholine.

ECT has been used successfully to treat major psychiatric disorders during pregnancy and has not been associated with significant complications in the mother or fetus. The decision to use ECT during pregnancy requires active involvement of the patient's obstetrician. Routine intubation or intensive fetal monitoring during ECT do not seem warranted based on the published literature. A delivery suite should be available for patients in the later stages of pregnancy in the unlikely event that an emergent delivery is required.

ECT course

A typical course of ECT consists of 6–12 treatments administered once daily, two or three times per week. There have been attempts to speed the ECT course by giving multiple treatments at a session (2–4 seizures per session). However, there is little evidence that this practice enhances clinical response and multiple treatments increase the risk of memory impairment. The number of treatments in an ECT course depends primarily on clinical response and side effects of treatment, particularly memory loss and confusion. Fixed courses of treatments for all patients are inappropriate because the response to ECT can vary greatly from patient to patient.

Once a stable degree of improvement is achieved, ECT treatments are usually discontinued, and the patient is started on maintenance treatment. All patients who respond to ECT require effective and aggressive maintenance treatment because there is a significant risk of relapse during the first 3–6 months following a successful ECT course. The maintenance treatment is usually an antidepressant medication that the patient has not failed in the past. In some patients, ECT is used as a maintenance treatment. When used for this purpose ECT is administered on a schedule of decreasing frequency starting with once weekly treatment followed by gradual tapering to once monthly treatment. Maintenance ECT is usually administered on an outpatient basis. Difficulties with this form of treatment include the usual side effects of ECT and inconvenience for patients and their families. Patients are not allowed to drive or operate complex machinery on days that they receive ECT, making transportation to and from the treatment center problematic. Despite these limitations, outpatient maintenance ECT is one of the fastest growing parts of ECT practice and is appropriate for patients who have failed multiple prior medications but who have a good response to an acute course of ECT.

ECT and psychotropic medications

There is little evidence that concurrent use of psychotropic medications enhances the beneficial effects of ECT, but certain medication effects could increase the adverse effects of ECT. For example, medications with significant anticholinergic effects (e.g. tricyclic antidepressants, antiparkinson drugs or low-potency antipsychotics) could compound the memory impairment associated with ECT. Some evidence suggests that benzodiazepines may diminish the beneficial effects of unilateral ECT, presumably by increasing seizure threshold. Similar concerns exist with anticonvulsants used for mood stabilization (e.g. valproic acid, carbamazepine, lamotrigine). Certain medications (bupropion, clozapine, amoxapine, and maprotiline) may predispose to prolonged seizures during ECT, but the evidence supporting this is limited. Lithium may increase the cognitive impairments of ECT and may be associated with spontaneous seizures and other neurological complications during ECT. Phenelzine, a monoamine oxidase inhibitor, has been reported to inhibit pseudocholinesterase and could prolong the apnea produced by succinylcholine.

For most patients, psychotropic drug use should be kept at a minimum during an ECT course. Severely agitated and psychotic patients can be treated with high-potency antipsychotic drugs during a course of ECT. Severely anxious patients can be treated with low doses of a shorter-acting benzodiazepine (e.g. lorazepam, alprazolam). For temporary sleep disturbances, zolpidem is a reasonable choice. To the extent possible, the use of anxiolytic and hypnotic medications should be minimized during an ECT course.

ECT mechanisms

In considering how ECT works, it is important to emphasize that the one constant across numerous studies is that the therapeutic benefits of ECT require repeated induction of generalized CNS seizures. Thus, considerable effort has been directed towards understanding how generalized seizures alter brain function. Unfortunately, most major neurochemical systems that have been studied show some alteration following ECT (or electroshock in animals), making it difficult to be confident of the role played by any one system.

Certain effects appear unlikely to be involved in the efficacy of ECT. For example, anesthetic medications have little to do with the therapeutic benefits. Similarly, there is no convincing evidence that ECT causes structural brain damage. The memory-impairing effects of ECT are also unrelated to the therapeutic benefits. Most innovations in ECT technique have been aimed at maintaining therapeutic benefits while eliminating, to the extent possible, the cognitive impairing effects of the treatment. The routine use of unilateral electrode placements, brief pulse stimulators, and titrated electrical doses are three notable examples.

It is presently believed that the therapeutic and adverse cognitive effects of ECT result from changes in neurotransmitter biochemistry, receptors, and post-receptor signaling. Leading candidates include the biogenic amine and muscarinic cholinergic transmitter systems. Because many psychotropic medications alter the function of biogenic amine transmitter systems (norepinephrine, dopamine, and serotonin), there has been interest in examining the effects of ECT on these systems. Some effects of ECT on biogenic amine systems are consistent with the effects of psychotropic medications (e.g. beta adrenergic receptor down regulation), but others are inconsistent with medication effects (e.g. increases in serotonin type 2 receptor binding). Other hypotheses suggest that changes in neuroendocrine systems, biochemical second messenger systems or CNS gene expression ultimately underlie the effects of ECT.

Another line of thought postulates that the anticonvulsant effects of ECT are important in the clinical benefits. Again, the mechanisms of these effects are not certain but could involve changes in the γ-aminobutyric acid (GABA), opioid, or adenosine transmitter systems. It is interesting that caffeine, an adenosine receptor antagonist, is sometimes used to prolong ECT seizures, suggesting the importance of the adenosine system in seizure termination. The anticonvulsant hypothesis of ECT is attractive given the effectiveness of certain anticonvulsants as mood stabilizers and could account for beneficial actions in both mania and depression. However, there is no direct evidence demonstrating that any neurochemical or neurophysiological effect of ECT, exclusive of a generalized CNS seizure, is critical for the clinical effects observed.

New directions: transcranial magnetic stimulation (TMS)

Despite its efficacy in major psychiatric disorders, there are substantial problems associated with ECT. This has prompted efforts to develop other somatic treatments that maintain the benefits of ECT, but diminish side effects. Among these, TMS is one of the most promising. TMS is based on the idea that the flow of electricity through a coil generates a magnetic field that penetrates the skull and stimulates underlying brain tissue. The TMS field strength is about 2 tesla, similar to the fields used in magnetic resonance imaging. TMS is more focal than electrical stimulation, being confined to a region with a diameter of several centimeters and penetrating the brain only a few centimeters below the skull.

TMS has been used experimentally to modify the function of the cerebral cortex reversibly and to study information processing in specific brain regions. This prompted studies to determine whether TMS could be used to treat patients with psychiatric disorders. At present, most information is available about the use of TMS in treating depression. While these studies are still preliminary, there is evidence that repetitive rapid-rate TMS (rTMS), involving multiple stimulations per session targeted to the prefrontal cortex, has therapeutic benefits without causing generalized seizures. Efforts are under way to define the optimal stimulus intensities (defined relative to motor threshold), frequency of pulses, number of pulses administered, and course of treatment. Using higher frequency (e.g. 20 Hz) or lower frequency (e.g. 1 Hz) pulses, it appears possible to activate or inhibit focal regions of cortex, respectively. Present evidence suggests that either higher frequency stimulation of the left frontal cortex or lower frequency stimulation of the right frontal cortex is beneficial in treating patients with non-psychotic major depression, with some studies reporting outcomes comparable to ECT. Effects on psychotic depression have been less favorable. Some evidence suggests that 1 Hz stimulation of the left temporoparietal cortex (presumably inhibiting function in the region) may be beneficial in treating refractory auditory hallucinations in patients with schizophrenia.

In addition to the use of sub-convulsive TMS, there is interest in determining whether magnetic stimulation can be used to induce generalized seizures. Because of its more focal field of stimulation, magnetic seizure therapy (MST) may provide a means of producing therapeutic seizures but with diminished cognitive side effects.

Summary

ECT is an extremely powerful treatment for certain psychiatric disorders (see *Pearls & Perils*). It is most useful in the management of severe mood disorders, psychotic disorders, and catatonia. In some cases ECT can be life saving. The beneficial effects of ECT require a generalized seizure, but certain characteristics of the electrical stimulus, particularly in non-dominant hemisphere ECT, are also important. The major risks of ECT include a small chance of death from cardiovascular complications and time-limited problems with memory loss and confusion. ECT is appropriate for treating psychiatric disorders in patients with concurrent medical and neurological disorders and may be preferred over certain psychotropic medications. In high-risk medical patients, particularly those with severe cardiac illnesses, a thorough understanding of the hemodynamic effects of ECT coupled with a careful analysis of the risk-benefit ratio is mandatory. Non-psychiatric physicians and psychotherapists can enhance the effectiveness of ECT by recognizing its

KEY CLINICAL QUESTIONS AND WHAT THEY UNLOCK

- *Has this patient been treated with ECT before? What was the response?*
  If yes and response was good, ECT may be a reasonable choice for treating a relapse. If yes and response was poor, it is important to understand whether the poor outcome was related to failure of the acute course of ECT, a problem with maintaining the benefits after ECT was discontinued, or side effects of the treatment. Many patients who report poor responses to ECT actually describe failures of maintenance treatment. Additionally, it is important to know what side effects were encountered during ECT and whether these influenced the perceived outcome. Understanding prior problems with ECT often suggests strategies to minimize discomfort that could be implemented with the first treatment in a course (e.g. prophylaxis with analgesics or antiemetics for headaches and nausea; careful attention to memory dysfunction in individuals previously experiencing significant confusion).
- *What factors place this patient at risk for complications/side effects from ECT?*
  Here the focus is on the pre-ECT medical evaluation with emphasis on neurological, cardiac, respiratory, and gastrointestinal findings that can influence the safety of general anesthesia. Understanding the cardiac effects of ECT is important in planning effective and safe courses of treatment for patients with underlying cardiovascular illnesses.
- *What is the current state of this patient's memory and cognitive function?*
  Because ECT is associated with memory loss and confusion, it is important to assess memory and cognitive function carefully at baseline, during and after a course of treatment. It is important to document baseline function because major psychiatric disorders can be associated with altered performance on a variety of cognitive tasks. Deteriorating memory function during a course of ECT requires strategies to diminish this effect (e.g. alteration in electrical dose, electrode placement, frequency of treatment, anesthetic medications, concurrent medications). The use of brief standardized tests can be helpful in monitoring changes in cognitive function over time (e.g. Mini-Mental Status Examination).
- *How has this patient responded to previous trials of antidepressant medications?*
  When selecting maintenance treatment following an acute course of ECT it is of major importance to have information about prior responses to psychotropic medications, including information about doses, duration of trials, side effects, and outcomes. Present evidence suggests that reinstitution of previously failed medications will not sustain remissions achieved with ECT. However, the ability to discern medication failures from inadequate treatment can be difficult without careful documentation.

efficacy, assisting with patient selection, and actively participating in efforts to minimize risks.

PEARLS & PERILS

- ECT is a safe and effective treatment for major depression, mania, catatonia, and acute worsening of psychosis in schizophrenia.
- ECT is administered under general anesthesia with muscle relaxation.
- The therapeutic effects of ECT require the repeated induction of generalized CNS seizures.
- There are no absolute contraindications to ECT. Patients with brain tumors, particularly those with focal neurological signs or evidence of increased intracranial pressure, are at risk for neurological decompensation.
- Each ECT treatment is associated with significant increases in blood pressure and heart rate. These effects need to be considered carefully when treating patients with cardiovascular illnesses.
- Confusion and memory impairments are time-limited side effects of ECT and do not contribute to the therapeutic benefits of ECT. The risk of memory impairment can be diminished by use of non-dominant hemisphere electrical stimulation.

Annotated bibliography

Abrams, R (2002) *Electroconvulsive Therapy*, 4th Edition, New York, Oxford University Press.
This book provides an excellent, well-referenced overview of ECT and is a must for any serious ECT practitioner. For primary care physicians, the book presents a good discussion of cardiovascular changes associated with ECT and the use of ECT in medically ill patients.

American Psychiatric Association, Committee on Electroconvulsive Therapy (2001) *The Practice of Electroconvulsive Therapy: recommendations for treatment, training and privileging*, 2nd Edition, Washington DC, American Psychiatric Association.
This book contains the recommendations of the American Psychiatric Association concerning the use of ECT. The rationale for specific recommendations are clearly outlined. This book is presently a bit out of date but still contains useful information.

Devanand, DP, Dwork, AJ, Hutchinson, ER, Bolwig, TG, and Sackeim, HA (1994) Does ECT alter brain structure?, *Am J Psychiatry* 151: 957–970.
This paper presents an excellent overview of the effects of ECT on the CNS. Based on a careful review of the existing clinical and preclinical literature, the authors conclude that there is no systematic evidence supporting the hypothesis that ECT alters brain structure.

CHAPTER 24

Practical Genetics for the Primary Care Physician

Alison J. Whelan, MD and Jennifer Ivanovich, MS

Introduction

Knowing about the influence of genetics on medical illnesses and how to discuss genetic risk and genetic testing with patients and families is a core skill for any clinician. The major focus of genetic research for the last 100 years has been the study of single genes and their effects. Over 1200 genes that cause single gene disorders have been identified, and genetic diagnostic testing is available for hundreds of Mendelian disorders. To date, clinically relevant genetic insights lag in psychiatric medicine compared to many other disciplines, reflecting that relatively few psychiatric diseases are Mendelian or chromosomal in nature. There are, however, many disorders with a psychiatric component that are classic Mendelian or chromosomal disorders.

Since many common psychiatric disorders are multifactorial and involve a significant genetic component, advances in genomics will improve understanding of psychiatric diseases over the next several years. Genomics is the study of all genes in the genome with an emphasis on gene function, the complex interactions between genes, and the role of genes in a variety of common disorders. This emerging field of genetics includes epidemiology, computational biology, protein expression studies, and population genetics. Genomic medicine will influence understanding of the epidemiology of many common, multifactorial disorders, alter the approach to risk stratification, allow development of novel drugs aimed at underlying genetic abnormalities, and lead to individualization of pharmacotherapy based on an individual's genetic make-up, which influences efficacy and side effects of therapy.

In this chapter, we provide an overview of the major clinically relevant concepts in genetics and genomics, describe common pitfalls in the clinical applications of genetics, and discuss the unique impact on families of diagnosing genetic disorders.

Relevance of genetic medicine in primary care

Genetic diseases were once considered to be rare disorders affecting a small percentage of the population. The discipline of medical genetics was likewise considered an outlying specialty with little integration into general medicine. The extensive media coverage of the Human Genome Project left general practitioners wondering how highly publicized genetic advances could be of value in their daily practice. Genetic medicine truly became relevant to primary care physicians in the 1990s when the genetic basis of some common illnesses, such as breast cancer and cardiovascular disease, was demonstrated.

In total, genetic diseases are not rare. Table 24.1 lists well-described single gene disorders, chromosomal abnormalities, and genetic associations, and it highlights the growing array of genetic disorders in every discipline. Consider the pediatric setting. Yoon and colleagues have estimated that 9–12% of all pediatric hospitalizations are related to birth defects or genetic conditions using 17 categories of single gene disorders or major structural anomalies. In comparison with other pediatric hospitalizations, their study group was three years younger, stayed three days longer on average, and experienced greater than four times the mortality rate.

Similar analyses have not been conducted among adult inpatients, but several factors suggest the prevalence of genetic disease among adults is even higher, though it more often goes unrecognized. First, children with some classical genetic disorders, which were once considered fatal or

TABLE 24.1

Selected genetic diseases of importance to the primary care physician

Continuum	Disease (incidence)	Common features	Inheritance	Testing
Reproductive (diagnostic)	Down syndrome (1 in 800)	Mental retardation, congenital heart defects, gastrointestinal abnormalities, late age dementia	Chromosomal trisomy	Chromosomal or FISH analysis on fetal sample obtained by CVS or amniocentesis
Reproductive (screening)	Neural tube defect (1 in 1,000)	Spina bifida, anencephaly, hydrocephalus	Multifactorial	Maternal α-fetoprotein screening used to detect pregnancies at increased risk. Fetal ultrasound used for diagnosis
Childhood	Neurofibromatosis (1 in 3,000)	Café-au-lait spots, neurofibromas, optic pathway gliomas, Lisch nodules, seizures, learning disabilities	Autosomal dominant	Clinical examination. DNA testing of NF-1 gene available but seldom needed
	Gaucher disease (1 in 1,000 in Jewish population)	Hepatosplenomegaly, thrombocytopenia, anemia, osteopenia	Autosomal recessive	Biochemical enzyme analysis of β-glucosylceramidase enzyme activity
	Fragile X syndrome (1 in 4,000 males; 1 in 8,000 females)	Mental retardation, enlarged testes, attention deficit hyperactivity disorder, mild autistic features (decreased eye contact, hand flapping and other repetitive movements)	X-linked (results from trinucleotide repeat mutation)	Direct DNA analysis of the FMR-1 gene
	Shprintzen syndrome (1 in 4,000)	Conotruncal heart defects, palatal abnormalities, learning disabilities, immunologic dysfunction, psychiatric disease	Deletion of chromosome 22q11 segment	FISH analysis of chromosome 22q11
	Mitochondrial diseases (1 in 1,000 adults and children)	Encephalopathy, seizures, migraines, ataxia, exercise intolerance, cardiomyopathy, diabetes	Mitochondrial or autosomal recessive (depending on gene involved)	Direct DNA analysis of multiple nuclear and mitochondrial genes
Adult	Early onset dementia (<5% of all Alzheimer disease)	Early adult onset of progressive dementia, cerebral cortex atrophy, amyloid plaque formation, intraneuronal neurofibrillary tangles	Autosomal dominant	Direct DNA analysis for PSN1, PSN2, and APP genes
	Huntington disease (1 in 15,000)	Progressive motor disability, cognitive decline, psychiatric disturbances	Autosomal dominant (trinucleotide repeat mutation)	Direct DNA analysis of trinucleotide repeats in HD gene
	Ehlers Danlos syndrome type IV (1 in 50,000 to 1 in 100,000)	Arterial, intestinal, and uterine fragility, increased risk for arterial rupture, aneurysm, dissection	Autosomal dominant	Biochemical studies of electrophoretic mobility of type III procollagen. DNA analysis of COL3A1 gene
	Multiple colon polyps (10–100 polyps)	Multiple adenomatous polyps identified in large bowel (excluding FAP)	Autosomal recessive	Direct DNA analysis of MYH gene
	Hemochromatosis (1 in 200–400)	Excessive iron accumulation, diabetes mellitus, skin pigmentation changes, arthritis, cardiomyopathy, cirrhosis or hepatic fibrosis	Autosomal recessive	Biochemical screening of serum transferrin-iron saturation and serum ferritin concentration. DNA testing of two common mutations in HFE gene

Continued

TABLE 24.1 (continued)

Selected genetic diseases of importance to the primary care physician

Continuum	Disease (incidence)	Common features	Inheritance	Testing
(risk association)	APOE	Increased risk for Alzheimer's disease associated with E4 allele. Possible increased cardiovascular disease risk associated with E4 allele	Association study	Currently, testing is not recommended
(risk association)	Factor V Leiden Thrombophilia (3–8% heterozygotes in US and Europe, 1 in 500 homozygotes)	Increased risk of venous thromboembolism	Single allele (heterozygotes) (modest increased risk) Two alleles (homozygotes) (very increased risk)	APC resistance assay or DNA based testing of Factor V gene for factor V Leiden allele
Population (newborn screening)	Galactosemia (1 in 30,000)	Feeding problems, failure to thrive, liver damage, sepsis in untreated children. Ovarian failure in treated females	Autosomal recessive	Biochemical measurement of galactose-1-phosphate uridyltransferase (GALT) activity
(carrier screening)	Cystic fibrosis (1 in 3,200 Caucasians)	Chronic lung infections, pancreatic insufficiency, absent Wolffian ducts structure in males	Autosomal recessive	Direct DNA analysis of 25 most common mutations in CFTR gene

associated with decreased life expectancy, are living well into adulthood. For example, nearly 40% of all children with Down syndrome have a significant congenital heart defect. With improved surgical interventions, the average life expectancy has improved, and more physicians are caring for adults with this condition. Second, understanding of the genetic basis of common disorders continues to expand. Nearly 10% of all people with colon cancer have a single gene mutation that places them at high risk to develop colorectal and other types of cancer. This incidence figure does not include the many at-risk relatives who should undergo earlier and more intensified cancer surveillance based on the family's genetic predisposition. Overall, single gene disorders are being found to account for an increasing percentage of chronic disease. More importantly, diseases with multifactorial etiologies are the most significant determinant of genetic disease prevalence among adults. Psychiatric illnesses, diabetes, and cardiovascular disease are primarily determined by multifactorial etiologies, with the genetic contribution varying among diseases and within a given disease among individual families.

Alzheimer's disease is prototypical of the complex underlying genetic basis of multifactorial disorders. For most individuals, Alzheimer's disease develops from a multifactorial process. The genetic contribution is significant, but it is far less than for highly penetrant, single gene disorders. For these individuals and their families, it is much more likely that primary care providers will be central to their genetic care. (See Case 24.1 and "Interpreting tests for multifactorial disease" for further discussion.)

The growing recognition of genetic and multifactorial disorders should encourage all clinicians to become familiar with the presentation and diagnosis of these disorders. Physicians must understand how the identification of a genetic disorder may impact delivery of care. First, diagnosis of a specific disorder delineates the immediate and long-term medical complications associated with the syndrome and allows initiation of medical management reflective of these risks. Second, recurrence risks for an individual's children, grandchildren or siblings may be addressed or refined using new genetic data. New genetic technology is increasingly available to aid in diagnosis and management. This is an important consideration for adults with genetic disorders for whom technology was not available during their childhood. Revisiting testing options should be explored with every adult with a known or possible genetic disorder. Finally, genetic advances may bring about new opportunities for disease prevention and health promotion. As an example, with the availability of breast cancer susceptibility gene testing, women at high risk to develop disease can be identified and begin prophylactic medical and surgical options to prevent disease.

John is a 45-year-old attorney for a large private firm. His mother was diagnosed in an early stage of Alzheimer's disease at 64 years of age. Her disease has progressed over the ensuing five years, leaving her completely dependent on the care of others and necessitating a move into a nursing care facility. There is no other family history of Alzheimer's disease or dementia. John's father died 20 years ago of an acute myocardial infarction.

John approaches his primary care physician about apolipoprotein E (ApoE) testing at the urging of his wife, who is a physician. He and his wife have recently read about the association between ApoE and Alzheimer's disease risk, and they wish for him to be tested. John admits he is reluctant to obtain this information, but he agrees with his wife that he should pursue testing before they make an important, upcoming financial decision.

Critical questions that should be addressed in this case are:
- Is Alzheimer's disease hereditary in this family and, if so, what are the medical and family history clues to hereditary disease?
- What risk does John have to develop Alzheimer's disease?
- Is genetic testing available? Would it be useful to John?

Alzheimer's disease is the leading cause of dementia in the elderly, with an estimated lifetime risk to develop disease of 15%. About 5% of families have hereditary disease resulting from a single gene mutation inherited in an autosomal dominant pattern. These mutations may occur in the PSN1, PSN2, APP, or Tau genes and are associated with an extremely high risk for early onset dementia, with lifetime risks approaching 100%. Hereditary disease is characterized by early age of onset and multiple affected generations with multiple

affected, closely related relatives. These families clearly have a "genetic disease" and typically receive genetic services from academic genetic centers.

The majority of families have more complex disease resulting from complex gene-environment interactions. The ApoE (apolipoprotein E) gene, found on chromosome 19, has three common alleles: E2, E3, E4. The ApoE4 allele is a risk factor for late onset familial Alzheimer's disease. The association between ApoE4 and Alzheimer's disease is dose dependent, as the association is stronger with an increasing number of E4 alleles. For Caucasians, the odds ratio ranges from 4 (single E4 allele) up to 15 (two E4 alleles), compared to the most common genotype (E3: E3). The ApoE4 allele is associated with a younger age of onset, and there appears to be a greater risk among women than men. In contrast, the E2 allele seems to have a protective effect in the development of disease. Given the *a priori* risk to develop disease, the calculated lifetime risk to develop Alzheimer's disease with an E4 allele is 29%.

John's needs might better be met by a thorough discussion with his primary care physician than with a geneticist, genetic counselor, or neurologist. He can be reassured his family history is not consistent with early onset autosomal dominant Alzheimer's disease. The primary care physician can discuss with John the limited predictive value of ApoE4 testing. The presence of an E4 allele confers a greater risk, but it is not highly predictive for Alzheimer's disease. For this reason, national professional genetic societies and Alzheimer's disease associations have recommended against presymptomatic testing of the ApoE4 allele. The primary care physician can work with John to clarify any misunderstanding of the predictive value of testing and address the stresses of his mother's illness with him and his family.

- Revisiting testing options should be explored with every adult with a known or possible genetic disorder.

When should a genetic diagnosis be considered?

Understanding the genetics of a disorder includes recognizing that the disorder may have a genetic component, gathering the relevant individual and family history, and interpreting the pattern of inheritance. Once these steps have been completed, consideration of diagnosis, risk estimates

in unaffected family members, diagnostic testing, and care plans can be considered. The physician caring for adults is disadvantaged by the difficulty in obtaining prenatal and early childhood history as well as by the lack of data on medical complications experienced among adults with hereditary disease. Some of these complications are reviewed below.

Medical history

Examples in the medical history that may prompt consideration of genetic disease include:
- Prenatal medical history:
  - decreased fetal movements
  - abnormalities in amount of amniotic fluid (e.g., oligohydramnios or polyhydramnios)
  - abnormal structure identified on ultrasound (e.g., cystic hygroma at 18 weeks' gestation).
- Childhood medical history:
  - one rare birth defect (e.g., encephalocele)

- two or more common birth defects (e.g., congenital heart disease and pyloric stenosis)
- ambiguous genitalia
- failure to thrive (not due to social or environmental factors)
- developmental delay or mental retardation.
- Adult medical history:
  - lack of menses in a young female
  - multiple miscarriages/pregnancy losses
  - unexplained neurologic decline (e.g., memory loss in a healthy 40-year-old)
  - early age of onset of a common disorder (e.g., colon cancer in a 34-year-old)
  - two or more rare diseases in a single individual.

Physical examination

The physical examination should include evaluation for dysmorphic features, i.e., features that fall outside normal standards or are distinct from the family appearance. It takes training to specifically characterize dysmorphic features, but an experienced clinician can often identify the presence of dysmorphic features if s/he is attentive. It is particularly useful to carefully scrutinize facial features, ears, hands, feet, nails, skin, and hair, noting variations that may be atypical. Several physical standards are available, making it easier to distinguish normal variation from abnormal trait. Standards for hand, finger, and foot length; interpupillary distance; palpebral fissure length; limb proportion; and penis and clitoris length are available to aid in diagnostic assessment. Growth standards for several specific genetic or chromosomal syndromes also exist. Qualitative features are more challenging to describe and are subject to greater rater variation. Qualitative traits such as blue sclerae, facial asymmetry, low set ears, unusual hair pattern, coarse facial features, weak cry, joint hyperextensibility, unusual sweating, velvety skin, or abnormal smelling urine may also prompt consideration of genetic disease. Review of previous photographs may be useful for identifying features that have become more distinctive or less obvious over time.

Family history

Interpretation of family history is an important component of any evaluation that considers possible patterns of inheritance. Since DNA-based analysis is limited to highly penetrant single gene disorders, family history assessment remains critical for stratifying disease risk and identifying individuals with an increased disease predisposition. However, gathering family history during an intake evaluation is often limited to a few targeted questions, limiting the ability to identify specific patterns. The importance of family history assessment cannot be overstated. Every health care provider should be able to obtain and interpret a detailed family history to answer the question "Is this person at significant increased risk for a genetic disorder?"

A positive family history is a well-established risk factor for psychiatric illnesses, including schizophrenia and affective disorders. While obtaining and analyzing a family history in a busy practice is challenging, limited studies have shown collection of family history data for common diseases is possible. The utility of a single family history tool in the identification of several diseases including cardiovascular diseases, diabetes, and several types of cancers has been demonstrated. The essential features of a screening family history tool are: self-administered, easy to understand, minimal time required for completion, multiple diseases and multiple generations are included, and ethnic heritage information is listed. A screening family history tool should be utilized by primary care physicians in order to assess family-based risk (Table 24.2).

In addition to the family history gathered at the initial visit, it is important to update family history information during follow-up visits. Acheson found that family practice physicians asked family history questions during only 22% of established follow-up visits. This low follow-up results in a failure to identify changes in family members' health, which might alter a person's risk stratification or the utility of new genetic technology that can be used to more precisely define risk.

Even physicians who regularly ask family history questions often have difficulty interpreting the reported history. Accurate interpretation and risk stratification of complicated pedigrees require genetics expertise, but a number of features in the family history should prompt consideration of genetic disease and subsequent genetic referral or further investigation. These include:

- multiple relatives affected with a similar disease consistent with a known pattern of inheritance (e.g., different types of cancer)
- multiple relatives affected with diagnoses that may share a common genetic etiology (e.g., behavioral disturbances and mental retardation)
- earlier age at diagnosis than the average age of onset (e.g., schizophrenia diagnosed at 14 years of age)
- multiple pregnancy losses (e.g., greater than two unexplained miscarriages)
- unexplained early or sudden death (e.g., healthy 22-year-old male dies suddenly with normal toxicology screening)
- consanguineous relationships within a family (e.g., offspring of consanguineous relationships will have higher risk for multifactorial and autosomal recessive diseases)
- ethnic background associated with an increased risk for disease (sickle cell anemia in African Americans, cystic fibrosis in Caucasians of northern European descent,

TABLE 24.2

Screening family history tool incorporated in the general patient intake form

1 Are you adopted?

❏ Yes   ❏No

   If yes, do you know your biological family history?

❏ Yes   ❏No→Please skip remaining questions

2 Are you a twin?

❏ Yes   ❏No

If yes,   ❏ Identical   ❏Same sex, unknown if identical   ❏Fraternal or non-identical

3 What is your maternal ethnic and religious background? _____

4 What is your paternal family ethnic and religious background? _____

5 Please list any type of birth defect, genetic condition, mental retardation, or serious illnesses such as cancer, diabetes, or mental illness in any family member biologically related to you.

Relative	Birth defects, genetic conditions, serious illnesses including age at diagnosis	Mother's side	Father's side
Mother			
Father			
Daughter(s)			
Son(s)			
Sister(s)			
Brother(s)			
Niece(s)			
Nephew(s)			
Grandmother			
Grandfather			
Aunt(s)			
Uncle(s)			
Cousin(s)			
Other			
Example—Aunt	Uterine cancer—48 years of age		

breast cancer in Ashkenazi Jews, thalassemias in Southeast Asians).

Genetics primer

Understanding the molecular genetic basis of a disorder is vital to understanding disease risk, selecting appropriate molecular testing, understanding the limitations of any test result, and determining the potential impact for other family members. Genetic disorders can be classified in one of three categories: chromosomal, single gene, and multifactorial; the emerging category of "oligogenic disorders" is classified with the multifactorial disorders.

Chromosomal disorders

Chromosomal disorders are disorders that result from numerical or structural alterations in one or more chromosomes. Chromosomal disorders cause a wide range of

prenatal and pediatric problems; some of these manifest psychiatric or behavioral concerns in children and others predispose to later-onset psychiatric disorders.

PEARLS & PERILS

- All chromosomal disorders are described by means of a standard set of abbreviations and nomenclature.
- When a chromosomal test is ordered or the test results are reviewed, it is important to ask:
  - What chromosome (or segment of chromosome) is duplicated or lost?
  - Is this specific chromosomal abnormality well described clinically and, if so, what current and future medical concerns should be addressed or screened for in this patient?
  - What is the likelihood that the patient's children and other family members will have the same or related chromosomal abnormality?

Routine chromosomal or karyotype analysis is used to evaluate the number and structure of the chromosomes. This analysis is most often performed using blood or amniotic cells, but it can be carried out on cultured skin fibroblasts or chorionic villi as well. Cells are induced to enter metaphase, fixed, and giemsa-stained for microscopic examination of the number and pattern of the chromosomes. Cytogeneticists examine the banding pattern to identify structural changes with a lower limit of resolution of 3–4 megabases. Structural chromosomal disorders include unbalanced chromosomal translocations, deletions, insertions, and duplications. These chromosomal alterations cause clinical disorders because they create genetic imbalance despite retaining the normal number of chromosomes. In contrast, aneuploidy is the loss or gain of a chromosome (e.g. trisomy 21 or Down syndrome). These major chromosomal disorders typically come to medical attention because of multiple congenital anomalies, with developmental and/or growth delays. While the major medical concerns and developmental delay are typically of concern in childhood, a growing number of people with major chromosomal abnormalities are living to adulthood. Evidence of an increased predisposition for adult-onset disorders, including psychiatric disease, is being documented. For instance, adults with Down syndrome have a higher frequency of depression and early onset dementia than the general population.

Microdeletion syndromes are increasingly being recognized as the molecular etiology of a number of well-described genetic syndromes. Each of these syndromes is caused by a deletion of a particular region of a chromosome that is too small to be identified on routine karyotype analysis but can be identified using fluorescent in-situ hybridization (FISH) with chromosomal analysis. A FISH probe—a small, fluorescent-tagged DNA fragment specific to the DNA sequence in the area of deletion—is hybridized to metaphase chromosomes. In normal individuals, the probe hybridizes to the appropriate sequence and a fluorescent signal is visible on each of the paired chromosomes. If the individual has the microdeletion, only one of the pair of chromosomes will have a fluorescent signal. While routine karyotyping is an appropriate general diagnostic test in individuals with multiple congenital anomalies, development delay, short stature or other concerns, FISH testing is appropriate only to confirm the diagnosis of a single disorder of concern. Since the FISH probe is specific for a single DNA segment, knowledge of the clinical features of the particular microdeletion syndrome is necessary to decide whether FISH testing would be useful. If a microdeletion is identified, heritability of the syndrome must also be discussed with the family. Individuals with a microdeletion have a 1:2 chance of passing on the abnormal chromosome, and the syndrome, to each of their offspring. Microdeletions often arise *de novo* in an individual, but it is important to note that many microdeletion syndromes have a variable clinical manifes-

tation. Hence, it is not uncommon for a parent of an affected individual to be undiagnosed but carry the deletion. Since diagnosis could have important clinical implications for the individual and their other offspring, the testing of parents should be considered in these disorders (see Case 24.2).

Subtelomeric microaberrations represent a unique group of syndromes resulting from alterations in the subtelomeric regions of chromosomes. Telomeres are gene-rich areas located near the ends of chromosomes, and cryptic rearrangements or deletions have recently been shown to occur in 4–10% of children with developmental delay or mental retardation and dysmorphic features. There is also some data to suggest other childhood neuropsychiatric disorders may be associated with subtelomeric microaberrations. Because insufficient data are available to discern whether particular clinical presentations are associated with subtelomeric microaberrations on particular chromosomes, a panel of 41 subtelomeric FISH probes has been developed and is available clinically. As additional data accumulate on these disorders, their frequency and the frequency of neuropsychiatric concerns in these disorders will become more clear.

Comparative genomic hybridization is a method for surveying the entire genome for microscopic deletions or insertions. After the entire genome of the test (patient) case is labeled fluorescently with one color, and a normal (control) genome is labeled with a different color, the two are mixed and then hybridized to normal metaphase chromosomes. A computer then detects areas where the two fluorescent signals are unequal, indicating a gain or loss of DNA in the test (patient) sample. This very powerful tool is utilized in research studies, but major technical limitations preclude clinical use at this time.

Mendelian disorders

Mendelian disorders are disorders caused by inheritance of mutations in a single gene located on a nuclear chromosome (in contrast to mitochondrial disorders). A brief review of Mendelian patterns of inheritance follows, with examples to illustrate practical considerations.

Autosomal dominant conditions are encoded by genes lying on the autosomes (chromosomes 1–22) and expressed in heterozygotes; i.e., individuals with one copy of the normal gene and one copy of the mutant gene show the clinical manifestations of the condition. For autosomal dominant disorders, there is a 50% chance of passing the mutant gene, and the disorder, on to each offspring. An affected individual with a negative family history may have developed the disorder because of a spontaneous new mutation. In many autosomal dominant conditions, penetrance and expressivity affect the clinical findings in a given individual. Penetrance is the proportion of individuals with a disease causing mutation that show clinical evidence of the disease. Although penetrance is an all-or-none phenomenon, there may be "age

Karen is a 20-year-old woman who was diagnosed with schizophrenia at 14 years of age. Her parents recently transferred her care from a child psychiatrist to an adult psychiatrist. Her new physician refers her for a medical genetics evaluation, as he is concerned that she may have an underlying genetic syndrome given her complex medical history and early onset of schizophrenia.

Karen has a history of a cleft palate, repaired at one year of age, and a ventricular septal defect, which required surgical intervention at three years of age. She had significant learning concerns but was able to complete high school. Upon evaluation by the medical geneticist, she is noted to have mild dysmorphic features, including a long narrow face, broad nasal bridge and tip, and slender, tapered fingers. There is no family history of learning concerns or birth defects. The geneticist is concerned about chromosome 22 deletion syndrome. Chromosomal testing using fluorescent in-situ hybridization (FISH) specific for chromosome 22q11 is ordered, and a microdeletion of one of the two 22nd chromosomes is identified. This testing confirms the diagnosis of Shprintzen syndrome, also known as velo-cardio-facial syndrome, based on the clinical history, dysmorphology examination, and chromosomal analysis.

The chromosome 22q11 deletion is the most common autosomal deletion, occurring in 1 in every 4,000 births. Nearly 90% of affected individuals share the same deleted chromosome region, encompassing an estimated 30 genes. The genes critical for distinguishing the phenotypic variation have not been elucidated.

The common clinical characteristics associated with Shprinzten syndrome include conotruncal heart defects, hypocalcemia, cleft palate, mild dysmorphic features including broad nasal root and tip, and slender, tapered fingers. Delays in motor and speech development, learning concerns, and mental retardation are common. Significant variability exists among affected individuals and families. Psychiatric disease, including bipolar disease and schizophrenia, is commonly noted in adults with Shprintzen syndrome, occurring more frequently among adults than children.

For Karen, the medical geneticist aided in her diagnostic assessment. After the diagnosis was made, the genetic counselor worked with Karen and her family to provide information about the clinical features and chromosomal basis of the disorder. Given that there was no family history of heart disease, cleft palate, learning disability or psychiatric disease, it was most likely that Karen's chromosome deletion arose *de novo*. As such, Karen's siblings would have little risk of having the same chromosome deletion. Karen's parents may consider chromosomal testing if they wish to confirm they do not carry the deleted chromosome and their other children are not at risk. The chance Karen could have an affected child, however, is 50%. Genetic counseling in this regard is complicated by the clinical variability that exists within and among affected families. If Karen wanted to know prenatally if a pregnancy was affected, chorionic villus sampling (CVS) or amniocentesis could be performed to obtain fetal cells for FISH analysis. This technology is limited by the inability to correlate the results with practical clinical information. The medical genetics team assisted Karen and her family by identifying her disorder, and providing education, counseling, and coordination of her health care.

dependent" penetrance, particularly in adult-onset disorders. In disorders with age-dependent penetrance (e.g., Huntington's disease), clinical signs and symptoms are typically absent in infancy and childhood but have an increasing probability of developing with increasing age. Understanding age-dependent penetrance is key to accurate risk assessment and counseling. Expressivity is a term used to describe the variable nature and severity of clinical manifestations. Understanding the range of variable expressivity in a given disorder is vital to diagnosis, prognosis, and accurate assessment of an individual's disease risk based on family history information (see Case 24.3).

Example: a newborn is diagnosed with tuberous sclerosis (TS) because of the presence of a cardiac rhabdomyosarcoma and cortical tubers identified on brain MRI. TS is an autosomal dominant disorder with variable expressivity and a new mutation rate of 30%. The child's parents have no known medical problems and assume their child has a new mutation. However, careful physical examination of both parents reveals that the father has diagnostic, albeit mild, findings of TS including ungual fibromas, skin pigmentation changes, and facial angiofibromas. With this information, the family is counseled about autosomal dominant inheritance. Importantly, they come to understand that future children have a 50% chance of inheriting TS and the father's siblings should consider screening for TS.

Autosomal recessive conditions are also caused by genes located on the autosomes, but only homozygotes (i.e., individuals in whom both copies of the gene are mutated) are affected. Expressivity and penetrance are typically less relevant in autosomal recessive disorders, although in some disorders, the severity of disease may be at least partially predicted by the underlying mutation(s). Generally, the family history is negative for disease. Parents of the affected individual are considered to be "carriers," with a mutation

Carol is a 38-year-old woman who is admitted to the hospital for evaluation of a possible stroke. Her symptoms include recent onset of progressive swallowing difficulties and hoarse voice. She has had four similar episodes over the last three years with gradual partial recovery from each. Previous neuroimaging studies revealed limited areas of non-specific white matter disease. A brain MRI was performed on admission and showed multiple areas of old infarction, including a subacute infarct of the right corona radiata and three new areas of infarct. Brain angiography was normal. She has no other medical problems and no history of hypertension, hypercholesterolemia or tobacco use.

Carol is married, with two healthy daughters, ages 12 and 10. She has three younger living siblings. Her only brother has a history of migraine headaches. Carol's mother is alive and well at 64 years of age. Carol's father died nearly 30 years ago at 42 years of age. He was diagnosed with multiple sclerosis. A paternal uncle also died at a young age with a diagnosis of multiple sclerosis.

Carol's physician raises the possibility of CADASIL, given her clinical history of early age infarcts and her father's (and uncle's) history of white matter disease. CADASIL is an acronym for Cerebral Autosomal Dominant Arteriopathy with Subcortical Infarcts and Leukencephalopathy. This highly penetrant disease is characterized by early onset of recurrent ischemic strokes, pseudobulbar palsy, gait disturbance, pyramidal signs, and sphincter incontinence. The mean age of onset is 45 years of age, and migraine headaches with aura is a common presenting symptom. No effective treatment is available, and the disease progresses until death, generally over a period of 10–15 years. The disease results from mutations in the NOTCH3 gene; the gene function is unknown. Clinical genetic testing of exons 3 and 4, where the majority of mutations exist, is available.

Consultation from the geneticist and genetic counselor is requested to aid in the diagnostic assessment, coordination of testing, and patient education. The geneticist and genetic counselor meet with Carol and her husband to review the differential diagnosis as well as the rationale, benefits, and limitations of genetic testing for CADASIL disease. A blood sample is obtained for genetic testing, and a mutation in exon 3 of the NOTCH3 gene is identified. The geneticist and genetic counselor work with the neurologist to provide Carol and her husband with the results of this analysis.

A more thorough review of the disease is provided, including a review of the clinical progression and genetic basis of the disease. In addition to her own medical outcome, Carol is concerned about the risk that her daughters have inherited the disease. Carol's children each have a 50% probability to have inherited the family mutation. In adult-onset disorders for which childhood interventions do not affect outcome, it is typically recommended that at-risk individuals not undergo presymptomatic testing until they are old enough to give informed consent.

The confirmation of a diagnosis and identification of a specific NOTCH3 gene mutation is of medical relevance to Carol's extended family. First, Carol's father's and paternal uncle's diagnoses of multiple sclerosis were incorrect. Their early-onset white matter disease is consistent with CADASIL. Second, presymptomatic genetic testing is now an option for Carol's adult family members to consider. Carol's siblings each have a 50% chance to have inherited the family mutation from their father. In contrast to Carol's diagnostic testing, presymptomatic testing provides information on disease predisposition to healthy individuals. Genetics education and counseling are often required, and always recommended, prior to presymptomatic testing of adult-onset disorders. The purpose of this intervention is to provide information about the features of the disease, available medical or surgical therapies, genetic basis and inheritance patterns, as well as the benefits and limitations of testing. The individual's rationale for testing and medical decision-making approach is explored. Potential medical and psychological consequences and benefits are examined in the context of the individual's personal life circumstances and available medical therapies.

in only one copy of the gene. Consanguineous matings are associated with increased frequency of autosomal recessive and multifactorial diseases because of the shared genetic background. However, in the majority of individuals with autosomal recessive disorders, there is no consanguinity. Parents of an affected individual have a 25% chance of having another affected child, and unaffected siblings have a two-thirds chance to be a carrier.

X-linked disorders are caused by genes on the X chromosome and may be dominant but more commonly are recessive. The mutation is typically passed from a "carrier mother" to 50% of her children. Expression is primarily seen in males because they have only one X chromosome.

Mitochondrial disorders

Mitochondrial disorders are caused by mutations in the mitochondrial genome. Mitochondria are cytoplasmic organelles that have their own small circular chromosome encoding 37 genes important in oxidative phosphorylation. Most cells contain at least 1000 mitochondrial DNA molecules. Mitochondria are replicated independently of the nuclear genome during mitosis and are randomly distributed to the daughter cells. Thus, if a cell contains a mixture of normal and mutant mitochrondrial DNA, during mitosis, by chance, a daughter cell may receive all normal, all mutant, or a mixture of mitochondrial DNA. The phenotypic expression is dependent on the relative proportion of normal and mutant mitochrondrial DNA in the tissue cells and reflects the variable expressivity associated with any mitochrondrial disease. The pattern of inheritance is distinct from autosomal dominant disorders as transmission is only maternal in origin; all children of affected females are at risk.

Multifactorial disorders

Multifactorial disorders are caused by the combined effects of multiple genes, each of which has limited individual impact on phenotype and environmental effects. Genetic epidemiologic studies suggest that schizophrenia, major depression, bipolar disorders, autism, panic disorders, addiction, substance abuse, and even some behavioral traits such as impulsivity are multifactorial disorders with significant genetic components. Studying multifactorial diseases is complicated by several factors, each of which seems particularly confounding in psychiatric disorders and explains, in part, why advances in psychiatric genetics lag behind other disciplines. Multifactorial diseases typically have significant variation in severity of symptoms and age of onset, which results in difficulty defining an appropriate phenotype and selecting the best population to study. These disorders vary widely in their etiologic mechanism so there may be a number of different biological pathways involved. Identifying the appropriate environmental factors is key and can be very complex in psychiatric disorders.

Example: family, twin, and other studies clearly indicate that alcohol dependence has strong genetic and environmental influences. It is clear that social norms and exposure to alcohol influence the triggering of the genetic susceptibility (i.e., if one lives in a society in which alcohol consumption is stringently limited either in availability or by strong social norms, a genetic predisposition to alcohol dependence is mitigated). In a society in which alcohol use is more prevalent, such as much of the United States, genetic susceptibility is more likely to emerge. However, within the United States, social norms vary tremendously, and a single individual likely has significant exposure to several norms (e.g., parental, familial, peer, and workplace). For every psychiatric disorder with a genetic component, current studies suggest a complex interaction between genes and environment, which may begin very early in life. Teasing out the relevant environmental influences is an epidemiologic challenge that must be met to truly understand the genetics of this disorder. A number of approaches are used to determine the relative role of environment and genetics and to identify specific environmental risk factors and susceptibility genes.

Family studies assess the proportion of affected relatives of a specific relationship (e.g., first degree, second degree, etc.) to a proband. These studies can suggest genetic susceptibility but, because families share a common environment, do not prove a genetic susceptibility. These studies provide information for empiric risk recurrence, which can be very useful to families and is discussed in detail in Case 24.4.

Twin studies have been very useful in studying complex diseases, and they have been used extensively in psychiatric genetics. Classical twin studies compare monozygotic with dizygotic twins. Since monozygotic twins arise from a single fertilized egg, they have essentially identical genetic

---

CASE 24.4

Jeanne is a 32-year-old, single woman who was diagnosed with stage II breast cancer at 30 years of age. She has completed her breast cancer treatment including mastectomy, chemotherapy, and radiation therapy. She has been disease-free for one year.

She presents to her primary care physician with concerns about her family history of bipolar disease. Her mother experienced her first manic episode at 33 years of age, when Jeanne was just three years old. Jeanne is especially concerned because she has been experiencing periods of depression and anxiety. She has been unable to stay in a steady relationship for over two years and has received poor performance reviews by her employer, where she was once on a fast-paced career track. Jeanne asks her primary care physician if she has bipolar disease. She feels destined to develop this disorder based on her personal experience and reading of the popular press. Her personal estimate of her lifetime risk for bipolar disorder is 98%.

Bipolar disease is a disease of affect, ranging from extreme elation (mania) to severe depression (see Chapter 8). Disturbances in thinking and behavior are common. The disease prevalence is estimated to be 1%, with an average age of onset in the early twenties. Twin and family studies have confirmed that a positive family history is a risk factor, with an early age of onset and the number of affected relatives associated with an increased risk. Risk estimates available from epidemiological-based research vary significantly. A child of an affected individual has an estimated 5–15% lifetime risk to develop bipolar disease. A monozygotic twin of an affected individual has a 40–70% lifetime risk to develop disease. Intensive research is under way to identify chromosomal regions and candidate genes that contribute to disease development in families with multiple affected individuals.

The primary care physician can offer Jeanne clinical reassurance. Her chance of developing bipolar disease is increased, but nowhere near as high as she believes. Clarifying her risk and offering referral to a psychologist seems most appropriate to address Jeanne's concerns. Her feelings of depression, new difficulties with relationships, and change in her work approach may be coincident with the completion of her breast cancer treatment. Jeanne may be addressing the chronic nature of her cancer diagnosis for the first time, as well as her feelings of loss and fears for the future. If necessary, a formal psychiatric assessment to either confirm or refute her suspicion may allow Jeanne to best address the underlying nature of the concerns she raises with her primary care physician.

material. Dizygotic twins have the same degree of relatedness as siblings and are expected to have approximately half their genetic material in common. If a disease is completely genetic, one would expect 100% concordance in monozygotic twins (i.e., all twin pairs would either both have the disease or both not have the disease) but dizygotic twins would differ. If a disease is completely environmental, one would not expect any more concordance between monozygotic than dizygotic twin pairs. For example, in depression 40% of monozygotic twin pairs are concordant compared with 20% of dizygotic twin pairs. From these data, an estimated heritability of 40% can be calculated, suggesting that genetics is an important susceptibility factor in this disease. One limitation of twin studies is the assumption that identical twins share more in their environment than dizygotic twins. Therefore, concordance studies comparing twin pairs who have been separated from an early age with twins who have been reared together can give additional evidence for a genetic component. These registries are small and rare but quite valuable.

A variation of twin studies that helps to tease out the effect of environment is adoption studies. In these studies, it is assumed that an individual carries his genetic material with him but leaves behind the shared environment. If the frequency of a disease in adopted individuals is similar to that seen in individuals who remain with their biological parents, then genetic factors are likely to be more important. Conversely, if the frequency of the disease in the adopted individuals is similar to that of their adoptive parents, then environmental factors are more likely to be important. For example, approximately 10% of adopted children who have a biological parent with schizophrenia develop schizophrenia, whereas only 1% of adopted children of unaffected parents develop schizophrenia. These studies give no indication of the genes involved, but they have been important first steps in determining whether more complex genetic studies should be undertaken. Evidence suggesting that very early environmental exposures may have a lasting impact advocates for caution in interpreting these studies, however.

Polymorphisms, i.e., variations in DNA sequence, are scattered throughout the genome. The most common are single nucleotide polymorphisms (SNPs), which occur at a rate of approximately 1/1000 nucleotides. SNPs occur when a single nucleotide in a genome sequence is altered. Large, population-based studies can be used to determine whether a particular polymorphism occurs more commonly in individuals affected with a disease than in the general population. Demonstration of such an association does not imply the polymorphism causes the disease, but it does suggest the polymorphism may lie in close proximity to a disease-associated gene. Association studies can lead to identification of candidate genes that lie in a region that can be studied for causative mutations.

Laboratory evaluations

Three primary types of laboratory studies are used in the evaluation of patients suspected of having hereditary disease: cytogenetic analysis, enzyme or primary metabolic analysis, and molecular/gene analysis.

Cytogenetic analysis

Cytogenetic analysis is used to examine the number and structure of the 46 chromosomes; it cannot detect single gene disorders. This type of analysis is most often used in the evaluation of individuals with dysmorphic features, major structural abnormalities, mental retardation, and multiple pregnancy losses. Detection of microscopic rearrangements and deletions has been greatly improved with the advent of fluorescence in-situ hybridization (FISH) technology as discussed previously.

Enzyme or primary metabolic analysis

Enzyme and metabolic analyses are used for the evaluation of inborn errors of metabolism and lysosomal storage diseases. Overlap between normal and heterozygote enzyme levels may exist, making carrier detection for autosomal recessive disorders problematic. Blood, urine or skin fibroblasts may be required for testing.

Molecular/gene analysis

DNA analysis remains primarily limited to the evaluation of single gene disorders, but it is the method of choice when available. Testing is most often performed using a sample of blood, making testing logistics straightforward.

Interpreting tests for Mendelian disorders

Genetic testing is available for hundreds of disorders. Understanding the molecular basis of the disease is important in order to decide when to do genetic testing and accurately interpret the results. Mendelian disorders may be monogenic (e.g., all neurofibromatosis is caused by mutations in the neurofibromin gene) or oligogenic [e.g., hereditary non-polyposis colon cancer can be caused by mutations in any of several genes involved in DNA repair (MLH1, MSH2, MSH6, etc.)]. At the DNA level, a disorder may be caused by a single allele (e.g., sickle cell disease is a monogenic, monoallelic disorder caused by a single base pair change that effects a substitution of valine for glutamic acid at position six of the beta-globin polypeptide) or multi-allelic (e.g., cystic fibrosis may be caused by more than 100 allelic mutations in the CFTR gene, making cystic fibrosis a monogenic, multi-allelic disorder).

Knowing these factors for any genetic disease allows the clinician to ask: What gene test(s) should be ordered? How complicated (and expensive) is the test? What does it mean if no mutation is found? Is it because this individual does not have the disease in question or because the currently available genetic testing lacks sensitivity and does not identify all disease-causing mutations? To best answer these questions and facilitate appropriate test selection and interpretation of results, one should request consultation from a geneticist and/or review information on the GeneTests website (www.genetests.org) as well as discuss the testing with individuals at the molecular diagnostic laboratory performing the test *prior* to ordering the test (Table 24.3).

Gene mutations themselves can be classified as single nucleotide substitutions, deletions, insertions or trinucleotide expansion disorders. The first three types influence the design (and cost) of diagnostic testing, and elucidation of types of mutations has led to better understanding of gene function. Trinucleotide repeat disorders have unique clinical characteristics that are a reflection of the underlying molecular defect and have important clinical implications. Huntington disease was the first trinucleotide expansion disorder identified. Many of these disorders are adult-onset, neurodegenerative disorders, and some have a psychiatric component. Examples include Fragile X, spinocerebellar ataxias, and myotonic dystrophy. The genes involved all have a nucleotide triplet (typically CAG) that is normally present in the DNA sequence as a repetitive sequence $(CAGCAGCAG_n)$ within the gene or its regulatory sequences. These trinucleotide sequences may vary in length in the population, but have an upper limit of normal. Individuals with the disease have a trinucleotide repeat length that exceeds a critical level. The size of the nucleotide expansion is correlated with severity and earlier onset of disease. Importantly, the expanded repeat is unstable, leading to possible further expansion of the repeat in the next generation, resulting in more severe disease.

The concept of increasing severity or earlier age of onset in subsequent generations is called "anticipation" and has been clearly proven only at the molecular level in this set of disorders. Understanding anticipation is important in counseling family members. A key point to remember is that while increasing repeat size correlates with increasing severity of disease at the population level, there is sufficient individual variability so that predicting severity or age-of-onset based on repeat size is, at best, a guess. A final point necessary for genetic counseling and test interpretation is a test result in the "premutation range." These repeat lengths are small enough that the individual has a normal functioning gene and is not at risk to develop the disease. However, the repeat length is in the unstable range, so the individual is at risk to have an affected child.

Interpreting tests for multifactorial diseases

Most multifactorial disease analyses are still at the research stage. For many diseases, multiple candidate loci or genes have been identified, but identifying alleles (variants or polymorphisms) within these genes, proving they are associated with disease, and finally determining the level of risk conferred by a particular allele are arduous tasks. When an allele is clearly shown to confer risk, it provides tremendous insights into the mechanism of disease and the development of targeted therapy. However, the value of such tests for medical decision making in individual patients must be carefully considered. For example, the apolipoprotein E (ApoE) gene has three common alleles, E2, E3, and E4, that are present in the population as six genotypes. Genetic epidemiologic data clearly demonstrate that inheritance of one ApoE4 allele is associated with an earlier onset and higher relative risk of Alzheimer's disease (AD). Inheritance of E2 alleles is relatively protective. Studies of Caucasian populations demonstrate that homozygotes for the E4 allele are 15 times more likely to develop AD than the general population. The risk appears to be higher in Japanese individuals and somewhat lower for Hispanic and African-American subjects.

While this relative risk is quite striking, the predictive value of ApoE allelotyping in an individual is limited. If an individual is identified to be homozygous for the E4 allele, the lifetime risk for AD is estimated to be 30–50%. ApoE testing is currently *not* recommended because the positive predictive value is quite low, the psychological burden of being at risk for AD may be substantial, and prevention through presymptomatic interventions has not been demonstrated. However, if additional AD susceptibility genes, together with ApoE status, provided greater predictive value, or if new therapeutic strategies were developed, ApoE testing might become a useful clinical test. Consideration of ApoE testing highlights several important concepts that should be considered when ordering any genetic susceptibility test. Relative risk may be dramatic, but positive and negative predictive values are more important in the care of individuals. There may be ethnic variation in both the frequency of the alleles and the degree of risk conferred by an allele, reflecting a different genetic background and perhaps differences in environment. Therefore, it is important to know whether the ethnic background of the patient has been adequately represented in population studies. Caution should be used in ordering susceptibility tests if early detection has not been shown to be of benefit, particularly in diseases that carry a substantial psychological burden. For all such diseases, the practitioner must have sufficient up-to-date knowledge about the disease as well as the test in order to appropriately and accurately counsel patients about potential risks and benefits.

It is almost certain that susceptibility genes will be identified for many common diseases, including psychiatric diseases, in the next several years. Panels of susceptibility genes (e.g., a cardiovascular risk profile, an Alzheimer's disease risk profile, an affective disorder risk profile, etc.) might soon be clinically available. For genetic tests, as for any test, the

TABLE 24.3

Medical genetics information resources

Resource	Sponsor	Information available
Genetests www.genetests.org	Roberta Pagon, MD, Peter Tarczy-Hornoch, MD, University of Washington	Database of clinical and research testing laboratories searchable by location, disease name, gene name, or protein product. Catalog of medical genetics clinical services searchable by location, service, or specialty. Expert-authored and peer-reviewed descriptions of 225 genetic diseases (GeneReviews). Illustrated glossary of terms and genetics teaching materials.
Online Inheritance in Man (OMIM) www.ncbi.nih.gov/omim	Dr Victor McKuzick, MD, Johns Hopkins University, National Center for Biotechnology Information	Database of genetic conditions including catalog of human genes. Nearly 15 000 disease-specific entries. Catalog of disease genes organized by genes (OMIM Morbid Map). Catalog of cytogenetic map location of disease genes (OMIM Gene Map).
Office of Genomics and Disease Prevention www.cdc.gov/genomics	Office of Genomics and Disease Prevention Centers for Disease Control	Information on policy, guidelines, and ethics related to genetics and society. Position papers and reports on the public health perspective of medical genetics advances.
National Human Genome Research Institute www.nhgri.nih.gov	National Human Genome Research Institute National Institutes of Health	Information on frequently asked questions about genetics and specific genetic disorders. Educational resources on the Human Genome Project, genetics teaching modules, and a glossary of genetic terms with downloadable illustrations. Information on policy and ethical issues including privacy, discrimination, social and cultural issues related to medical genetics.
Genetic Alliance www.geneticalliance.org	The Genetic Alliance	Database of national genetic support groups searchable by disease or organization name. Healthcare insurance information for individuals with genetic disease. Disease-specific database searchable using the Disease Infosearch™ tool.
Genetics in Primary Care Training Program genes-r-us.uthscsa.edu/resources/genetics/primary_care.htm	Genetics in Primary Care National Newborn Screening and Genetics Resource Center	Genetics training modules which use representative patients seen in primary care.
Genetics Societies Homepage genetics.faseb.org/genetics	Federation of American Societies of Experimental Biology	Links to seven recognized professional genetic societies including American Society of Human Genetics and American College of Medical Genetics.
National Society of Genetic Counselors www.nsgc.org	National Society of Genetic Counselors	Database of genetic counselors searchable by location, institution, name or specialty. Consumer information about genetic counseling.

The clinical utility of genetic laboratory studies depends on the question being asked and the given clinical context: diagnostic, predictive/presymptomatic or reproductive/family planning. Consider a 29-year-old woman who has clinical features consistent with dementia and a three-generation paternal family history of early-onset dementia in multiple relatives consistent with hereditary dementia. Molecular genetic testing is available. A variety of questions may be raised by the patient, her family, and her physicians. Consideration of several of these questions helps illustrate the role, benefits, and limitations of molecular testing.

Question 1: Does the patient have a diagnosis of hereditary dementia? In this situation, genetic testing provides little additional information beyond what is clinically obvious and offers minimal value in her personal diagnostic assessment. In contrast, genetic laboratory studies are more useful when a diagnosis is not absolutely certain. For an 18-year-old man who is diagnosed with a pheochromocytoma, testing may identify a cancer predisposition syndrome that is the underlying basis for his presenting illness.

Question 2: What is the disease-causing mutation in this family with hereditary dementia? Genetic testing is of significant utility in answering this question. Identifying the specific mutation does not provide the patient with much additional clinical information, but it is of critical importance in offering presymptomatic testing to at-risk relatives. To be

most informative, an affected family member (a known mutation carrier) is tested first so the specific family mutation can be identified. If a mutation is not identified in an affected relative, presymptomatic testing cannot be offered to family members. If a mutation is identified, molecular genetic testing can be used to determine the genetic status of at-risk relatives.

Question 3: The 32-year-old sister of the young woman with dementia is currently 12 weeks pregnant. What is the likelihood the fetus inherited the family mutation for early-onset hereditary dementia? This risk can be calculated as 25%. (There is a 50% chance that the mother inherited the mutation x 50% chance that the fetus inherited the mutation.) More definite risk can be identified using prenatal genetic analysis, but this involves significant ethical issues. Prenatal diagnostic testing for adult-onset disorders is often limited and, in some laboratories, not offered because there is an ethical concern regarding the performance of presymptomatic testing on an individual (the fetus) without consent. Prenatal testing is more often available for diseases when there is no available treatment, onset occurs in childhood, penetrance approaches 100%, and the couple is strongly considering pregnancy termination. Use of genetic testing for reproductive planning is not always this complex, but ethical concerns, family choice, and current status of testing and treatment always should be considered carefully.

thoughtful practitioner should consider the pretest probability of disease, the positive and negative predictive value of the test, the utility of a positive or negative test in medical decision making, and most importantly, the needs and interests of the individual patient (see Case 24.5).

Risk assessment and genetic counseling

The term "genetic counselling" was credited to Sheldon Reed, who used it in the late 1940s to describe the provision of genetic services to families, including the need to address psychosocial sequelae associated with hereditary disease. Genetic counselors are allied health professionals who typically work with geneticists, perinatologists, and obstetricians; they may also work side by side with neurologists, oncologists, surgeons, and cardiologists. Genetic counselors are masters-level trained professionals with extensive training and coursework in medical and molecular genetics, cytogenetics, developmental biology, embryology, teratology, biostatistics, epidemiology, counseling, communication, and ethics.

In 1974, the American Society of Human Genetics defined the practice of genetic counseling including a non-directive tenet that has continued in today's practice. A non-directive approach was appropriately advocated because genetic counselors primarily work with families making family planning decisions. The non-directive approach has remained an important tenet given the lack of data to identify

the most appropriate medical approach (e.g., ovarian cancer surveillance among women with hereditary breast cancer). While there exist some differences, non-directive counseling is likened to patient-centered care. As genetics expands, the scope of genetic counseling is also evolving, but the central goal remains helping patients understand genetic information in order to aid personal and medical decision making.

An additional important component of genetic medicine is deciding how genetic professionals and primary care physicians should work together to provide genetic medicine. For many individuals with or at-risk for disease, their needs are best addressed in the primary care setting. However, there are always families who benefit from the formal genetic assessment and genetic counseling offered in a specialty genetics clinic.

CONSIDER CONSULTATION WHEN...

- Individuals with a "rare" genetic disorder seek counsel on the long-term medical complications (e.g., Turner's syndrome).
- Individuals with a suspected genetic condition cannot be diagnosed by the primary care physician.
- Individuals request extensive genetics education and counseling (e.g., hereditary dementia).
- Individuals require complex genetic testing (e.g., spinocerebellar ataxias or mitochrondrial diseases).

TABLE 24.4

Components of risk assessment and genetic counseling

Component	Description
Evaluate medical/family history	Collect detailed medical history including medical records prior to evaluation. Obtain three-generation pedigree prior to evaluation. Collection of medical records on affected family members may be required in advance to verify reported diagnoses
Provide genetics education	Review the clinical features, genetic basis, inheritance pattern, recurrence risk data, available prophylactic medical and surgical therapies, and diagnostic or predictive genetic testing options Communicate laboratory screening test or genetic test results, including positive predictive value of a given test result
Establish clinical care network	Inform all caring physicians of genetic diagnosis including short- and long-term medical implications Assist with obtaining physician referrals and insurance coverage for intensified surveillance, if indicated Update patient and physicians on new developments that may impact long-term medical management Serve as a resource center for caring physicians with questions about specific diagnoses

Encourage health promotion	Encourage healthy lifestyle changes that may reduce risk
	    Smoking cessation class
	    Scheduled exercise programs
	Promote body awareness and self-examinations
	    Breast self-examination
	    Skin examination
	    Blood pressure checks

Address psychosocial issues	Address psychosocial issues associated with hereditary disease, identifying mechanisms for adaptation and personal control Encourage psychological counseling with psychologist or psychiatrist if psychological distress associated with a given syndrome negatively impacts daily activities
Coordinate genetic testing	Collect genetic testing information including specificity and sensitivity of testing technique, laboratory that performs the analysis, specimen processing requirements and testing charges Obtain informed consent to conduct the testing

For adults with, or at-risk for, common diseases with a genetic component, the focus of genetic counseling should be:

- to identify the patient's understanding of the disease etiology and processes
- to advance understanding of accurate disease risk perception
- to assist with adaptation to disease risk
- to promote a healthy lifestyle and disease surveillance practices
- to advocate feelings of personal control and well-being.

Several components of the genetic counseling process are required to achieve this focus and are listed in Table 24.4. Two components require further discussion. Establishment of a clinical care network—a team of physicians and health care providers who will collaboratively provide care reflective of genetic liability—is an essential component in the care of adults with genetic disease. For the genetic counselor, this requires not only providing the patient with personally meaningful information necessary for self-advocacy but also informing primary care providers of the associated increased risks for disease, intensified surveillance practices, or prophylactic medical and surgical options, when available. It is common for genetic counselors to play a pivotal role in securing appropriate medical services for affected individuals long after genetic counseling has been offered. The coordination and explanation of genetic testing are other key components, but they are often perceived by physicians unfamiliar with the practice as the *only* components. As noted previously, the utility of genetic testing information varies depending on the context and clinical question. Families may benefit from genetic assessment and educational information without pursuing genetic testing, even when it is available.

Psychological factors associated with presymptomatic testing

Presymptomatic, predictive genetic testing, whether for highly penetrant single gene disorders or for disease associations, is being offered more commonly for medical management purposes. Huntington's disease was the first adult-onset disorder for which presymptomatic genetic testing was offered. Testing was conducted under extensive pre-test education and psychological evaluation protocols with post-test assessment. Presymptomatic Huntington's disease testing was the test case for the ethical scrutiny of the advances brought about by genetics research. Studies began to evaluate the psychological sequelae associated with presymptomatic prediction of disease and have continued with the institution of testing for hereditary cancer and other degenerative neurologic diseases.

Overall, these studies have shown a decrease in distress levels for both carriers and non-carriers following testing. For individuals who did not pursue testing, psychological distress has remained the same or increased. These results suggest what is often observed in the clinical setting: knowing the results, whether good or bad, is easier to adjust to than the gray cloud of uncertainty. Furthermore, pre-test emotional state is more predictive of post-test outcome than the results of the testing. Overall, significant psychological disturbance has not been identified with presymptomatic genetic testing.

Although these results are encouraging, interpretation should be considered cautiously for several reasons: most studies have followed participants for less than three years following testing; the highly motivated individuals who participated in these studies may not be representative of the majority of people seeking predictive testing; and the research protocols included intensive, carefully monitored counseling and support, which may not be replicated in clinical settings. Furthermore, it is unknown whether similar results would be found for individuals seeking association testing, in which the predictability of disease is less certain.

Genetic discrimination

Professional medical societies, patient-focused disease organizations, and the popular media have appropriately raised concerns regarding the possibility of genetic discrimination, defined as the use of genetic information (genetic testing or family history information) in underwriting decisions. In the early 1990s, a flurry of legislation was introduced around the United States prohibiting genetic discrimination. Not all states enacted such laws and for those that did, protection varied dramatically.

Despite the flood of legislative activity there has been only cursory evidence to suggest discrimination is a reality. Hall and Rich found no well-documented cases of insurers requesting presymptomatic genetic test results, either before or after non-discriminatory laws were passed. Highly publicized media reports along with the growing legislative efforts sends a mixed, contradictory message to patients with no evidence to document the risk. Health professionals have done little to clarify the issue, continuing to advise patients

to seek genetic information outside an insurance company's purview. Consequently, individuals who could use genetic information to alter their medical decision making or family planning decisions have forgone testing over fear of discrimination. Likewise, patients seeking genetic testing directly by paying "out-of-pocket" have done so with a false sense of security, believing that only the ordering physician would have access to the results. Ironically, patients have sought testing for reasons related to medical decision making but have done so in a way that limits the dialog and coordination of care among their physicians.

Unlike any other medical evaluation, genetic testing has become almost mystical, clouded by the fear of genetic discrimination. Individuals seeking genetic information are challenged to wade through the hype and fear surrounding genetic testing in order to make decisions that are most appropriate for their given situation. While a reasonable degree of concern about genetic discrimination is appropriate, fear of such discrimination should not prevent individuals from considering testing that may have significant medical relevance.

Annotated bibliography

Ensenauer, RE, Reinke, SS, Ackerman, MJ, Tester, DJ, Whiteman, DAH, and Tefferi, A (2003) Primer on medical genomics part VIII: essentials of medical genetics for the practicing physician, *Mayo Clin Proc* 78: 846–857.
This is part of an excellent series of articles on medical genomics that is directed toward the primary care physician and non-genetics specialist. Areas of review include: history of genetics and sequencing the human genome, methods in molecular genetics, microarray experiments and data analysis, expression proteomics, bioinformatics, molecular genetics in clinical practice, the evolving concept of the gene, clinical applications of microarrays, gene therapy, pharmacogenomics, and ethical and regulatory issues. The entire series of articles is listed in Tefferi, A and Spelsberg, TC (2004) Primer on medical genomics: the end of the beginning, Mayo Clin Proc 79: 659–660.

Harper, P (in press) *Practical Genetic Counseling*, 6th Edition, Oxford, Butterworth-Heinemann.
This text is often used by genetic counselors and medical geneticists but is highly valuable to primary care physicians. An introduction of the principles of genetic counseling, calculation of genetic risks, and basic principles of Mendelian, non-Mendelian, and chromosomal syndromes is provided. Brief descriptions of the genetic basis of numerous genetic conditions and common diseases are provided including schizophrenia and affective psychoses.

Khoury, M, Burke, W, Thompson, E (eds) (2000) *Genetics and Public Health in the 21st Century. Using genetic information to improve health and prevent disease*, Oxford University Press, New York.
This text defines a framework for the integration of genetics into public health. Topics reviewed include population genetic screening, evaluation of genetic testing, delivery mechanisms of genetics services, and the ethical, legal, and social issues associated with new advances in medical genetics.

King, R, Rotter, J, Motulsky, A (eds) (2002) *The Genetic Basis of Common Diseases*, 2nd Edition, New York, Oxford University Press.

This excellent text provides an extensive description of the genetic features of common diseases. Introductory chapters review the approach to studying complex common diseases. Chapters on cardiopulmonary diseases, immunologic and infectious diseases, gastrointestinal and endocrine disorders, rheumatologic diseases, cancer and neuropsychiatric disorders are included. The genetic and epidemiologic evidence, the biological basis of genetic susceptibility, as well as the clinical application of genetic information, are provided in each chapter.

Yoon, PW, Scheuner, MT, and Khoury, MJ (2003) Research priorities for evaluating family history in the prevention of common chronic diseases, *Am J Prev Med* 24(2): 128–135.

This article reviews the use of family history tools in stratifying risk for common diseases and identifying individuals with increased disease susceptibility. The authors review the critical research issues necessary to validate a family history tool that would be useful in the public health setting. This article summarizes a workshop convened to assess the validity of family history in the prevention of common diseases. This journal issue contains additional articles written from the workshop including family history assessment of cardiovascular disease, diabetes, asthma, and cancer.

CHAPTER 25

Adolescent Issues

John N. Constantino, MD and Richard E. Mattison, MD

Introduction

Although many of the problems of adolescents are related to the developmental tasks of the adolescent period, primary care physicians should be cognizant of the rates of psychiatric disorders in this age group and of their associated serious dysfunction. The most recent epidemiological studies have found rates of psychiatric disorders in general adolescent populations of 15–20%. Whereas some disorders, such as attention-deficit/hyperactivity disorder (ADHD), may persist from childhood, other diagnoses often have their onset during adolescence. These include affective disorders, anorexia nervosa, and substance abuse.

It is often assumed that adolescence is a time of significant turmoil, however, research has demonstrated that the majority of teenagers negotiate this period of development with fairly minimal social, academic, or familial disruption. Given the 15–20% rate of psychiatric disorders in this population, signs of serious life dysfunction during adolescence should be carefully evaluated.

This chapter first briefly reviews the major developmental tasks of adolescence. Next, the physician's role in the assessment of adolescent psychopathological conditions is considered. This is followed by a discussion of the evaluation and care of major psychiatric disorders of adolescence. Finally, issues pertaining to teenagers with chronic medical disorders and accompanying psychopathological conditions, as well as issues related to teenagers with physical symptoms but no established medical basis, are also discussed.

Developmental tasks and problems in adolescence

Struggles with issues of identity and self-esteem are common in adolescence. The physical and psychological transitions from dependency on the family to autonomy (and reproductive competency) are central developmental tasks of adolescence. The process is, in part, driven by cognitive development (including acquisition of the capacity for formal operational and abstract thinking) and by the physiological phenomenon of puberty.

Children initially develop their identities in the context of their families. Ideally they achieve a sense of uniqueness and importance as individuals and a sense that they are connected in stable relationships with family members. In adolescence, the individual develops personal standards to replace those of family members and forms an identity based on his or her perceived place in the societal context beyond the family. Adolescence is often seen as a time of conflict, and indeed it is only through conflict in the real world that many adolescents achieve sufficient understanding of themselves to develop their own standards. The common problems of adolescents can often be related to basic issues of independence and the formation of a personal identity. For example, a parent's intrusion into an adolescent's physical or social domain may be met with resentment because it is perceived as overt nonrecognition of his or her independence. Adolescents may withdraw or insist on being left alone when they perceive a threat to their autonomy. Conversely, adolescent delinquency often clashes with norms that represent authority and control.

Physicians can try to help parents understand their adolescent's transition into adulthood in such terms, and they can help parents understand their own reactions to their adolescent's emerging autonomy. At the same time, parents need to set limits on the basis of ensuring safety, which may help prevent harmful consequences of judgment errors. Recent research indicates that in stressed or high-risk environments, it may be more difficult (if not impossible) for parents to walk the fine line of compromise between restriction and the provision of freedom. For example, efforts to protect adolescents from various forms of victimization or violence may necessitate difficult decisions about restrictions on social or peer-related activities that are important for normal development. Less-than-stable family structures add greatly to the difficulties associated with striking a reasonable balance.

Office assessment

Time constraints in the primary care practice environment result in a tendency to under-diagnose psychiatric disorders and therefore to under-refer when they are present. Nevertheless, it often falls upon the primary care physician to determine whether an adolescent has psychological symptoms of a transient nature or of a more fully developed psychiatric disorder, which requires exploration. The reality for most physicians is that there is a limited amount of time per patient, certainly not the hour or more that is usually necessary to adequately assess a teenager's or a parent's complaints about possible psychiatric conditions. Some physicians solve this dilemma by setting aside a regularly scheduled block of longer appointment times for adolescents about whom they are particularly concerned.

Another approach is the use of established screening instruments to help evaluate an adolescent's or a parent's concerns. Such an empirical approach can be practical and effective, and it uses the physician's limited time wisely. The Child Behavior Checklist is a widely used quantitative rating scale which measures the severity of problem behaviors by parent and/or teacher report. It identifies clinical cutoff scores for anxious/withdrawn behaviors, thought disorder, social problems, attentional problems, aggressive/delinquent behavior, and social competency. For internalizing disorders, self-report measures may be even more revealing than parent-report assessments: examples include depression inventories such as the Beck or the Reynolds, and the Yale-Brown Obsessive Compulsive Scale; these can be quickly added to a clinical assessment when the respective conditions are suspected. Using well-validated screening measures, a physician can assess the extent to which an adolescent's behavior deviates from population norms and thereby confirm suspicions that an adolescent's problems are indeed serious enough to require referral to a psychiatrist or other mental health professional.

Primary care physicians should also develop a concise interview to assess adolescents who present with behavioral or emotional problems. It is critical to determine whether or not suicidality, homicidality, psychosis, maltreatment, and/or substance abuse impairment are present. Risks for pregnancy and sexually transmitted disease should be assessed, and the physician should also briefly ascertain an adolescent's general functioning in the school setting as well as with friends and family. Finally, physicians should develop effective referral techniques and recognize that adolescents commonly fail to keep initial mental health appointments; follow-up and perseverance are important aspects of the process.

Specific psychiatric disorders in adolescents

Attention-deficit/hyperactivity disorder (ADHD)

The knowledge base regarding ADHD is growing steadily. It is now known that most children with ADHD do not outgrow the disorder (Box 25.1). The cardinal symptoms may change over the course of development. The symptom of hyperactivity may diminish to fidgetiness, which unfortunately in the past often led to the conclusion that adolescents were outgrowing the disorder (possibly related to the onset of puberty). Additionally, the childhood presentations of impulsivity and poor concentration may transform. Impulsivity in adolescence may reveal itself as poor frustration tolerance and wide mood swings with subsequent explosive anger. Poor attention and concentration may become exemplified by poor organization or planning abilities. Furthermore, accumulating complications, such as poor self-esteem, poor school performance, increasing conduct or drug problems, and strained relationships with peers and family, can add to the burden of a teenager living with ADHD.

Thus teenagers with ADHD and their families can be informed by primary care physicians that chances are good that a teenager who still has ADHD will probably have to contend with symptoms into adulthood. Some further prediction is also reasonable. The adolescent who has responded to treatment in a supportive, stable family and has not developed compromising secondary problems most likely has a good chance to continue an optimal course. In contrast, the teenager with ADHD who has coexisting symptoms of conduct disorder has a considerably worse prognosis. Indeed, such patients often have a course (followed by approximately 25% of individuals with ADHD) toward considerable life dysfunction and development of an antisocial personality disorder or complicating substance abuse. Clearly, when a physician encounters the latter struggling teenager with ADHD, the treatment plan must be intensified, with appropriate warning to the parents about the poor predictors and the parents' need to sustain if not increase their treatment efforts. Consequently, a family physician must have an established network of mental health professionals who are especially skilled in the total care of youth with ADHD and in the support of these children's families (an example of an effective national parent support network is Children and Adults with Attention Deficit Disorders or CHADD).

The primary care physician should direct a different type of attention to the child with ADHD who appears to be entering adolescence successfully; the approach is analogous to that for a child with diabetes who is entering adolescence with the disorder under good control and who desires the

Box 25.1 Attention-deficit/hyperactivity disorder

DIAGNOSTIC CRITERIA

A. Either (1) or (2):

1 Six (or more) of the following symptoms of *inattention* have persisted for at least six months to a degree that is maladaptive and inconsistent with developmental level:

Inattention

- often fails to give close attention to details or makes careless mistakes in schoolwork, work, or other activities
- often has difficulty sustaining attention in tasks or play activities
- often does not seem to listen when spoken to directly
- often does not follow through on instructions and fails to finish schoolwork, chores, or duties in the workplace (not due to oppositional behavior or failure to understand instructions)
- often has difficulty organizing tasks and activities
- often avoids, dislikes, or is reluctant to engage in tasks that require sustained mental effort (such as schoolwork or homework)
- often loses things necessary for tasks or activities (e.g., toys, school assignments, pencils, books, or tools)
- is often easily distracted by extraneous stimuli
- is often forgetful in daily activities.

2 Six (or more) of the following symptoms of *hyperactivity-impulsivity* have persisted for at least six months to a degree that is maladaptive and inconsistent with developmental level:

Hyperactivity

- often fidgets with hands or feet or squirms in seat
- often leaves seat in classroom or in other situations in which remaining seated is expected
- often runs about or climbs excessively in situations in which it is inappropriate (in adolescents or adults, may be limited to subjective feelings of restlessness)
- often has difficulty playing or engaging in leisure activities quietly
- is often "on the go" or often acts as if "driven by a motor"
- often talks excessively.

Impulsivity

- often blurts out answers before questions have been completed
- often has difficulty awaiting turn
- often interrupts or intrudes on others (e.g., butts into conversations or games).

B. Some hyperactive-impulsive or inattentive symptoms that caused impairment were present before age seven years.

C. Some impairment from the symptoms is present in two or more settings (e.g., at school [or work] and at home).

D. There must be clear evidence of clinically significant impairment in social, academic, or occupational functioning.

E. The symptoms do not occur exclusively during the course of a pervasive developmental disorder, schizophrenia, or other psychotic disorder and are not better accounted for by another mental disorder (e.g., mood disorder, anxiety disorder, dissociative disorder, or a personality disorder).

Code based on type:

- *attention-deficit/hyperactivity disorder, combined type*: if both criteria A1 and A2 are met for the past six months
- *attention-deficit/hyperactivity disorder, predominantly inattentive type*: if criterion A1 is met but criterion A2 is not met for the past six months
- *attention-deficit/hyperactivity disorder, predominantly hyperactive-impulsive type*: if criterion A2 is met but criterion A1 is not met for the past six months.

Coding note: for individuals (especially adolescents and adults) who currently have symptoms that no longer meet full criteria, "in partial remission" should be specified.

From American Psychiatric Association (2000) Diagnostic and Statistical Manual of Mental Disorders, 4th Edition, Text Revision, Washington, D.C., American Psychiatric Association.

appropriate transfer of care to increased self-management. The teenager's understanding of ADHD should be ascertained. Ideally, the adolescent has reasonable knowledge that ADHD is a chronic neurobiological disorder that is helped by medicine and appreciates the cardinal symptoms of ADHD and the common secondary problems they may cause.

The teenage patient may have already developed practical methods to deal with problems that the medicine cannot address. Commonly, such an adolescent is curious about other steps to limit or decrease the use of medicine (much like children with other chronic medical disorders). Such a teenager should be referred to an appropriate mental health professional for a brief course in self-management of ADHD's symptoms; for example, the teenager must learn to identify situations that lead to impulsive behavior and develop techniques to prevent potentially embarrassing outcomes. If possible, the goal is to establish circumstances when self-management techniques could modify medication needs. This foundation will serve the adolescent well into adulthood and the assumption of full responsibility of managing their ADHD. As an adolescent reflects on the future, a healthy understanding of personal strengths and weaknesses, taking into account the symptoms of ADHD, also helps in early career planning.

Advances in the treatment of ADHD are continuing. In general, medication is still considered necessary but not sufficient, with comprehensive treatment planning still needed as a constant consideration. Stimulants remain a drug of choice. When indicated, they are now used more chronically (including into adulthood) and comprehensively (covering the entire day). The emphasis is on the constant maintenance of high-quality functioning to permit normal development. Adolescents, in particular, have increased homework and often need the benefit of increased concentration through a late afternoon dose to successfully complete home assignments, which may in turn affect their overall school grades and overall success. Also, interpersonal relationships are vitally important, and an adolescent's uncontrolled impulsivity and hyperactivity may sabotage family and extracurricular peer activities. Thus any trial discontinuation of a teenager's medication must be carefully monitored, not only with respect to academic functioning but to overall psychosocial functioning as well. Adolescents often appreciate the long-acting, once-a-day preparations for the stimulants (available for both methylphenidate and dextroamphetamine).

A new addition to the pharmacologic armamentarium for ADHD is atomoxetine, a non-stimulant norepinephrine reuptake inhibitor with downstream influences on dopaminergic functioning. Atomoxetine has been extensively tested in adults and children with ADHD. It is a safe, generally well-tolerated, non-controlled substance, that provides round-the-clock continuous symptom relief with once-per-day dosing. It is clearly superior to placebo in patients with ADHD; its efficacy in comparison to stimulant medication is currently under investigation.

Bupropion is a safe, well-tolerated antidepressant, which has also been shown to be effective for the treatment of ADHD in controlled clinical trials. Medicines such as desipramine and clonidine are better than placebo in treating ADHD, but they are generally not as effective for concentration as a stimulant. Desipramine may more help the adolescent who has ADHD with anxiety or depressive symptoms, whereas clonidine may particularly assist the adolescent who has ADHD with more serious overactivity or aggressivity. However, desipramine may produce cardiac complications (and even associated sudden death), and sedation can be troublesome with clonidine. The use of these drugs in combination with stimulants is not yet well understood.

What should a primary care physician do, given this array of medication selections, when monitoring an adolescent who was previously stable on methylphenidate but who is now destabilizing? In such cases beyond general maintenance, consultation is the best policy. For example, a teenager whose symptoms are stable while taking a stimulant may start to show some depressive signs, which in reality are situationally related and not at the magnitude of a major depression. Addition or substitution of another medication could actually further complicate the teenager's condition (by destabilizing the ADHD or creating new side effects), but a brief course of psychotherapy could correct the problem. The dictum of medication simplicity should always be followed instead of quick polypharmacy. Unless a physician has extensive experience with the wide range of medications for ADHD, consultation with a child psychiatrist for any new complication is indicated, much as it would be in the treatment of any other medical disorder with which the physician has experience primarily in monitoring the stable, uncomplicated condition. Often, when an adolescent who has previously uncomplicated ADHD experiences a change in symptoms, the issue is not medication but some other facet of the disorder that must be addressed in a nonmedication manner.

Finally, the monitoring of ADHD by primary care physicians has been improved by the development of good empirical rating instruments (such as the Conners rating scales), which help measure the status of a teenager's symptoms. Such information is especially important with regard to school functioning. A parent typically cannot supply sufficient valid feedback about his child's school functioning, which must be obtained directly from teachers. Such teacher checklists (with either a general or ADHD-oriented focus) can be gathered twice a year—at the end of the first grading period and at the beginning of the fourth grading period—to monitor a teenager's initial adjustment and then to be sure that the stable status was maintained. Because of multiple teachers in secondary school, it is advisable to have a major subject teacher from the morning and one from the afternoon complete such forms.

Affective disorders

The primary care physician commonly encounters depressive symptoms in adolescents and must be able to distinguish transient or situational depressive states from the more dysfunctional major depressive disorder (MDD) and dysthymic disorder (see Chapter 8). Early occurrence of a depressive disorder in childhood or adolescence may indicate the beginning of a more pernicious course of affective disorder than an initial onset in adulthood. For example, childhood dysthymic disorder may take an average of several years to dissipate, and youth with MDD (despite high rates of recovery from initial episodes) appear to be at high risk for recurrence or for the eventual development of bipolar disorder (which includes episodes of mania). Additionally, a youth with a depressive disorder is at higher risk for suicidal behavior. Thus early identification and intervention are important.

In a large randomized controlled trial, the selective serotonin reuptake inhibitor (SSRI) fluoxetine was shown to be superior to placebo in the treatment of MDD in children and adolescents. In contrast, children and adolescents with MDD do not respond to tricyclic antidepressants (TCAs) better than to placebo. Lithium appears to be effective in teenagers who develop bipolar disorder (manic-depressive illness), but it also entails careful baseline and follow-up laboratory evaluations. In addition, the efficacy of anticonvulsant mood stabilizers and atypical neuroleptics for adolescents with bipolar disorder is under active investigation, following up on promising findings from case series and open trials.

Despite the bright prospects for effective psychopharmacologic intervention for many psychiatric disorders, it is important to exercise caution in extrapolating the results of adult treatment studies to the treatment of children and adolescents. An historical example of this is the fact that randomized, controlled trials of tricyclic antidepressants in the treatment of major depressive disorder in children and adolescents have been uniformly negative, despite the overwhelmingly positive results of such studies in adults. More recently, enthusiasm about the use of SSRIs to treat depression in adolescents—advanced by a successful published randomized controlled trial involving fluoxetine—has had to be tempered by (as yet unpublished) negative results of FDA trials involving paroxetine and venlafaxine in children and adolescents. These unpublished studies have additionally revealed the possibility of modest but statistically significant increases in suicidal ideation among adolescents treated with either of these specific agents, in comparison to placebo controls. Such findings have resulted in widely publicized warnings and safety recommendations, which, themselves, need to be put into perspective, since many individual adolescent patients seem to have benefited from these medications. Pending peer-reviewed publication of confirmatory studies, many practitioners have adopted the stance of avoiding the initiation of treatment with the specific SSRIs that generated these warnings (paroxetine and venlafaxine), but continuing their use among patients who appear to have improved without adverse effects as a result of their use.

Research into the efficacy of nonmedication treatments for adolescents has shown that cognitive-behavior therapy (CBT) is an effective treatment for MDD. In CBT, an adolescent is taught to identify depressive thought patterns that he may automatically engage and then to develop new, more positive ways of thinking and acting; parents can then reinforce such advancements. Studies have also begun to contrast the effectiveness of antidepressant medication alone, CBT alone, and combined therapies, much as has already been accomplished for adults with major depression.

Thus physicians who suspect a depressive disorder in an adolescent should optimally refer the youth to a psychiatrist for confirmation. They could consider initiation of a trial of an SSRI and/or CBT, after ruling out the presence of suicidal ideation or substance abuse.

Intimately related to depressive illness in adolescents is the topic of suicide, since the two conditions are often associated (see Chapter 29). Suicide attempts and completions

both markedly rise during adolescence, and completion rates in male teenagers have increased in recent years. (Overall, suicide is a leading cause of death in adolescents, along with accidents, and violence.) Male adolescents more commonly complete suicide; female adolescents more commonly attempt suicide; and completion is more common in Caucasians than in minority populations. The higher rate of male teenagers who complete suicide is probably related to the availability of firearms (their most common method) and drugs or alcohol (a common associated factor). Among adolescents who attempt suicide, up to 50% make a repeat attempt (especially during the two years after the initial attempt), and there may be an increased long-term risk for death by suicide.

In the instance of a suicide attempt by a teenager, immediate referral to an emergency room is indicated until the situation can be adequately assessed. Several factors raise the level of concern, including whether there has been a previous attempt, the seriousness of attempt, the presence of a recent disciplinary crisis or humiliation, access to drugs or firearms, a lack of family support, a history of violence, and the presence of a psychiatric disorder (not only depression, but also conduct disorder [CD], personality disorder, or substance abuse). After assessment, the primary care physician should make sure that a follow-up appointment with a mental health professional is kept. The chance of a repeat attempt is high, and follow-up appointments are notoriously not kept. Therapeutic programs for recent adolescent suicide attempts emphasize family involvement and increasing the youth's coping and problem-solving strategies.

Finally, whereas symptoms of depression and suicidal behavior cause family physicians to consider affective illness, one other common adolescent complaint—school refusal—should also raise a physician's concern about the possible presence of a depressive illness. Refusal to go to school may be related to pure truancy, to an ongoing struggle with a poorly treated learning disability, or to some stress at school, especially one involving peers. However, if a youth has previously been functioning reasonably well at school and then not only does not want to go to school but also declines usually enjoyable family or peer activities, further assessment for depression is indicated. In such cases, other depressive symptoms usually are readily elicited. It is important to prevent school absence from becoming chronic, because the secondary issues (teacher irritability with the student, embarrassment in explaining the situation to peers, and loss in steady course achievement) only compound the problem.

Anxiety disorders

In the past, anxiety symptoms or disorders were often thought to be short-term. However, longitudinal studies have begun to indicate that anxiety disorders in youth can continue as adult anxiety disorders (see Chapters 9 and 10) or evolve into other adult disorders, especially depressive disorders. Thus child and adolescent anxiety disorders cannot be considered routine or short-lived and must at least be monitored.

SSRIs and cognitive-behavioral therapy are emerging as the treatments of choice for anxiety disorders in adolescents. In cognitive-behavioral therapy for specific phobias, the young patient is gradually exposed to the phobic situation, first in thought and then in actuality. This process is supplemented by relaxation techniques and positive reinforcement by the family.

Clomipramine, fluvoxamine, and other SSRIs have been shown to be very effective in children and adolescents with obsessive-compulsive disorder (OCD). Cognitive-behavioral intervention (which has proven helpful in adults with OCD) is now being studied in youth to complement medication. Teenagers are educated to understand symptoms of OCD as an intrusive process with accompanying anxiety that can be combated with a variety of symptom-reducing strategies. As with other adolescent psychiatric disorders, a primary care physician's role in managing OCD should probably be limited to monitoring OCD medication after a psychiatric consultant has stabilized the patient.

Finally, in the area of anxiety disorders, physicians must be aware of the symptoms of posttraumatic stress disorder (PTSD). This disorder entails a form of re-experiencing a traumatic (potentially life-threatening) event, accompanied by symptoms of autonomic hyperarousal and chronic avoidance of stimuli associated with the trauma, all of which persist beyond the one-month period following the event. If an adolescent has experienced a traumatic event (including physical or sexual abuse), a physician should first ensure that the teenager is openly discussing the trauma with close loved ones or qualified counselors. Such open communication may reduce the risk of later development of PTSD. If open communication about the event with loved ones does not occur, early referral to a mental health professional should be made. As with other anxiety disorders in youth, CBT is typically implemented for treatment (focusing on gradual discussion of the trauma).

Additionally, in a related matter of long-term management, a teenager who has experienced a trauma (such as child abuse) and has apparently recovered, still needs occasional brief reassessment for long-term symptoms of PTSD. Such an adolescent may still be at risk for PTSD or another psychopathological disorder, and abused children may show problems with mood control or interpersonal relationships.

Other psychiatric disorders

Youth with conduct disorder (CD) are problematic for all clinicians. Too often their courses are chronic and treatment-resistant. Consequently, a tendency for a primary care physician to give up early may often prevail; that is, any youth with

symptoms of CD may too quickly be thought to have a poor prognosis (Box 25.2). Therefore, in adolescent patients with symptoms of CD, physicians must be sure that certain basic steps have been accomplished early. Any success may help reduce the considerable morbidity—not only psychiatric but also medical—for which these children are at risk (premature death, injuries secondary to violence, sexually transmitted diseases, and substance-abuse sequelae).

An adolescent with an acute onset of symptoms of CD must be vigorously assessed, especially for physical or sexual abuse. Such a youth must also be evaluated for neurological disease, substance use, another experience of environmental violence, major depression or mania, and paranoia or psychosis. Swift diagnosis and proper intervention may lead to considerable improvement, as well as to the prevention of further deterioration and consolidation of the symptoms. Indeed, late-onset CD appears to have a better prognosis than early-onset CD. A teenager's history may also reveal that what appears to be acute is actually occurring in the context of another chronic psychiatric disorder, especially ADHD or a learning disorder. Such teenagers may have gone through grade school in precarious balance with these disorders, only to have their fragile equilibrium disrupted by entrance into the junior high or middle school atmosphere and its demands—especially those that are of a social nature or peer-related. Thus the updating of previous treatment plans may serve such youth well and also prevent early symptoms of CD from progressing into a more chronic and disabling condition.

More commonly, physicians have young patients who have chronic rather than acute conduct disturbances. Such youth and their families require constant support from primary care physicians and especially need to participate in available treatment programs. Emphasis should be placed on the external provision of limits and boundaries. The reexamination of school curriculum may reveal that a learning disorder in an adolescent is not being sufficiently addressed and must be further remedied by the school to diffuse the teenager's increasing frustration and anger. Some research has also shown the success and cost-effectiveness of after-school programs that emphasize prosocial activities for at-risk youth, such as sports to promote teamwork and good sportsmanship. Typically, structured programs and other therapeutic interventions can be successful for CD while they are in effect, but the benefits dissipate when the intervention program ends. Therefore, a chronic disease model of treatment is most appropriate for this condition. Specific interventions with promising results in initial controlled trials are multisystemic therapy (MST), as well as pharmacological agents to reduce aggression. The latter include stimulant medications, lithium, and the atypical neuroleptic, risperidone.

Eating disorders have their peak ages of onset during adolescence, with anorexia nervosa's average age of onset at

Box 25.2 Conduct disorder

A. A repetitive and persistent pattern of behavior in which the basic rights of others or major age-appropriate societal norms or rules are violated, as manifested by the presence of three (or more) of the following criteria in the past 12 months, with at least one criterion present in the past six months:

Aggression to people and animals

1 often bullies, threatens, or intimidates others
2 often initiates physical fights
3 has used a weapon that can cause serious physical harm to others (e.g., a bat, brick, broken bottle, knife, gun)
4 has been physically cruel to people
5 has been physically cruel to animals
6 has stolen while confronting a victim (e.g., mugging, purse snatching, extortion, armed robbery)
7 has forced someone into sexual activity.

Destruction of property

8 has deliberately engaged in fire setting with the intention of causing serious damage
9 has deliberately destroyed others' property (other than by fire setting).

Deceitfulness or theft

10 has broken into someone else's house, building, or car
11 often lies to obtain goods or favors or to avoid obligations (i.e., "cons" others)
12 has stolen items of nontrivial value without confronting a victim (e.g., shoplifting, but without breaking and entering; forgery).

Serious violations of rules

13 often stays out at night despite parental prohibitions, beginning before age 13 years
14 has run away from home overnight at least twice while living in parental or parental surrogate home (or once without returning for a lengthy period)
15 is often truant from school, beginning before age 13 years.

B. The disturbance in behavior causes clinically significant impairment in social, academic, or occupational functioning.

C. If the individual is age 18 years or older, criteria are not met for antisocial personality disorder.

Specify type based on age at onset:

- *childhood-onset type*: onset of at least one criterion characteristic of conduct disorder prior to age 10 years
- *adolescent-onset type*: absence of any criteria characteristic of conduct disorder prior to age 10 years.

Specify severity:

- *mild*: few if any conduct problems in excess of those required to make the diagnosis and conduct problems cause only minor harm to others
- *moderate*: number of conduct problems and effect on others intermediate between "mild" and "severe"
- *severe*: many conduct problems in excess of those required to make the diagnosis or conduct problems cause considerable harm to others.

From American Psychiatric Association (2000) Diagnostic Statistical Manual of Mental Disorders, 4th Edition, Text Revision, Washington, D.C., American Psychiatric Association.

14 and bulimia nervosa's at 19 (see Chapter 15). Enhanced awareness of these illnesses by both physicians and the public, combined with improved treatment approaches, appear to be making an impact on outcome. Longitudinal studies of anorexia nervosa (currently more substantial than studies of bulimia nervosa) now provide primary care physicians with more information that they can use to advise families with teenagers who have anorexia nervosa. The majority of patients recover or improve, although approximately 20% develop a chronic course and about 5% develop a course that leads to death. Eating habits return to normal in over 40% of patients, and weight is regained in 60%. The majority of all patients experience normal educational and employment careers, but in contrast, only a minority achieves marriage or successful partnerships. Poor prognostic factors include bulimia nervosa, greater loss of weight, and chronicity.

Specific medical issues of a patient with anorexia nervosa may confront the physician. At the initial examination, certain medical conditions must be ruled out (such as brain tumors, diabetes, adrenal disease, malabsorption syndrome,

and regional enteritis), although the highly unusual eating habits and beliefs of anorexia nervosa are usually telltale. Additionally, the medical state of a teenager with anorexia nervosa may necessitate hospitalization for a number of serious complications, such as dehydration, electrolyte imbalance, or disturbances in cardiac condition. Hospitalization may also be necessary because of suicidal symptoms, failure to respond to outpatient treatment, or an unworkable family situation. An important first inpatient step is for the staff to make eating and exercising decisions for the patient until weight has gradually restabilized.

Multifaceted outpatient treatment plans for adolescent eating disorders appear to be productive (after the initial goal of weight stabilization has been gradually achieved). The physician's important role is often to monitor weight and any medical complications that may arise. Other common components of comprehensive programs include individual psychotherapy, group therapy, and family intervention tailored to specific needs. Finally, no medication is yet specific for anorexia nervosa, but SSRIs are helpful in bulimia nervosa. If major depression or OCD is present as a comorbid disorder, it is very important to implement specific intervention for the co-occurring condition.

Drug and alcohol use by teenagers is common (see Chapter 14). For example, over 90% of high school seniors have used alcohol, and over 45% have used marijuana. Daily usage in this age group for these two drugs is 4% and 3%, respectively. Thus a primary care physician should approach substance use much like sex education. Sensitive discussion and inquiry must be routine, and the physician should have a prevention protocol. The reduction of risk and harm is an important goal that can be achieved with emphasis on the vulnerability to dependence or the escalation to a more serious drug, contraction of human immunodeficiency virus (HIV) or sexually transmitted diseases, impulsive suicide, and death by car accident (40% of such deaths are associated with alcohol).

Screening is particularly important, because substance use is often missed. Although the instruments available for screening (including serum and urine toxicology screens) are reasonably sound, clinical assessment by the individual physician is equally important. If use is acute, the observed changes are much like other acute behavioral and emotional changes in adolescents, and acute environmental problems or the early onset of another psychiatric disorder must be ruled out. The converse is also true; that is, if there is any acute behavioral or emotional change in an adolescent, substance use must always be ruled out with a drug screen that assesses the suspected drugs. The possibility of dependence should also be ascertained; signs of dependence include daily use, withdrawal symptoms relieved by use, evidence of tolerance, subjective acknowledgment of lost control over use, and daily life revolving around drug activities and drug-using peers.

The adolescent's physician can make a difference in a teenager at-risk for or just beginning to use substances. Indeed, postponement of use until the late teens may reduce the chance of eventual addiction. Preusage warning signs should be noted, especially any history of substance use in the family and the presence of CD, and responded to with early education of the teenager and the family. Establishment of acute use should lead to aggressive intervention against causative situational problems or any psychiatric disorder. Identification of poor prognostic factors (that is, early and frequent use) can lead to intensive individual and group intervention attempts by trained professionals. If use becomes more serious, with accompanying life dysfunction and resistance to outpatient intervention, then a residential treatment program may be necessary.

Issues in general medical disorders

Although the majority of children with chronic medical disorders do not have psychiatric disorders, they are twice as likely to have psychological problems as children without such medical disorders, especially when the more general concept of psychological distress is considered. Thus the primary care physician commonly (either directly or indirectly) observes anger, anxiety, or sadness in adolescents with chronic medical disorders. Such teenagers may be more at risk for anxiety and depressive disorders.

Psychological problems in adolescents with chronic medical disorders can partly be understood through consideration of the unique obstacles of their developmental stage. Teenagers with either longstanding or newly diagnosed medical conditions face increased struggles (compared with the average healthy teenager) as they negotiate independence, peer acceptance, sexual growth, establishment of self-identity, and the demanding future of adulthood. Thus a fluctuation in a previously stable child with a chronic medical illness must first be evaluated by the physician for its relationship with any of several adolescent developmental tasks. The same is true for children with developmental disorders (e.g., mental retardation or an autism spectrum condition) as they make the transition through adolescence.

As a teenager and his family begin to face a chronic illness, thorough psychological assessment can be very important. Indeed, the initial participation of a psychiatrist may even be advisable, since some research (for example, with asthma patients) has shown the eventual reduction of long-term use of medical services when such a multidisciplinary approach is used. Additionally, recent research with newly diagnosed young patients with diabetes has demonstrated that past psychiatric illness or the development of an adjustment disorder within a few months of the initial diagnosis of diabetes increases the risk of patients for developing later psychiatric disorders. The following risk factors for psychological problems should also be considered in a teenager with a newly diagnosed medical disorder: relation of the illness to environmental exposure (such as trauma) or genetic factors, a prolonged diagnostic period or initial misdiagnosis, physical deformity or disability, and the degree of negative prognosis.

Thus in the initial assessment, previous or ongoing psychopathological conditions in the adolescent and his family should be noted, as well as their patterns of coping with previous distress. Communication and education about the illness with the teenage patient and the family is essential at the beginning, as is thoroughly addressing their initial questions. Early misunderstanding or serious reactions must be dealt with expeditiously, especially to prevent the development of noncompliance. The patient and the family must be educated to recognize distress in themselves and to clearly assess their coping abilities. This establishment of a healthy working relationship with the adolescent and the family allows the medical care team, often led by a primary care physician, to provide for the psychological needs of the youth and the family swiftly and consistently.

With this appropriate baseline, specific future deviations may be more readily understood and addressed. That is, initial understanding of the "baseline" strengths and weaknesses of an adolescent with a medical disorder and his or her family, plus an appreciation of accompanying developmental tasks, helps a physician monitor and respond to any occurrence of psychological distress or temporary noncompliance. For example, brain involvement (secondary to either the disorder or the treatment) alerts the physician to more closely monitor school progress, because the occurrence of poor performance or absenteeism may be related to neuropsychological impairment. The physician may have to assist the family in ensuring that the school staff understands and plans for a teenager with such neurobiological compromise.

Finally, in addition to adolescents with chronic medical disorders, primary care physicians commonly face young patients with physical symptoms, such as recurrent abdominal pain, that are without an identifiable medical basis. The approach may be straightforward when an acute, stressful situation is identifiable along with relatively minor physical symptoms. However, more problematic is a prolonged or severe medical situation that has already generated an extensive and costly but negative workup and has also produced secondary psychological disruption that has progressively affected school, peer activities, and the family.

Research has not clearly shown how to handle such situations. However, close collaboration between a primary care physician and a psychiatrist appears important. As general principles, the physical symptoms should be acknowledged, monitored, and reasonably treated by the family doctor, who should also promote the necessity of psychiatric consultation. At the same time, the mental health professional should work to prevent further psychological deterioration as well as to identify and treat more basic individual or family psychopathological disorders. Frequent communication among the professionals is essential. Such a coordinated effort with these challenging young patients and families should begin as early as possible in the course of the illness to prevent the development of secondary psychological sequelae that may over time become more debilitating than the original physical complaints.

Conclusion

Fortunately, the great majority of teenagers negotiate their developmental transition through adolescence well. A primary care physician who observes turmoil in the life of a teenager must be suspicious of a psychiatric disorder, which occurs in about one-fifth of children in this age group (see *Pearls & Perils*). The crucial role for family physicians treating adolescents with psychopathological conditions is to properly screen and refer such teenagers to mental health professionals, a procedure that is currently not sufficiently accomplished. Physicians should give emphasis to their evaluation and referral techniques more than their practices of prescribing psychiatric medications, since the use of medicines in adolescent psychiatric disorders (with the possible exception of ADHD) is complicated and should be conservative.

Primary care physicians should not underestimate their potential (through aggressive initial inquiry and action) to limit the progression of psychopathological disorders in teenagers who are abused, who present with acute symptoms of CD or substance use, or who develop a chronic medical disorder.

PEARLS & PERILS

Adolescent issues

- Although most children do well during the transition through adolescence, there is a 15–20% prevalence rate of psychiatric disorders in this age group.
- Many of the less dysfunctional, common problems of adolescents can be understood through their relationships to the major developmental tasks of independence and identity formation.
- The time constraints of primary care practice often lead to both underdiagnosis and under-referral of teenagers with psychiatric disorders.
- Doctors who care for teenagers should give emphasis to their skills and techniques in the early detection, referral, and collaborative monitoring of adolescents with psychiatric disorders, rather than in the prescribing of psychiatric medications.
- The majority of children with ADHD do not outgrow the cardinal symptoms, and a large proportion continue to benefit from medication through adolescence (and quite likely adulthood) as part of their overall treatment plan.
- When depression, maltreatment or substance abuse is suspected, it is of paramount importance to assess adolescents for the presence of suicidal ideation and to secure emergency psychiatric evaluation if it is present.
- Primary care physicians can often prevent the progression of a conduct or addictive disorder through the aggressive identification of the earliest symptoms of these disorders.
- In an adolescent with a newly diagnosed chronic medical disorder, a physician's thorough baseline understanding of and response to the youth's and the family's psychological states may eventually decrease the amount of subsequent needed medical service and the development of psychopathology.

Annotated bibliography

Emslie, GJ *et al.* (2002) Fluoxetine for acute treatment of depression in children and adolescents: a placebo-controlled, randomized clinical trial, *J Am Acad Child Adolesc Psychiatry* 41(10):1205–15.
A groundbreaking study of the benefits of SSRIs for depressed children and adolescents.

Hacker, DJ (1994) An existential view of adolescence, *J Early Adolesc* 14(3):300–327.
This is a remarkable synthesis of the existing psychological literature on adolescence, in which basic developmental tasks are defined and a practical framework for understanding and interacting with adolescent patients is derived.

Kazdin, AE (2000) Treatments for aggressive and antisocial children, *Child Adolesc Psychiatr Clin N Am* 9(4):841–58.
This is a comprehensive and authoritative review of intervention strategies for children and adolescents with conduct problems.

Reiff, MI *et al.* (2003) Attention-deficit/hyperactivity disorder evaluation and diagnosis: a practical approach in office practice, *Pediatr Clin North Am* 50(5):1019–48.
A thorough review and synthesis of best practices for assessment of ADHD in clinical practice. (See also the guidelines of the American Academy of Pediatrics (www.aap.org) for an excellent review of specific practical recommendations for the diagnosis and treatment of ADHD.)

CHAPTER 26

Psychiatry and Old Age

Eugene H. Rubin, MD, PhD

Introduction

The population of adults over the age of 65 is rising dramatically in the US. In the year 2000, there were about 35 million Americans age 65 and older; this number will double to about 70 million by 2030. There were about 4.3 million Americans age 85 and older in 2000; this will increase to almost 9 million by 2030 and to near 20 million by 2050. In this chapter, key geriatric principles and their application to psychopathology in the elderly will be discussed.

Selected demographics of aging

There is no uniform definition of "old." Currently (and subject to change), 65 may be considered "old" in terms of eligibility for Medicare. The minimum age necessary to receive full social security benefits, however, is being delayed beyond age 65. Although physicians attend to many ill people between the ages of 65 and 70, most in this age range are reasonably healthy. Their health status more closely resembles people in their 50s than those in their 80s. An important indicator of geriatric health is the capability to function independently. This ability changes substantially between the ages of 65 and 85. This difference between the "younger old" and the "older old" is reflected in the percentage of people who reside in nursing homes; only about 1% of people between the ages of 65 and 74 need this level of assistance, compared with about 19% of those 85 and older. The elderly are a heterogeneous group regarding most aspects of life from financial comfort to physical health; however, physical human frailties catch up with many people in the mid to upper 80s.

As a physician's patient population ages, the percentage of that population who are women increases. For every 10 men age 65 and older, there are 13 women in this age range. Among people age 85 and older, there are 23 women for every 10 men. Seventy-five percent of men age 65 and older have living spouses, compared to 43% of women in this age range. Only about 13% of women age 85 and older still have spouses, compared with about 50% of men.

Money is a major concern for many older people. Although some are wealthy, about 10% of people age 65 and older are living at or below the poverty level. Another 27% have incomes that are between the poverty level and twice the poverty threshold. (In 2002, the federal poverty threshold for individuals age 65 and over was an annual income of less than $8,700.) It becomes very difficult to purchase medications when one can barely afford room and board. These financial concerns become all the more compelling when considering that a 65-year-old adult, on average, will live 16–19 more years and an 85-year-old person will live about six more years.

The aging body

Even though over 70% of people age 65 and older describe their health as good, very good, or excellent, many are inconvenienced by painful or function-limiting conditions. About half of people age 70 and older have arthritis, about 40–45% have hypertension, and 20–25% report heart disease. Hearing and vision impairments are common and can interfere with social contact. About 15% report significant depressive symptoms. Cognitive impairment becomes increasingly common with age, and one-third or more of those age 85 and older have dementia. Heart disease is by far the most common cause of death, accounting for over one-third of all deaths. Cancers and stroke account for another one-third.

Anatomical and functional changes occur in every organ system with aging. Age-related changes in liver and kidney function, together with a decreasing percentage of muscle and increasing percentage of fat, change how the body handles drugs (discussed below). Visible changes occur in the skin. Pulmonary and cardiac reserves decrease. Aging of organs is probably related to several factors, including genetically programmed cell changes, acute and chronic environmental damage, and the influence of disease.

Like other organs, the brain undergoes age-related changes, although the relative contribution of normal aging versus disease is often unclear. Some brain atrophy occurs in cognitively intact very old people although the amount varies considerably among individuals. Neurons in different brain regions have varying degrees of susceptibility to genetic age-related changes or environmental damage. Various microscopic deposits accumulate in the aging brain. The amount of lipofuscin increases but has no known clinical correlates. Other age-related neuroanatomical changes such as Lewy bodies, Hirano bodies (cytoplasmic inclusions in certain neurons), granulovacuolar degeneration, tangles, and plaques may occur in certain regions in small amounts in successful aging, but they occur in much larger amounts with diseases such as Alzheimer's disease or Parkinson's disease. The degree of accumulation of these changes in truly healthy aging is a subject of scientific debate. Aging is also associated with changes involving certain CNS transmitter systems. The degree to which such changes are a natural by-product of aging versus the result of pathological processes is unknown. Neurotransmitter, neuroreceptor, and post-receptor age-related changes are important since they may explain why the elderly are more sensitive to certain centrally active medications.

Obvious changes occur in physical and mental abilities with aging. Top athletes in their seventies, although still capable of remarkable achievements, usually cannot compete with top athletes in their twenties. Changes in brain function result in diminished maximal performance, although such changes do not usually interfere with most everyday activities. The degree to which these changes in brain perform-

ance are a result of inevitable aging processes versus age-related diseases is difficult to determine. Certain skills change more than others. The ability to learn new information while simultaneously being distracted diminishes with age. Memory recall is more sensitive to aging than memory recognition. Timed motor tasks requiring visuospatial processing are age sensitive. It is common for elderly people to report increased difficulty in rapidly recalling names. Increasing dependency on notes and calendars occurs. These changes are usually reported to be a nuisance, but they do not interfere with the ability to be productive at work or home. If cognitive changes interfere with daily activities, the possibility of an incipient dementia needs to be entertained (see Chapter 12).

General principles of geriatric psychiatry

One important principle of geriatric psychiatry is that diagnosis is more complicated with elderly patients. Cognitive disorders are common in very old patients and can interfere with patients' remembering and reporting symptoms. Patients often have multiple medical illnesses with accompanying behavioral pathology that can make the diagnosis of primary psychiatric disorders difficult. Lack of energy, poor appetite, and sleep difficulties are non-specific symptoms associated with many chronic disorders, such as renal failure, heart disease, arthritis, and diabetes. These symptoms can also occur as part of a major depression, and deciding whether such symptoms result from a chronic medical illness or major depression can be hard. In addition, elderly patients are often taking multiple medications. Some drugs have psychiatric side effects, and little is known about the additive behavioral toxicity of drug combinations. Confusion, anxiety, agitation, mood changes, personality changes, and psychotic symptoms are not uncommon side effects of polypharmacy in the elderly. People whose brain functions are already compromised from illnesses such as dementia or delirium are even more sensitive to CNS drug toxicity.

Diagnosis is further complicated by the possibility that psychiatric disorders may present differently in elderly patients than in younger patients. For example, young or middle-aged adults with depression are often symptomatic most of the day nearly every day over weeks or months. Symptoms of depression in the cognitively or medically impaired elderly may not be as persistent; symptoms may persist only a few hours a day and may not occur every day. Although such a pattern of symptoms does not fulfill strict DSM-IV criteria for a major depression, this pattern may be a common presentation in the older, medically ill patient. The geriatric psychiatrist should be knowledgeable of the strict diagnostic criteria, but also should use common sense when considering psychiatric diagnoses.

Some psychiatric disorders are strictly age-related. Dementia of the Alzheimer's type (DAT) is rare in people under the age of 50, but its incidence increases dramatically with age; it is one of the most common disorders of octogenarians. Such an age-associated pattern suggests a relationship between CNS aging and disease pathophysiology. Many psychiatric disorders have an age of onset in young or middle life. Some of these disorders with earlier onset are chronic or recurrent with symptoms continuing into old age. The elderly patient with a history of early-onset recurrent depression is likely to continue to have depressive episodes in later life. In both chronic and recurrent disorders, symptoms may be influenced by age, concurrent medical disorders, and medications. In addition, there may be age-related changes in pharmacological responsivity and side effects of treatments. Sometimes, an illness that has a typical onset early in life presents for the first time in late life. Examples include late-onset major depression, bipolar disorder-manic episode, anxiety disorders, and schizophrenia. Interestingly, the pathophysiologies of these disorders may be different when symptoms occur for the first time late in life, compared with initial presentation earlier in life. There may be age-related structural damage of CNS regions that results in the psychiatric symptoms. This will be illustrated below in a discussion of late-onset depression.

Another common geriatric principle is the need to simplify pharmacological regimens whenever possible. Such simplification often leads to clinical improvement and allows more accurate psychiatric diagnosis and treatment planning. Elderly patients are often under the care of several physicians and are ingesting a large number of medications. Additionally, elderly patients may continue to take medications prescribed years earlier without re-evaluation for their need. Elders often self-medicate with over-the-counter medications such as non-steroidal anti-inflammatory agents for pain and antihistamines for sleep. A patient's pharmacological history should be periodically reviewed and, whenever possible, gradual simplification of the pharmacological regimen should be attempted. Medications may be no longer necessary, or one agent can successfully serve the function of several. When discontinuing medications, a gradual taper with careful monitoring is recommended. As medications are withdrawn, psychiatric symptoms may disappear or patterns of symptoms may become clearer, allowing for more confidence in making diagnoses. Should psychopharmacological intervention be necessary, simplified drug regimens decrease the risks from medication interactions. When psychopharmacological agents are initiated, risk-to-benefit ratios should be re-evaluated often. Knowledge about the natural history of the disorder coupled with this risk-to-benefit evaluation is useful when deciding the duration of psychopharmacological treatment.

Another important geriatric principle that applies to geriatric psychiatry is the need to monitor patients' functional abilities. The physical abilities of elderly patients can deteriorate rapidly if they are unnecessarily restricted to bed. If patients are not encouraged to be mobile, muscle atrophy can

occur quickly. Elderly people can fall easily when weak. With falls come fractures. Patients with a history of falling or unsteadiness can develop a "fear of falling" syndrome that further restricts their mobility and may lead to further weakness and increased risk of fractures. Fractures can result in nursing home placement. Therefore, it is important to maximize an elderly patient's mobility and monitor the influence of psychiatric treatment on activities of daily living. Similarly, cognition can be adversely affected by medical illnesses and pharmacological treatment, and cognitive status should be monitored as changes in treatments are made. Decreased function can also be secondary to hearing and vision difficulties, and even slight improvement helps patients to regain their abilities to converse, listen, watch television, and participate in activities. Simple interventions can improve function and can make major differences in the health of elderly patients.

> - In elderly patients, psychiatric diagnoses are often complicated by behavioral symptoms associated with medical disorders and medications.
> - Complicated drug regimens are common in the elderly and can confuse both the patient and the physician.
> - The patient's ability to function in activities of daily living should be monitored when treating psychopathology.

PEARLS & PERILS

Pharmacological principles of geriatric psychiatry

When using psychotropic medications in the elderly, the following four pharmacological considerations require special attention: pharmacokinetic changes with age, pharmacodynamic changes with age, medication-illness interactions, and medication-medication interactions.

Pharmacokinetic changes

Pharmacokinetics involves the physical handling of drugs by the body, including their absorption, distribution, metabolism, and elimination. Although pharmacokinetics can be complex, some basic, practical concepts are helpful for everyday patient management. These concepts involve three pharmacokinetic terms: half-life, volume of distribution, and clearance.

Most psychotropic medications are handled by processes that follow first-order kinetics. This means that drugs accumulate or are eliminated in a manner proportional to the amount of drug present; that is, the same proportion of drug is eliminated per unit time regardless of the amount of drug.

The time it takes to eliminate half the amount of drug is called the "half-life" of the drug. For drugs following first-order kinetics, the half-life is the same for 1,000,000 units of drug to decrease to 500,000 and for 10 units to decrease to 5 units. Some drugs such as alcohol are metabolized by processes following zero-order kinetics, which means that the same AMOUNT of agent is metabolized per unit time independent of the initial amount; that is, the body processes the agent at the same rate independent of the amount of agent in the plasma. The term "half-life" would not apply to drugs handled by zero-order kinetics. For a drug like alcohol, which follows zero-order kinetics, it would take ten times longer to drop from a concentration of 20 to 10 units/volume as it would to drop from a concentration of 2 to 1 unit/volume. (If this were a first-order kinetic process, the time would be the same.)

The time to reach steady-state plasma levels depends on an agent's half-life, assuming its metabolism follows first-order kinetics. When a medication is taken repeatedly, approximately half of the final steady-state level accumulates in the first half-life, 75% in two half-lives, 88% in three, 94% in four, and about 97% in five half-lives. Half-lives of many psychotropic drugs increase substantially with patient age. In some individuals, agents with long half-lives, such as diazepam or fluoxetine, can take weeks before reaching their final steady-state plasma level. Information about a drug's half-life can be found in standard references and can be useful in patient management.

All drugs are distributed to fat, muscle, and water. The proportion of a drug that accumulates in each of these different compartments depends on the chemical characteristics of the drug, such as its fat solubility. Many psychotropic drugs (with notable exceptions, such as lithium and risperidone) are highly fat soluble. At steady state, fat-soluble drugs have a relatively low concentration in plasma and high concentration in fat. Volume of distribution (VOD) is defined as the volume that would be required to account for the total amount of drug in the body if the concentration were the same as in plasma. A compound that is highly fat soluble would have a low plasma concentration, and therefore, a large volume of plasma would be required to account for the total amount of drug in the body. Such a drug would have a high VOD. Conversely, a low VOD suggests that the agent is not highly concentrated in fat deposits but is more water soluble and would have proportionately higher concentrations in the plasma. With aging, the percent of the body that is fat increases; therefore in elderly people, more agent accumulates in body fat at steady state. This increase in VOD of fat-soluble agents directly increases the half-life of the drug as discussed below.

Clearance is perhaps the most important pharmacokinetic parameter. It is defined as the volume of plasma that would be totally cleared of active drug per unit time. Active drug is usually cleared by hepatic metabolism, renal elimination, or both. Clearance is the critical pharmacokinetic parameter in determining plasma steady-state levels. With aging, blood flow to the liver and kidneys can change. Also, certain liver enzymes work less efficiently in the elderly. Diminished clearance increases both a drug's half-life and plasma steady-state concentrations.

The relationships between these three key pharmacokinetic parameters (half-life, VOD, and clearance) are illustrated in two clinically useful pharmacokinetic equations:

1 Half-life is proportional to VOD divided by clearance
2 Steady-state plasma concentration is proportional to dose per time divided by clearance.

The influence of aging on the pharmacokinetics of psychotropic drugs can be understood using these two equations. Although the effect of aging on the pharmacokinetic parameters of individual drugs should be verified in pharmacology references, many psychotropic drugs are highly fat soluble and are metabolized by liver enzymes that become less active with age. With such agents, the VOD increases and clearance decreases with age. From Equation 1, it is apparent that half-life substantially increases in this situation. Furthermore, it can be seen from Equation 2 that the steady-state plasma concentration increases to a degree inversely proportional to the clearance. Therefore, patients develop higher steady-state plasma levels unless the dose is proportionately lowered. Neither half-life nor VOD directly influences the final steady-state plasma level; however, an increase in half-life means that it will take longer for steady-state levels to be reached. The practical consequences of these pharmacokinetic changes are that, in the elderly, drugs may continue to accumulate for long periods of time and dosage may need to be substantially lowered in order to maintain an appropriate plasma level. If a drug's clearance is decreased by half, the final concentration will double unless the dose is decreased.

PEARLS & PERILS

- The accumulation and elimination of most drugs follow first-order pharmacokinetics.
- Clearance of many drugs decreases with patient age as a result of changes in hepatic and renal function.
- Since the percent of body fat increases with patient age, the volume of distribution of fat-soluble drugs increases with age.
- Half-life is proportional to the volume of distribution divided by clearance.
- The half-life of a drug can increase substantially with patient age. Therefore, both the time to reach steady-state levels and the time to eliminate a drug can be much longer in older patients.
- Since the final steady-state level of a drug is inversely proportional to clearance, smaller doses may be sufficient in order for elderly patients to attain plasma levels similar to younger patients.

Pharmacodynamic changes

Pharmacodynamics deals with the responsivity of tissue to a given concentration of drug. Such responsivity may be involved with the therapeutic effects of the agent or with its side effects. If with age, the sensitivity related to a drug's side effects increases and the responsivity related to its therapeutic efficacy decreases, then the risk-to-benefit ratio changes in a disadvantageous direction. The mechanisms underlying pharmacodynamic changes may involve receptors, cell membranes, post-receptor coupling, or genomic control. With aging, some drugs may have increased effects at the same concentration, while others may demonstrate decreased effects. Increasing sensitivity to the development of long-term side effects can also occur, as exemplified by the increased incidence of tardive dyskinesia in elderly patients exposed to antipsychotic agents.

Medication-illness interaction

Elderly people are more likely than their younger counterparts to suffer from chronic illnesses. Such illnesses can influence the risks of utilizing psychiatric medications. For example, liver disease or renal disease may change the clearance of medications. The presence of arthritis may make it more difficult for a patient to tolerate movement disorders that might be caused or exacerbated by some antipsychotic agents. Patients with disorders influencing gait or balance may be less able to tolerate the orthostatic blood pressure changes of certain antidepressants or antipsychotics.

Some cardiac disorders increase the risk from tricyclic antidepressants. Medications with sedative potential, including certain antianxiety agents, antidepressants, and antipsychotics, may increase confusion in cognitively impaired patients or result in falls, especially in the frail elderly. Weight gain resulting from certain psychiatric drugs may increase risks of cardiovascular disease, especially in elderly individuals with hypertension, diabetes, and elevated cholesterol. Repeated re-evaluation of risk-to-benefit ratios of psychopharmacological interventions is a key principle of geriatric psychiatry.

Medication-medication interaction

Many elderly people take multiple medications. A large number of drug interactions involving two agents have been reported; complexity expands when three or more drugs are prescribed. Specific pharmacologic interactions involving complicated regimens are difficult to study, and therefore it is important to be aware of the possibility of such interactions. In general, it is preferable to use as few medications as possible. Medications accumulate for longer periods of time in the elderly, and newly added medications can interfere with the clearance of the other prescribed drugs and change

their steady-state levels. Risk can be kept to a minimum by being alert to these possibilities, carefully monitoring the patient, and measuring plasma levels when appropriate. Increasing data is accumulating about the involvement of cytochrome P450 systems and drug interactions (see Cozza *et al.*).

Psychopathology in the elderly

The evaluation of psychiatric symptoms in the elderly is a several-step process and includes obtaining a complete history; performing physical, neurological, and psychiatric examinations; developing a differential diagnosis; and ordering appropriate laboratory, radiological, and psychological tests. With these data in hand, a working diagnosis can be made. Certain illnesses, such as dementia and delirium, commonly present for the first time in old age. Other illnesses, such as major depression, mania, and schizophrenia, usually have an earlier onset, and it is important to know whether recent symptoms represent an initial episode or relapse of prior episodes. Recurrent episodes often resemble earlier episodes after controlling for the potential age-related interactions discussed previously. Treatments that were effective with earlier episodes are likely to work again, as long as the appropriate pharmacokinetic and pharmacodynamic principles are considered in order to adjust the dose when prescribing psychoactive medications.

Different pathophysiological mechanisms may underlie disorders that typically have an early onset when the initial presentation occurs late in life. Patients who have early-onset illnesses are more likely to have a family history of the illness, suggesting that the mechanism in early-onset disease may involve genetic predilection. Initial presentation of the same illnesses late in life can be associated with anatomic abnormalities involving specific brain regions. In other words, genetics may lead to biochemical abnormalities in specific brain regions in young individuals, whereas anatomic lesions in the same regions may produce the same symptoms in the elderly.

Late-onset depression

Depression illustrates many of the concepts discussed in the previous section. Depression can be an episodic or chronic illness. A person may experience only one or two episodes of depression during his life, or the illness may reoccur with painful frequency. Symptoms of depression may arise at any age (see Chapter 8); attributing these symptoms to depression may be more difficult when other illnesses are present, however. Physiological symptoms of depression such as diminished appetite, poor sleep, and fatigue can occur as a result of many illnesses. A diagnosis of depression in the elderly requires both the physiological and psychological symptoms. Patients with recurrent depressions often recognize their earliest symptoms and are able to accurately predict the return of the full syndrome. Early symptoms, such as a characteristic pattern of awakening or a specific type of low self-esteem, can be very distinct to such patients. These early or prodromal symptoms are clinically important, since rapid pharmacological intervention may prevent the progression to more dangerous symptoms.

When depression occurs for the first time late in life, especially when there is no family history of major mood disorders, it may be associated with brain pathology such as infarcts or white matter abnormalities, particularly involving the left frontal lobe and striatum. These two regions have been shown in studies using positron emission tomography (PET) to have abnormal blood flow in young patients with familial depression. A careful neurological examination is important in the evaluation of elderly patients with new-onset illness, and appropriate radiological tests may also be indicated.

Depression is highly associated with specific CNS diseases such as Parkinson's disease. This association may be secondary to the involvement of the striatum in Parkinson's disease, since this region may also be involved in depression. When depression is associated with CNS illnesses or neuroanatomical damage, standard treatments are still often effective.

Major depression may also occur in patients suffering from chronic debilitating medical disorders (see Chapters 27 and 28). The mechanism of this association is not known. In some cases, the medical disorder may lower the threshold for developing depression in a genetically predisposed person. Alternatively, depression and the medical disorder may share similar predisposing risk factors. The major stress of a debilitating illness may also be involved in the development of a depressive syndrome. Major depression associated with diseases such as diabetes may be chronic unless treated. It is a mistake to assume that major depression is an understandable response to the illness and therefore needs no treatment. Depression associated with chronic medical disorders often increases the morbidity and mortality of the medical disorders. It is, therefore, important for the general practitioner to be able to recognize and treat geriatric depression. Depression associated with chronic illnesses usually responds to standard treatment.

PEARLS & PERILS

- Different pathophysiological mechanisms may cause the same clinical syndrome in older vs. younger patients.
- Anatomical lesions in specific parts of the brains of elderly patients can lead to a psychiatric syndrome that, in younger patients, may be related to genetic or biochemical factors acting in the same brain regions.

Depression and dementia of the Alzheimer type

Several of the geriatric principles discussed earlier in this chapter are further illustrated by a review of the interaction of major depression and dementia of the Alzheimer type (DAT). DAT is a very common, progressive illness of elderly people that gradually strips them of their memory, thinking abilities, orientation, personality, self-care abilities, and autonomy (see Chapter 12). Insight and understanding are often impaired early in the disease process. Patients with DAT may not be aware of any difficulties, whereas their families are distraught about their loved ones deteriorating before their eyes. Many patients with mild DAT exhibit no depressive symptoms. They describe themselves as active, interested in life, and enjoying their senior years. They may report that their memory skills are not as good as before but that they are getting along just fine. Sleep is satisfactory, and appetite may be described as "too good." They appear content and have no thoughts of death or suicide. Their loved ones indicate that they are no longer very active and have little ability to remember recent information but seem happy and unaware of what is happening. This type of history is consistent with DAT without major depression.

Other elderly patients exhibit the symptoms of a major depression without any evidence of cognitive difficulties. For example, a patient may have a history of excellent health until a marked change in behavior and activities develops. She becomes discouraged and disinterested in her busy schedule of activities. Crying and talking about being worthless and a failure become common. When the patient is reminded about being on many committees, running the lay ministry at church, and volunteering twice a week at the food pantry, she dismisses these accomplishments as being insignificant. Her sleep patterns change substantially. She loses interest in food. The patient begins to talk about joining deceased relatives. Memory may be reported as being unchanged. The patient can describe past events in detail without difficulty. She can accurately describe details of a recent vacation, as well as all the travel arrangements, to four European countries. On testing, she remembers recent and past details well. She balanced her checkbook the week before and brought a well-organized stack of papers to an accountant for tax return preparation the previous month. Such a patient clearly has a major depression without evidence of DAT.

Many patients, however, fall between these two extremes. They develop not only clear-cut symptoms of classic depression but also cognitive impairment that interferes with short-term and long-term memory and orientation. Such patients demonstrate diminished interest and abilities to take care of themselves. When this pattern of symptoms occurs, it is important to obtain an accurate history of the patient's cognitive status prior to the development of the depressive syndrome from knowledgeable collateral sources. If it becomes evident that the patient did not have subtle signs of deterioration prior to the development of depression, it is likely that the patient is suffering from a major depression and that the cognitive impairment is a result of the depressive disorder. This conclusion is strengthened when the history reveals that the patient had previous episodes of a cognition-impairing major depression. Aggressive treatment usually leads to improvement of both affective and cognitive symptoms. Cognitive impairment associated with an episode of major depression has been referred to as "dementia of depression" and is often reversible. The long-term prognosis remains to be clarified, and it is not clear whether patients with this syndrome have an increased risk for eventually developing DAT.

Another common scenario is illustrated by the following history. A 70-year-old patient and his family report a two-year history of increasing memory and thinking difficulties. Items are lost, messages forgotten, and chores remain undone. The patient demonstrates increasing word-finding problems. His computational abilities are compromised. He becomes lost occasionally and no longer has the ability to perform tasks that were routine a few years previous. His concentration and interest have gradually diminished in parallel with cognitive changes, and he has become increasingly more passive and withdrawn. The patient has exhibited brief periods of crying and low mood only during the last several months, well after cognitive deficits were noticeable. Such symptoms had never occurred earlier in his life. These "sad" periods last several hours and respond to a change in activity, such as going shopping with his spouse.

Over the last month, these symptoms have occurred on about half the days. During these "bad days," the patient experiences feelings of worthlessness. His interest in activities, although gradually diminishing over the last several years, is significantly lower. His sleep is more disrupted during these bad periods, and his appetite is diminished. The patient admits to increased thoughts about death if asked during such a day. This constellation of symptoms suggests the possibility of a depressive episode in addition to DAT.

It is likely that symptoms of depression are modified by DAT, so it may be difficult for patients with dementia to consistently maintain the psychological symptoms of depression over long periods of time. Symptoms of depression may be fragmented and easier to interrupt by a change in activity. It is important to inquire about a prior history of depression because, if such a history exists, the likelihood is greater that the symptoms represent a depression in addition to the dementia. If both the psychological and physiological symptoms of depression exist for the same several-hour periods during a week or more in a month and such a pattern did not exist several months previously, pharmacological and psychotherapeutic treatment may be warranted. For a diagnosis of depression concurrent with DAT, it is important to be convinced that several of the following psychological symptoms of depression are present: dysphoria, crying spells, low self-esteem, guilt, death thoughts, or suicidal ideation. Diminished interest, decreased energy, and deteriorating concentration are symptoms common in DAT in the absence of concurrent depression. Assuming that these three symptoms alone suggest the presence of major depression could lead to the unnecessary use of antidepressants. Elderly patients, especially those with cognitive impairment, may be at increased risk for side effects from antidepressant medications. Careful use of the pharmacological principles discussed previously coupled with frequent patient monitoring is necessary when managing depressive symptoms with medications. Longitudinal evaluation of specific target symptoms is useful in determining treatment efficacy. Treating DAT with a cholinesterase inhibitor and education may also help concurrent depressive symptoms. Mild depressive symptoms may also respond to counseling and exercise. However, if depressive symptoms are disabling, more aggressive treatment with medications, counseling, and possibly electroconvulsive therapy may be warranted.

Depression and suicide in the elderly

Depressive disorders are associated with substantial morbidity and increased mortality. Even in the medically healthy, depression is associated with increased difficulties involving work, school, and family. Patients suffering from medical diseases together with a concurrent depression have a more difficult course and poorer prognosis than patients with the same medical disorder without a concurrent major depression. In addition, depressed patients with or without concurrent medical illnesses have increased mortality resulting from an increased rate of suicide. Most people who take their own lives suffer from psychiatric illness at the time of death. Depression is the most common psychiatric illness associated with suicide. Alcoholism, with or without concurrent major depression, also is associated with increased risk of suicide.

The majority of elderly patients who commit suicide have an active depression at the time of their deaths. The depression may not be dramatic in presentation; common symptoms in suicidal depressed elderly patients include recent decreases in activity, insomnia, and weight loss. The presence of a function-impairing medical illness is common. Although the majority of those age 60–65 who take their own lives have experienced prior depressive episodes, only a minority of depressed octogenarians who commit suicide have a prior history of depression.

Suicide rates vary as a function of both age and gender. Far fewer women commit suicide than men. The rate of suicide in women peaks at about age 50 and then very gradually decreases. In contrast, suicide rates in men demonstrate a sharp increase beginning in the mid-60s. Elderly white men have the highest rate of suicide. White men age 85 and older have a suicide rate in excess of 65/100,000 per year in contrast to a rate of less than 10/100,000 per year for women of the same age. Elderly African-American men also have a much higher suicide rate than African-American women. The suicide rates in the white population are substantially higher than in the African-American population.

Elderly patients contemplating suicide frequently give hints that they are thinking about death. They usually admit to their thoughts when they are directly asked. Screening for depression, including specific inquiry regarding suicidal ideation, should be an important part of every geriatric examination. A high percentage of both young and elderly patients who commit suicide had recently visited their primary care physicians and were suffering from symptoms of major depression at the time of that visit. In fact, over 45% of these people had visited their primary care doctors the week before they committed suicide, and at least 70% did so within the month before they died.

When an elderly patient talks about suicide, the discussion warrants a quick response. When a depressed elderly man talks about suicide, he may act without further warning. When depressed elderly people make suicide attempts, they are frequently successful. When they do not succeed, they are often seriously wounded both physically and psychologically. The preferred methods for suicide among the elderly are shooting, hanging, and overdosing. Most elderly people who attempt suicide fully intend to die; their attempts are usually not cries for help.

- Major depression is the most common illness associated with suicide.
- Elderly white men are a high-risk group for suicide.
- About 70% of people who complete suicide visited their physicians within the month prior to taking their lives; many were suffering from major depression at that time.

PEARLS & PERILS

Some patients suffering from chronic debilitating medical disorders believe that suicide makes sense for them. However, it is imperative for the physician to determine whether such thinking is being influenced by a concurrent depression. Even depressed suicidal patients with terminal illnesses may respond to antidepressant treatment and are pleased that they did not harm themselves when depressed. They appreciate an opportunity to take care of final tasks. Certainly, there are also many patients suffering with painful, functionally debilitating disorders who consistently believe in their right to take their own lives and who are not depressed. The role of the physician with such patients can be very difficult.

Physicians need to let their patients know their own beliefs and allow another physician to take over a patient's care if requested. Some patients will request a physician's assistance in dying. Such assistance has complicated ethical, moral, and legal implications.

Chronic psychosis and the elderly

Psychotic symptoms, including delusions, hallucinations, and formal thought disorders, are not uncommon in the elderly. Patients may also have negative symptoms including passivity, withdrawal, poverty of thought content, and poverty of speech. New-onset psychoses in the elderly represent a heterogeneous group of disorders. A percentage of patients have "true" schizophrenia with later onset than usual. These patients may have a similar genetic diathesis and family history as those with younger onset. Another group of patients may have a schizophrenia-like illness related to anatomical changes in specific brain regions. Abnormalities on magnetic resonance imaging (MRI) occur often in elderly patients with psychopathology. If these lesions influence the circuitry that is related to schizophrenia, it is conceivable that schizophrenia-like symptoms can occur. A third group of elderly patients with late-onset psychosis includes those with DAT who exhibit psychotic symptoms out of proportion to the typical cognitive deficits. Psychotic symptoms can also occur in people with mania, psychotic depression, or delirium.

Age of onset and family history contribute important diagnostic information. If a patient has had symptoms for decades, he is likely suffering from schizophrenia. Schizophrenia is often chronic, with symptoms lasting throughout middle and late life. Over time, some patients develop an increase in negative symptoms and diminution of overt psychotic symptoms. Acute psychotic exacerbations can occur and can be associated with decreased compliance with antipsychotic medication. About one-half of younger patients have a favorable long-term outcome in terms of active psychotic symptoms, but only about one-fourth of patients demonstrate improvement involving socialization skills.

When patients with early-onset schizophrenia reach old age, active pharmacological treatment should be reevaluated in terms of current symptoms. Older-generation antipsychotic medications can have side effects that are poorly tolerated in the elderly, including sedation, falls, orthostatic blood pressure changes, anticholinergic toxicity influencing peripheral organs (bladder, heart, eyes, and mouth) and central nervous system function (cognition), acute movement disorders, and chronic movement disorders. Elderly people are very susceptible to parkinsonian side effects including bradykinesia, tremor, and rigidity, which can hamper mobility and initiate a downward cycle of decreasing ability to function with activities of daily living. Tardive dyskinesias are common in elderly patients chronically exposed to older-generation antipsychotic medications. Severity can range from mild to severe. The social consequences of mild dyskinesias, such as lip smacking, can lead to decreased socialization. Severe dyskinesias can interfere with swallowing, communicating, walking, and breathing. Newer-generation antipsychotic medications are effective and more easily tolerated than the older agents. The prevalence of acute and chronic movement disorder side effects is decreased. Some of these newer agents may increase glucose levels and be associated with significant weight gain, however. Such side effects can increase risks for cardiovascular disease. The potential consequences of these effects need to be considered when examining risks and benefits.

Elderly patients can develop *de novo* symptoms resembling those that typically occur in early-onset schizophrenia. The prevalence of schizophrenia in the families of elderly patients with new-onset schizophrenia-like disorder is about halfway between that occurring in families of the early-onset patients and families of those without psychiatric illness. There are several interpretations of these data, including the possibility that elderly patients with new-onset disorder represent a heterogeneous group—some with as high a genetic risk as early-onset patients and others with much lower genetic risk.

The premorbid history of elderly patients with new-onset psychosis is also heterogeneous. Some have no unusual premorbid features. About half, however, have a history suggestive of schizoid or schizotypal personality disorder. These patients often are loners, are less likely to marry, and have had less socioeconomic success.

New-onset psychotic disorder occurs more often in elderly women than elderly men even after correcting for the increased proportion of women in the elderly population. This is in contrast to early-onset psychotic disorder in which the illness occurs at least as often in men as women. The age of onset of paranoid schizophrenia may be later than other subtypes of schizophrenia, and as age of onset increases, there is an increasing ratio of women to men with this form of schizophrenia. It is possible that the increased proportion of women in the elderly population with new-onset illness may be a continuation of the gender-age relationship observed in the cases with earlier onset.

Patients with moderate to severe DAT often demonstrate psychotic symptoms (see Chapter 12). These symptoms can include delusions and hallucinations. In DAT, psychotic symptoms may be more fragmented than those observed in patients with schizophrenia. Some patients in the early stages of DAT also demonstrate psychotic symptoms, which may overshadow the more subtle difficulties with memory, orientation, and judgment. Dementia with Lewy bodies (DLB) can also cause hallucinations and delusions (see Chapter 12). Because schizophrenia can lead to cognitive deficits and both DAT and DLB can have significant psychotic symptoms, it can be difficult to distinguish between these disease entities. A thorough longitudinal history from a knowledgeable collateral source is important in determining whether subtle progressive cognitive deterioration preceded the psychotic symptoms. If so, a dementia is more likely involved. Longitudinal follow-up with careful cognitive assessments may help clarify the diagnosis. It is also possible for patients with late-onset schizophrenia to develop an Alzheimer-type dementia as they age.

Psychotic symptoms in the elderly can be painful and debilitating. Despite the risk of significant side effects, many patients with late-onset schizophrenia improve with antipsychotic medications and attention to social intervention. Lower doses may work well in the elderly, and the risk-to-benefit ratio should be closely monitored. Patients with recurrent exacerbations of severe psychotic symptoms usually require continued therapy. Because late-onset psychoses have different etiologies, the natural history of these symptoms may vary depending on pathophysiology. Psychotic symptoms related to DAT may also improve with the use of the antipsychotic medication; however, there is increased risk from these medications in elderly patients with DAT. Antipsychotic medications can have substantial side effects in people with DLB. A careful evaluation of the degree of disability and discomfort caused by these symptoms should be balanced against the potential risks from medications.

Summary

Psychopathology is common in elderly patients but often it is not recognized. Cognitive impairment can be hidden behind a smile. Affective symptoms may not be detected unless the clinician asks specific questions. Patients with multiple somatic complaints may have psychiatric illness exacerbating or mimicking medical disorders. When symptoms are revealed and appropriate diagnoses made, treatments are typically effective. Recognizing and treating such symptoms have the potential to decrease morbidity and mortality.

In this chapter, general geriatric and pharmacological principles have been reviewed and selected psychiatric topics that demonstrate certain of these principles have been discussed. When providing psychiatric treatment, it is important to ensure the safety of the psychiatrically ill elderly patient. If there is a risk of suicide, hospitalization can be life saving. Prior to pharmacological management, simplification of current treatment regimens may help clarify the cause of psychiatric symptoms and minimize risks from drug interactions. Many of the new psychiatric medications are simpler and safer to use than earlier generations of psychotropic medications. It is recommended that outpatient visits include evaluation of suicidality, affect, function, and cognitive status. The primary care physician should consider consultation with a psychiatrist when there is uncertainty regarding the evaluation of safety issues pertaining to psychopathology, when the diagnosis is unclear, when there is concern about treatment issues, or when the patient does not improve or continues to deteriorate after treatment has been implemented.

Annotated bibliography

Arana, GW, Rosenbaum, JF, Hyman, SE, Labbate, LA, Fava, M (2005) *Handbook of Psychiatric Drug Therapy*, 5th Edition, Philadelphia, Lippincott Williams & Wilkins.
A concise and excellent psychopharmacology text.

Coffey, CE and Cummings, JL (eds) (2000) *The American Psychiatric Press Textbook of Geriatric Neuropsychiatry*, 2nd Edition, Washington, DC, American Psychiatric Press.
This up-to-date, excellent text contains basic reviews of CNS function and assessment as well as chapters addressing geriatric psychiatric disorders.

Cozza, KL, Armstrong, SC, and Oesterheld, JR (2003) *Concise Guide to Drug Interaction Principles for Medical Practice: Cytochrome P450s, UGTs, P-Glycoproteins*, 2nd Edition, Washington, DC, American Psychiatric Publishing, Inc.
A useful book dealing with an increasingly important topic of drug interactions.

Jacobson, SA, Pies, RW, and Greenblatt, DJ (2002) *Handbook of Geriatric Psychopharmacology*, Washington, DC, American Psychiatric Publishing, Inc.
A useful text addressing psychiatric drugs in the elderly.

Spar, JE and La Rue, A (2002) *Concise Guide to Geriatric Psychiatry*, 3rd Edition, Washington, DC, American Psychiatric Publishing, Inc.
This pocket-size, 352-page book is of high quality and is an excellent concise text.

CHAPTER 27

Psychiatric Disorders Associated with General Medical Conditions

Nuri B. Farber, MD and Kevin J. Black, MD

Introduction

In this chapter the focus turns from the consideration of specific psychiatric disorders to the complex issue of evaluating and treating psychiatric illness that appears in conjunction with other medical conditions. Given the continuing evolution of our understanding of the psychiatry-medicine interface, several key concepts are highlighted in order to establish a framework for understanding future developments. Special attention is given to the occurrence of psychiatric disorders in the context of neurological, endocrine or chronic medical illness. In addition, puerperal disorders are discussed.

General guidelines

Importance of diagnosing psychiatric disorders

Patients who exhibit unexplained physical symptoms are said to be "somatizers." As discussed in Chapter 17, somatization, in addition to being the main manifestation of somatization disorder, can also be present in several other psychiatric disorders (e.g., major depression, generalized anxiety disorder, panic disorder). While the occurrence of somatization in patients without medical illnesses has been recognized and diagnosed for decades, studies are just now beginning to show that certain physical complaints in patients with a medical illness can be a reflection of a psychiatric disorder. For example, evidence is now accumulating that unsubstantiated (i.e., no confirming evidence from exam or laboratory studies) complaints of lower extremity pain, gastrointestinal dysfunction (e.g., nausea, vomiting,

diarrhea, constipation, pain, bloating), and occasionally impotence in a patient with diabetes mellitus may be symptoms of a mood or anxiety disorder instead of being secondary to 'neuropathy.'

Thus, whenever the clinician is confronted with a physical complaint that has an atypical symptom profile or is inconsistent with objective evidence, (s)he should evaluate the patient for psychiatric illnesses associated with somatization. Establishing the presence of a psychiatric disorder in a somatizing patient is important for several reasons:

1 Evaluation—the realization that somatic complaints are symptoms of a psychiatric disorder and not indicators of worsening physical health decreases the need to submit the patient to invasive tests, which may subject the patient to significant risks and costs often with only minimal beneficial consequences.

2 Treatment—comorbid psychiatric disorders can significantly affect the clinical treatment of general medical conditions. For example, hypoglycemic symptoms (e.g., dizziness, headaches) in a diabetic patient currently symptomatic with major depression are unreliable indicators of poor metabolic control. In this instance the physician must rely on laboratory values (e.g., serum glucose) instead of symptoms in determining the appropriate medical regimen for glucose control. In cases where major depression is unrecognized, the physician or the patient may make inappropriate medication changes that could have adverse consequences.

Appropriate diagnosis allows the institution of treatment directed at the underlying psychiatric illness. With treatment, improvement or resolution of the psychiatric syndrome and any associated somatic complaints typically occurs. However, in cases where the psychiatric disorder goes undetected, the somatic symptoms typically persist, sometimes subjecting the patient to an unfavorable outcome.

3 Prognosis—appropriate treatment of the psychiatric disorder often leads to its remission and the resolution of the associated signs and symptoms. With improvement in mental state, patients usually return to their previous level of functioning and are much better able to comply with appropriate medical treatment (e.g., consent for surgery, exercise regimens, dietary restrictions). Not unexpectedly, the presence of a psychiatric illness can also have a substantial impact on the overall prognosis of patients with chronic medical illnesses. Studies indicate that, in patients with coronary artery disease, the presence of major depression presages a worse cardiac outcome (i.e., myocardial infarction, angioplasty, coronary artery bypass graft, death). Although the reason for the increased morbidity and mortality in this subgroup of patients is not known, the higher prevalence of ventricular tachycardia in patients with major depression could account for their poorer outcome. Major depression appears to be associated with poorer outcomes in other chronic medical illnesses (end-stage renal disease, diabetes mellitus, cancer) as well, but studies are still needed to better define the risk. It remains to be determined whether effective treatment of the psychiatric disorder will alter the course of the comorbid medical illness.

4 Financial considerations—the recognition and treatment of psychiatric disorders associated with somatization in patients with chronic medical illness typically lead to a reduction in health care costs and an increase in productivity by avoiding unnecessary tests and medication and by improving the health of patients (Box 27.1).

BOX 27.1

Importance of diagnosing psychiatric disorders in patients with general medical conditions

1 Somatization is a common symptom of several psychiatric disorders.
2 Psychiatric disorders probably account for the majority of neuropathic symptoms in patients without objective indications of neuropathy.
3 Psychiatric conditions can modify the clinical presentation of medical illness.
4 Appropriate psychiatric diagnosis should result in decreased morbidity and mortality either from the effective treatment of the disorder or from the decreased use of unneeded diagnostic procedures.
5 Appropriate psychiatric diagnosis leads to an overall decrease in the cost of health care delivery.

If no psychiatric disorder can be found after careful evaluation[1] and neither a neurological nor other medical disorder can be discovered to account for the symptom, the clinical process responsible for the unexplained somatic symptom often eventually surfaces during careful follow-up and usually turns out to be non-psychiatric in nature. It is important that such patients be followed carefully over time with an open mind regarding psychiatric, neurological, and medical disorders. Finally, it should be emphasized that emerging clinical data indicate that the presence of a well-described and validated psychiatric disorder (*e.g.*, major depression, somatization disorder) probably accounts for the symptoms in a significant number of patients who previously have been diagnosed with one of several poorly validated syndromes (e.g., chronic fatigue syndrome, multiple chemical supersensitivities).

Diagnosing mental disorders in patients with general medical conditions

Throughout this textbook, a medical model approach to the evaluation and treatment of the major psychiatric illnesses has been emphasized. Nowhere is the medical model more important than in diagnosing and treating mental illness in medically ill patients. In this group of patients, the physician must be adept in evaluating general medical and psychiatric illnesses and in determining whether the given signs or symptoms are manifestations of a "medical" or a "psychiatric" process, or both. While this determination is conceptually simple, in practice it can sometimes be exceedingly difficult. For example, complaints of poor appetite in a patient with cancer could be secondary to a cachectic state, drug-induced nausea, or a major depressive episode. Similar difficulties can arise when evaluating poor energy, insomnia, or any of several other physical symptoms.

When evaluating a physical symptom that is part of a patient's general medical condition, the practitioner should first elicit the characteristics of the symptom in detail. Particular attention should be paid to timing of onset and offset of the symptom, aggravating and ameliorating factors, and the presence or absence of any associated symptoms. For example, complaints of insomnia in a patient with congestive heart failure could be secondary to paroxysmal nocturnal dyspnea, diuretics, or major depression. The occurrence of awakening after a couple of hours of sleep would be more consistent with the first two causes while onset of insomnia in the early morning (e.g., 5 a.m.) with an inability to fall back

---

[1] Given the potential ramifications, the physician should always resist the temptation of invoking a psychiatric disorder, such as major depression, to explain a somatic complaint without first having performed a complete and in-depth psychiatric evaluation.

asleep argues more for major depression. Special emphasis should be given to the physical signs or symptoms that are not manifestations of both psychiatric and medical illness. In the above example, reports of orthopnea or the presence of edema would favor paroxysmal nocturnal dyspnea. Poor appetite would suggest, however, that major depression might be more likely. In difficult cases, interviewing outside sources and following the patient over several weeks often prove helpful.

In contrast to physical signs and symptoms, psychological signs and symptoms, since they are not typically a direct manifestation of medical illness, are much better indicators of the presence of a psychiatric disorder and do not pose as great a diagnostic dilemma. However, psychological signs and symptoms confront the physician with a new challenge: determining whether the psychological symptom is pathological or normal. For some psychological manifestations (e.g., expansive mood, delusions, hallucinations), the determination is relatively easy. In contrast, depressive symptoms (e.g., low mood, loss of interest) tend to pose conceptual problems for physicians and patients alike because they are understandable (i.e., "I'd be depressed too if . . ."). As in other fields of medicine, severity and duration, and not understandability, are usually the critical factors in determining whether any given response is pathological or not. For example, the normal ("understandable") response to the stress of a cardiovascular treadmill test includes tachycardia and hyperventilation (in order to meet increased cardiac demand). In patients with an abnormal cardiovascular system, the understandable response still occurs but it typically appears at a lower level of cardiovascular stress. After the stress is discontinued, it takes a longer time for the cardiovascular system to return to baseline. Furthermore, as the severity of the abnormality in the cardiovascular system increases, decreasing amounts of cardiovascular stress are needed to produce the same degree of cardiovascular response. Higher demands on the system lead to the appearance of other signs and symptoms (e.g., T-wave changes on the electrocardiogram, blood-flow changes on thallium scans, angina, chest pain, diaphoresis) that are more obviously pathological since they are not "understandable." Thus, the presence of signs and symptoms (i.e., phenotype) of a pathological state in an organ is a function of both the amount of stress placed on that organ (i.e., current environment) and the current level of organ functioning. An organ's current level of functioning is, in turn, a property of the organ's initial capacity (i.e., genotype) modified by past non-genetic events (e.g., level of conditioning, previous ischemic events).

The same reasoning can be applied to psychological responses to mental stress. Thus, a complaint of sadness could be a normal reaction to a devastating illness. However, if the sadness continues unabated or worsens with time (i.e., present for most of the day, nearly every day for at least two weeks) and becomes associated with dysfunction (i.e., se-

vere distress or impairment in social or occupational functioning), it is considered abnormal. Depending on the presence or absence of other signs and symptoms, the pathological response is characterized as either an adjustment disorder or major depression. (For specific diagnostic criteria, see Chapter 8.)

In addition to low mood, anxiety and worry are two other psychological responses often ignored because they are "understandable." Psychological signs and symptoms like suicidality, guilt, and worthlessness tend not to pose problems for most clinicians and are readily accepted as pathological because of their severity. However in some circumstances (e.g., debilitating and progressive neurological illnesses), even suicidality may be considered by many to be a rational, normal, and understandable reaction. While this is possible, such patients should be carefully evaluated for psychiatric disorders like major depression and treated for these disorders, if present.

After ascertaining the presence or absence of each diagnostic criterion, the physician should re-evaluate the patient's medical status, including a review of the medical problems, medication, pertinent exam findings, and laboratory values. Following this approach should allow the physician to make accurate diagnoses in the majority of patients. However, even after extensive evaluation in which no stone has been left unturned, the diagnosis will remain unclear for some patients. In such instances, the physician may elect to consider the presence or absence of a previous personal or family history of psychiatric illness. Given the strong familial pattern seen in most major psychiatric disorders and the knowledge that patients with previous psychiatric dysfunction are at higher risk for future psychiatric problems, medically ill patients with a positive family or past personal history of a psychiatric disturbance are probably at greatest risk for developing a comorbid psychiatric condition. In cases where such an individual has several signs and symptoms suggestive of a psychiatric disorder but does not meet the specific syndromal criteria, close follow-up is warranted. However, the physician might opt for empirical treatment in those patients with significant morbidity (e.g., inability to function at work, death thoughts) where conservative management might pose unwarranted risks. Referral to a psychiatrist might also be useful in deciding whether or not to treat a specific individual.

By following the above approach, physicians should be able to correctly evaluate most instances of psychiatric disorders that appear in the context of a general medical condition (see *Pearls & Perils*). However, the inherent difficulty in determining the presence of specific criteria sometimes results in the physician being unable to either substantiate or rule out the presence of a psychiatric syndrome. Re-evaluating these patients over time (e.g., once every couple of weeks) often clarifies the diagnosis. However, some patients might warrant being treated empirically.

Evaluating medically ill patients for psychiatric disorders

- Diagnosis is often complicated by the overlap of signs and symptoms between the two disorders.
- Ascertain the presence or absence of each diagnostic criterion for the psychiatric disorder under consideration.
- Ascertain the severity of the medical illness to help guide interpretation of whether the somatic sign or symptom in question is psychiatric or medical in origin.
- Look for the presence or absence of signs and symptoms that are not associated with the patient's medical illness but that occur in a psychiatric disorder (e.g., psychological signs).
- Patients with a family or past personal history of psychiatric illness are typically those at highest risk for psychiatric illness.

treated helps to eliminate pressure from the patient for immediate symptom relief (Box 27.2).

BOX 27.2

Treatment guidelines

1 If the patient has severe symptoms or is suicidal or psychotic, refer to a psychiatrist.
2 In general, treat the disorder as if it occurred in isolation.
3 Be vigilant for drug-drug and drug-illness interactions.
4 If no response after 2–3 weeks, increase dose if appropriate.
5 If still no response 2–3 weeks later, consider psychiatric referral.
6 Avoid the use of other non-essential psychiatric medications (e.g., benzodiazepines for insomnia).

Treatment

While double-blind placebo-controlled studies examining the treatment of major depression in patients with specific comorbid medical illnesses are sparse, available evidence indicates that antidepressants are safe and effective for major depression in these populations. Treatment is generally straightforward and follows the guidelines used to treat the psychiatric disorder in the absence of a comorbid medical condition. (See specific chapters in psychopathology section for treatment guidelines.) However, the choice of a specific therapeutic agent and dose must take into account the patient's medical history and other medications. Because most, if not all, patients with a general medical condition and a comorbid psychiatric disorder take at least two (and probably three or four) different medications, the potential for drug interactions exists.

The general rule is to be vigilant for drug-drug interactions (pharmacokinetic and pharmacodynamic) and to simplify the medication regimen as much as possible in order to decrease the risk of a clinically significant interaction. Given the potential for drug-drug interactions, clinicians should resist the temptation to prescribe medications that relieve specific symptoms but do not treat the underlying psychiatric disorder (e.g., benzodiazepines for insomnia[2] or for major depression-associated anxiety). Educating patients about their psychiatric illness and explaining that their symptoms (e.g., insomnia, anxiety) will start to improve after the first week or two of treatment and resolve as their illness is

A major consideration in selecting therapeutic agents for patients with coexisting medical illnesses involves the metabolism of the agents and the potential interactions with drugs being used to treat the medical disorder. The cytochrome P450 (CYP) system is the main route of metabolism for most therapeutic agents. In humans, the P450 system consists of at least 40 different enzymes (several of which are subject to genetic polymorphism) that are grouped into 12 different families. The approximately dozen enzymes responsible for drug oxidation belong to three families (CYP1, CYP2, and CYP3). Fortunately for physicians, most drugs are substrates for one of two enzymes (CYP2D6 and CYP3A4). Several drugs can either induce or inhibit CYP enzymes thus leading to the potential for drug-drug interactions. While most interactions are not clinically significant, several, like the terfenadine-ketoconazole interaction, can be disastrous. Over the past decade a large effort has been made to better characterize these interactions and new information about specific drugs and their interactions is becoming available almost daily. Several electronic databases accessible on the internet or downloadable to a computer or handheld device (Table 27.1) allow physicians to stay up to date. The availability of these electronic resources has lessened the value of textbook-based sources because textbook information is often out of date by the time it is published.

The clinician should also be vigilant for pharmacodynamic interactions. The ability of psychiatric drugs to interact with several different receptor systems increases the chance that a significant pharmacodynamic interaction will occur. Monoamine oxidase inhibitors (MAOIs), tricyclic antidepressants (TCAs), and antipsychotics are the most notorious in this regard. Table 27.2 lists the more common pharmacodynamic interactions that occur with psychiatric medications.

---

[2] Similar to the use of antipyretics to control the fever seen with infections, there are some data, albeit weak, that the use of sedatives to relieve the insomnia of major depression might even be counterproductive.

TABLE 27.1

Internet-based drug-drug interaction resources

Source	URL
Indiana University, Department of Medicine	http://medicine.iupui.edu/flockhart/
Clinical Pharmacology Matters	http://cpip.gsm.com/
Mental Health Connections, Inc.	http://mhc.com/Cytochromes/
Physician Desk Reference	http://www.pdr.net/pdrnet/librarian
Arizona Center for Education and Research on Therapeutics	http://www.qtdrugs.org

Pharmacodynamic interactions

Purported mechanism	Interaction
α_1-Adrenergic receptor blockade	Potentiation of antihypertensives
clozapine low potency antipsychotics risperidone TCAs	– prazosin (especially)
Dopamine reuptake blockade	Interference of antipsychotic action
buproprion	– dopamine receptor antagonists
H_1 Histamine receptor blockade	Potentiation of sedation
clozapine	– alcohol
olanzapine	– antiepileptic agents
quetiapine	– antihistamines
low potency traditional antipsychotics	– benzodiazepine
risperidone	Potentiation of weight gain
TCAs	– agents that alter caloric intake
Inhibition of monoamine degradation	Serotonergic syndrome
MAOIs	– meperidine
	– serotonergic TCAs
	– SSRIs
	Hypertensive crisis
	– sympathomimetics
	– high tyramine (various food
	– products)
Membrane stabilization	Potentiation of arrhythmias
TCAs	– Type 1a antiarrhythmic
Muscarine receptor blockade	Potentiation of constipation,
clozapine	urinary retention,
olanzapine	accommodation
low potency traditional antipsychotics	– anticholinergic drugs
TCAs	

Psychiatric considerations in the neurological patient

Many neurological illnesses have psychiatric features, including psychosis, mania, depression, anxiety, and personality change. Reviewing all psychiatric complications of all neurological illnesses is beyond the scope of this chapter, and helpful reviews for specific conditions are listed in the Bibliography and Annotated bibliography. The present discussion will focus primarily on depression, which (after delirium and dementia) is the most common reason for psychiatric referral in patients with neurological illness (see Table 27.3).

Diagnostic considerations

As discussed above, considerable skill is required to distinguish depressive symptoms from the effects of general medical illness and treatment. In hospitalized patients, "NPO" orders, nursing evaluations at midnight, and confinement to bed make it difficult to diagnose poor appetite, insomnia, and anhedonia (loss of interest or pleasure in nearly all activities), respectively. However, injury to the brain adds an additional level of diagnostic confusion. Brain lesions can cause psychiatric illness, but they can also cause other neurobehavioral syndromes that either mimic or hide signs of depression. The following patient history illustrates two such neurobehavioral syndromes.

Mr F, a 35-year-old man with no prior psychiatric illness, presents with sudden left hemiplegia. Arteriography shows a complete dissection of the right internal carotid artery. He has signs consistent with infarction in the territory of the right middle cerebral artery. A week later, a nurse alerts the physician to repeated crying spells, sleeplessness, poor appetite, and comments about death that might indicate suicidality. The patient expresses reasonable disappointment in his loss of health but has sensible plans for working around his new disability. He appears surprised at questions about depression, and he steadfastly maintains that his mood is "good." His orientation and short-term memory are normal. However, affect is somewhat blunted. Although he can correctly identify emotional coloring that the examiner adds to a neutral sentence, he is unable to repeat a neutral sentence with any significant emotional modulation.

This patient was unable to put emotional coloring ("prosody") into his verbal communication using pitch, inflection, gesture, and facial expression. This phenomenon

TABLE 27.3

Medical conditions associated with psychiatric disorders

Secondary anxiety
Adrenergic agonists
Alcohol/sedative withdrawal
Caffeine
Hypoglycemia
Hypoxia
Secondary catatonia
Bilateral infarcts of
   anterior cerebral arteries
   globus pallidus
   thalamus
   brainstem
Hypothalamic tumors
Neuroleptic toxicity
Phencyclidine (PCP) and
   ketamine intoxication
Secondary depression
HIV infection
Huntington's disease
Multiple sclerosis
   (especially temporal lobe plaques)
Parkinson's disease
Reserpine or alpha-methyl-dopa
Stroke
   prefrontal cortex (left hemisphere)
   basal ganglia (left hemisphere)
Wilson's disease
Secondary mania
Adrenergic agonists
Choreiform illnesses
Corticosteroids
Encephalitides
Orbitofrontal and brainstem
   tumors
Right orbitofrontal or subcortical
   brain injury

Secondary obsessive-compulsive disorder
Bilateral globus pallidus lesions
Carbon monoxide poisoning
Manganese poisoning
Post-encephalitis lethargica
Sydenham's chorea
Secondary panic disorder
Parkinsonism
Secondary personality change
Dementia of the Alzheimer type
Diffuse head injury
Epilepsy (limbic focus; controversial)
Focal head injury (frontal and temporal lobes)
General paresis (neurosyphilis)
Secondary psychosis
Acute intermittent porphyria
Dopamine agonist intoxication
Epilepsy (especially limbic focus)
LSD and other hallucinogen use
Lupus cerebritis
Metachromatic leukodystrophy
Neurosyphilis
Phencyclidine (PCP) and ketamine intoxication
Stroke
   subcortical
   right parietal cortex
Wilson's disease

Adapted from Csernansky *et al.*, 1997 (permission granted).

has been called motor (or expressive) aprosodia and has been observed with strokes in the nondominant anterior operculum (analogous to Broca's area in the dominant hemisphere). Although there is controversy as to the validity and localization of lesions associated with aprosodia, it can be observed in some stroke patients. The importance for psychiatric diagnosis is that some patients are unable to look and sound sad even when they feel sad. Thus, a patient with motor aprosodia may say he or she is sad but not appear sad, leading the physician to underestimate the likelihood of major depression. On the other hand, "flat affect" in a patient with motor aprosodia (or parkinsonism) may be mistaken for major depression when none is present. In short, the ability of stroke patients to show emotion must be specifically assessed before one can meaningfully interpret their affect.

Second, this patient denies several objective signs of depression that were observed by his nurses. This may indicate anosognosia for depression. Anosognosia originally referred to a lack of awareness of hemiplegia. However, the term can also describe unawareness of visual, tactile, cognitive, or emotional deficits following brain injury. Patients can have anosognosia for one type of deficit while remaining aware of another. Clearly one cannot claim that a patient *feels* sad if he denies it. However, major depression is a syndrome, not a symptom. Occasionally stroke patients who deny sadness still exhibit anhedonia, insomnia, anorexia, and crying, and talk of suicide or hopelessness. In such cases, the stroke often involves the right parietal lobe. Since a DSM-IV major depressive episode can be diagnosed using observable signs of depression even when there are no self-reported symptoms, these patients can be said to have anosognosia for depression.

Some may question why a diagnosis of depression need be made if the patient is unaware of the illness. (Though to be fair, the same point could be asked regarding diagnosing hemiplegia when the patient is unaware of it.) However, major depression predicts higher morbidity and mortality in stroke patients, and treatment may improve rehabilitation outcome even when patients do not recognize their depression. Also, patients with this fascinating presentation respond to antidepressant medications in typical fashion. The importance of anosognosia for depression can be summarized in this unsurprising way: patients with brain damage may not be able to reliably describe their own symptoms, including mood symptoms. Several studies support this hypothesis by showing poor correlation of self-report and observable signs of depression in stroke patients. Fortunately, the best solution is simply part of good medical practice — for confident diagnosis the physician may need diagnostic information not only from the patient but also from direct observation of the patient's behavior. Such observations may be made by the physician, hospital personnel, family members or other caretakers. The point is that the usual psychiatric examination must be expanded in order to adequately assess patients with known brain lesions (see Box 27.3). However, the additional effort required is often modest.

BOX 27.3

Recommendations for diagnosing depression in patients with focal brain lesions

1 Before relying on depressive symptoms or signs from the patient interview:
   - rule out fluent aphasia
   - rule out motor aprosodia
   - assess memory.
2 Always gather diagnostic information from third parties (e.g., family, nurses).
3 Require a full depressive syndrome, including adequate duration (for instance, the DSM-IV "A" criterion for a major depressive episode). Specifically:
   - individual symptoms or signs known to be directly caused by the primary illness (independent of depression) should not be counted toward the diagnosis of depression (e.g., fatigue in patients with multiple sclerosis or anorexia in many cancer patients)
   - crying or apathy alone should not be diagnosed as a major depression
   - even a complete depressive syndrome that is present on a single interview, or for only a week or so, should not be confidently considered major depression.

Adapted from Black, 1995.

In a case like the one previously described, the need for a thorough psychiatric assessment is clear. However, there are many neurological patients in whom major depression is obvious. Prospective studies show a high prevalence of major depression in certain neurological illnesses. In stroke, for instance, about 20% of patients meet criteria for a major depressive episode, and another 20% show milder, subsyndromal depressive symptoms. The same proportions hold for Parkinson's disease. These numbers reflect cross-sectional prevalence; over the entire course of the illness the percentages are even higher. Huntington's disease, epilepsy, and multiple sclerosis are other neurologic illnesses with a high prevalence of significant depression.

The previous case shows how specific neurobehavioral syndromes can interfere with diagnosis. Some neurological diseases can produce specific depressive symptoms or signs independent of any other evidence of major depression. For example, multiple sclerosis commonly causes fatigue whether or not sadness, guilt, insomnia, suicidality, or loss of interest is also present. Parkinson's disease is another example, discussed in detail below. Because of such difficulties, many approaches have been suggested to help with the diagnosis of major depression in patients with neurological disease. At the extremes, some researchers prefer to ignore causation of symptoms and count all depressive symptoms, while others exclude all symptoms that could be caused by the primary illness. Different strategies may be appropriate for different purposes, and increasingly, data are available to compare diagnostic schemes in specific disease populations.

For clinical purposes, we favor the following diagnostic approach. The first requirement is a careful assessment, including information from third parties as appropriate, by a clinician who is well acquainted with the neurological disease in question. Second, symptoms or signs that are commonly produced by the illness in the absence of depression, such as limited facial expression in Parkinson's disease, are excluded. The remaining symptoms are used to diagnose or exclude a major depressive episode by DSM-IV criteria. Justification for this strategy derives from the observation that, in many neurological illnesses, the symptom profile and course of depression are similar to those of idiopathic major depression.

Population studies clearly suggest that some illnesses directly cause depression. However, in a single individual, it is usually impossible to definitely know the cause of a psychiatric illness. For instance, there is no reason to think that a stroke protects the patient from the usual risk factors for major depression, such as a personal or family history of depression. For this reason, several authors have argued that it is more defensible to stop after diagnosing a major depressive episode and note the possibility that it is caused directly by the neurological illness, without definitively specifying the cause. However, the DSM-IV Committee felt that it was more clinically useful to diagnose either "major depressive disorder" or "mood disorder due to a general medical condition," using the physician's best judgment of etiology based on the overall clinical picture. For certain illnesses, the latter diagnosis is clearly defensible, as discussed below. However, we also recommend the use of the more modest DSM-IV diagnosis "mood disorder not otherwise specified." In any case, depressive symptoms call for clinical attention and treatment.

Some mood studies in neurological populations have discussed "minor depression," referring to depressive symptoms that do not meet criteria for a major depressive episode. Minor depression defined in this way is more highly correlated with disability and is more persistent than major depression. In some patients minor depression appears to be a normal reaction to the loss of health, whereas in others it presages a later major depression. Further studies of these milder, subsyndromal depressive symptoms are needed, including treatment studies. In DSM-IV, minor depression can be classified as a "mood disorder not otherwise specified."

Major depression is a serious complication of neurologic illness. Stroke patients with depression actually have higher mortality than non-depressed stroke patients; they also have a worse rehabilitation outcome. Studies of patients with stroke, multiple sclerosis, and Parkinson's disease all show that major depression strongly predicts cognitive impairment even after controlling for age, disability, and severity of illness. Depression also can be responsible for somatic complaints. In addition, major depression carries with it its own risk of death and a great deal of suffering. One physician wrote that depression "is probably more unpleasant than any disease except rabies" (Price, 1978). For all these reasons, effective treatment of depression is important in neurological patients.

Treatment considerations

Treatment studies in several neurological populations have shown that major depression usually responds to antidepressant medication or ECT. (For most neurological illnesses, treatment studies utilizing psychotherapy are unfortunately lacking.) However, many neurological patients appear to be especially sensitive to treatment side effects. Tricyclic antidepressants (TCAs) cause important side effects via their antagonism at several receptor types, including α_1-adrenergic (hypotension), muscarinic cholinergic (confusion, dry mouth, impaired visual accommodation, urinary retention, constipation), and H_1-histaminic (sedation), among others. Among the TCAs, nortriptyline and desipramine are generally better tolerated. Bupropion probably has an increased risk of producing seizures in patients with brain lesions, head trauma, or prior seizures. Selective serotonin reuptake inhibitors (SSRIs) are generally well tolerated, although efficacy data is still limited for several important illnesses. Other later-generation antidepres-

sants, such as venlafaxine and mirtazapine, are also widely used. Electroconvulsive therapy can be safely used in most neurological patients, often with gratifying results. However, since there are special considerations for ECT in several illnesses (Parkinson's disease, multiple sclerosis, epilepsy, brain tumors, and myasthenia gravis, among others), ECT should be performed by a psychiatrist with special expertise in using ECT in this population. In general, the recommendations listed in Box 27.2 apply to neurological patients with major depression. If patients do not respond within about six weeks of treatment, psychiatric consultation should be considered, and the diagnosis of major depression should be reviewed.

In spite of effective treatment, studies of depression in neurologic patients continue to show that many patients with major depression are undertreated. There seem to be two reasons for this: (1) major depression is not diagnosed in many patients, and (2) major depression is not adequately treated once diagnosed. To address the first problem, given the high prevalence of depression in patients with neurological disorders, the physician should routinely screen for depressive symptoms. At a minimum, each patient with known brain disease should be asked about persistent sadness. This could be accomplished using a simple self-report questionnaire, such as the Beck Depression Inventory or one of the questionnaires adapted for use in specific illness populations. Such screening is imperfect as it measures low mood instead of assessing the presence of a major depressive episode. It does identify, though, people who might have major depression.

As to the second problem, undertreatment of diagnosed depression may reflect an erroneous impression that major depression in these patients is somehow "appropriate." This may arise in part because the term "depressed" in lay language commonly refers to mild and transient sadness. Naturally no one is expected to feel happy about serious illness, and ordinary sadness may be normal or beneficial. However, when symptoms co-occur such that the full syndrome of major depression is present, the response is no longer "appropriate" but instead produces dysfunction (i.e., morbidity) and mortality in severe cases. Thus, physicians should actively treat major depression no matter how "understandable" it may seem. Another cause of undertreated major depression is the use of very small doses of antidepressants (e.g., daily doses of amitriptyline 25 mg or fluoxetine 5 mg). Small doses may be required initially for tolerability or chronically in patients with markedly impaired pharmacokinetic clearance. Still, as a general long-term strategy low-dose antidepressants offer only side effects without proven benefit for major depression.

Etiological considerations

As discussed in the first section of this chapter, there is an increased prevalence of major depression in nearly all serious medical conditions. This is popularly attributed to expected sadness in the face of life difficulties, such as serious illness. However, the facts are not that simple. For instance, the majority of patients with a stroke feel some sadness and disappointment, but only a minority experience major depression. Thus, the commonly heard statement, "I'd be depressed, too, if I had their illness" is only true for the symptom of depression (sadness) and not for the major depressive syndrome. Additionally, although some might contend that major depression is a normal response to illness, this argument fails to explain the presence of poststroke mania and psychosis.

There is some evidence that "life stress," including nonpsychiatric illness, may influence the timing of a major depressive episode in predisposed individuals. Along these lines, patients diagnosed with stroke, multiple sclerosis or Parkinson's disease have a higher risk of major depression after their illness is diagnosed if they have a personal or family history of major depression prior to diagnosis. On the other hand, there is increasingly strong evidence that major depression in certain illnesses is directly caused by the brain lesion. It should not be surprising that injuring the organ of emotion can cause mood disorders, but many people react skeptically to this notion, probably because of the mind-body duality ingrained in our culture. Some of the evidence that some major depression is directly caused by certain neurological illnesses is reviewed in Box 27.4.

BOX 27.4

Evidence for direct causation of depression in certain neurological illnesses*

1 Depression is more prevalent in these conditions than in equally disabling conditions that do not affect the brain.
2 Depression is strongly predicted by lesion location within the brain.
3 Extent of disability is not strongly predictive of depression.
4 Depression has different demographics in these patients than in the general population.
5 Depression can develop before symptoms of the primary illness (but later in life and more often than expected for idiopathic major depression).
6 Brain function is different in neurological patients with vs. without depression.
*Data support one or more of these statements for each of the following illnesses: multiple sclerosis, Huntington's disease, Parkinson's disease, Wilson's disease, stroke, traumatic brain injury, and primary dystonia.

The fact that some illnesses contribute directly to causing a major depressive episode is an unfortunate experiment of nature, but it offers hope for better understanding the pathophysiology and neuroanatomy of idiopathic major depression. For instance, observations that major depression is often associated with Cushing's disease and hypothyroidism led to important studies of cortisol and thyroid dysregulation in severe idiopathic depression. Secondary depressions have also helped to validate new biological findings in idiopathic major depression (see Chapter 8).

Special neuropsychiatric issues in Parkinson's disease

In several neurological illnesses, major depression presents diagnostic and treatment considerations similar to those seen in depressed patients without a general medical illness. Parkinson's disease (PD) warrants a more detailed discussion because it is an increasingly common illness that offers a number of exceptions to this general rule.

The most common psychiatric complication of PD is major depression. There are several diagnostic issues specific to PD. Some patients with PD experience pathological crying, i.e., involuntary tears in the absence of sadness; this symptom can respond to initiation of dopamimetic medication. Pathological laughter is less common in PD. Apathy or fatigue also can present as the predominant symptom in PD in the absence of a major depressive syndrome. Although there is little direct information about treatment of these symptoms in PD, a trial of dopamimetic treatment is reasonable for either. More typical PD symptoms can also be misinterpreted as depressive symptoms. These include facial hypomimia ("masked facies"), internal tremor without other evidence of anxiety, or akathisia or tremor that the patient identifies as "anxiety."

One less common situation that should be distinguished from a prolonged, steady major depressive episode occurs in patients whose depressive symptoms are essentially limited to motor "off" periods. These patients also tend to have levodopa-induced dyskinesias and a long history of levodopa treatment. As a group, off-period depression patients have high rates of psychiatric comorbidity including dopa-induced psychosis, dementia, and past major depression. "Off" depression in these patients generally requires adjustment of dopamimetic treatment rather than traditional antidepressant therapy. The same appears to hold true for off-period anxiety (including off-period panic attacks), which is even more common.

After consideration of these diagnostic issues, depression in PD still differs from idiopathic major depression. Depressed patients with PD are less likely to have self-reproach, delusions, and hallucinations; less likely to complete suicide; and more likely to have substantial anxiety and a chronic course. Men and women have similar rates of depression in PD, compared to the higher risk to women of major depression in general.

Major depressive episodes in PD generally do not respond to the dopaminergic drugs typically used for the motor manifestations of parkinsonism, although this assertion is based on limited evidence. Psychostimulants such as methylphenidate have unproven efficacy. However, when a mild major depressive episode occurs in a patient who requires increases in antiparkinsonian medication to better treat motor signs, it may be appropriate to defer antidepressant treatment until the clinical picture is more stable. Certainly, close follow-up is needed. This wait allows the physician to accurately interpret any treatment-emergent psychiatric side effects, and mood does improve during this interval in some patients. Further direct study is needed, since the dopamine D_3 receptor-preferring agonist pramipexole is an effective antidepressant in non-parkinsonian patients with major depression, and preliminary reports suggest that other dopamine agonists may also be effective in that population.

On the other hand, moderate to severe major depression is often the patient's most disabling problem, and vigorous treatment of depression is indicated. There is little treatment efficacy data for antidepressants in PD. However, paroxetine is currently being tested in a multicenter study supported by the NIH. Since anticholinergics have some efficacy in treating parkinsonism, physicians may be tempted to choose a tertiary amine TCA such as imipramine or amitriptyline. However, in most patients, doses adequate for antidepressant effect produce confusion or other significant anticholinergic side effects, and the risks outweigh the small motor benefit conferred. Newer antidepressants are usually better tolerated. At present, SSRIs are the most commonly prescribed antidepressant medications in the US. SSRIs have indirect antidopaminergic effects, but these are usually relatively insignificant clinically, compared to the effects of the primary disease and its treatment. Mirtazapine is also used widely and is well tolerated in patients with PD.

All antidepressants are relatively contraindicated in patients who are taking the monoamine oxidase inhibitor selegiline, due to occasional occurrence of the "central serotonin syndrome," which can be life-threatening. The serotonin syndrome can include confusion, rigidity, pyrexia (elevated body temperature), myoclonus, and autonomic instability. Often the antidepressant may be more important to the patient's overall health than the selegiline, and discontinuation of selegiline (with adjustment of other antiparkinsonian medication and an appropriate wait before beginning the antidepressant drug) can resolve the treatment dilemma. In other cases, ECT or psychotherapy may be used instead of an antidepressant medication, depending on the severity of the depression and other factors. However, sometimes the clinical situation dictates a need to prescribe both selegiline and an antidepressant; this should be undertaken only with close monitoring by the physician after carefully weighing the risk-benefit ratio for the individual and obtaining informed consent. In fact, despite an FDA warning, many patients with PD take an SSRI with selegiline, and the serotonin syndrome is rarely reported. A relatively noradrenergic antidepressant, such as desipramine or mirtazapine, may be more prudent in this situation, though this is speculative.

ECT can be helpful in selected patients suffering with both Parkinson's disease and a major depressive episode. In fact, ECT has been shown to produce short-lived improvements in motor signs even in non-depressed parkinsonian patients. However, there is a high rate of interictal delirium in depressed parkinsonian patients undergoing ECT, so special care is necessary when using ECT in this population. Interestingly, this complication of ECT is also frequently seen in patients with primary pathology of the caudate nucleus. At our center, ECT is started at a frequency of twice per week in parkinsonian patients.

Psychosis is a common complication of dopaminergic therapy in patients with Parkinson's disease or diffuse Lewy body disease. The first step in treating psychosis is careful diagnosis. Attention, orientation or level of consciousness are often impaired, and the usual diagnostic evaluation for delirium should be pursued first (see Chapter 11). Unnecessary medications should also be eliminated, especially those with psychoactive effects. If symptoms persist after ruling out delirium and reviewing all medications, anticholinergics should be eliminated, followed by elimination or reduction of amantadine and then dopamine agonists, if necessary. Levodopa generally has a better therapeutic index than these agents with respect to psychosis. If these steps are ineffective, patients with psychosis may respond to a reduction in dosage of levodopa. This response can take two weeks, however, and some patients cannot tolerate a lower dose because of their motor symptoms and signs. Patients with PD are extraordinarily sensitive to the acute motor side effects of antipsychotics, and severe worsening of parkinsonism is often observed with typical neuroleptics, and to a significant extent with risperidone and olanzapine. Remarkably, the first complete randomized controlled trial of any antipsychotic in Parkinson's disease patients was not reported until 1999. It showed that clozapine provided adequate treatment of psychosis in PD even if antiparkinsonian medication dosages are increased. Although use of clozapine involves significant expense, weekly blood draws, and a risk of agranulocytosis, it may represent the best treatment option for selected patients. Numerous open label studies support the use of quetiapine. Typical doses for both clozapine and quetiapine for psychosis in PD are 12.5–100 mg nightly, much lower than doses used in schizophrenia. Further data are needed for aripiprazole and ziprasidone.

Detailed discussion of other psychiatric complications of PD are beyond the scope of this chapter. These complications include dementia in PD and other parkinsonian illnesses, social phobia and other anxious syndromes, treatment-induced mania or disinhibition, treatment-induced complex stereotypies ("punding"), and REM sleep behavior disorder.

The etiology of psychiatric symptoms in PD has been studied. Several large-scale case-control studies have shown that the excess incidence of major depression in PD actually begins prior to the first motor signs. Thus depression in PD cannot be entirely a psychological reaction to symptoms or diagnosis. Most of this excess occurs during the five years preceding the first movement abnormality, suggesting that in some PD patients, depression is most likely a specific consequence of neurodegeneration. Similarly, anxiety disorders are common in patients with PD, even before the development of parkinsonian motor symptoms. The excess prevalence of anxiety begins at least 20 years prior to diagnosis of PD. Social phobia is very common and may relate to observations of abnormal dopaminergic function in young, otherwise healthy people with social phobia. Several other psychiatric complications of PD are also demonstrably caused, at least in part, by the illness or its treatment. For instance, disinhibition often shows a typical dose-response relationship to dopamine agonist therapy, and under blinded conditions, off-period changes in mood precede rather than follow changes in motor symptoms.

Summary

Major depressive episodes are common in illnesses that cause brain lesions and are largely a direct effect of lesions in areas involved with emotional physiology, rather than an appropriate emotional response to illness. These patients require careful, thorough clinical assessment to achieve accurate psychiatric diagnosis. Major depression in several neurological disorders confers a worse prognosis (at least if untreated). Although major depression generally has a rewarding treatment response, it is commonly unnoticed or undertreated. Thus, major depression should be actively sought and treated in these patients. Psychiatric consultation is recommended for any of the indications in Box 27.3.

Psychiatric disorders in patients with a chronic medical illness

Major depression

The occurrence of major depression in patients with a chronic medical illness has been the subject of much study. A good broad review was written by Popkin and Tucker in 1992. More focused reviews of major depression in specific conditions such as end-stage renal disease, diabetes mellitus,[3] and coronary artery disease are listed in the Bibliography. Additional information on the occurrence of major depression in diabetes mellitus and coronary artery disease can be found in Chapter 28.

Major depression is known to be a common comorbid complication of several chronic medical illnesses (see Box 27.5). Compared with a point prevalence[4] of 3–5% for major depression in the general population, patients with end-stage renal disease (5–8%), coronary artery disease (18–25%), and diabetes mellitus (15%) are at increased risk for major depression. Patients with malignancy or acquired immunodeficiency syndrome (AIDS) also have an elevated risk of major depression. Although the risk for major depression in other chronic medical illnesses is not as clear, it might be reasonable to conclude that patients are at greater risk of developing major depression whenever chronic medical illness is present. However, the picture is not that simple because certain chronic illnesses appear to have a substantially increased risk of major depression. Whereas malignancy in general probably has a prevalence of major depression similar to that seen in other chronic illnesses, there is wide variation among the different specific types of cancer. In contrast to lymphoma where only about 1% of patients develop major depression, 50% of patients with pancreatic cancer develop the syndrome. This predilection for major depression in patients with pancreatic cancer, combined with the observation that some patients develop major depression *prior* to the diagnosis of pancreatic cancer, suggests that major depression in some patients is not just a reaction to the illness but rather a part of it.

BOX 27.5

Chronic medical conditions commonly associated with major depression

- Coronary artery disease.
- Diabetes mellitus.
- End-stage renal disease.
- Human immunodeficiency virus.
- Malignancies, particularly pancreatic.
- Myocardial infarction.

---

[3] While diabetes mellitus is an endocrine disorder, we will discuss it with the other chronic medical conditions and not with endocrine disorders because the approach to evaluating and treating psychiatric illness in diabetes mellitus is much more similar to that of other medical conditions.

[4] Point prevalence is defined as the percentage of patients who meet criteria for a given illness at *one point in time* and is different from lifetime prevalence, which is the percentage of patients who meet criteria for a given illness *any time* during their lives.

Specific issues with treating major depression in patients with coronary artery disease

In situations where major depression presents in patients with coronary artery disease, clinicians should keep in mind that TCAs have Type 1a antiarrhythymic effects. The ability of TCAs to slow cardiac conduction combined with the higher prevalence of ventricular tachycardia in these patients argues against their use in patients with coronary artery disease, especially in the immediate post myocardial infarction (MI) period. However, TCAs have been safely used in this population and in cases of severe major depression with suicidality and lack of response to other medications, they might constitute appropriate treatment. Electroconvulsive treatment might be another option in this severely ill group. Use of a TCA should also be avoided in patients with a greater than grade I A-V conduction block. SSRIs, which lack type 1a effects and do not antagonize α_1 adrenergic receptors, would be more appropriate as front-line agents. Supporting this view, a recently completed study found that sertraline, one of five SSRIs on the US market, did not adversely affect cardiovascular outcome when used in patients with a recent MI or with unstable angina. However, the physician should bear in mind that subjects in this study did not receive sertraline until an average of one month after an MI and were not severely medically ill. In addition, significant but uncommon adverse events might have been missed since only 400 patients were studied.

While sertraline appears to be relatively free of significant toxicity in this patient group, this might not be the case for all agents in this class because several SSRIs substantially inhibit one or more of the CYP enzymes. Of the five available SSRIs (citalopram,[5] fluoxetine, fluvoxamine, paroxetine, sertraline) sertraline and citalopram appear to inhibit CYP enzymes the least and thus could be reasonably expected to produce fewer instances of drug-drug interactions. However, for any specific drug or specific CYP enzyme another SSRI might be better. For example, several antihypertensives are metabolized by CYP2D6. If a patient were only on an antihypertensive, then fluvoxamine, which does not inhibit CYP2D6, would be the best choice among the SSRIs. The exact role of antidepressants from other classes in the treatment of major depression in this subpopulation of patients remains to be determined. The ability of venlaflaxine to cause a dose-dependent increase in heart rate, blood pressure, and cholesterol levels might limit its use in this patient population.

[5] Citalopram consists of equal amounts of both optical isomers. Escitalopram is composed of only the biologically active optical isomer. Its therapeutic and side effects have not be shown to be different from those of citalopram. For purposes of this chapter it is not considered as a different agent.

Specific issues with treating major depression in patients with diabetes mellitus

Several studies have shown efficacy for antidepressants in the treatment of major depression in patients with diabetes mellitus. In the past, TCAs have been favored, especially for severe cases, but their hypotensive effects could be problematic in this patient group. It was originally thought that TCAs might exhibit antidiabetic effects through a direct effect on the adrenergic system as well as through indirect effects of ameliorating major depression. In the only double-blind placebo-controlled study to date, improvement in major depression associated with nortriptyline treatment appeared to lower glycosylated hemoglobin levels. However, nortriptyline appears to directly elevate glycosylated hemoglobin and cancel out the indirect benefits from the improvement in major depression. Thus, the use of TCAs in patients with major depression might have minimal overall effects on elevated glycosylated hemoglobin, despite effective treatment of major depression. SSRIs probably lack direct adverse consequences on glycosylated hemoglobin because of their more selective pharmacology, and thus they might lower glycosylated hemoglobin by improving depression.

Fluoxetine was recently shown in a double-blind placebo-controlled trial to improve major depression in subjects with diabetes. However, only a trend level (P = .13) effect on lowering glycosylated hemoglobin was seen, possibly as a result of a small sample size. Further studies with larger numbers of subjects will be needed in order to determine whether SSRIs have a beneficial effect on glycosylated hemoglobin. For now, SSRIs are considered front-line agents because they are better tolerated than TCAs. Based on pharmacokinetic concerns, sertraline and citalopram are probably the preferred SSRIs for this patient group. Studies are still needed to evaluate whether fluoxetine's greater tendency (as compared to other SSRIs) to cause anorexia and weight loss is clinically relevant in the routine treatment of major depression in patients with diabetes mellitus. MAOIs are relatively contraindicated in patients with diabetes mellitus given their ability to cause severe hypoglycemia. Finally, clinicians should remember that diabetic patients with major depression require close monitoring of their glucose status, since caloric intake and physical activity varies depending on depressive state.

Specific issues with treating major depression in patients with end-stage renal disease

The bulk of the literature regarding the treatment of major depression in patients with end-stage renal disease consists of case reports. One small open-label study suggested that a good response occurred in the majority of patients receiving desipramine at about half the typical dose. Blood levels were found to be in the lower end of a therapeutic range in most of these patients. A similar result was found in patients on hemodialysis. These findings contradict the results of two other studies evaluating desipramine blood levels in patients with decreased renal function, as well as predictions of blood levels based on pharmacokinetic principles.[6] Until more definitive studies are done, it would be safest, when prescribing desipramine in this patient population, to use a low dose initially and adjust upward if indicated by serum levels.

In contrast, the use of nortriptyline appears to follow pharmacokinetic predictions and does not require dose adjustment in patients with end-stage renal disease. While the effective dose of most TCAs may not differ in patients with end-stage renal disease, the drugs should, nevertheless, be started at a low dose and increased slowly in order to prevent orthostatic hypotension in this patient group. As always, serum levels should be routinely monitored. Regarding SSRIs, paroxetine, like desipramine, does not follow pharmacokinetic predictions and should also be used at half the normal adult dose. The dose of fluoxetine does not need to be adjusted. In the case of sertraline and fluvoxamine, until clinical data are available, one should probably use low initial doses and adjust upward if clinical status warrants. While patients with end-stage renal disease tolerate SSRIs better than TCAs, the ability to check serum levels and adjust doses as needed in a timely manner suggests that TCAs might be more appropriate agents in cases of moderate to severe major depression where one might not be able to wait 2–4 weeks to see whether a patient is responding to an SSRI before adjusting the dose upwards.

Specific issues with treating major depression in patients with cancer

While there is a relative dearth of studies on the use of antidepressants in patients with malignancy, available evidence indicates that these drugs can be efficacious. TCAs are the best studied and are sometimes used as front-line agents given the propensity of SSRIs to cause nausea, anorexia, and weight loss. Nortryptiline or desipramine would probably be preferred agents because of their better side-effect profiles. Venlafaxine might prove useful for those who cannot tolerate the side effects of TCAs. Bupropion should not be used in patients at risk for seizures (e.g., those with CNS lesions). The weight gain associated with mirtazipine has made it a favorite with some physicians for the treatment of the depressed cachectic patient.

---

[6]If greater than 95% of the drug is metabolized (i.e., less than 5% excreted unchanged by the kidney), then there would be only a minimal decrease in the clearance of the drug in patients with compromised renal function. In such cases, serum levels would not change significantly and there should be no need for adjustment of dose.

Dysthymia

Dysthymia is a mood disorder in which the signs and symptoms are chronic but never reach the intensity of major depression (see Chapter 8 for further details). Dysthymia can present as a comorbid illness in patients with a chronic medical illness. In this context, dysthymia has been most thoroughly studied in patients with diabetes mellitus; however, even here the knowledge base is scant. In addition, it is not entirely clear whether the term "dysthymia," as applied to patients with medical conditions, represents a separate and distinct mood disorder, a mild variant of major depression, or a normal response to a stressful situation. In general, one should be suspicious of subclinical major depression in any patient with dysthymia and should consider instituting antidepressant treatment empirically in severe cases. Further conclusions and recommendations about dysthymia should be drawn with great care until the exact nature of dysthymia in medically ill patients is clearer.

Generalized anxiety disorder

Even though anxiety is the hallmark of generalized anxiety disorder, it is also a common manifestation of major depression, and the clinician should always rule out major depression as a cause (see Chapters 8 and 9). Generalized anxiety disorder has been most studied in association with diabetes mellitus, irritable bowel syndrome, and esophageal spasm syndrome. However, these avenues of research are in their infancy, and information is sparse at best. One interesting fact is that the symptoms of generalized anxiety disorder usually precede the onset of intestinal symptoms in irritable bowel syndrome, suggesting that it might be etiologically related to this gastrointestinal disorder. As discussed later in this chapter, anxiety is also seen in several endocrine disorders, though it is unclear whether it occurs in isolation or in the context of generalized anxiety disorder or major depression.

Treatment of generalized anxiety disorder is the same whether or not the disorder is associated with a medical condition and consists of pharmacotherapy with buspirone or benzodiazepines (see Chapter 9). Because the symptom of anxiety can be the initial presenting symptom of a major depressive episode, the clinician should always be vigilant for the potential manifestation of major depression. Such a change in diagnosis would dictate a change in treatment.

Panic disorder

Although anxiety occurs commonly in medically ill patients, comorbid panic disorder, as defined by DSM-IV, appears infrequently. Panic disorder can be seen in diabetes mellitus, but more commonly it occurs in patients with irritable bowel syndrome and esophageal spasm syndrome. The primary care physician typically encounters panic disorder, not as a true comorbid process however, but rather masquerading as angina in a person *without* coronary artery disease. Prompt recognition and appropriate treatment of panic disorder prevents the patient from undergoing potentially dangerous diagnostic procedures and being prescribed inappropriate medications. The treatment of panic disorder is the same whether or not the disorder is associated with a medical condition, and the reader is referred to Chapter 9 for more specific information.

Psychiatric disorders in the puerperium

The puerperium is a period of dramatic physiologic changes that has long been associated with psychiatric disturbances. Three syndromes are currently recognized: postpartum ("baby") blues, postpartum depression, and postpartum psychosis (see *Pearls & Perils*). Issues concerning the management of gravid patients with psychiatric disorders will not be addressed here. This topic has recently been reviewed in an excellent chapter by Newport and colleagues.

PEARLS & PERILS

Puerperal disorders

1 Postpartum blues are normal and do not need specific treatment.
2 Postpartum depression is pathological and must be treated, like any major depressive episode.
3 Postpartum psychosis is a serious disorder and needs immediate psychiatric intervention.
4 The postpartum period is considered to extend to the end of the fourth week postpartum.
5 Typically, initial symptoms become apparent within the first two weeks postpartum for the majority of patients.

Postpartum blues

Postpartum blues is a mild and transient syndrome. It typically begins in the first postpartum week. The major symptom is low mood, though mothers also report other affective symptoms (e.g., irritability, insomnia, anxiety, and fatigue). Given that postpartum blues occurs in 25–85% of mothers, the syndrome is usually considered a normal sequela of birth. It is assumed that abrupt changes in hormone levels occurring in the early postpartum period have a role in the syndrome. There is only minimal impact on the mother's ability to care for herself and her infant. No specific treatment is needed and the syndrome usually resolves on its own within two weeks.

Postpartum depression

Like the postpartum blues, postpartum depression typically

begins shortly after birth. Fifty percent of patients with postpartum depression develop symptoms within the first two weeks after delivery.[7] In contrast to the blues, the symptoms and signs of postpartum depression are not transient and worsen with time until a full major depressive episode develops. Without treatment, the episode lasts for approximately seven months. The mothers (perhaps 10–20% of all pregnant women) who go on to develop postpartum depression might be individuals who are at greatest risk for developing major depression in general. Much thought and study have been invested in determining the cause(s) of and risk factors for postpartum depression. Unfortunately, this research has been characterized by problems with diagnostic validity, definition and design, and consistent results have been the exception rather than the rule.

Given the current state of knowledge, it seems prudent that during the first month postpartum, clinicians closely follow patients with a family history of major depression or a past personal history of either major depression or postpartum depression. Severe cases of postpartum depression in which hopelessness or suicidality are present should be referred to a psychiatrist. Mild to moderate depression usually can be treated with antidepressants by the primary physician as long as the mother is not breast-feeding. Because women in the postpartum period can be sensitive to medications, antidepressants should be started at half of the usual dose and increased as tolerated by the patient and as indicated by their clinical state.

Most, if not all, antidepressants are excreted into breast milk, raising concern for the effects of these agents on the breast-feeding infant. In cases where women suffering from postpartum depression do not wish to discontinue breast-feeding, referral to a psychiatrist is indicated in order to aid in the assessment of benefits and risks of psychotherapeutic drug use and for the possible use of psychotherapy. In the past decade several case series have been published regarding the use of SSRIs in this population. No adverse effects were reported in infants for fluvoxamine, paroxetine, and sertraline, which suggests that these agents probably can be administered safely to breast-feeding mothers. Appropriate risk/benefit decisions should be made on a case-by-case basis, however. In case series, fluoxetine has been linked to colic and decreased amounts of weight gain in breast-fed infants, possibly because of its longer half-life. Citalopram has been associated with behavioral changes in infants, also.

---

[7] While a minority of patients develop a depressive syndrome up to a year after childbirth, it is doubtful that these cases are related to parturition. It seems wise for both investigative work and clinical care to adopt some arbitrary line to demarcate the end of the puerperal period. Although six weeks would be consistent with obstetrical practice, four weeks, as proposed in DSM-IV is probably better, since it should improve the homogeneity of the sample while still capturing the vast majority of patients.

Other than the SSRI class, tricyclic antidepressants have been studied the most. Of the TCAs, nortriptyline appears to carry the least risk for the infant. When used, nortriptyline should be prescribed as a single dose at bedtime, and the mother should be instructed to skip the nighttime feeding. These two practices should minimize exposure to the infant by decreasing the amount of nortriptyline in the breast milk. Nefazodone has been associated with drowsiness and lethargy in a case report involving a single infant. Since data on the safety and pharmacokinetics of other antidepressants (venlafaxine, buproprion, mirtazipine) are sparse, these should be reserved for cases where SSRIs and TCAs are contraindicated.

Postpartum psychosis

Postpartum psychosis, although occurring in only 0.1–0.2% of births, is a severe sequela of pregnancy. Like other puerperal disorders it strikes typically within two weeks after delivery. The psychosis occurs usually in the setting of either depression or mania and it is not unusual for a postpartum episode to be the initial presentation of bipolar disorder. Exacerbations of schizophrenia are rare in the immediate postpartum period. Instead, patients with schizophrenia tend to have psychotic exacerbations at least one month after giving birth and thus would not be considered under DSM-IV to have a postpartum psychosis. Given the severe nature of psychosis and its impact on mental functioning, immediate referral to a psychiatrist is almost always indicated. For the protection of the mother and the infant, psychotic patients typically need inpatient psychiatric treatment.

Treatment and outcome depend upon the underlying disorder, with most patients having a course similar to that of bipolar disorder. When lithium is indicated the mother should be encouraged to forego breast-feeding since lithium levels are measurable in the nursing infant and in some cases have been twice that of the mother's. Use of anticonvulsants in breast-feeding mothers is problematic given that anticonvulsants may produce apoptotic neuronal death in the developing brain. With respect to prognosis of the mother, a substantial minority (40% with a median follow-up of 11 years in one study) have no further psychiatric sequelae. Twenty-five percent of patients suffer a relapse following a subsequent (but not necessarily the next) pregnancy, while the remaining 35% develop a recurrence of psychiatric illness before their next pregnancy. Therefore, patients with a history of postpartum psychosis (as well as those with a family history of bipolar disorder) should be observed closely during the first month postpartum for the emergence of this syndrome.

Given the documented risk of developing a postpartum psychosis in patients with bipolar disorder, psychiatric referral during pregnancy should be obtained in these patients in order to insure close monitoring during the postpartum period. In addition, since lithium, valproate, and carbamazepine all have teratogenic effects and should be discontinued during some parts of pregnancy, close monitoring by a psychiatrist is required, and strong consideration should be given to the re-institution of prophylactic treatment immediately after parturition. Finally, given the abrupt changes in volume status and drug clearance that occur in the immediate postpartum period, the physician should monitor the patient and follow drug levels closely, especially when prescribing lithium. Newport and colleagues have recently reviewed the pharmacokinetic and treatment issues that arise during pregnancy and lactation.

Psychiatric manifestations of endocrine disorders

The ability of endocrine disorders to produce psychiatric disturbances has been recognized since the early days of medicine, and a further understanding of their associated psychiatric manifestations should enhance our understanding of idiopathic psychiatric disorders. Unfortunately, little systematic research had been done in recent decades, and thus this area has not benefited from the improved diagnostic and research techniques of modern psychiatry. Despite the lack of progress, endocrine disorders warrant separate discussion in order to highlight two points: (1) in contrast to psychiatric disorders in other medical conditions, "psychiatric" treatment in this population is aimed initially at correcting the underlying enodocrinologic abnormality; and (2) except for neurological disorders, endocrine dysfunctions offer the best evidence for "secondary" psychiatric disorders and show great promise for further research.

Psychiatric manifestations of endocrine dysfunction include anxiety, major depression, mania, psychosis, dementia, and delirium (Table 27.4). Often the CNS effects of endocrine dysfunction can be the initial and most clinically obvious indicator of the hormonal disturbance. A complete discussion of the precise details of each endocrine disorder is beyond the scope of this chapter, and the reader is referred to a review by Reus (1986) and Table 27.4 for further details. For illustrative purposes, disorders involving the thyroid gland will be the focus of this section.

Hyperthyroidism

The mental effects of hyperthyroidism can vary from mild (fatigue, anxiety, irritability) to moderate (excitability, emotional instability) and severe (mania, psychosis). Delusions and hallucinations, typically visual, can also occur alone or in conjunction with a manic state. Typically, severely affected patients also have physical signs of hyperthyroidism (e.g., elevated pulse, a fine hand tremor, and hot dry hands), but their presence is often missed on initial evaluation when the

TABLE 27.4 Psychiatric manifestations associated with endocrine disorders

Endocrine abnormality	Psychiatric manifestations
Adrenal	
Cushing's syndrome	anxiety, delirium, major depression, mania, psychosis
Addison's disease	catatonia, delirium, dementia, major depression, psychosis
Parathyroid	
hyper-	anxiety, delirium, major depression, mania, psychosis
hypo-	anxiety, delirium, dementia, major depression, mania, psychosis
Pituitary	
acromegaly	major depression
hyperprolactinemia	major depression
hypopituitarism	delirium, dementia, major depression
Thyroid	
hyper-	anxiety, delirium, major depression, mania, psychosis
hypo-	anxiety, delirium, dementia, major depression, mania, psychosis

physician is confronted with the behavioral and cognitive signs of CNS dysfunction in a psychotic and hyperactive individual who appears manic. In such cases, the most obvious clue that the CNS dysfunction is caused by a general medical condition is age. Onset of psychosis or mania after age 35 or 40 suggests that the psychosis may be secondary to a general medical condition. In such cases, the physician should be vigilant for features that would indicate a non-psychiatric cause and pursue a complete work-up to exclude other causes (see Tables 27.3 and 27.4).

Although hyperthyroidism is typically associated with manic-like activated states, some patients develop a syndrome consisting of psychomotor retardation and apathy that is much more reminiscent of a major depressive disorder. Still others have a syndrome akin to generalized anxiety disorder. Delirium is a rare presentation of hyperthyroidism, occurring in less than 5% of cases, but given that delirium is an indicator of a medical emergency (in hyperthyroid patients it typically heralds the impending onset of a thyroid storm), its presence must be considered in any patient with recent onset of CNS dysfunction. The presence of fluctuating impairment on bedside cognitive tests of orientation (person, place, time) and attention (serial sevens and months backwards in order) suggests that a patient is delirious and that a general medical condition or medication side effect is

likely to be the cause of the psychiatric signs and symptoms (see Chapter 11 for more details). Delirium can be thought of as "acute brain failure" akin to acute renal failure. Both reflect organ dysfunction caused either by the inability of the body to maintain the homeostatic environment needed for proper organ function (e.g., decreased blood flow, hypoxia) or by a process intrinsic to the organ (e.g., nephritis, trauma, meningitis, seizures). Both are medical emergencies since, if the abnormality cannot be found quickly and corrected, death of the organ or individual may ensue.

Hypothyroidism

Typically, one envisions the behavioral disturbances associated with *hyper*thyroidism (activated, manic-like) to be the opposite of those produced by *hypo*thyroidism (a hypoactive retarded state similar to that seen in major depression). While decreased energy, poor concentration, weight gain, anhedonia, and poor mood are all common in hypothyroidism, a wide variety of signs and symptoms can be seen that overlap substantially with those seen in hyperthyroidism (e.g., anxiety, irritability, and agitation). If unrecognized and untreated, "myxedema madness," in which delusions and hallucinations occur, can develop. In its final end state, dementia is present. Delirium is a rare consequence and usually only appears in those patients who develop hypothyroidism acutely, such as after thyroidectomy.

Thus, the signs and symptoms of mental dysfunction associated with hypo- and hyperthyroidism overlap significantly. This phenomenon extends to most other endocrine abnormalities with a variety of different psychiatric disorders being associated with any one endocrine disorder. Whether the ability of an endocrine disorder to produce many different psychiatric syndromes reflects poor diagnostic techniques, genetic predisposition, the complex interaction between the neuronal and endocrine systems, or a combination of these is not known. Data emerging from basic research indicate that hormones, via several different mechanisms, can have direct effects on the functioning of neurons. The knowledge that mild endocrine abnormalities exist in patients considered to have a primary psychiatric disorder and that these abnormalities disappear with routine psychiatric treatment suggests that CNS function can alter endocrine systems. Thus, the relationship between CNS and endocrine functioning is probably bi-directional. Furthermore, the anatomical evidence for a complex intertwined web of projection pathways between diverse limbic brain areas and the hypothalamus, combined with the location of hormone receptors in several areas of the CNS, indicate that the concept of a simple serial feedback mechanism controlling endocrine function is probably oversimplistic. Instead, there appears to be a highly complex relationship that governs the normal and abnormal functioning of these two systems and probably accounts for the diverse clinical pattern.

Diagnosis and treatment

Until a clearer picture of this complex relationship is available, the general rule is to determine, to the extent possible, which system (endocrine or nervous) is the primary cause of the signs and symptoms. As is the case with diagnosing mental disorders in patients with chronic medical illnesses, clues such as age of onset, family history, and the presence or absence of non-overlapping signs and symptoms can be used to determine whether the primary pathology is psychiatric or endocrinologic. Treatment is aimed initially at correcting the primary disorder. Thus, hypothyroid patients with secondary depressive-like sequelae are given thyroid supplementation and are not initially treated with antidepressants. The only definite exception occurs in the case of an agitated, psychotic but non-delirious patient where antipsychotics, benzodiazepines, and inpatient hospitalization are used to prevent physical harm. With appropriate endocrinological treatment, mental functioning typically improves over time as endocrine function returns to normal. However, it is not uncommon for patients to continue to have significant psychiatric symptoms in spite of normalized endocrine function. Whether the continuing presence of mental dysfunction in these cases represents persistent CNS dysfunction, a comorbid psychiatric process, or a mild subclinical endocrine abnormality is unknown. Little can be done in the first scenario; however, further pharmacological manipulation might lead to additional improvement in the latter two scenarios. Although clinical data are lacking in such cases, it is reasonable to assume that the patient's past medical history or family history might offer clues to whether the adjunctive use of psychiatric medications (e.g. antidepressants) or further endocrine manipulation (e.g., additional thyroid supplementation in a previously hypothyroid patient, who is presently biochemically euthyroid) would be more likely to lead to further improvement.

Prognosis

Prognosis depends upon the specific endocrine disorder, but in general, physical stigmata usually resolve upon the successful treatment of the endocrine abnormality. In contrast, psychiatric manifestations tend to be more resistant to treatment and can persist even after the biochemical indices have normalized. A definitive conclusion on whether there will be residual impairment cannot be reached for several months since improvement in mental functioning can lag behind the successful treatment of the endocrine disorder. In addition, the chance for a full recovery of CNS functioning decreases as the duration of symptoms increases. For example, hypothyroid patients with delirium, when they are appropri-

ately diagnosed and treated, have a high recovery rate (80%), probably because they are treated soon after the onset of hypothyroidism. In contrast, hypothyroid patients who have been symptomatic for over two years rarely show improvement in mental functioning (see *Pearls & Perils*).

PEARLS & PERILS

Endocrine disorders

- In general, any psychiatric presentation can be seen with any endocrine disorder.
- There is typically little correlation between the severity of the endocrine disorder or its physical signs and the presence or severity of the mental changes.
- It is not uncommon for the mental changes to be the first indication of endocrine dysfunction.
- Except in cases of psychosis, initial treatment is targetted at the underlying endocrine disorder.
- In cases of continued psychiatric symptoms where treatment of the endocrine disorder has been maximized, adjunctive psychiatric medications can be used.
- The longer the symptoms have been present, the poorer the prognosis.

Conclusion

In this chapter, we have tried to make several crucial points about psychiatric illness in the general medical patient. First, diagnosis is important because psychiatric illness in general medical patients is common and usually treatable. For instance, major depression is generally underdiagnosed, yet effective treatment can relieve suffering, possibly improve medical outcomes, decrease medical costs, reduce physical complaints, and prevent suicide. Delirium, also referred to as "mental status changes" or acute confusional states, indicates a severe underlying general medical illness. Delirium can cause psychotic or depressive symptoms; if these symptoms are misdiagnosed as depression, the physician has missed an important indication of the seriousness of the underlying medical condition.

Second, diagnosis of psychiatric illness, although sometimes straightforward in these patients, commonly requires exceptional clinical skill. A thorough psychiatric assessment is required, followed by careful consideration of the symptoms and signs. Deciding whether or not symptoms result from the underlying nonpsychiatric illness requires knowledge of both the primary illness and the psychiatric side effects of medical treatment. Thus, psychological symptoms can be especially important. Accurate psychiatric diagnosis can be especially difficult in patients with coarse brain disease.

Third, treatment of psychiatric disorders in general medical patients generally follows established treatment recommendations for the disorder when it occurs in the absence of other medical conditions. However, drug-illness and drug-drug interactions can make treatment difficult. Referral to a psychiatric specialist is sometimes needed.

Finally, the cause of psychiatric disorders in the medically ill appears to be heterogeneous. In many chronic illnesses, major depressive episodes probably represent typical major depression, perhaps triggered by the loss of health and increase in life stress. Other conditions (such as certain endocrine and neurological illnesses, or the postpartum state) bring a markedly elevated risk of major mental illness. In some cases, the reason for this high risk is still unknown, but in others, there is substantial evidence that the psychiatric disorder is caused by direct pathological effects of the illness on brain functioning.

Psychiatric complications of nonpsychiatric illnesses are common and often add further suffering to an already difficult situation. They can also cause additional morbidity or even death. They certainly are not "normal." Accurate diagnosis and adequate treatment of delirium, major depression, generalized anxiety disorder, panic disorder or psychosis in this population not only provide a rewarding challenge to the clinician's skill, but also greatly improve patients' quality of life.

Annotated bibliography

Gjerdingen, D (2003) The effectiveness of various postpartum depression treatments and the impact of antidepressant drugs on nursing infants, *J Am Board Fam Pract* 16:372–82.
This article is a recent review of the literature on the treatment of postpartum depression.

Popkin, MK and Tucker, GJ (1992) "Secondary" and drug-induced mood, anxiety, psychotic, catatonic, and personality disorders: A review of the literature, *J Neuropsychiatry Clin Neurosci* 4(4):369–385.
This article is a broad review of "secondary" psychiatric disorders undertaken by members of the DSM-IV task force. Although there has been substantial advancement in several areas since its writing, it still is probably the best brief review on this subject.

Preskorn, SH (1999) Antidepressant options in primary care, *Clinical Cornerstone* 1(4):31–55.
This article reviews the basic and clinical pharmacology of antidepressants for the primary care practitioner and discusses interactions with other drugs.

Reus, VI (1986) Behavioral disturbances associated with endocrine disorders, *Ann Rev Med* 37:205–14.
This review briefly discusses the psychiatric manifestations of Cushing's syndrome, Addison's disease, hyperparathyroidism, hyperthyroidism, hypothyroidism, hyperprolactinemia, and hypopituitarism. Its continued utility 20 years after its writing is an indication of the scarcity of investigation that is occurring in this area.

Yudofsky, SC and Hales, RE (2002) *The American Psychiatric Publishing Textbook of Neuropsychiatry and Clinical Neurosciences,* 4th Edition, Washington, DC, American Psychiatric Publishing.
This textbook provides a good general review of the psychiatric aspects of neurological as well as endocrine disorders.

CHAPTER 28

The Impact of Psychiatric Disorders on Medical Illness

Kenneth E. Freedland, PhD, Robert M. Carney, PhD, and Patrick J. Lustman, PhD

Introduction

The previous chapter discussed the evaluation and treatment of psychiatric disorders that occur in conjunction with general medical conditions. This chapter describes the effects that psychiatric disorders have on the incidence, course, and outcome of general medical conditions. Most of the research in this area has focused on the impact of depression on specific medical illnesses, and this chapter follows suit. Other psychiatric conditions are discussed where there is enough evidence to warrant their inclusion. The chapter begins with a discussion of general issues surrounding research on the impact of psychiatric comorbidity on medical illnesses and continues with a closer look at some of the specific medical illnesses that have been studied.

General issues

Psychiatric comorbidity in general medical illnesses

If the prevalence rates of a psychiatric disorder and a general medical condition are both high enough, many individuals will have both conditions by chance, even if they are completely unrelated to one another. However, the prevalence of comorbid depression in chronically medically ill patients is too high to result from chance alone. Consequently, it is necessary to consider the nature of the relationship between depression and medical illness.

It is tempting to assume that because depression is more common in medically ill patients than in demographically similar but medically well individuals, it must be *due* to the medical illness. Certainly, major medical illnesses are significant stressors that can contribute to the onset, persistence, or recurrence of depression in vulnerable individuals, and some medical conditions can affect brain function in ways that contribute directly to psychopathological states. However, depression can co-occur with medical illness for other reasons as well. In fact, many individuals become depressed before (in some cases, long before) the onset of medical illness.

According to recent findings from the National Comorbidity Survey Replication (NCS-R), the typical age of onset of major depressive disorder, at least in younger birth cohorts, is between adolescence and early adulthood. In contrast, most of the chronic medical conditions in which there are high rates of comorbid depression, such as coronary heart disease (CHD) and stroke, are relatively rare until middle or old age. Major depression is a chronic or recurrent disorder in many cases. Many patients start having major depressive episodes years or even decades before they develop any chronic medical illnesses, and by the time they are diagnosed with a condition such as CHD, they may have had multiple depressive episodes or a long history of chronic, unremitting depression. Since Axis I comorbidity is common in major depression, some of these patients will also have had other problems such as an anxiety or substance abuse disorder long before they ever develop a chronic medical condition such as CHD.

The temporal sequence between acute medical events and psychiatric conditions must also be considered. For example, both major depression and subsyndromal depressive disorders are common in patients who have been hospitalized for an acute myocardial infarction (MI). In some cases, the MI precedes, and apparently precipitates, the depressive episode. In many other cases, however, the patient was already depressed at the time of the acute MI. It has been estimated that this temporal pattern occurs in almost half of the cases of post-MI depression. An acute MI and its aftermath might worsen or prolong a preexisting depressive episode, but it cannot have played a role in the onset of the episode.

There is only limited evidence that the impact of comorbid depression on the course and outcome of medical illnesses depends on the temporal relationship between the two disorders. There is stronger evidence of "dose-response" relationships between the severity and chronicity of depression and the risk of adverse outcomes in some medical illnesses. In short, the impact of depression seems to depend more on its severity, and perhaps on its frequency or chronicity, than on whether its onset preceded or followed the onset of the medical illness.

Compound comorbidity

As mentioned previously, most of the research on the effects of psychiatric comorbidity on general medical conditions has focused on specific illnesses. However, there are high rates of comorbidity among some of these illnesses. For example, diabetes is a major risk factor for coronary artery disease (CAD), and many cardiac patients have diabetes. These medical comorbidities affect some of the same outcomes that are influenced by psychiatric conditions. Therefore, it is important to adjust for medical comorbidity when studying the effects of psychiatric disorders on outcomes in populations defined by a particular medical condition, such as in research on depression in post-MI patients.

Another implication of compound comorbidity is that psychiatric disorders may affect the development, course, and outcome of multiple medical conditions in individual patients. One way this might occur is if the psychiatric condition has physiological or behavioral effects that transcend specific medical illnesses. Depression, for example, has been shown to decrease adherence to treatment regimens in a number of different medical illnesses. Therefore, being depressed could simultaneously affect adherence to diabetes self-management and to medications for heart disease in patients who have both conditions. Alternatively, psychiatric conditions might alter the relationships between comorbid medical conditions. For example, major depression accelerates the clinical onset of CHD in women with diabetes. When depression is identified in women who already have both diabetes and CHD, this triple conjunction might be traceable, at least in some cases, to an earlier catalytic effect of depression on the progression from diabetes to CHD.

Finally, patients suffering from multiple medical conditions may be more vulnerable to depression than are patients with only one medical illness. For example, in a recent study of patients hospitalized for an acute myocardial infarction, the odds of having major depression increased as the number of comorbid medical conditions increased.

The medical patient's perspective on psychiatric comorbidity

- Some medically ill patients are unaware of being depressed or anxious, even when their psychiatric problems are clinically significant, and some believe that such problems should not be disclosed or treated.
- Some patients are uninformed about the medical risks associated with health-related behaviors such as smoking or physical inactivity; similarly, some are unaware of the risks associated with comorbid depression in medical conditions such as myocardial infarction.
- Patients who are currently depressed or anxious are much more likely than nondepressed, nonanxious patients to attribute their medical illness (at least in part) to stress, depression, anxiety, anger, or other emotional problems.
- If present, such attributions can be used to help motivate medically ill patients to accept treatment for their depression or anxiety; if absent, other potential benefits of treatment (e.g., improved sleep, decreased fatigue) can be highlighted.

PEARLS & PERILS

Types of effects of psychiatric comorbidity

Numerous cohorts of medically well individuals have been followed to determine whether psychiatric symptoms or disorders increase the risk of developing medical illnesses. We now have evidence that certain psychiatric conditions do increase the risk of developing specific medical illnesses. However, there has been more research on the effects of psychiatric comorbidity in patients who are already medically ill. The universe of potential effects is similar across medical illnesses. They include (1) worse medical risk factor profiles, (2) higher risks of medical morbidity and mortality, (3) more severe functional impairment, (4) worse adherence to medical treatment and to risk factor modification, and (5) higher utilization of medical services.

Some of these effects have been documented in prospective epidemiological studies. For example, longitudinal studies of initially healthy, young adult cohorts have shown that depression and other negative mood states increase the risk of developing certain medical conditions later in life. Other relationships are less readily amenable to prospective research and have been documented primarily in cross-sectional studies. This inevitably raises "chicken and egg" questions. For example, there is a strong correlation between depression and functional impairment in patients with heart disease. It is possible that functional impairment is depressogenic. It is also possible that depression exacerbates functional impairment. Indeed, functional impairment is a diagnostic criterion for major depression and for many of the other psychiatric disorders defined in DSM-IV. There might also be a reciprocal relationship between depression and functional impairment.

Despite these uncertainties, there is evidence that depression can cause functional impairment both in medically ill and in otherwise healthy individuals. Some of the best evidence comes from a 1995 study by a team of researchers at the RAND Corporation who followed nearly 1,800 adult outpatients with depression, diabetes, hypertension, a recent MI, and/or congestive heart failure (CHF) over a period of two years. They found that depression had substantial and long-lasting effects on multiple domains of functioning and quality of life that equalled or exceeded the effects of the chronic medical illnesses.

In addition to studying the effects of psychiatric disorders on medical morbidity and mortality, researchers are also trying to identify the mechanisms underlying these relationships. For example, although it is now well established that depression increases the risk of mortality after an acute MI, we do not yet know how it exerts this effect. A number of possible physiological and behavioral pathways are currently being investigated.

Suicide

Serious medical illness is a risk factor for suicidal ideation and behavior, and major depression is one of the most powerful predictors of suicidality in the context of cancer, heart disease, stroke, and other medical conditions. Consequently, detection and treatment of depression is one of the most important steps that clinicians can take to reduce the risk of suicide in medically ill patients.

Clinical trials

There have been very few large, multicenter clinical trials testing whether treatment of psychiatric comorbidity can improve the course or outcome of medical illnesses. Some trials have attempted to influence health outcomes by modifying health behaviors rather than psychiatric disorders. In the landmark Diabetes Control and Complications Trial, for example, patients with insulin-dependent diabetes were trained to follow an intensive diabetes management regimen. Compared to traditional therapy, intensive management delayed the onset and slowed the progression of diabetic complications. Similarly, in the Diabetes Prevention Program Trial, individuals at risk for Type 2 diabetes were randomly assigned to a lifestyle modification program, metformin, or a placebo. Both the lifestyle intervention and the medication reduced the incidence of diabetes, but the former was more effective than the latter. Other trials have focused on psychiatric disorders such as depression in cardiac patients.

The evidence is still quite limited that treatment of psychi-

atric disorders in medically ill patients can alter the course or outcome of the medical illness. Consequently, at this point, the most important reason to treat psychiatric comorbidity in medical patients is still to alleviate the distress, impairment, and adjustment problems associated with the psychiatric disorder. The possibility that reducing psychiatric comorbidity might improve medical outcomes makes treatment all the more important, but this should not be the principal rationale for psychiatric intervention, at least not until there is more evidence to justify treating patients for this reason.

Psychiatric comorbidity in specific medical illnesses

Diabetes mellitus

Several epidemiological studies have shown that depression is a risk factor for incident type 2 diabetes. The most recent findings are from the National Health and Nutrition Examination Epidemiologic Follow-up Study. The incidence of diabetes over a 15-year follow-up period was about 7 per 1000 person-years among individuals with high levels of depression on the initial examination, compared to about 3.5 among those with lower levels.

The estimated prevalence of depression in patients with diabetes has varied widely across studies, due to differences in sample characteristics, methods of assessment, and case definitions. Although actual estimates have varied even among studies that have utilized structured psychiatric interviews to determine DSM-IV diagnoses, the odds of having depression are consistently twice as high in diabetic patients as in nondiabetic comparison groups. When averaged across studies, the estimated point prevalence of major depression in diabetes is approximately 10%. The average prevalence of clinically significant depressive symptoms in diabetes, as assessed by self-report questionnaires, is about 25%.

As in many medical illnesses, depression is associated with poor adherence to medical treatment in diabetes. Adherence to dietary recommendations and to glycemic control regimens is significantly lower in depressed than nondepressed patients. Whether depression has comparable effects on adherence in insulin-dependent and non-insulin-dependent diabetes is controversial. Nevertheless, the weight of evidence suggests that depression interferes with adherence in both types of diabetes.

Poor adherence hastens the onset of serious diabetic complications, and depression plays an important role in this problem. Depression is associated with hyperglycemia and is a moderately strong predictor of diabetic complications including retinopathy, nephropathy, neuropathy, macrovascular complications, and sexual dysfunction. As noted previously, depression accelerates the clinical onset of coronary heart disease in women with diabetes.

It is possible that depression could also lead to complications by interfering with the intensity or quality of diabetes care. However, a recent study of a national sample of over 38 000 outpatients with diabetes treated at Veterans Health Administration facilities found that depression and other forms of psychiatric comorbidity did not interfere with the quality of prescribed diabetes care. Substance use disorders were an exception, however. Patients with these disorders were less likely to receive foot or retinal examinations than were other patients.

There have not yet been any large, multicenter trials of treatments for depression in diabetes. However, single-center controlled clinical trials at Washington University have demonstrated that conventional treatments including cognitive-behavior therapy and fluoxetine can improve not only depression but glycemic control as well.

Coronary heart disease

Several longitudinal studies have shown that symptoms of depression in initially healthy cohorts predict the subsequent development of CHD. Some of these studies have focused specifically on the incidence of MI, while others have also examined other expressions of incident CHD such as coronary revascularization. In most of these studies, the relative risk (RR) ratios for depressive symptoms have ranged from about 1.5 to about 2.0. One study has also reported an odds ratio (OR) of 4.5 for major depression as a predictor of incident MI.

These findings have generated controversy about whether depression plays a role in the development of coronary atherosclerosis. Depression could predict incident MI and other manifestations of CHD without being atherogenic, if coronary atherosclerosis evolves for reasons unrelated to depression and if depression accelerates the onset of clinical events in patients who already have significant coronary artery disease. Depression might be thrombogenic but not atherogenic, or it might accelerate diagnosis and revascularization by heightening awareness of angina pectoris. On the other hand, it is also possible that depression *does* play a role in the development of coronary atherosclerosis, perhaps via its association with other risk factors such as cigarette smoking. The only way to resolve this question is to conduct a longitudinal study with repeated assessments of the coronary arteries. Advanced, non-invasive imaging technologies such as cardiac MRI might make this possible at some point. For now, we may not know how depression increases the incidence of CHD, but we know that it does.

The estimated point prevalence of major depression in patients with CHD is approximately 15%, and the prevalence of minor depression is about the same. These rates do not differ very much across clinical stages of CHD. For example, the rates are about the same among patients hospitalized for an acute MI as they are in individuals with newly diagnosed coronary disease who have never had an acute coronary event. They do, however, differ according to the patient's background characteristics. Major depressive episodes are more common among younger patients, females, and patients with a past history of depression. Also, patients who have residual symptoms from a previous episode are at increased risk of having another major depressive episode.

The prognostic importance of depression has been established in patients with newly diagnosed coronary disease, in patients hospitalized for acute coronary events (myocardial infarction or unstable angina), and in patients recovering from coronary artery bypass graft (CABG) surgery. One of the first studies in this area was conducted at Washington University in the late 1980s. It showed that major depression doubles the one-year risk of cardiac events in patients with newly diagnosed coronary disease. Two of the earliest studies of post-MI patients were conducted in Canada; major depression predicted decreased survival with adjusted hazard ratios of approximately 4.3 during the first six months after the infarction and about 3.6 over the first 18 months. Depressive symptoms, as measured by the Beck Depression Inventory, had an even stronger effect on 18-month survival. These findings have been replicated in more recent studies and have been joined by reports that depression predicts mortality after CABG surgery.

Depression is associated with a number of major and minor risk factors for CHD, including diabetes, hypertension, smoking, obesity, and physical inactivity. It also interferes with modification of some of these risk factors. For example, it hinders smoking cessation and participation in exercise programs. However, these factors have been included as covariates in the studies that have identified comorbid depression as an independent risk factor for cardiac morbidity and mortality in patients with coronary disease. This suggests that the prognostic importance of depression is not attributable, at least not entirely, to its impact on traditional cardiac risk factors.

These findings have spawned a search for physiological mechanisms linking depression to adverse cardiac outcomes. Cardiovascular autonomic dysregulation is one of the leading candidates. Depression is associated with relatively low heart rate variability (HRV) and high blood pressure variability (BPV) in cardiac patients. Both low HRV and high BPV have been shown to predict mortality in similar patients. Studies have recently begun to emerge on other potential mechanisms as well, including pro-inflammatory and pro-coagulant processes. However, much more research will be needed before a comprehensive model of the pathways linking depression to CHD morbidity and mortality is established.

Depression alters not only survival but also symptom severity, daily functioning, and quality of life in patients with heart disease. For example, a large study of Veterans Administration outpatients found that high scores on a depression screening questionnaire predicted more frequent angina, more angina-related physical limitations, less satisfaction with treatment for heart disease, and lower health-related quality of life.

So far, only two large, multicenter clinical trials of treatments for depression in cardiac patients have been conducted. The Enhancing Recovery in Coronary Heart Disease (ENRICHD) study was a multicenter clinical trial of treatment for depression and/or low perceived social support in post-MI patients. Nearly 2,500 patients were enrolled within 28 days of hospitalization for an acute MI and randomly assigned to usual care or to cognitive-behavior therapy for up to six months. Patients who were severely depressed at enrollment or whose depression did not respond adequately to the cognitive-behavioral intervention were also treated with sertraline. There was significantly greater improvement in depression and social support in the intervention than in the usual care arm, although the between-group differences were quite modest. There was no difference between the groups in reinfarction-free survival, the trial's primary medical endpoint, during several years of follow-up.

The Sertraline Antidepressant Heart Attack Randomized Trial (SADHART) was a randomized, double-blind, placebo-controlled clinical trial in which 369 patients hospitalized for an acute myocardial infarction or unstable angina who met the DSM-IV criteria for major depression were randomly assigned to a flexible dosage of sertraline or placebo for 24 weeks. There were no significant differences between the groups at 24 weeks on safety outcomes such as changes in left ventricular ejection fraction. There was also no between-group difference on the Hamilton Rating Scale for Depression (HRSD). However, in a subgroup with severe, recurrent major depressive disorder, treatment was associated with a small but significant improvement as determined by the HRSD scores. Ratings on the Clinical Global Impression Improvement (CGI-I) scale more clearly favored the sertraline arm. Although the trial was not large enough to evaluate the effects of sertraline on medical endpoints, there was a promising trend towards fewer cardiac events in the sertraline than in the placebo arm. Furthermore, a SADHART substudy showed that treatment with sertraline is associated with reductions in platelet and endothelial biomarkers.

Despite intensive treatment, the patients in the intervention arms of these two trials improved little more than did those in the control arms, and their odds of survival were no better. Further research is needed on the outcomes associated with the treatment of depression in patients hospitalized for an acute MI or unstable angina.

Congestive heart failure

There has been much less research on psychiatric comorbidity in patients with CHF than in other cardiac patient populations. Nevertheless, there is growing evidence that depression is a common comorbid condition in patients with heart failure and has a number of undesirable consequences. There is also evidence that depression is a risk factor for incident CHF in medically vulnerable individuals (e.g., hypertensive patients). Alcoholism is also a risk factor for CHF because alcoholic cardiomyopathy is a direct cause of heart failure.

The prevalence of comorbid major depression in CHF is similar to the rates documented in other cardiac patient populations. However, it varies dramatically among subgroups defined by age and level of functional impairment. We have found the prevalence to be very low in elderly patients with mild (i.e., New York Heart Association [NYHA] Class I) CHF and extremely high in younger patients with severe (NYHA Class IV) CHF. Approximately two-thirds of the latter patients suffer from major depression. The prevalence increases along with NYHA class, but the increase is much steeper in younger than older patients.

There is growing evidence that depression is a risk factor for mortality in patients with CHF. The risk appears to be higher among patients with major depression than among those with milder forms of depression. There has been little research on the mechanisms underlying this effect, but cardiovascular autonomic dysregulation is a leading candidate. It plays a critical role in the progression of heart failure, and it might be exacerbated by depression.

Stroke

Two large epidemiological studies have established that depression is a risk factor for stroke, particularly for ischemic cerebrovascular accidents. A 13-year follow-up of Baltimore participants in the Epidemiological Catchment Area study revealed that individuals with a history of major depression were 2.6 times more likely to have a stroke than were other participants after adjusting for other risk factors. Antidepressant medications at baseline did not mitigate this risk. In the NHANES-I Epidemiologic Follow-Up Study, self-reported depressive symptoms predicted the incidence of stroke over an average of 16 years of follow-up, with a relative risk of 1.7. The risk was particularly high among African-American participants, with a relative risk of 2.6.

Major depression and subsyndromal depressive disorders are slightly more common in patients hospitalized for stroke than in those hospitalized for acute MI. The estimated prevalence of each disorder averages around 19% across studies. Some studies have suggested that patients with left frontal or left basal ganglia lesions are especially likely to develop major depression during the first two months after the stroke, and some have shown a strong correlation between the proximity of the lesion to the left frontal pole and the severity of depression. However, other studies have failed to replicate these findings. Furthermore, the cumulative 12-month incidence of depressive disorders is higher after stroke than after acute MI, but this difference disappears after adjustment for sex, age, and severity of disability. In short, the role of brain dysfunction in the etiology of post-stroke depression remains controversial.

Depression increases functional impairment and slows functional recovery in stroke patients, just as it does in other medical patient groups. One of the distinctive effects of depression on long-term recovery from stroke is that it increases the risk of falls, and thereby indirectly increases the risk of hip fracture and other injuries. Length of stay in post-acute rehabilitation facilities is no longer for depressed than nondepressed patients, but the efficiency of rehabilitation is lower among depressed patients. In other words, nondepressed patients tend to achieve greater functional recovery through rehabilitation than do depressed patients. Depression is also a risk factor for mortality in stroke patients. Depending upon the study, depression assessed during or soon after hospitalization for stroke roughly doubled or tripled the risk of mortality over the following year.

There have been several randomized, placebo-controlled trials of antidepressants for post-stroke depression. Evidence for the efficacy of nortriptyline is fairly consistent. In contrast, trials of fluoxetine have produced mixed results. Citalopram has shown promise in a small, placebo-controlled trial.

Cancer

Psychiatric comorbidity in cancer is a complex topic. There are many different types of cancer, and there are vast differences within and among types of cancer in symptoms, treatment, prognosis, and central nervous system effects. These factors can interact with depression and other psychiatric problems in multiple ways.

Whether depression is a risk factor for cancer incidence is not yet clear. Some of the strongest evidence in favor of this hypothesis comes from a prospective study of nearly 5,000 elderly subjects which found that symptoms of depression predicted cancer incidence. The effect of depression was stronger among nonsmokers than smokers, suggesting that depression was not merely a proxy for smoking. Other studies have failed to find any relationship between depression and cancer incidence. Approximately one out of every three cancer patients has mild to moderate depression, and about one out of every four has major depression. Intense pain, rapid progression of cancer, and poor prognosis are prominent risk factors for severe depression, regardless of the specific type of cancer.

Despite several negative findings, there is growing evidence that depression and hopelessness predict more rapid progression of cancer and shorter survival after diagnosis of cancer. For example, a Finnish Cancer Registry study found a "dose-response" relationship between the severity of hopelessness and the risk of cancer mortality. The mecha-

nisms underlying these relationships are not yet known. Some of the possibilities that are being investigated include reduced adherence to medical treatment regimens and reduced tolerance for painful, disfiguring, or otherwise burdensome treatments; neuroendocrine dysfunction; and decreased immunocompetence.

In 1989, David Spiegel and his colleagues at Stanford University published the results of a small clinical trial in which women with metastatic breast cancer were randomly assigned to supportive group therapy or to usual care. The women who received the intervention survived an average of 37 months, compared with only 19 months for the women who received usual care. This study generated considerable controversy and interest in replicating its findings. Including the original study, there have now been ten published trials. Five of the studies found a modest survival advantage for patients who received a psychosocial intervention, and five found no effect on survival. The findings have been more consistently favorable with respect to other outcomes such as reductions in emotional distress and pain, and improvements in psychosocial functioning and quality of life. Whether or not psychosocial interventions affect survival, they have become an important form of adjunctive care for cancer patients.

It is difficult to conduct antidepressant treatment trials in cancer patients because of the barriers created by the illness and its treatment, as well as by competition from clinical trials of experimental cancer therapies. Nevertheless, a number of small, controlled clinical trials have been conducted. Several agents, including fluoxetine, desipramine, paroxetine, amitriptyline, and mianserin have been tested, with generally favorable results. In addition to reducing depression and improving health-related quality of life, antidepressants have been successfully used as adjunctive therapy for pain.

Conclusion

Depression and other forms of psychiatric comorbidity are very common in medically ill patients. However, clinical depression should not be regarded as a "normal" reaction to medical illness. In many cases, it should not be regarded as a reaction to medical illness at all, since the onset of depression often precedes rather than follows the onset of medical illness. Regardless of its etiology, depression has a number of adverse effects on the course and outcome of chronic medical illnesses such as diabetes, heart disease, stroke, and cancer. The effects range from emotional distress and functional impairment, to decreased survival. Most of the research on the prognostic importance of depression in medical illness has focused on all-cause mortality, but depression is also one of the most important risk factors for suicidality in medically ill patients.

Treatment of comorbid depression has been shown to have

a variety of collateral benefits, although evidence that it can prolong survival is still quite limited. Treatment can improve the patient's mood, functioning, quality of life, and adherence. While many questions remain to be answered about comorbid depression in medically ill patients, there is a growing consensus that treatment of depression should be an integral part of these patients' medical care. Increasing evidence supports the use of carefully selected antidepressants and/or cognitive-behavior therapy for medically ill patients with comorbid depressive disorders. More efficacious treatments are still needed, since some patients fail to respond to existing therapies. Nevertheless, the majority of depressed, medically ill patients can benefit from intervention.

Annotated bibliography

Biological Psychiatry (2003) 1 August, 54(3).

This special issue on mood disorders and medical illness includes contributions from many of the leading researchers in the area. The reviews were prepared for a Consensus Conference on "Recognizing and meeting the needs of patients with mood disorders and comorbid medical illness," convened in November 2002 by the Depression and Bipolar Support Alliance.

CHAPTER 29

Suicide

Richard D. Wetzel, PhD and George E. Murphy, MD

Definition of terms

Suicide refers to a death caused by actions of the deceased with the intention to end his or her own life. People who die by their own hand usually intend their death, although a few are the victims of their own ignorance of pharmacology or a miscalculation that others would rescue them. In practice, a competent authority (coroner/medical examiner) must recognize and certify that the death resulted from suicide.

Attempted suicide refers to acts, resulting in actual self-damage, of an individual who tries unsuccessfully to cause his own demise or more often who intends others to believe that he was attempting to kill himself. Suicide threat refers to communications ("I want to die") or actions that do not cause bodily harm (holding a gun to one's head). The linguistically unfortunate term "parasuicide" has been used in the clinical literature to refer to all forms of non-lethal suicide behavior.

Suicide attempts

It has been widely recognized since the work of Stengel and Cook that suicide and attempted suicide are not identical phenomena. They are separate, but overlapping behaviors. Some who attempt suicide do go on to commit suicide if adequate management fails. A solid understanding of suicide cannot be obtained solely from the study of living people who threaten or survive attempts. Compared to people completing suicide, attempters are younger, much more likely to be female, more impulsive, more likely to be reacting to an immediate social stress, and psychiatrically less homogeneous. Personality disorder is more common in this population than it is in those who complete suicide.

Suicide attempts may be instrumental acts, i.e., attempts to die or to manipulate the environment, or expressive acts to reduce internal distress, anger, and depression. What people call a suicide attempt is usually not that at all. Rather, a suicide attempt is frequently a drastic form of communication—a cry for help. But sometimes the behavior signals serious trouble, including the wish to die. Nine out of ten identified acts of deliberate self-harm occur by overdose with medication. Sublethal, often trivial, amounts of medication are the rule, as are provisions for rescue. More than one-half of these events come to a physician's attention only later or not at all. The second most common method for attempting suicide is wrist cutting.

In suicide, as in most other human activities, a carefully planned effort is more likely to succeed than an impulsive one. The more carefully planned the attempt, the more serious should be the concern for the individual's safety. Attempts at suicide that are perceived as manipulative often elicit anger from physicians and their staff. It may be helpful to consider this kind of attempt as caused by an absence of the appropriate socials skills to communicate or to obtain what one wants from others more gracefully and effectively.

All suicide attempts should be taken seriously, in the sense that they should cause concern and provide the opportunity to examine for psychiatric illness, especially evidence of major depression or substance abuse, either alone or comorbid with a personality disorder. Age is an important factor to consider, also. Suicide attempts after the age of 40 must be regarded with great caution. By that age, most people have found better ways to handle all but the weightiest problems. They are more organized and less impulsive. The acts become more dangerous both physically and psychiatrically. Survival may be by accident or unplanned intervention. Even a medically trivial act may be a practice run for the real thing. The physician should take no chances.

The lifetime risk of suicide in people who attempt suicide is 12–15%, well above the risk of suicide in major depression or any other psychiatric disorder. If the physician is not certain the patient is safe, a psychiatric opinion should be secured. At least one-third of all suicides have a history of deliberate self-harm. The vast majority of people with a history of suicide attempt who later complete suicide have only one known prior attempt.

DIAGNOSIS

Table 29.1 Features associated with suicide attempts in which there is a true intent to die

Discriminating features

1 Concurrent depression and/or alcoholism.
2 Specific detailed plan.
3 Actions based on a plan.
4 Clear intent to die; no plans for rescue.
5 Serious medical consequences.

Consistent features

1 Male.
2 Older.

Variable features

1 Social stressors, especially in people with active substance abuse or in teenagers.

PEARLS & PERILS

- Suicide and attempted suicide are separate but overlapping behaviors.
- A suicide attempt may represent a true attempt to die, an attempt to manipulate the environment, or an act to reduce internal distress.
- All suicide attempts should be evaluated carefully by an adequately trained mental health professional.
- Patients who attempt suicide should be screened for major depression, substance abuse, and personality disorder.

Suicide threats

Roughly two-thirds of those who commit suicide communicated their thoughts regarding suicide in one or more ways. Few informants in these cases regarded the communications as manipulative in intent, however alarming and unwelcome the content. Often individuals unwittingly express thoughts that have been preoccupying them. Individuals who threaten suicide without harming themselves are much like those who actually attempt suicide. The average age is slightly higher and the female to male ratio is higher. Some evidence suggests that they may, on average, be more ill psychiatrically.

What is the goal?

In our society, physicians and mental health professionals are expected to detect and prevent suicidal behavior in their patients. Prevention of suicide depends on the recognition of patients that should be the focus of special concern and further evaluation. The goal is not to predict suicidal deaths accurately. Borum and colleagues pointed out that the goal is to identify patients in situations and circumstances that require intervention and clinical management until the situation improves sufficiently. The risk for violence towards self or others waxes and wanes. Risk factors that can be modified should be identified and treated.

PEARLS & PERILS

- The goal is not to predict suicidal deaths accurately.
- The goal is to identify patients in situations and circumstances that require intervention and clinical management until the situation improves.

Methods for studying suicide

Research on those who survive suicide threats or attempts is accomplished through both interviews and psychological testing. Research on people who completed suicide has been done with three different methods, which yield somewhat different results. The primary method is the "psychological autopsy." Since the deceased cannot be interviewed, other informants must be used. A reconstruction of the emotional state and behavior of the person prior to the death is made based on interviews with many friends and relatives. This is usually supplemented with review of medical records, conversations with health care professionals and evaluation of the physical evidence. This process can be done by researchers or by representatives of the coroner/medical examiner. To our knowledge, this procedure was first used for research purposes on community samples in St Louis in 1958 by Robins and colleagues and in Los Angeles for medical-legal purposes in selected cases at the same time by Litman and colleagues. The Los Angeles group coined the phrase "psychological autopsy." Studies on the psychological autopsy procedure have shown satisfactory reliability and validity.

A second method used to examine suicide involves longitudinal studies of people with specific psychiatric or medical disorders. These usually have been carried out at major research centers, which may attract the most ill or refractory patients. In general, these studies report very high rates of suicide. The shorter the length of follow-up, the higher the percentage of deaths due to suicide. A third method utilized in some countries involves using registry studies and combining national records of death with national records of psychiatric or medical disorders. In general, these studies show relatively lower risk of suicide in the disorders examined. They also show that the presence of more than one disorder increases the risk of suicide.

While each kind of study is informative, it is our belief that the psychological autopsy studies of broad-based community samples are foundational.

Recognition of suicide risk

The recognition of the need for concern and further evaluation can come about in one of several ways—from profiling (recognizing that the patient's clinical and social situation is like that of people who commit suicide), receiving communications about suicide from the patient or his family and

friends, or assessing threats (recognizing the telltale patterns of behavior and communication seen in most people shortly before a suicide occurs). These approaches offer valuable insights into suicide. This recognition of suicide risk should be followed by appropriate preventive behavior.

General profile of those who commit suicide

Ninety to ninety-five percent of people who commit suicide worldwide are suffering from psychiatric illness at the time of the fatal act. Two psychiatric illnesses account for 80% of these deaths: major depressive disorder (MDD) and substance abuse disorder (especially alcoholism) (Table 29.2). Two-thirds or more of people who commit suicide communicate their suicidal thoughts to others in advance of the act,

TABLE 29.2 Selected diagnoses in community studies of suicide

	N	Any affective disorder %	Alcohol abuse or dependence%	Schizophrenia spectrum %	Substance abuse/ dependency %	No psychiatric illness %
Robins, Murphy, et al. USA (1959)	134	45	30	2	25	6
Dorpat and Ripley USA (1960)	114	30	27	12	31	0
Barraclough, et al. United Kingdom (1974)	100	70	15	3	19	7
Beskow Sweden (1979)	270 ♂	45	31	3	37	4
Hagnell and Rorsman Sweden (1979)	28	50	18	7	NR	7
Chynoweth et al. Australia (1980)	135	55	20	4	34	2
Mitterauer Austria (1981)	94	63	30	5	45	0
Kapamadzija, Biro, and Sovljanski Yugoslavia (1982)	100	75	41	3	41	0
Shafii et al. USA (1985)—teens	21	76	38	NR	62	5
Rich, Young, and Fowler USA (1986)	283	44	54	3	56	5
Arató, et al. Hungary (1988)	200	63	20	9	20	19
Brent et al. USA (1988)—teens	27	63	33	0	37	7
Runeson Sweden (1989)—teens	58	28	21	17	28	5
Brent et al. USA (1993)—teens	67	49	24	0	27	11
Asgård Sweden (1990)	104 ♀	59	7	3	12	9
Henriksson, et al. Finland (1993)	229+	66	43	10	NR	2
Lesage et al. Canada (1994) ≤ 35	75	60	24	9	23	12
Cheng Taiwan (1995)	116	88	44	7	45	2
Shaffer et al. USA (1996)—teens	120	67	26	4	42	9
Conwell et al. USA (1996)	141	47	56	16	63	10
Foster et al. Ireland (1997)	118	36	43	7	44	14
Appleby et al. (1999) England ≤ 35	84	25	33	19	NR	24
Vijayakumar and Rajkumar India (1999)	100	25	34	4	36	12
Cavanagh et al. Scotland (1999)	45	47	13	4	31	2
Phillips et al. China (2002)	519	40	7	7	NR	37
Totals	3332	1698	970	218	896	388
	100%	51.0%	29.1%	6.6%	37.0%	11.6%
		25%-88%	7%-54%	2%-12%	19%-56%	0%-37%

usually more than once to more than one person. One-half consult a physician within a month of their deaths. People who have been under psychiatric care are more likely to communicate their intent than those who have not been under psychiatric care.

Most people with MDD who kill themselves are underdiagnosed and/or undertreated by the physician. In a Finnish national study by Isometsä *et al.*, it was noted that 60% of the Finnish suicides suffering from major depression were on antidepressants if treated by psychiatrists, but only 16% if treated by other medical professionals. Only 3% had received ECT. The potential exists for physicians and other concerned people to sharply reduce the suicide rate.

All but a small fraction of those who commit suicide suffer from psychiatric illnesses. Epidemiological studies show that only about one-fourth of the adult population in the United States has or had a psychiatric disorder and is at risk for psychiatric illness. Therefore, three-fourths of the population are not candidates for suicide at any time. That narrows the field, but not enough.

Diagnostic correlates of suicide

Psychiatric disorders

Affective disorders

Depressive disorders (major depressive disorder and bipolar disorder) have been recognized as the primary illnesses associated with suicides studied worldwide. About one-half of people who commit suicide are clinically depressed when they take their lives. (Some of these people may also be ill with comorbid psychiatric disorders.)

Suicide in major depressive disorder occurs chiefly in response to internal cues. Recent major disruptions involving social issues do not significantly exceed the norms of the age-adjusted population. Suicide in widowhood is somewhat more common than expected, but the recent death of a spouse is not associated with increases in suicides. Ill health may contribute to suicide risk in older people, but the rate is not dramatically inflated. The incidence of cancer increases with age, and therefore it is found to be present with some frequency among older people who commit suicide. However, equally common is an unwarranted conviction of harboring a malignancy, which should be understood as a symptom of depression.

Without salient external cues, the impetus to suicide can be seen as stemming chiefly from the combination of misery and hopelessness that are common features of depression. Sleepless nights bring neither rest nor escape from mental pain. Loss of interest and impaired concentration void escape through distraction. Guilt inflates worthlessness, and psychomotor agitation precludes rest. Hopelessness intrudes and then prevails, and the biological imperative of self-preservation is breached. Thoughts of death arise early in the course of most depressive episodes. Unchecked, they

progress to consideration of self-destruction. Suicide notes by depressed people speak of internal rather than external concerns (see *Pearls & Perils*).

PEARLS & PERILS

Cues to consider major depressive disorder

- Depression does not always walk in the door self-identified. It can develop insidiously in patients under treatment for other complaints.
- Psychomotor agitation and retardation are diagnostic signs. Medication effects (such as akathisia or oversedation) as well as major depression should be considered.
- Newly developed irritability, demanding behavior, and poor compliance with medication may be signs of depression.
- The facial appearance of sadness or tearfulness calls for directed inquiry regarding depressive syndrome. Physicians readily recognize the mood, but they may miss the diagnosis.
- Unplanned weight loss or a complaint of poor appetite or insomnia should cue the physician to inquire about other symptoms of depression. Do not treat symptoms in isolation until depression has been ruled out.
- Not every depressed patient relates to feeling depressed. Synonyms include feeling sad, blue, down in the dumps, and feeling "blah." Mood disturbance should not be ruled out without trying those probes.

It is quite unusual to find suicide associated with the manic phase of bipolar disorder when mood is characteristically up. But in some, mood may shift quickly into depression. Also, some patients have mixed episodes of illness with simultaneous symptoms of mania and depression, including querulous mood along with excited behavior and poor judgment. The depth of depression may be very difficult to assess. Many people with affective disorder who commit suicide also have comorbid conditions, including substance abuse and physical illness.

Alcoholism and substance abuse

Alcohol abuse and dependence have been diagnosed in 13–56% of suicides, with a mean of 29% across 25 studies. Overall, substance abuse (including that of alcohol) has been diagnosed in 37% of over 3300 suicides. In contrast to people suffering from a primary depression who complete suicide, recent disruption in significant interpersonal relationships occurs in at least a third of the cases involving substance abuse disorders. To be sure, personal, social, legal, and vocational troubles are the identifying consequence of these disorders. Whereas one-half of people suffering with alcoholism who commit suicide experience the loss of a close interpersonal relationship in the last year of their lives, two-thirds of these events take place in the prior six weeks. This is different from the presuicidal experience of patients with depression. Moreover, the fear or expectation of such an event is equally as common as an actual loss among people who are alcoholic.

These disruptions in interpersonal relationships and threatened disruptions are not the only risk factors involved with suicide in people with substance use disorders. Nearly everyone (96%) in a series of 50 suicides by people suffering from alcoholism was still drinking excessively. More than four-fifths had communicated suicidal thoughts or acts. Three-fourths were experiencing a comorbid major depressive episode. Nearly three-fourths had little or no social support. More than one-half had significant health problems; one-half were unemployed; and more than one-third were living alone. These findings strongly distinguished this population from alcoholics who had not committed suicide as well as from people who committed suicide when suffering solely from depression. The recent experience of loss among alcoholics who commit suicide is precisely paralleled by that of abusers of other substances who commit suicide. Given the overall similarities of substance abusers of whatever preference, it is likely that the basis for suicide is the same in all of them. There is considerable overlap between alcohol and drug abuse. The Epidemiological Catchment Area Study noted that 21.5% of alcoholics also had a drug abuse or dependence diagnosis. In people with drug abuse or dependence, 47.3% had an alcohol use disorder as well.

Factors associated with increasing risk of suicide in this group are cumulative. Loss or threatened loss of a close interpersonal relationship is important, especially when other social support is weak or absent. Subacute and chronic risk factors include continued substance abuse, a history of suicidal communication (including suicide attempts), a comorbid depressive syndrome, poor or no social support, substantial health problems, unemployment, and living alone. They are easily tracked in an alcoholic patient. As the number of such factors climbs to three or more, risk of suicide becomes greater, and the need for evaluation, intervention, and management becomes more urgent.

Physicians are reluctant to acknowledge character flaws in their patients and commonly equate substance abuse with weak character. Thus, they avoid making the diagnosis. The behaviors that serve to identify substance abuse are often known to them but not named for what they are. Again, recognizing the disorder is primary.

Schizophrenia

Schizophrenia has been identified in about 5–7% of cases in community studies of suicide. It is not a major risk factor in community series, but the lifetime risk for suicide in those afflicted with schizophrenia may be as high or higher as that for affective disorder. It is a significant contributor to suicides among those who had been hospitalized for a psychiatric disorder.

The majority of people with schizophrenia who take their own lives are young, often better educated than the average, and previously had high expectations for their future. (Some studies indicate a risk for suicide throughout the course of the illness.) After one or two psychotic episodes, an awareness of a limited future dawns. Depression and suicide attempts become a part of the picture. The suicide usually appears to have been impulsive, if only in the lack of verbal warning. It often occurs when the patient is on leave from the hospital during a remission of psychotic symptoms. It is difficult to justify on humanitarian grounds continued restrictive hospitalization when psychosis remits, although some small risk of suicide exists. Vigorous treatment of a complicating depressive syndrome may be protective and improve the quality of life for those suffering with this unfortunate disorder.

Panic disorder and generalized anxiety disorder

A number of follow-up studies involving people with panic disorder have identified an excess of suicides, although this diagnosis is very low among suicides studied retrospectively in the community. Panic disorder is commonly found to be associated with other Axis I disorders, either as an antecedent or as a complication. Prominent among these Axis I disorders are affective disorder and substance abuse disorder. Henriksson and colleagues found 17 of 1397 suicides in a one-year time span in Finland had a prior diagnosis of panic disorder. All had another psychiatric disorder at the time of their death, either a depressive disorder or a substance abuse disorder. The authors concluded that "suicide in people with panic disorder is associated with superimposed major depression and substance abuse, and with personality disorders." They suggested that the symptoms of panic disorder may be obscured by the symptoms of depression at the time of death.

Panic attacks or more generalized anxiety may increase when depression supervenes, but among actual cases of suicide it is the depression, and not the anxiety, that has taken the center stage. The depression must be recognized and treated; symptoms of the panic disorder should also be treated. When substance abuse complicates the picture, the risk factors are those previously described for substance abuse.

Delirium and dementia

Delirium and dementia contribute in a small way (1–2%) to illnesses associated with suicides. Distorted perceptions are the hallmark of delirium. Sometimes the visions (hallucinations) are terrifying. Perceiving the approach of a fearsome monster or the room to be wildly aflame, the patient who is delirious may leap through a window in a vain attempt to escape. If the ensuing fall proves fatal, it has more in common with accidental death than with suicide. Delirium is a dangerous state and calls for serious protective measures — impenetrable screens or unbreakable glass in the windows — while the source of the delirium is sought. An accumulation of medications, each by itself innocuous, is often the cause. (See Chapter 11.)

Poststroke dementia is often associated with depression. Depression is the risk factor for suicide in these cases and should be recognized and treated.

Personality disorders

Borderline personality disorder and antisocial personality disorder account for nearly all of the suicide mortality in this group, but they are usually associated with other psychiatric disorders. Substance abuse (including alcohol) is the most common complication, which, in turn, may be complicated by a depressive episode. A history of suicide attempts is common in both antisocial personality disorder and in borderline personality disorder. Indeed, suicide attempts and threats comprise one of the criterion symptoms of borderline personality disorder. Disruptions in the social sphere (such as rejection, abandonment, or arrest) may be a precipitating factor. But without comorbidity with other psychiatric disorders, the risk of a fatal outcome is slight.

People with personality disorder may be less able to tolerate depression. They may also act more impulsively.

Lifetime risk of suicide in psychiatric disorders

Guze and Robins summarized the follow-up studies of patients with depression and showed that the median percent dead by suicide was 19%. They estimated that 15% of all patients with depression would die by suicide. That figure has been widely quoted in the literature, but the estimate is problematic. If, in fact, 15% of all people with depression committed suicide, the number of suicides would be much greater than the 30,000 suicides that occur in the United States annually. Assuming that one-half of the 30,000 suicides (i.e, 15,000) are people with depression and that one in seven depressed people commits suicide (14%), that would suggest there are 105,000 people at risk with depression. This is well below the estimated population prevalence for depression. If 5% of men and 10% of women in the United States have depression, there would be conservatively more than 15,000,000 people with a lifetime history of depression. This analysis suggests a much lower lifetime risk of suicide in depressed people. Murphy and Wetzel, using this logical approach with alcoholism, estimated that the lifetime risk of suicide in alcoholics was about 3% to 4%.

Harris and Barraclough performed an exhaustive review of 152 English language follow-up studies and reported the number of suicide deaths associated with different psychiatric disorders. Some of the results are listed in Table 29.3. Inskip, Harris, and Barraclough used more sophisticated mathematical modeling procedures to estimate the lifetime risk of suicide in patients with affective disorder, alcoholism, and schizophrenia. They concluded that 7% of patients with alcohol dependence, 6% of patients with depression, and 4% of patients with schizophrenia would eventually die as a result of suicide. Suicide risk is particularly high close to the time of diagnosis for schizophrenia and affective disorder. However, using their models, the suicide risk for alcohol dependence is similar throughout the lifetime of the disorder.

The genetics of suicide

Most studies of people who attempt and those who complete suicide have found increased rates of suicide in their families. The size of the increase seems to be greater than one would expect simply from the increased risk of suicide resulting from psychiatric disorders. Haberlandt reported a low concordance rate for suicide in monozygotic twins (18%), but no concordance pairs in fraternal twins. Roy looked at 176 additional twin pairs. Combining data with other studies including Haberlandt's, he found that 17 of 129 monozygotic twins (13%) were concordant for suicide while two of 270 fraternal twins (<1%) were concordance for suicide. These data would seem to suggest a genetic contribution, but the gene or genes involved clearly are not controlling or fully penetrant.

An adoption study done in Denmark, showed that adoptees who committed suicide had a significantly higher percentage of biological relatives who die by suicide (4.5%) than the relatives of matched adoptees who had not committed suicide (0.7%). The members of the adoptive families did not have an increased risk of completed suicides.

The aggregation of suicides in some, but not all, families with a psychiatric disorder suggests a number of possibilities:

1 There is a familially transmitted variant in the disease, such as degree of severity, that increases risk.
2 There are different forms of the disease with differing levels of risk.
3 There are other familially transmitted host characteristics (e.g., personality) that interact with the disease to increase risk.

Results from the adoption studies seem to indicate that some of the familial factors are genetic.

Non-psychiatric disorders

Cancer and other life-threatening diseases

Suicide occurs in patients with cancer. Since these patients die while under a physician's care, many may escape the medical examiner's attention. Of course, a complicating depression affects the tolerability of the suffering and the attractiveness of the alternative. Depression should be treated

TABLE 29.3

Excess mortality in psychiatric and behavioral disorders

Group	Sex	Number of studies	Number of subjects	Observed suicides	Expected suicides	Standardized mortality ratio
Dysthymia	Both	3	48,515	1405	117.7	11.9
Alcoholics	Males	18	40,017	559	114	4.9
Alcoholics	Females	10	3,308	63	3.5	—
Reactive psychosis	Both	2	21,762	1,067	70	15.25
Mixed drug abuse	Both	4	3,140	103	7.9	13.1
Anxiety disorder	Females	1	6,655	65	10.7	6.1
Anxiety disorder	Males	1	3,256	86	13.3	6.5
Schizophrenia	Males	8	13,634	607	62	9.8
Schizophrenia	Females	6	9,424	200	24.9	8.0
Affective disorder—NOS	Males	10	3,488	165	8.9	18.5
Affective disorder—NOS	Females	11	5,660	154	6.6	23.3
Mental retardation	Both	4	2,591	1	2.4	0.4
Opioid abuse	Males	4	4,037	24	4.3	—
Opioid abuse—HIV	Both	2	2,013	9	0.1	—
Tobacco	Males	1	18,415	80	44.3	1.8
Tobacco	Females	2	11,541	30	16.4	1.8
Neurosis	Males	2	2,740	30	15.1	2.0
Epilepsy	Both	4	3,470	25	5.6	4.4
Self-poisoning	Both	4	3,349	251	6.4	39.1
Attempted suicide	Both	3	1,667	216	5.2	41.9
Psych. inpatients	Both	3	25,111	298	26.7	11.2
Any psychiatric care	Males	3	20,994	127	14.4	8.8
Any psychiatric care	Females	3	21,255	85	6.6	12.9

Adapted from Harris and Barraclough (1998)

vigorously, not only to relieve suicidal thoughts but also to make the patient more comfortable overall. Of equal or greater concern is the patient who mistakenly believes he or she has cancer. This conviction is nearly always a manifestation of a depressive episode, and it may be the presenting symptom. Risk assessment in depression is discussed earlier in this chapter.

Acquired immunodeficiency syndrome

Among dreaded diseases, acquired immunodeficiency syndrome (HIV/AIDS) ranks at or near the top. Its diagnosis initially was reported to be associated with an increased risk of suicide—over 60 times that of the general population, an obvious overestimate; these reports were poorly done or poorly controlled. A review of the literature, adjusting for age, sex, and race shows that the rate of suicide is between 1.5–2 times that expected in the general population.

Starace reported that suicidal acts are not more frequent in individuals with HIV/AIDS compared to HIV seronegative people showing the same "at risk" behaviors; the prevalence is higher only when compared with the general population. Dannenberg and colleagues compared the mortality due to suicide among 4147 HIV-positive military service applicants and 12,437 HIV-negative applicants disqualified from military service for other medical conditions. Ten suicides were seen among the 70-month follow-up. Suicide rates in both groups (49/100,000 in HIV +) were marginally higher than those for the US general population, after adjustment for age, race, and sex. The investigators concluded that HIV-positive individuals do not appear to have a significantly increased risk of death from suicide in the months following HIV screening in this study population.

Major depression may develop in patients with HIV. The rates of depression in HIV-infected patients have been found to be relatively high (20 to 30%) in research using depression rating scales. Studies of people infected with HIV that used structured diagnostic interviews yield rates of current major depression ranging from 6% to 11%. Risk factors for depression in patients with HIV infection include a personal history of either depression prior to infection or a personality disorder prior to infection. The rate of depression is higher in people reporting perceived lower social support. Suicidal ideation is related much more closely to the presence of depression than to HIV infection.

It has been thought that even the possibility of receiving the diagnosis of human immunodeficiency virus (HIV) can precipitate suicide. Van Haastrecht and colleagues studying Dutch drug injectors over a four-year interval found that notification of HIV-positive status did not appear to lead to a sudden and significant rise in suicide or overdose mortality. The vulnerable patient receiving very bad news may be at risk. The bad news itself does not seem to create the vulnerability. Because male homosexuality is a risk factor for HIV/AIDS, it is important to consider whether homosexuality is associated with increased risk of suicide. National or statewide data do not exist on the frequency and correlates of completed suicide in gay and lesbian people in the general population, including youth. Many believe that there is a relationship between suicidal behavior and homosexuality in adolescence. Much of the literature that has given support to this hypothesis is poorly controlled. Shaffer and colleagues found no evidence that suicide is common among gay youth or that, when suicide does occur among gay teenagers, it is a direct consequence of stigmatization or lack of support. No community study of suicide has shown that homosexual youths or adults have an increased risk of suicide.

Other disorders

Huntington's disease is associated with increased risk of suicide. Several studies indicate that the risk of suicide is 2–3 times as high as expected. Both acute and chronic renal insufficiency carry an increased risk of suicide, most likely mediated by a comorbid depression, a disorder to which sufferers from both illnesses are prone.

Age-associated risk of suicide

Conwell and colleagues noted that young people who commit suicide are more likely to have substance abuse problems or psychosis. The middle-aged more often had alcohol problems while the elderly more often had depression.

Adolescent suicide

Adolescents who commit suicide have much higher rates of substance abuse than other adolescents. Carlson and colleagues suggested that substance abuse was the most significant contributor to the increase in the national suicide rate in adolescence (from 2% of all suicides to 7%). Brent and colleagues also found high rates of substance abuse. However, they concluded that "affective disorder is the most significant and predominant risk factor for adolescent suicide." They also noted the importance of bipolar spectrum disorder.

Controlled studies also show that almost all adolescents who commit suicide have long histories of adaptational difficulties. Conduct disorder is seen in many. In an exception to the usual rule, Brent and colleagues found that conduct disorder conveyed a higher risk of completed suicide in the absence of an affective disorder. Adolescents completing suicide were more likely than controls to have a possible or probable personality disorder. Marttunen and colleagues divided adolescents who commit suicide into three groups: those with alcohol dependence, those with depressive disorder, and others. Those with alcohol problems were more likely to have interpersonal separation (43% versus 0% in the depressed). They were more likely to have problems with the law or discipline (50% versus 11%) and were more likely to be unemployed. Consistent with studies of adult suicide, recent interpersonal loss was more common among victims with alcohol abuse than among victims suffering from depression.

Comparing adolescents who commit suicide to adolescents hospitalized for suicide ideation, Brent and his associates observed that the dead adolescents were more than twice as likely to have guns in their homes (74.1% versus 33.9%).

Suicide in young adults

The most common psychiatric disorders in people who complete suicide under age 30 are substance abuse disorder and affective disorders. Rich and colleagues observed there were three significant differences in stressors in younger suicides. They were less likely to be ill, more likely to be unemployed, and more likely to have legal difficulties. Younger people may be more impulsive in their suicides.

Suicide in late life

Risk factors for late-life suicide differ somewhat from those observed earlier in life. In addition to affective disorder, risk factors include conjugal bereavement, medical illness, and living alone. In contrast, family discord and legal and financial problems are the most common stressors associated with suicide in young adults. According to Henriksson and colleagues, depressive syndromes were observed in 74% of suicide victims age 60 or older. Alcohol dependence or abuse was less common than in younger suicides.

Suicidal communications

Many people contemplating suicide tell others about their intent before they kill themselves. Such communications deserve careful evaluation. According to some reports, suicidal patients are aware that they are thinking about suicide, but not of how often they speak of it to friends and family.

Once concern is aroused, it is highly useful for the clinician to obtain as much information as possible from informants about recent communications and behavior. The reaction of family and friends to these communications is equally important information. The absence or presence of concern and social support may increase or decrease the likelihood of suicide. Robins and his associates found that at least 68% of men and 74% of women had communicated their intent to commit suicide at least once. These findings have been replicated in subsequent psychological autopsy studies. For example, Isometsä and colleagues examined 571 cases of suicide in Finland in which the patient visited a health care professional within 28 days of their suicide; almost one-half visited psychiatric professionals. Of the 571, 100 had seen the health professional on the day of their death. In 128 cases (22%), the issue of suicide was discussed with the health professional. There was an association between having a history of attempted suicide and communicating an intent to commit suicide (30% versus 15%). Patients seen in psychiatric settings were more likely to communicate their suicide intent. Women who committed suicide were more likely to communicate their intent than men (32% versus 18%). The investigators state, "One cannot always expect the person in danger of suicide to express such intent spontaneously." They suggest that health care professionals engage in the active and comprehensive examination of depression and suicide thoughts. This is principally a matter of asking questions (see *Key clinical questions*).

KEY CLINICAL QUESTIONS AND WHAT THEY UNLOCK

- *Have you had thoughts of death?*
- *Have you wished you were dead?*
- *Have you thought of taking your life? If so, what have you specifically thought of doing?*
- *What preparations have you made for dying?*
- *What preparations have you made to prepare others?*
- *What preparations have you made to obtain the means?*
- *What preparations have you made to have the opportunity?*
- *When will you do it? Under what circumstances?*
- *Have you decided to proceed to do it?*
  Answers to these questions assist the treatment team to better understand the nature of the patient's suicidal thoughts and details regarding the patient's specific plans.

If the patient is evasive or unconvincing, the family should be interviewed as well. The physician should pay serious attention to any gut feelings. It is wrong to suppose that, by inquiring, the physician can plant the idea of suicide. Thoughts of death are ubiquitous—"nearly universal"—in depression.

Threat assessment

The base rate for suicide is low in the population; the best actuarial prediction will always be that suicide will not occur. Even in patients with major depression, a family history of suicide and a history of significant suicide attempt, the base rate is very low. This does not mean that one can ignore assessing the risk of suicide in specific cases. As reviewed by Borum and colleagues, threat assessment research has changed the way in which mental health professionals have thought about and conducted assessments of violence potential. So far, it has primarily been applied to the prevention of homicide. However, it is equally applicable to the prevention of suicide. Suicide can be thought of as a form of targeted violence in which the target is the self. There has been a shift away from thinking of violence as an innate, unchangeable characteristic of the individual towards thinking of violence as dependent on the situation and circumstances, subject to change and intervention and varying in the degree of severity.

It has been recognized for years that increased risk of suicide can be inferred from patterns of behavior similar to those seen in completed suicides shortly before their deaths. Suicidal intent is demonstrated in a number of ways. The intent to commit suicide may be demonstrated by a previous unsuccessful suicide attempt; the more severe the medical consequences, the greater the intent that may be inferred. Trivial attempts are no guarantee of the patient's safety, however. While the majority of suicides die on their first attempt, a history of suicide attempt is the strongest predictor now identified. The victim may put his or her affairs in order—arranging finances, papers, creating or modifying a will, and making preparations for a funeral or funeral service. The victim may hint at his intent to family and friends so that they will not be too shocked and disturbed when the suicide occurs. The victim may exercise final opportunities to give advice and counsel to family and friends on the conduct of the rest of their lives or similar matters. The victim may consider the means that will be used in causing the death and make special efforts to obtain the means or to prepare the means. The victim may make special efforts to ensure a good opportunity for his or her demise. This may include inquiring about others' schedules or plans. It may include a trip to a secluded place where the event may take place.

Gut feelings that not all is well should not be ignored. Whatever leads to concern about one's patient, a reasonable and thoughtful evaluation should result.

Preventing suicide

Suicide risk changes over time. Appropriate management gets the patient through periods of greatest risk in the safest way acceptable while beginning longer term treatment. Detective novels about murder focus on means, motive, and opportunity. Short-term, acute prevention of suicide should focus on these as well. In particular, severely suicidal patients should not have the means or the opportunity to commit suicide. Prevention efforts in jails that focus on increased staff awareness as well as removing means and opportunities from the environment have been highly successful. Removal of firearms from the premises is an essential first step when the person at risk is not confined.

The key to preventing suicide on a long-term basis usually involves successful treatment of the underlying psychiatric illness. That in turn calls for prompt and accurate diagnosis. Most people who have committed suicide while under medical care have had illnesses that were undiagnosed, underdiagnosed, and undertreated. Depressed mood has been recognized but not translated into a diagnosis of depressive disorder. Instead, only symptoms have been treated, particularly insomnia and anxiety. Hypnotics and anxiolytics do not relieve depression. Even in cases where antidepressants have been prescribed, the dosage has been subtherapeutic by any standard in many cases. Although treatment failures occur even when depression is diagnosed and treated aggressively, those people with untreated or undertreated depression most often become suicide statistics.

A majority of patients with suicidal thoughts can be safely treated as an outpatient. It is a matter of clinical judgment in deciding the most appropriate treatment setting. When choosing an antidepressant, the physician should consider its potential as an agent of self-destruction. All tricyclic antidepressants (TCAs) are toxic. A week's supply at full therapeutic strength can prove fatal if taken in a single dose. That risk is reduced when a responsible family member controls the medication. Serotonin-selective reuptake inhibitors (SSRIs) are less toxic than TCAs and have fewer side effects in most patients. Idiosyncratic intolerance is a common cause of noncompliance with the prescribed medication regimen. Dosage must be monitored closely in the early weeks of treatment. Effective management of antidepressant therapy is not as difficult as many primary care physicians suppose. It involves appropriate doses and careful follow-up. Becoming very familiar with two or three antidepressants, as opposed to superficial familiarity with a large number, can be helpful.

A 1990 report by Teicher and colleagues of six cases involving emerging or reemerging suicidal preoccupation in patients receiving fluoxetine implied that the drug was responsible. Subsequent comment has been mostly nonconfirmatory. As is true of other SSRIs, fluoxetine is a useful and widely accepted antidepressant with a low side-effect profile. At the time of this writing, the FDA is examining the issues involved in the treatment of depression and suicidal behaviors and is encouraging manufacturers of many antidepressants to issue a warning statement, recommending that patients treated for depression be closely monitored. Careful follow-up is an important part of the treatment of depressed patients.

Early in the course of antidepressant treatment, individual patients occasionally experience marked anxiety or agitation. This also happens in untreated patients. Family and patients should be warned to immediately contact the treating physician should these or other marked changes in symptoms occur.

It is difficult for people who are mentally healthy to understand a person's decision to take his own life. Suicides usually are not the result of psychosis. But with deepening depression, there often comes the conviction that life is futile and that suffering will never end. People at risk may agree to rational arguments to the contrary, but the half-life of that acquiescence is unknown and variable. This is especially true since depressive symptoms vary in severity at different times of the day. One must not suppose for a minute that he or she has actually talked a patient out of suicidal thoughts for all time. At the same time, talking with a depressed patient is helpful. Some formal psychotherapies (cognitive, behavioral, and interpersonal) have demonstrated benefit in depressed outpatients. These therapies may be beyond the scope or interest of the primary care physician, but referral to an experienced practitioner is worth considering. In severe depression, psychotherapy alone should not be used to prevent suicide. Patient compliance with all aspects of the therapeutic regimen is important and dependent on good physician-patient communication and consistent follow-up by the health care team.

The physician should keep informed as to the development and urgency of the patient's suicidal ideation or plan. The intensity of suicidal thoughts waxes and wanes within an episode of depression. To some extent, it varies as a function of the severity of symptoms, but it can increase even when other symptoms appear to be unchanged or improving. With any level of suicidal thoughts, the physician should insist that the family remove all firearms from the dwelling. The patient who has evolved a fully lethal plan and secured the means for its execution should be hospitalized immediately under intensive psychiatric observation. A course of electroconvulsive therapy (ECT) is the quickest and surest way to reverse suicidal intent. It should be followed by vigorous pharmacotherapy. When the diagnosis or optimal treatment is in doubt, the physician should refer a depressed patient to a psychiatric specialist.

The frequency of suicide sharply increases in the weeks immediately after discharge from inpatient psychiatric treatment. The change from daily contact to monthly appointments may feel like abandonment to the patient. Depressive symptoms often recur, and if the physician is hard to reach, despair may ensue. The primary care physician may assist in the close professional support needed for the recently discharged patient.

The bottom line in preventing suicide among people with substance abuse disorders is to stop the drinking or other substance abuse behavior. Most of the social stressors that are found among the suicides in this population are directly attributable to the consequences of substance abuse. Currently, most substance abuse treatment involves outpatient treatment, and every physician should identify a treatment program to which he or she is comfortable referring patients. Alcoholics Anonymous (AA) is sometimes helpful and always worth trying. Patients should be advised to visit several chapters before deciding whether and where to continue. The tone, social level, and orthodoxy vary considerably, and a good social fit is necessary for continued participation.

When social support is poor or absent, loss or threats of loss (equally as potent) may be decisive. The period of greatest danger probably lasts no more than the months around the event, so hospitalization, day hospital program, or other supportive measures may be helpful in providing the needed protection. The depressive syndrome commonly encountered in people with severe alcoholism deserves careful evaluation and treatment. It often remits spontaneously with detoxification and the associated improvement in the patient's social situation. When it does not, it must be treated vigorously. Substance abusers are often uncooperative and noncompliant, so protective efforts do not always prevail. However, it is far better to try and fail than to fail to try (see *Pearls & Perils*).

PEARLS & PERILS

- Although most patients with thoughts of suicide usually tell the physician when asked, they rarely volunteer that information. The physician should ask gently, but it is important to ask.
- Patients with a fully lethal plan and the means to accomplish it at their disposal are at high risk and should be hospitalized without delay in a secure psychiatric facility.
- The physician should insist that the family remove all firearms from the home even when the patient has low levels of suicidal ideation.
- Too many physicians look for an explanation for depression, and having found one, fail to treat the depression. The diagnosis is the diagnosis and calls for vigorous treatment.
- Having another psychiatric diagnosis is not protective. Depression can and does complicate many other diagnoses (for example, substance abuse or panic disorder) and brings with it the risk of suicide.

A few people with suicidal thoughts do not have a psychiatric disorder. Strong support and attentive palliative care may help ameliorate the situation. Since psychiatric illnesses are so common in the suicidal patient, a patient with suicidal thoughts should be carefully evaluated before concluding that a psychiatric disorder is not playing a role.

The literature seems clear: failure to diagnose, undertreatment, and lack of social support by physician, family, and friends allow for too many suicides.

Annotated bibliography

Borum, R, Fein, R, Vossekuil, B, and Berglund, J (1999) Threat assessment: defining an approach for evaluating risk of targeted violence, *Behav Sci Law* 17(3):323–37.
This is an excellent, clear, and easy-to-understand presentation of current views of threat assessment.
Isometsä, ET (2001) Psychological autopsy studies—a review, *Eur Psychiatry* 16(7):379–85.
This is a reader-friendly review of the findings of almost all of the reported psychological autopsy studies.
Murphy, GE (1992) *Suicide in Alcoholism*, New York, Oxford University Press.
The case histories of 50 people with alcoholism who committed suicide comprise the core of this book. Each story is different, but there are many features in common. The methodology of the research is described, as are the risk factors for suicide derived from this study and compared with other populations.
Robins, E (1981) *The Final Months: a study of the lives of 134 persons who committed suicide*, New York, Oxford University Press.
This is the first systematic community study of suicide and details the first case histories of its victims. The findings of this work, completed in 1958, have been replicated numerous times.

CHAPTER 30

Forensic Issues

Melissa Swallow, MD, Sean H. Yutzy, MD, and Stephen H. Dinwiddie, MD

OUTLINE

Introduction

Although the primary care physician's exposure to the legal system is limited, the occurrence of psychiatric illness in patients broadens the scope of potential medicolegal issues for the treating physician. Many physicians regard any intrusion of law into medicine as being at best an inconvenience and at worst a disaster, but the physician who adheres to the principles of good medical practice using a pure advocacy model of patient care will have little trouble meeting any challenges that the adversarial system produces.

Forensic psychiatry lies at the interface of medicine, psychiatry, and the law. Uniquely qualified to act as an expert consultant to the legal system, the forensic psychiatrist's most prominent role is to assess an individual's thoughts, feelings, and behaviors *as these relate to a specific legal issue.* Thus, forensic psychiatrists might be requested, for example, to evaluate the mental state of individuals involved in either criminal proceedings or civil litigation. Rather than usurping the role of the judge or jury by addressing the ultimate legal question — whether it be insanity at the time of a crime, nature and degree of emotional damages sustained by a plaintiff in a civil suit, competence to waive a specific legal right, or another of the myriad of such issues — the forensic psychiatrist lends expertise to the court and attempts to provide a thorough and unbiased opinion on which the legal system can rely when reaching a disposition.

In reading this chapter, the practitioner should be aware that the issues are described broadly and the details of statutory and case law vary among jurisdictions. Similarly, the examples and discussion in this chapter should not be taken as legal advice, but rather provide a conceptual framework for practitioners to appreciate issues that cross the boundaries of medicine, psychiatry, and the law. When necessary, specific legal consultation should be sought.

Civil commitment

Principle

Civil commitment is a legal mechanism allowing dangerous, psychiatrically ill individuals to be involuntarily hospitalized. The specific criteria for commitment vary from state to state, and the reader is advised to become familiar with his or her jurisdiction's specific criteria and procedure.

Historically, civil commitment has been derived from two separate concepts. The first is *parens patriae*, the doctrine that the sovereign (or the state) has a responsibility to his subjects analogous to the parent's duty to her children, i.e., the state can intervene in order to protect the well-being of its citizens — in this case by providing for detention and treatment of mentally retarded and mentally disordered individuals deemed to be in need of such services. This concept is rooted in English law and was intended as a means to protect those who could not protect themselves. The second concept is that of the police power of the state, the power by which a safe and orderly society is maintained. These two principles might be broadly characterized as "medical" and "legal," respectively, in that the first implies that citizens may justifiably be held against their will primarily if in need of treatment, while the second implicitly holds interests in the individual's liberty, reserving civil commitment for those found to be both mentally disordered and substantially disruptive of society, i.e., presenting a danger either to themselves or to others. The legal principle of civil commitment involves striking a balance among an individual's autonomy, upholding the *parens patriae* doctrine (intended to protect the individual) and enforcing the police power of the state (intended to protect society).

This shifting balance between individual and societal interests is reflected in the evolution of civil commitment laws in the United States. During the early and middle twentieth century, the *parens patriae* justification for involuntary admission dominated. However, by the 1970s physical liberty was seen as a greater social good than prevention of suffering, and civil commitment became primarily based in the state's police power. Civil commitment was seen as analogous to incarceration and, required due process rights typically given to criminal defendants such as the right to counsel, to a hearing, and to question witnesses.

Each state sets its own statutes for civil commitment criteria, but the basic criteria are similar, requiring the presence of a serious psychiatric illness causing either a danger to self or others *or* (at least in some states) evidence that the individual's illness substantially interferes with the ability to provide self-care. Other states allow for commitment when a person is noncompliant with treatment, which is likely to result in deterioration in the person's mental state, or lacks the capacity to refuse treatment. Additionally, some states allow for outpatient commitment, requiring an individual to be compliant with office visits, medication, and other treatment. Finally, many states have Sexually Violent Predator laws that allow for the civil commitment of those with "mental abnormalities" or personality disorders that are "more likely than not to engage in predatory acts of sexual violence" (Missouri Revised Statutes, 2003). These statutes are grounded more in the police power of the state than in the *parens patriae* doctrine.

As the philosophical basis for civil commitment has shifted to the stricter "dangerousness" standard, many jurisdictions have separated the clinically related but logically independent question of involuntary treatment from the issue of commitment. That is, because the specific legal principles guiding consent to treatment are different from the concepts justifying commitment (see below), a separate procedure to determine whether the individual's refusal of treatment can justifiably be overridden must be held. This distinction is often puzzling to clinicians, since empirically it is known that virtually all such treatment refusals are incompetent, and the need for an additional review often leads to lengthier hospitalizations.

Discussion

In Case 30.1, the psychiatrist recognizes that his patient has a serious psychiatric illness that interferes with his ability to recognize the need for treatment. A strong case can be made that because of the patient's paranoia and incapacity to recognize his need for medical and psychiatric treatment, he will be unlikely to care for himself if released from the hospital. Therefore, release would result in potentially life-threatening congestive heart failure due to hyperthyroidism. While the psychiatrist, as a physician, can testify to this medical opinion, judicial decision-makers may prefer testimony from medical experts with specialized knowledge of the other relevant medical disorders. The primary care physician likely would have the option of choosing whether to appear in court, but should be aware of the obligation to advocate for the patient's best medical interest. Before appearing at the civil commitment hearing, the physician should review the issues and laws with the involved parties,

---

A 54-year-old single male with a long history of rheumatic heart disease, hyperthyroidism, and paranoid schizophrenia was involuntarily detained on the petition of the attending psychiatrist. Around age 30 the patient experienced the onset of hyperthyroidism, which was relatively well controlled medically with propylthiouracil. He had refused medical and surgical ablation. He had stopped his antithyroid medication on two occasions, both resulting in admission to the intensive care unit for life-threatening congestive heart failure due to hyperthyroidism.

His psychiatric history included six previous psychiatric hospitalizations, the last five hospitalizations occurring shortly after he had stopped taking his antipsychotic medications because he "felt fine." On those occasions, he had experienced a rapid recurrence of paranoia and command auditory hallucinations to strike out at strangers because he believed they were part of the conspiracy to kill him.

A week prior to admission, the patient informed his family that he no longer had any medical problems, stopped taking his antipsychotic and antithyroid medicines, and began to develop suspiciousness and paranoia. The patient was brought to the emergency room and was initially noted to be calm and cooperative. When seen in the emergency room, he admitted hearing voices commanding him to hurt people in red shirts because they were part of the plot to kill him, and said he did not know whether he could continue to control himself because the voices were so loud. He was involuntarily admitted after he refused hospital admission and became angry when offered medication. After admission, the patient was suspicious and paranoid but calm, and denied auditory hallucinations, suicidal or homicidal thoughts. He had a mild tremor and moderately elevated free T4 but consistently refused both antipsychotic and antithyroid medication because he was convinced that the pharmaceutical company had "adulterated the medicine with rat feces."

Over the next several days, the patient was noted to be withdrawn, but ate and slept well. He talked loudly to himself but continued to deny auditory hallucinations. The psychiatrist was aware of the lack of explicit suicidal or homicidal behavior and had to decide whether the patient met the criteria for extended involuntary psychiatric hospitalization.

CASE 30.1

the treating psychiatrist and the attorney involved in the case.

Several points are important to review. First, physicians may be concerned about a potential breach of confidentiality or violation of the patient's testimonial privilege. The civil commitment process is an exception to both as long as the action taken is in the furtherance of the detention. Second, it is always helpful to review the specific language of the civil commitment statute so that the relevant legal points can be directly addressed in testimony. Third, the physician's opinion must take into consideration his level of comfort and expertise with the medical facts. Generally, the physician can give an opinion regarding any or all of the following issues: (1) the presence or absence of a mental illness as defined by the jurisdiction in statutory language or case law; (2) the potential for exacerbation or recurrence of an underlying psychiatric illness; (3) the presence or absence of a medical illness; (4) the potential for exacerbation or recurrence of a medical illness; (5) the seriousness of both the psychiatric and medical illnesses; (6) the potential interplay between the psychiatric and medical illness; (7) the patient's capacity to recognize the need for treatment; (8) opinions on other medical issues; and (9) hypothetical testimony using the facts of this case or other cases to base opinions on potential outcomes.

Competency and informed consent

Principle

The legal concept of competency is a broad one that applies to both civil and criminal issues, so it is vital to clarify the specific issues for which competency is being questioned. Competency can be questioned on purely legal grounds (e.g., the individual is underage or has previously been adjudicated incompetent on the issue) or may be questioned based on clinical evaluation demonstrating that because of mental illness the individual lacks *capacity* to fulfill the requirements for a specific competency at the time.

Competency for criminal matters may apply to any stage of a criminal proceeding. For example, one must be competent to stand trial, to be sentenced for conviction of

a crime, or to be executed. Although the defendant is presumed to be competent until proven otherwise, the prosecuting attorney, defense attorney or even the judge may raise the question of competency when events dictate. If a competency examination is requested, a psychiatrist will assess for the presence of a mental disease or defect that impairs the defendant's ability to understand the criminal proceeding and to assist in his or her own defense. If, based on clinical evaluation, a defendant is found incompetent to stand trial, treatment for the purpose of restoration to competency is typically ordered. Under exceptional circumstances, such restoration may prove to be impossible within a reasonable time, in which case the defendant cannot be tried, but must either be civilly committed (if dangerous) or released.

Civil competencies include competency to consent to admission, to consent to treatment, or to refuse treatment. The legal concept underlying accepting or refusing treatment is that of informed consent (see Case 30.2). The concept of informed consent requires three elements: (1) information, (2) voluntariness, and (3) competency. The element of information has several interpretations, and the precise language varies among the jurisdictions. A significant number of jurisdictions adhere to a professional standard wherein the sufficiency of the information provided to the patient to make a decision is judged by what most physicians provide their patients. However, one of the more widely accepted paradigms is known as the "reasonable person" (patient) test, which is described as the information a reasonable person would need to know in order to make an informed decision. This information typically includes: (1) the nature of the illness, (2) the nature of the medication (or procedure) along with its risks, benefits, and side effects, (3) alternative treatments and their risks, benefits, and side effects, (4) the risks and benefits of no treatment, and (5) time to ask any questions that the patient deems necessary.

The second element of informed consent is voluntariness. Coercion may invalidate the process of consent. The third element is competency, and here a brief aside is necessary. In law there is a fundamental presumption that all individuals are competent to conduct their affairs unless there is a special consideration present, such as juvenile status or a previous

A 55-year-old man with a long history of diabetes, alcoholism, and schizophrenia came to the emergency room with a large soft tissue abscess on his neck. Physical examination revealed the individual to be in overall deteriorated condition, with a 3cm by 3cm fluctuant mass immediately adjacent to the trachea but posterior to the right jugular vein. His entire neck was tender to palpation and any movement. He was febrile (103°F), with elevated white blood cell count and blood glucose level.

While sitting alone, the patient was noted to carry on a conversation with himself. When the physician inquired about incising and draining the lesion, the patient responded with the following comment: "No way I'm letting you near me with a knife so that you can kill me for my money." The patient further stated that he had only come to the emergency room at the behest of the voices. A request was made for the consulting psychiatrist to come to the emergency room and declare the patient incompetent so the treatment refusal could be overridden.

CASE 30.2

formal adjudication of incompetency (by a judge and not a physician). Physicians may consider the issue of mental competency when reviewing a medical situation, but they are in fact opining on an individual's medical *capacity* to provide valid informed consent. That is, they are considering whether a mental illness interferes with the patient's capacity to comprehend the risks and benefits of the proposed treatment, alternatives, or no treatment and voluntarily make a decision.

Discussion

Although most physicians are generally aware of the elements of informed consent, not all are aware that when the patient refuses a procedure or medication, the same basic elements apply. If a competent individual understands the information (from a reasonable-person perspective, where applicable) related to a particular procedure or medication and voluntarily declines, in legal theory the refusal is valid and should be honored. When less serious issues are disposed of by informed refusal, few problems arise. However, if serious or life-saving treatments are being refused, a thorough review of the situation by all interested parties, including family, second-opinion physicians, various committees, lawyers, and judges, may be needed. In critical situations, of course, emergency treatment may generally be given unless there is reason to believe that such interventions would have been competently refused (e.g., based on prior instructions or faith).

In this example, a question is raised as to the individual's competency (medical capacity) to provide a valid informed refusal, since he appears to be refusing the procedure because of a paranoid psychotic misperception. Psychiatric consultation is most appropriate; although a psychiatrist cannot make the legal determination that the patient is in-

competent, a psychiatrist will be able to examine the individual and evaluate for the presence of mental illness that might impair the patient's ability to arrive at an informed decision. If the consultant opines psychiatric (medical) incapacity, steps to override this refusal should be based on consideration of the regulations and laws of the state, the best medical interest of the patient, his prior wishes (if relevant), and the gravity of the medical situation.

Guardianship and conservatorship

Principle

Although the specific tests for guardianship or conservatorship vary, in general guardianship can be established if as a result of a medical condition, including mental illness, the individual is unable to receive or process information in order to provide for the basic necessities of life, such as food, shelter, safety, and emergency procedures. Conservatorship may be established if as a result of a medical condition, including mental illness, the individual is unable to receive or process information in order to care for basic financial affairs.

Discussion

All physicians are aware that they have an obligation to advocate for the best interest of their patients. Here, this obligation properly impelled the physician to initiate a process that inadvertently upset her patient. One way to approach the situation would be to suggest that the patient obtain legal counsel to advocate for her interests. Furthermore, the physician should inform the patient that the physician has an obligation to advocate for the patient's best medical interest and that she will continue to fulfill this obligation.

A 65-year-old widowed woman, living independently has a history of coronary artery disease, hypertension and a family history of Alzheimer's disease. She had been medically stable taking multiple medications over the last year, except for a minor complaint about forgetfulness. The physician had noted some minor problems with memory, but the patient had been able to articulate her need for medication, as well as list doses and complicated schedules. One month ago she voiced a concern that somebody had broken into her house and stolen or "rearranged" her furniture. The police were summoned but did nothing. During a more recent office visit she related that people were rearranging her furniture, which she had confirmed by placing a hair between various pieces of furniture and the wall and observing that the hair had fallen to the floor the following day. While the patient could articulate the list of her medications, she appeared somewhat suspicious of her "need for all that medication."

The physician expressed concern about the patient living alone, and the patient allowed her to contact her family who lived in another state. The patient's daughter voiced a surprising amount of concern, and two days later an attorney contacted the physician's office, stating that the family had retained him to file a petition to have the patient declared incompetent. He wanted to know if the physician would fill out a form to that effect. The physician divulged no information about the patient but agreed to consider the material. On review, she noted that in addition to a guardianship affidavit there was a conservatorship affidavit.

The next day the patient called the physician and was quite distraught. She explained that the family had descended on her and was trying to take control of her person and assets. She related to the physician that she thought the family could hardly wait to get their hands on her $500 000 bank account. The patient pleaded with her physician to assist in her plight.

CASE 30.3

Once the patient has retained proper legal representation, the physician's role may evolve in several ways. The patient's attorney might ask for the physician's assistance in considering whether guardianship and conservatorship are medically indicated. The physician may refuse this offer if she wishes to remain completely neutral in this matter and not risk jeopardizing the physician-patient relationship.

If the physician considers proffering a medical opinion, she should be aware of the statutory language and relevant case law for the jurisdiction. She should also ensure that the patient releases the physician to discuss freely her medical findings and opinions with the patient's attorney. As part of this process, the patient should be informed that the physician will be formulating an opinion as to the patient's best medical interest and that this opinion may not support the patient's wishes and indeed might undermine her legal case. The patient should be made aware that she would be waiving confidentiality and testimonial privilege if she wishes her physician to testify, and that once formal opinions are formulated and expressed, they will be subject to the applicable discovery process (for example, affidavit, interrogatories, report, deposition, hearing, trial, and other procedures).

A judge, who typically considers the physician's medical opinions in the broad context of a general guardianship determination, determines the need for a guardian. Medical testimony is often given great weight in determining that full guardianship is needed, which would be a finding by the court that the patient is incompetent to handle all her affairs. The conservatorship issue is similar, but narrower in that only ability to handle finances is considered, but the issue is often litigated aggressively because of the substantial monies typically involved.

- Physicians have a fiduciary obligation to advocate for the best medical interests of their patients in all aspects of care.
- Details of statutory and case law vary among jurisdictions. Physicians should familiarize themselves with specific pertinent criteria and procedures for their jurisdictions. This is especially important in cases where the physician is testifying in a court proceeding.

PEARLS & PERILS

Confidentiality and privacy

Principle

The ethical obligation of a physician to keep information divulged by patients secret can be traced back to the Hippocratic oath. The premise of confidentiality is intended to promote full disclosure by the patient so that the physician can provide the most effective treatment. Current ethical codes such as those of the American Medical Association or the American Psychiatric Association emphasize confidentiality in the doctor-patient relationship. However, this obligation is not absolute. For example, if a patient poses a substantial danger of harm to self or others, confidentiality may ethically be breached, if necessary, to protect the target of the danger. By the same reasoning, some conditions are held to be so potentially harmful to society that reporting may be mandated by law, such as child abuse, elder abuse, certain communicable diseases, or gunshot wounds; indeed, failure to report may lead to civil or even criminal sanction.

Some legal situations may also negate confidentiality, such as in the course of court-ordered examinations, civil commitment proceedings, or civil litigation when an individual puts his mental state at issue such as in emotional distress or malpractice cases. Similarly, in an emergency, confidentiality may be breached when the information provided is in the best interest of treating the patient. The federal government formally addressed the issue of privacy with The Health Insurance Portability and Accountability Act (HIPAA) of 1996. The original impetus for the law was to provide continuous health insurance upon change of employment. The law expanded "... to improve portability and continuity of health insurance coverage in the group and individual markets, to combat waste, fraud, and abuse in health insurance and health care delivery, to promote the use of medical savings accounts, to improve access to long-term care services and coverage, to simplify the administration of health insurance and for other purposes."

HIPAA contains three main rules. The Transaction Rule sets standards for electronically transmitting claims and payments. The Security Rule establishes rules to protect health information. Finally, the Privacy Rule establishes guidelines for the use, disclosure, and protection of all Protected Health Information (PHI).

The Privacy Rule deserves particular mention. It requires 'covered entities' (providers, insurers, or administrators who engage in electronic transmissions) to comply with specific requirements that cover privacy polices by (among other things) designating privacy officers, providing procedures for patients to see or amend their records, and notifying patients of privacy policies. Penalties exist for failure to comply with the guidelines. Interpretation and implementation of HIPAA is currently ongoing.

Discussion

One of the exceptions to confidentiality and privacy is an emergency situation. In Case 30.4, the patient clearly posed an imminent danger to himself and others, and required sedation and treatment of his psychosis. The Privacy Rule does not require patients' consent for communication between health care providers. This nightmare scenario highlights the dangers associated with a mistaken and unreasonable adherence to the Privacy Rule.

A 39-year-old man was escorted to the Emergency Department by police after he was found wandering in traffic, yelling obscenities and shaking his fists at passing cars. Upon arriving in the Emergency Department, the man swung his fist at the triage nurse, missed, and hit an elderly man in the head, causing injuries requiring sutures. The psychiatric consultant noted that the patient was agitated, pacing the room, and incoherently speaking of a conspiracy between the state hospital, the police, and the CIA. Staff were able to ascertain that the patient had been previously hospitalized at another facility and treated for schizophrenia, but no other pertinent information was available and the patient had not been treated previously at the present facility.

Because this was an emergency situation, the consultant determined that the patient's confidentiality could be breached, but family informants could not be contacted. Personnel at the outside hospital where the patient had previously been treated refused to release medical records because of new privacy policies. The consultant clarified to the medical records supervisor that only information regarding the patient's previous medical illnesses and allergies to medications was needed. She again refused to release any information without the state hospital's privacy form completed and signed by the patient.

While the outside hospital was being contacted, the patient began screaming, banging his head against the hard tile floor, and attempting to barricade the door of the seclusion room with his body. He was given an intramuscular injection of an antipsychotic drug for sedation, but rapidly developed respiratory distress and profound hypotension, and ultimately was admitted to the ICU. Later, family members informed hospital staff that the patient had been warned never to take that particular antipsychotic medication after previously having a severe allergic reaction to it.

Criminal responsibility

Principle

Serious crimes are in general composed of two elements, both of which must be proved beyond a reasonable doubt in order for conviction. The first, obviously, is the commission of a wrongful act (actus reus). It must also be shown, that at the time of the commission, the defendant also had a wrongful state of mind (mens rea). For example, one individual might cause the death of another. Under some circumstances, this act might be a crime—but not always. It might be praised, for example, in the case of a soldier who kills an enemy during wartime or a police officer who shoots a criminal in order to save a hostage's life. It might be excused based on self-defense, or because of heroic but unsuccessful surgery, or because it was an unavoidable accident. Or it might be condemned but punished more lightly if it stemmed from recklessness rather than malice.

The basis of the legal concept of "insanity" is that moral responsibility for the act is held to be negated because of profoundly impaired reasoning ability: when the mental processes of an individual are profoundly disturbed, simple fairness dictates that the individual should not be held to the same standard of responsibility as the ordinary citizen.

Several legal tests for insanity have been proposed, but the basic principles are broadly similar: The individual must suffer from a mental disease or defect severe enough to impair the ability to appreciate the wrongfulness of the behavior. Psychiatrists are often involved in evaluating a defendant's mental state *as it existed at the time of the alleged crime.* Although not convicted of any crime, those found not guilty by reason of insanity typically are committed to secure forensic psychiatric hospitals, where most stay for longer

A 50-year-old man with porphyria and no criminal record was in an automobile accident while vacationing in a neighboring state. The patient was unconscious when taken to the hospital, and a barbiturate was used as part of the anesthetic induction used for emergency treatment. The patient complained of abdominal discomfort at discharge and later continued to report abdominal pain and dark urine. In addition, he began demonstrating erratic behavior and frank paranoia.

After discharge he went to a local park, sat down on a bench and fell asleep. A park ranger came by and notified him that he could not sleep on the bench. The patient was noted to be well dressed but incoherent in his conversation and bizarre in his interaction. The conversation escalated into an argument, and the patient took a swing at the park ranger, who pulled his gun. The patient advanced on the park ranger, who fled. The police were summoned and, after an extended brawl, the patient was detained in custody and five police officers were treated in the local emergency room for bruises and bites. The patient was legally processed and five counts of first-degree assault were brought against him. He was transferred from the jail to the hospital as a prisoner because of his unstable medical condition. He was eventually discharged and noted by the family to seem "normal." The patient retained counsel to defend him against his legal charges. The attorney contacted the patient's treating physician in his home state about the patient's long history of porphyria. The lawyer then informed the physician that he would like him to review the state statutes on sanity, case law, medical records, and police reports and consider offering an opinion on insanity.

periods of time than they would have in prison had they been convicted of the charged crime.

Discussion

Although the charges described in Case 30.5 may be disposed by several more expedient avenues, prosecutorial discretion occasionally requires a full sanity evaluation and sometimes trial. In potential cases where an underlying medical illness can be documented by laboratory testing and the disease is outside the usual evaluation and treatment role of a psychiatrist, a general medical physician may be invited to proffer an opinion. Often attorneys avoid using the patient's treating physician for a variety of reasons, including the inherent bias to advocate for his patient's best interest, lack of medicolegal sophistication, possible hidden concern on the part of the treating physician that he may be the eventual target of a malpractice suit (because of the original incident), causing perversion of subsequent testimony, and other reasons. However, in cases where the presence of an unusual medical "mental illness" is central, the attorney may feel strongly that not only should an independent medical expert testify but that the treating physician should also play a significant role in assisting the trier-of-fact (judge or jury) in deciding the case. Although the treating physician usually has the option not to participate (citing possible interference with physician-patient relationship), he should always consider the fiduciary obligation to advocate for the patient's best medical interest.

In cases where the treating physician elects to become involved, he should expend every effort to gain as complete an understanding of the entire process as possible. After obtaining a formal release from his patient to speak to the attorney, the physician can begin this educational process. The attorney will be able to provide the physician with all the available relevant information, including the statutory language and case law. However, the physician should be aware that the attorney represents the best legal interest of the patient and not the interests of the physician. Should the physician develop any concern or question about any issue related to his role, he may wish to retain his own counsel.

Working with the patient's attorney will probably give rise to a number of potential issues of interest, but the core request by the attorney is for the production of medical and perhaps medicolegal opinions. Medical opinion is considered here to be all the medical knowledge, information, and inferences that a physician can offer to assist the trier-of-fact in understanding the medical issues related to the case but not including a direct statement containing the ultimate medicolegal opinion on insanity (that is, the examiner's opinion as to whether the patient was insane at the time of the crime). However, before arriving at any "formal" medicolegal opinions to be expressed and rendered to the court, the physician may find review of several considerations helpful.

If a medicolegal opinion on insanity (criminal responsibility) is requested, the following general issues might be considered—though each case has its own unique considerations. The patient should be made aware that the treating physician is willing to consider offering an opinion about the medical and perhaps medicolegal aspects of the case for a legal determination regarding responsibility (insanity). Generally, the patient needs to agree for the physician to proceed after those involved give consideration to the following subset of preliminary issues. Confidentiality has to be waived either directly by the patient, through court appointment, or by other methods applicable in the jurisdiction. Testimonial privilege has to be waived directly by the patient, directly through judicial order, directly through the fact that it is a criminal proceeding, or by methods applicable in the jurisdiction. The patient should be aware that there is no guarantee that the physician will be helpful, and that any opinions, whether helpful or harmful, may become part of the public record. The physician should also consider (and disclose) the possible deleterious effects of harmful legal opinions on the overall physician-patient relationship. Because of such conflicts, it is generally better for a professional with no prior treatment relationship to undertake such an evaluation.

The examining physician should review and understand the applicable statutory language and case law governing the insanity defense in that jurisdiction. This may be involved and entail learning legal interpretation of special language as opposed to routine medical knowledge. This legal definition must then be applied to the facts of the case, which usually requires review of all available medical records pertaining to his patient's medical illness (and behavior) before the alleged assault, as well as the patient's medical status and behavior immediately before, during, and after the incident. Unlike a typical medical history, interview alone may not be sufficient; in order to understand the defendant's behavior, it is often necessary to interview individuals who observed the patient's behavior at the time of the incident and when he had prior exacerbations of illness (porphyria in the case example). Other documentation of the defendant's behavior can often be found in police reports, jail records, crime scene photos, and (in the case of assault or murder) even in treatment records or reports of the postmortem examination of the victim.

After this review, an examination of the patient is usually undertaken in which the defendant's complete history is usually reviewed, as in any other medical evaluation; however, the majority of the examination is typically spent also considering the patient's medical and psychiatric status at the time of the incident and whether or not the legal test was met.

Formal medicolegal opinions should be based on careful consideration of the relevant medical, legal, and psychiatric facts, so that the physician may provide an opinion at the level of certitude articulated by the legal profession as "reasonable medical certainty"—a phrase that has been defined variably by the courts and should be ascertained for that particular jurisdiction at the beginning of the case.

Malpractice

Principle

Professional malpractice is considered a tort, i.e., a civil (as opposed to a criminal) wrong; rather than punishing the wrongdoer, the goal is to "make the victim whole," i.e., compensate him or her for the damage caused by the defendant's actions. Generally, for a successful malpractice action, four elements must be demonstrated, often referred to as the "four Ds" (Simon and Gold, 2004).

The first, Duty, is the responsibility of physicians to treat patients according to prevailing standards of good medical practice. Obviously, this implies the formation of a physician-patient relationship. This need not be explicitly set out, as long as the physician acts in a way that would reasonably be taken to indicate a treatment relationship has been formed. The second "D" is Deviation. During the performance of their duties, physicians may deviate from the generally accepted standard of appropriate medical practice through an act of commission or omission. In some cases this may be intentional, but generally occurs through negligence. How this "standard of care" is determined varies by jurisdiction, although there appears to be a trend away from local toward national norms. It may be established in court by a variety of ways, such as reference to standard texts or articles, package inserts or instructions for drugs or devices, evidence of deviation from facility policies and procedures or guidelines set by professional societies, and so forth, but it is most commonly based on peer testimony.

The third required "D" is Damage, generally an adverse or undesired outcome of treatment. However, because unsatisfactory outcomes are not always avoidable and do not necessarily indicate poor care, a causal link must be shown between the fall below the standard of care and adverse outcome. Thus, the final "D" is that the bad outcome was Directly caused by (or Due to) the improper act(s) of omission or commission by the treating physician. All four elements must be present to a preponderance of the evidence ("more likely than not") to establish malpractice (see Case 30.6).

CASE 30.6

A 64-year-old, employed man was admitted to the hospital with abdominal pain, which he said had started three weeks earlier. It was described as intermittent and diffuse, vaguely localized to the lower right quadrant, not helped by nonprescription analgesics but temporarily relieved by drinking alcohol. He added that he had been drinking more heavily over the last four months, following the death of his wife after 44 years of marriage. He denied any other gastrointestinal symptoms, but reported a laparotomy 20 years earlier after shooting himself twice in the abdomen. He stated he had then been depressed over the death of his 15-year-old son and had been admitted to the psychiatric service where he was given "some kind of shock treatment," but he did not see a psychiatrist after discharge.

His family history was significant for a brother who had intentionally electrocuted himself. The patient stated he was concerned about being able to pay for hospitalization. When asked whether he had other problems or concerns, he reported insomnia "for months," loss of appetite with a 15 lb weight loss, feeling "down in the dumps," low energy, and occasional "crying jags." He had thoughts about not wanting to be around since he was "the only one left," and when directly asked about thoughts of suicide responded, "Yes, before coming in but . . . no, not while I am here in the hospital."

Physical examination revealed the patient to be under his ideal body weight and to have vague, diffuse lower and right-lower quadrant abdominal tenderness without point or rebound tenderness. There was an old laparotomy scar from the bullet removal, but the examination was otherwise negative. The next day's nursing notes described the patient as sullen and withdrawn, crying on several occasions. Clinical examination of the patient continued unchanged; admitting labs were normal. The following day, the attending physician's partner rounded on the patient and wrote, "The patient is melancholically depressed and must have psychiatric consultation because of suicidal thoughts before being discharged." Nursing notes documented that the patient talked about missing his wife, stated that there was really little point in his continued living with this pain, and complained of feeling "hopeless and completely fatigued." Radiologic and endoscopic studies were negative, and a surgical consultant opined that the pain was probably from "depression with somatic abdominal pain." The attending physician noted the patient "will need formal psychiatric evaluation for depression and suicidality before discharge."

The patient accepted the positive news from the attending physician that there was nothing "physically wrong." The patient was initially reluctant to be discharged but agreed after being told that a longer hospital stay had been denied by his insurer. He was scheduled to be seen as an outpatient the following week. The next day the physician was informed by police that this patient had been discovered dead early that morning, apparently from a self-inflicted gunshot wound.

Discussion

Requesting a consultation is a medical decision undertaken at the discretion of the attending physician, based on the circumstances of the case and the best medical interest of the patient. When failure to obtain consultation would be below the prevailing standard of good medical practice (in the view of a similarly trained and reasonably prudent medical practitioner), then a legal duty to obtain appropriate consultation exists. If consultation is not obtained and if as direct result of this deviation below the standard of good medical practice a legal damage results, then the case may be legally actionable.

Justification for psychiatric consultation in Case 30.6 could be based on (1) current diagnosis of depression; (2) elevated risk for suicide (based on, among other factors, prior attempt, recent loss, increased alcohol use, active depression, suicidal ideation, and—as it turned out—access to a firearm); and (3) the physician's (and partner's) opinions that the patient needed evaluation for depression and suicidality before discharge.

In this example, as is not uncommon in malpractice actions, two of the "Ds"—duty and damages—appear to be clearly established, at least for the attending physician. Whether the failure to obtain consultation was negligent (or falls below the standard of care) and, if so, whether such failure caused the patient's suicide is less clear and thus could become issues for a jury to determine.

Conclusion

Primary care physicians should be aware that the principles underlying concepts of professional negligence (malprac-

tice), informed consent, and competency extend throughout medical practice. In matters such as civil commitment or criminal responsibility, the expertise of a psychiatric or forensic psychiatric specialist is required; however the principle of patient advocacy may lead to the need for assistance from primary care practitioners in some legal determinations.

Finally, physicians should always be cognizant of the theme underlying these issues and guiding the physician-patient relationship: the fiduciary obligation of physicians to advocate for their patients' best medical interest in all aspects of care.

Annotated bibliography

Gutheil, TG and Appelbaum, PS (2000) *Clinical Handbook of Psychiatry and the Law*, 3rd Edition, Philadelphia, Lippincott, Williams & Wilkins.
This textbook provides excellent information for the general psychiatrist, primary care clinician, and other medical providers.
Rosner, R (2003) *Principles and Practice of Forensic Psychiatry*, 2nd Edition, New York, Oxford University Press Inc.
This is a high-quality comprehensive textbook geared toward forensic psychiatrists.
Simon, RI and Gold, LH (2004) *Textbook of Forensic Psychiatry*, Washington DC, American Psychiatric Publishing, Inc.
This is an excellent introduction to forensic psychiatry for the general psychiatrist.

CHAPTER 31

Ethical Issues in Psychiatric Practice

Stephen H. Dinwiddie, MD, Melissa Swallow, MD, and Sean H. Yutzy, MD

Introduction

Sophistication in identifying ethical issues and the skill to resolve conflicts between competing responsibilities are core attributes of the effective medical practitioner, regardless of specialty. Psychiatrists must deal with many of the same challenges and problems that face physicians in other areas of medicine. In addition, clinical dilemmas may become even more complex when the patient suffers from a significant psychiatric disorder that may affect his or her judgment, decision-making capacity, and desires.

The medical model of psychiatry

The medical model of psychiatry, discussed in greater detail in Chapter 1, is an approach to the care of patients that emphasizes attention to reliable diagnosis as a basis for treatment selection and prognosis. Adherents of this model emphasize that accurate clinical assessment and application of knowledge regarding the cause, course, and optimal treatment of psychiatric illness, as for any disorder, is central to the role of the physician. Furthermore, such knowledge is best obtained by rigorous, well-designed scientific study, without deference to any particular psychological theory in the absence of empirical support of its validity and utility. Although such "tough-mindedness" has been criticized as being uncaring and unsympathetic, Guze (1970) has pointed out:

> Scientific skepticism is in no way incompatible with compassion for the sick or disabled. In fact, it is the desire to help patients that causes one to be frustrated by the lack of definite knowledge about what really helps and what does not. There are few things more humanitarian than the effective use of knowledge to relieve suffering . . .

We suggest that those clinical decisions most likely to benefit the patient are those that are most accurately informed—and made with a clear understanding of the nature and extent of the physician's obligation to the patient. We believe that a reasonable starting-point in analyzing any clinical question that appears to have embedded ethical issues is to frame it pragmatically: Whose interests are at stake? Which of the available treatment interventions are most likely to have the intended effect while enhancing the patient's autonomy to the extent feasible? To what extent will that course of action impact other important figures in the patient's life, and how will that affect the patient?

Paternalism, autonomy, and beneficence

The patient-physician relationship has historically placed substantial ethical constraints on the physician's behavior. By virtue of training and experience, the physician has ready access to information about the patient's condition and is in a position to best understand the implications of the disease and treatments to be offered. Professional standards impose an obligation on the physician to act in the patient's best medical interest and forbid the practitioner from benefiting from this relationship by placing his or her self-interest ahead of the patient's. The patient, on the other hand, does not have equivalent restrictions and is free to accept or reject the physician's advice, even though disregarding it may lead to continuing health problems or death.

The freedom to make health care decisions for oneself is considered to be a more important social value than optimal medical treatment. But the concept of autonomy in making medical decisions presupposes that the patient is able to rationally choose between treatment alternatives; the prospect of a patient basing health care decisions on delusional material would certainly be disturbing to most physicians. Thus *autonomy* cannot mean simply that decision-making power must be completely vested in the patient. It also implies that the decision-making process should be logical and its outcome consistent with the patient's beliefs and values. Rather than simply dictating treatment decisions to the patient or ceding all responsibility for treatment choices, it would seem that the physician has responsibility to work with the patient to ensure that choices are made rationally, even if the ultimate decision is one with which the physician might not agree. Deferring to the patient's choice without regard to the way it was made might not be sufficient, and psychiatric consultation may be sought if the patient appears to be acting against values previously expressed. Such decisions might be made because the patient has insufficient information to rationally make a choice, or they might indicate the presence of an underlying mental illness distorting the reasoning process.

In extreme cases, such as demonstrated danger to self or others, there are social mechanisms such as guardianship or involuntary commitment and treatment that allow for substituted medical decision-making for individuals so mentally ill that they are judged unable to make rational choices. But while impairment of ability to consent to treatment can be quite dramatic, as in the case of the psychotic patient who responds to hallucinatory commands forbidding him to cooperate, more subtle degrees of impairment are certainly possible. Where is the line drawn? Should the consent of a patient with depression who assents to electroconvulsive therapy (ECT) because she is convinced it will cause her death be honored? Has a cancer patient who agrees to chemotherapy only because his spouse insists he do so truly acted voluntarily? Does it matter if he has always been a passive, easily led individual? Autonomy in making medical (or any other) decisions is not an all-or-none characteristic. Based on a variety of factors that may include the presence or absence of symptoms of psychiatric illness, personality style, store of knowledge, information-processing ability, and pre-existing attitudes, patients show a range of ability to actively participate in the process of deciding to undergo (or refuse) treatment. Even when the psychiatric condition is not severe enough to warrant involuntary commitment to a psychiatric facility, the physician may have an obligation to vigorously advocate for a course of treatment judged to be in the patient's best medical interest.

Irrational treatment refusal is only one side of the coin. Although concern about impaired decision-making arises most often when the patient refuses treatment that the physician believes is indicated, autonomy is also undermined when the patient assents to treatment without truly being able to participate in the decision-making process.

The physician is inclined to act expeditiously, particularly when the patient is acutely suffering. Under some circumstances, such as need for emergency treatment, it is inappropriate clinically and ethically to delay. But when there is time to reflect, one might ask whether (or when) such an exercise

in medical paternalism is justifiable. If treatment is imposed, how can the physician be sure that it is the patient's goals and not the physician's that are being furthered? Conversely, is it reasonable to believe that a patient whose decision-making ability is obviously impaired by medical or psychiatric illness can truly act autonomously? An authoritarian approach to treatment selection by the physician surely undermines the social value of respect for autonomy—but harm to the patient may result from an exaggerated and unrealistic deference to the patient's stated wishes. It might even be argued that adequate treatment of psychotic states or severe mood disorders, though instituted without all the elements of informed consent present, might well ameliorate the patient's irrational thought processes, thus enhancing rather than detracting from the patient's freedom.

Such ambiguities have led to the suggestion that rather than conceptualizing the physician-patient relationship primarily in terms of paternalism versus autonomy, the physician's main duty to the patient should be seen as one of beneficence, that is, an obligation to act in a way that will most benefit the patient. While acting in a beneficent manner often involves fostering and strengthening the patient's autonomy, it is conceivable that there are circumstances that would force the physician to act in a more paternalistic way. But while overt psychiatric illness may affect the patient's ability to consent to treatment, its mere presence does not negate this capacity any more than its absence guarantees it. A patient's capacity to consent may vary over time and is influenced by a multitude of emotional and intellectual factors, and the effect of mental illness—if any—on this capacity can be determined only by careful examination. Ultimately, the decision as to how forcefully to persuade a reluctant patient (or to decline to treat an incompetently assenting one) must, in this view, be based on the physician's assessment of likelihood, imminence, and severity of harm with or without treatment, combined with an understanding of the patient's values and goals.

More importantly, the obligation to act beneficently requires the physician to also be aware of personal preconceptions and ideals and to understand his or her own motives when recommending treatment. Respect for the individual requires sufficient self-knowledge that there is a reasonable assurance that the physician's recommendation stems from a balanced, objective reasoning process rather than being an unexamined imposition of the physician's personal values without reference to those of the patient.

This objectivity is needed especially in the case of the patient who may develop an unrealistically favorable view of the physician, discount any risks or reservations about treatment, and passively comply with the physician's advice. Conversely, though the physician should not try to use the patient's dependency to coerce agreement with a course of action the physician favors (for personal reasons), there is nothing wrong with the physician explicitly stating his or her own belief and the bases for that belief concerning optimal treatment. Especially in a pluralistic society where many strongly-held personal beliefs may influence the patient's attitudes toward a given course of treatment, a partnership dedicated to the patient's well-being, where both parties are actively informed of each other's values and goals, appears to be the most efficient vehicle for protecting and furthering the patient's interests.

Balancing risk and benefit

One of the duties of beneficence is highlighted when considering treatment options for psychiatric illness. Arguably the most drastic intervention, involuntary hospitalization and treatment, should carry with it a clear benefit, potentially setting the stage for ongoing treatment of a life-threatening illness when less intrusive means fail. Of course, the risks are also great. Overt disregard of the patient's treatment refusal carries with it potential harm, including discrimination by employers and insurers, and limitations of civil rights ranging from restriction of the ability to buy a firearm to restriction of freedom of movement.

It is well recognized that somatic treatments in psychiatry, as in other areas of medicine, carry with them potential risks and side effects, such as tardive dyskinesia, development of dependence on anxiolytics, use of prescribed drugs in attempted or completed suicide, confusion and memory disturbance from ECT, and so on. Less widely recognized are potential adverse outcomes from psychotherapy, which may include changes in attitude and behavior toward family members or other significant figures in the patient's life. For example, one not uncommon outcome in marital therapy is the conclusion (by one or both members of the couple) that dissolution of the relationship is preferable to its continuation. Although the patient may see such changes as positive, or at least that the losses in terms of changed relationships are counterbalanced by improvement in other areas of the patient's life, the possibility of an overall worse outcome nonetheless exists.

Even the act of diagnosis, a necessary and fundamental aspect of treatment, can potentially lead to harm. Misdiagnosis can lead to inadequate or harmful treatment, but even a correct diagnosis may lead to discrimination by employers or insurers and stigmatization by society. Reliance solely on diagnostic classification may also lead to routinized forms of care (or denial of care), with insufficient attention paid to the individual's manifestations of illness and response to treatment. More subtle forms of harm may also arise from misuse of diagnostic categories, such as absolving a patient of responsibility for his or her acts solely based on the presence of a given diagnosis.

As in any other area of medicine, the fact that therapeutic efforts may be ineffective or even cause more rather than less suffering in specific cases does not mean that treatment must be ineffective or fundamentally flawed. However, it is the physician who is most informed of the nature and likelihood of any risks and who is best able (with due regard for the patient's attitudes and values) to choose the optimum balance between risk and benefit. In the case of diagnosis, it is particularly important to realize that assigning a diagnosis may have unintended and possibly deleterious effects; the patient, family, or society may focus on the label rather than on the patient's characteristics, strengths, and needs.

Dual agency and the exploitation of patients

Because of the demands and expectations placed on them by society, psychiatrists, perhaps more than other medical professionals, run the risk of dual agency. Although professing that he or she is acting solely in the patient's interests, the psychiatrist may have another, less overt motive. The ability to involuntarily hospitalize patients, for example, has been criticized for this reason, the argument being that rather than acting as a caregiver, the psychiatrist is acting as an agent of the state to control a citizen's behavior, as a sort of unofficial policeman. Supporters of this position argue that individual autonomy (in the narrow sense of physical liberty only) should not be abrogated on the basis of mental illness but only if a crime has been committed. This is, however, a distinctly minority view. Though there has been a shift in recent years toward greater judicial oversight of the commitment process and an emphasis on dangerousness rather than illness *per se*, there is general agreement that the ability to detain some mentally ill individuals is a legitimate and necessary part of psychiatric practice.

Other forms of dual agency are potentially more problematic. Psychiatrists may interview individuals for a variety of reasons other than treatment. Such evaluations include, for example, assessment of criminal responsibility, competency to stand trial, emotional damages in tort litigation, or fitness for military duty. The nature of the psychiatric interview, which often entails the establishment of a significant degree of interpersonal rapport, may be misinterpreted as a therapeutic intervention. Conversely, the treating professional may be asked by the legal system to give testimony as to causation of mental illness, which requires substantially different techniques and sources of information, as well as radically changing the nature of the physician-patient relationship. In such cases, there is an obligation on the part of the psychiatrist to inform the individual in advance of the nature and purpose of the evaluation and that the information obtained may be used in a way that will not further the individual's interests. Particularly in the case of the treater-expert, because of the many (and frequently unanticipated) conflicts and their potential for undermining the pre-existing therapeutic relationship, it is preferable not to mix these two very different roles.

There has been a trend toward more conflicts of interest as systems for the delivery of health care have evolved. Physicians are increasingly regulated and reviewed, with payment for certain classes of procedures limited. Particularly for physicians employed by or contracting with organizations that use managed care arrangements, there is pressure to withhold rather than provide care. Whereas the patient may be led to believe that his medical interests are paramount, the physician may experience pressure to minimize cost, to the patient's detriment.

A more egregious violation of the physician's duty is sexual exploitation of patients or former patients. Although it is almost universally believed that such relationships, arising from the intense nature of the therapeutic situation, are a violation of trust, exploitive, and inherently unethical, it has been estimated that between 5% and 10% of therapists have engaged in sexual contact with a patient at some time. This rate accords with estimates of the prevalence of sexual contact between patients and primary-care physicians.

A number of other forms of exploitation can occur, as well. Short of sexual contact, probably the most egregious violations of the physician-patient relationship include taking financial advantage of the patient, for example by entering into business relationships or by using "insider" information from the patient to play the stock market. Other forms of financial exploitation include the physician using his influence with the patient to help a relative get a job, accepting large gifts or bequests, or providing medically unnecessary services.

The treating physician may also be tempted to be overly controlling with patients who are easily influenced, justifying such behavior on the basis of benevolence, or overly punitive of patients who are noncompliant or seen as uncooperative. Merely revealing the existence of a treatment relationship (for example, letting it be known that the psychiatrist is treating a celebrity) may be exploitive, as well as a violation of confidentiality.

Confidentiality

"What I may see or hear in the course of the treatment or even outside of the treatment . . . I will keep to myself . . ." goes the Hippocratic oath. The patient who withholds information relevant to the treatment process out of fear of further dissemination obviously undermines the therapeutic relationship. Particularly in psychiatric treatment, where information about behaviors that are illegal or memories or thoughts that might be painful or shameful may be divulged, there is great reason to safeguard patients' privacy.

However, while it is an important part of the treatment relationship, confidentiality between the patient and the physician is not absolute (see *Pearls & Perils*). The psychiatrist may find it necessary to breach confidentiality to prevent greater harm under some circumstances, such as when a patient presents a substantial likelihood of harming himself or someone else. In addition, reporting certain behaviors (child abuse, elder abuse) or medical conditions (certain communicable diseases, gunshot wounds) may be mandated by law.

PEARLS & PERILS

When confidentiality is a concern

- During communication with peers (presentations, case conferences, "curbside consults"), sensitive information may be inadvertently disclosed.
- In cases where treatment is provided by several practitioners, information may be inappropriately shared, thus increasing risk of further disclosure.
- Only minimum necessary information should be disclosed to third-party payers and reviewers.
- Treatment of minors is particularly problematic in that parents or guardians may feel entitled to information the patient does not wish to share.
- In child custody evaluations and/or court testimony, there is the risk that sensitive or damaging information may be publicly disclosed.
- Although testimony in court may require confidentiality to be abridged, care should be taken to minimize disclosure of unnecessary information.
- Concerned family members may legitimately wish to know details of the patient's diagnosis, prognosis, and treatment, but their wishes cannot supersede the patient's desire for confidentiality.
- Electronic databases may be vulnerable to unauthorized access, thus placing privacy of patient information at risk. Practitioners should ensure that proper security safeguards are in place and followed.
- Warning an endangered third party may require that patient confidentiality be breached in order to safeguard the potential victim's safety.
- The duty to protect confidentiality does not end with the patient's death.

Recognition of the ongoing erosion of patient privacy (for example, compulsory review of treatment by third-party payers) has led to some reform and statutory protection. Some examples include laws regulating release of information about substance abuse and treatment, and, more recently, broader privacy protection under the HIPAA regulations (see Chapter 30). However, it should be remembered that legal regulation and ethical duties do not necessarily run parallel, and the psychiatrist may find it necessary to take steps to prevent inappropriate disclosure even when proper legal forms have been followed. For example, if treatment records are subpoenaed, the psychiatrist may (after confirming that the patient does not wish the information divulged) try to quash the subpoena or request that the records be reviewed *in camera* rather than simply acquiescing to disclosure.

Failure to address with the patient issues of when or if confidentiality might be breached can imperil the treatment relationship. If the possibility is not addressed early in treatment before such issues arise, the patient may feel betrayed if the physician, whom the patient had considered an ally, is compelled to disclose information (for example, by warning a third party of danger posed by the patient). Of course, if a situation arises in which the patient's privacy must be compromised, the conflict can be worsened by concealing (or attempting to conceal) the fact that a breach had occurred.

Provision of care by multiple caregivers is another situation in which breaches of confidentiality may occur. This is, of course, not uncommon in psychiatry, where a patient may be seen for pharmacological treatment by a psychiatrist, for individual psychotherapy by another mental health professional, and perhaps in family or group therapy by a third. Again, while protection of confidentiality under such circumstances has been recently addressed at the federal level, it is important to keep in mind that the primary purpose of the exercise is to protect the privacy of the patient, rather than to unthinkingly follow one's recollection of regulations. Treatment is facilitated by free exchange of information, but all caregivers must ensure that such exchanges are permissible and done with due respect for privacy.

A kindred conflict may occur when the same individual functions in more than one role, such as providing both individual and family therapy to the same patient. In this case, steps must be taken to safeguard against the possibility that information provided in individual sessions might inadvertently be disclosed to family members. It is also possible for the duty to maintain confidentiality to conflict with what is perceived to be civic duty. For example, there is a misperception (which may be distressingly commonplace) that in line with the responsibility to protect potential victims, there is a corresponding obligation to report past crimes. In fact the opposite is true; not only is there no such legal requirement, but such a breach of confidentiality clearly violates a duty to the patient. A practice of such disclosure, if commonplace, could potentially affect the entire profession, undermining any trust in the therapist's assurances of privacy.

Perhaps the most emotionally difficult situations arise when dealing with family members who wish to know details of the patient's illness, prognosis, and treatment. Providing such information may be of great comfort to the family and can be most helpful to the patient. However, if the patient objects, the family's wants or needs cannot supersede the patient's wishes. This duty to maintain confidentiality may hold even after the patient's death. While disclosing information may help assuage family members' grief, there is always the possibility that the knowledge will later be misused.

Minors (or those adjudicated incompetent and who have a guardian appointed) cannot consent or refuse release of information about treatment under most circumstances. Nonetheless, particularly in the case of the adolescent, the issue of dual agency may arise, with the patient wishing the psychiatrist to conceal information to which the parents may feel they have a right. An even more complex situation may arise in the setting of a custody dispute, where parents may disagree about releasing treatment information or where one parent may wish it released as a tactic to undermine the other parent's legal position rather than to further the child's interests.

Under some circumstances, conflicts over confidentiality are inherent in the nature of the clinician's responsibilities. For example, psychiatrists working in the justice system may be called upon to treat criminal defendants in order to restore them to fitness for trial or to offer opinions about future dangerousness in the case of insanity acquittees. In such cases, where treatment is legally mandated and results communicated to the court, profound limitations on confidentiality are unavoidable.

Such conflicts indicate that psychiatrists must often try to reconcile many competing responsibilities—to the patient, to family, possibly to health care organizations, and to society. Careful consideration of multiple parties' interests and the psychiatrist's duty to each is often necessary to clarify which courses of action are allowable and, when conflicts cannot be reconciled, how best to protect the patient's interests.

The difficult patient

Patients may provoke a number of feelings in the treating physician. When those feelings are of anger and frustration, care may suffer because the physician wishes to avoid seeing the patient or becoming more involved in his or her treatment. Conversely, some patients (such as celebrities or family members of colleagues) may evoke in the treating physician a desire to provide exceptionally good or solicitous care (the "VIP syndrome").[1] Whether the physician strives too much or not enough, objectivity may be eroded, with consequent impairment in the physician's ability to provide optimal care.

Particularly in the case of patients perceived as resistant, antagonistic, or otherwise overtly uncooperative with

---

[1] This behavior is troubling not only because deviations from routine care have the potential for undermining systems put into place to prevent complications, but also because of its ethical implications: If the physician has the obligation to strive for optimal care in all cases, how can making extra effort for "special" patients be justified?

treatment, care may be hindered by the physician's reluctance to stay closely involved in the patient's treatment. In such cases the possible contribution of psychiatric illness cannot be ignored. This is not to say that treatment noncompliance is a mental illness, but feelings of frustration, disappointment, or anger at a patient are not necessarily illegitimate and should be considered a clinical indication for more thorough psychiatric assessment. For example, patients with somatization disorder may be quite demanding of both time and patience, and patients with substance-related problems may feign pain or anxiety complaints. Individuals with obsessive-compulsive disorder (OCD) may require much reassurance about trivial physical complaints. Less commonly, patients with unusual physical complaints may on closer examination prove to be suffering from delusions stemming from any of a variety of psychiatric syndromes.

It is easy to attribute noncompliance or otherwise not complying with the physician's recommendations to the presence of a personality disorder—all too often merely medical shorthand for identifying a disliked patient. Such an appellation may make the physician feel better but simply renaming the problem does little to address the very real problems such patients have, often leading to a sort of therapeutic nihilism. This is doubly problematic in that many disorders of personality are in fact quite amenable to treatment. Instead, we advocate first reframing the problematic behaviors *as clinical problems*—barriers to treatment as deserving of appropriate evaluation and intervention as any others. Once a diagnosis is made, treatment may be substantially improved not only because the underlying psychiatric condition can be addressed (thus clarifying and ideally simplifying the clinical situation), but also because the reason for the previous conflicts in treatment can be clarified for both parties. Ideally, at that point the patient and the physician can then explicitly agree on the nature of subsequent treatment.

Specific problematic areas

Physician-assisted suicide

Generally, those who support physician-assisted suicide (PAS) frame their case in terms of autonomy, arguing that rational patients are allowed to refuse life-sustaining treatment and should likewise be allowed the choice to end their lives more directly. They further note that physicians have been able to withhold futile treatment and that any distinction between hastening death by withholding treatment and actively assisting in the process is at best subtle.

Those who oppose PAS argue that although patients may accept or decline treatment, the principle of self-determination is not equivalent to a right to receive assistance in actively terminating one's life. Whereas it is permissible to provide treatment that also increases the risk of death ("the

principle of double effect"), purposefully taking life is a contravention of basic principles of medicine. Legitimizing this activity might undermine trust in the medical profession by obscuring the motives of the physician, who might be seen as interested in taking, rather than preserving, life. Opponents also argue that once PAS is allowed, a "slippery slope" could result, with increasing latitude in determining who should be assisted in dying (with or without adequate consent), and point to historical examples to substantiate such concerns.

Proponents argue that sufficient safeguards could prevent such slippage and that psychiatric evaluation could be used to ensure that patients requesting PAS were rational and competent to do so. We are unaware of any empirical studies that would justify such optimism. There have been no investigations as to what it might mean to be "competent" to request PAS, nor are there data on the accuracy or reliability of psychiatric assessment of such competence. On the other hand, there is substantial evidence that depressive illness in medically ill individuals is commonly overlooked, thus raising the possibility that a treatable intercurrent disease might often be missed. If mental competency and absence of contribution from treatable psychiatric illness are, necessary conditions for PAS to be allowed, it would seem that until there is adequate study of the accuracy and reliability of clinical judgment about such issues, debate over whether or not to allow PAS is premature unless it is acknowledged that the risk of clinical error of assessment of such issues is unknown.

Even if such concerns could be addressed, a number of concerns regarding the inherent accuracy of medical judgment remain. A decision about PAS requires "judgment calls" about at least three issues: (1) that the underlying medical condition could cause intolerable pain (note the inherently subjective determination of "intolerable"), (2) that no less drastic intervention would adequately relieve such suffering, and (3) that the patient's reported anguish is in fact caused by the condition and not caused or exacerbated by another, potentially treatable condition. Hence the physician asked to assist in a patient's suicide is faced with the task of determining the degree of the patient's suffering, its cause, and its prognosis, all to a very high standard of accuracy, in the absence of external validators such as laboratory tests to exclude psychiatric disease that could be complicating the clinical situation. Under such circumstances, physicians might be tempted either to justify their misgivings about the procedure by overdiagnosing psychiatric illness (thus subjecting the patient to unneeded, possibly intrusive treatment) or to act on feelings (either the physician's, the patient's, or the family's) of hopelessness and frustration and agree too precipitously. Given both the dearth of empirical information about rates of error of assessment and the inherent subjectivity of many of the necessary judgments, it is difficult to see how such a procedure can be justified in practice.

Treatment boundaries

The role of the physician is inherently artificial because of the asymmetry of the obligations and power of the treater and the patient. In psychiatry, given that emotional issues are often more directly relevant to treatment, there is a correspondingly greater need to remain cognizant of the limits of the therapeutic relationship. Even subtle behaviors can make the nature of the relationship ambiguous and therefore undermine treatment.

The common theme in violation of professional boundaries is exploitation of the patient. Extreme examples of violation of such boundaries, such as financial or sexual exploitation of the patient, have been noted above and may indicate a blatantly predatory stance on the part of the therapist. But probably more commonly, even egregious boundary violations tend not to appear *de novo*. Instead, emotional vulnerabilities on the part of the therapist may be inappropriately brought into the treatment setting, exemplified by behaviors such as inappropriate (but not overtly sexual) physical contact; excessive, unexamined acquiescence to the patient's expressed needs (e.g., scheduling of sessions at inappropriate frequencies or times); gift-giving; and role reversal, that is, disclosing to the patient material such as relationship difficulties, psychological conflicts, concerns about work, and so forth—in essence transforming the patient into the therapist and *vice versa*.

Thus, profound violations of boundaries often seem to represent the ultimate outcome of a gradual erosive process that may start with inappropriate meetings (outside of the office for "sessions" at meals, in cars, or at the patient's home) or having the patient perform services for the therapist, not infrequently combined with increasingly obvious evidence of role reversal. The problem may originate in perfectly legitimate, unmet emotional needs of the therapist—but meeting them in such a tremendously inappropriate manner is a grave violation of one's professional responsibility.

Organ transplantation

The need for donor organs continues to outstrip supply. How should a resource-intensive procedure that carries with it the potential for saving lives and substantially improving quality of life be offered to those who need it? On what basis should patients be chosen to receive transplants? Should psychosocial factors be weighed in such decisions, and, if so, what role should the psychiatrist play in the determination of suitability for transplantation?

If such a role exists for psychiatrists, they must be careful to avoid the issue of double agency. That is, before evaluation, patients should be informed of the nature and purpose of the interview and made aware that the information elicited could impact their acceptance as candidates for organ transplantation. Such disclosure should minimize the chance that the patient might misperceive the consultation as being purely therapeutic in nature.

More importantly, as with the issues surrounding physician-assisted suicide, basic empirical issues with direct bearing on ethical issues remain unaddressed. Whether or not basic fairness allows one to deny organ transplantation to patients with severe, treatment-resistant mental illness (a purely ethical issue), mental illness may be proposed as a relative contraindication to transplantation because of presumed associated risk of noncompliance with immunosuppressive therapy (a reasonable presumption but little examined despite being amenable to empirical study). It is not unreasonable to suggest that under conditions of great scarcity, resources should be allocated based on need and likelihood of success. However, what is meant by "success" may not be clearly defined: immediate survival, long-term functional outcome, quality of life, length of survival after transplantation, or some amalgam of all of these?

In fact, relatively little attention has been paid to the impact of specific psychiatric conditions on outcome. Even less has been paid to the effect of personality traits on compliance and psychosocial outcome (see Chapter 19), though such factors might be expected to play at least as great a role as overt psychiatric disorders.

The impact of alcohol and other substance dependence on whether a patient is judged suitable for liver transplantation is of particular interest, since the psychiatrist may play a more prominent role in the decision about transplantation. A brief analysis of the debate shows how empirical data might shape ethical debate. Individuals with cirrhosis from excessive alcohol use and/or hepatitis resulting from unsafe drug injection practices represent a large subgroup of those in need of liver transplantation. The case has been made that people who have developed cirrhosis because of such behaviors should be held responsible for their illness and assigned a lower priority for transplantation. Such ranking appears to penalize those who have significantly contributed to their health problems over a long period as opposed to those whose behaviors did not. However, such a formulation ignores the substantial variability in the natural history of addictions, which is one of relapse and remission, and not uncommonly characterized by spontaneous improvement and long-term abstinence. Despite concerns about the recurrence of alcohol or other drug abuse, there is little evidence to show that outcome in this group is substantially worse than for other conditions, particularly if the individual has remained abstinent for a period of time (typically 6 months) before the transplant. Moreover, the formulation of addiction as being a moral (rather than medical) issue has long been abandoned by the field and denial of access to this kind of care based on diagnosis is implicitly a choice to assign different values to diseases with the same endpoint (organ failure) based on undisclosed moral judgments.

Administrative versus clinical responsibilities

The physician who accepts a medical administrative position in a health care organization almost by definition occupies an ambiguous space. Medical expertise is a requirement for the position, but so is loyalty to the organization. The physician-administrator may have substantial—but not sole—responsibility for the organization's strategic plan and must support it. But whenever limited resources must be allocated (as is always the case in medicine) some patients' needs will not be met within that organization, and the physician-administrator may find it necessary to advocate for the organization's goals and deny the requests of a subordinate physician who is advocating for the patient's best medical interests. In the case of psychiatrists, this may be even more frustrating; in the setting of a general medical center, psychiatric services and psychiatric patients are often not accorded the same priority as medical or surgical services, and the psychiatrist-administrator must be content with relatively little influence over policy decisions. Where psychiatric services are a major or perhaps sole focus of the health care organization (for example, in state mental health facilities), medical leadership may not be supported by nonmedical administrators, who must answer to political and bureaucratic authorities.

On the other hand, the physician-administrator may be in a particularly privileged position as far as his ability to change policy. In our experience, identification and correction of clinically significant system problems can result in more cost-efficient care delivery. Moreover, the physician-administrator is far better equipped to identify and implement policies and procedures that encourage the use of evidence-based treatment approaches.

With administrative responsibilities comes an obligation even greater than that imposed on other physicians to take appropriate steps when confronted with an impaired colleague. This is a responsibility of all physicians, but in practice the emotional cost of such a confrontation often deters action. Thus, coworkers may grumble to each other but otherwise do little. The clinician-administrator, on the other hand, is mandated to investigate and take appropriate action where indicated not only because of the same ethical duty to protect patients from impaired caregivers, but also because of the additional responsibility to ensure appropriate levels of competency and care among staff. Such intervention is often emotionally painful to both the administrator and the putatively impaired professional. However, we would argue that psychiatric knowledge should be of particular value here, not only because many such impairments are a result of psychiatric illness or substance abuse, but also because psychiatric clinical skills should enable the administrator to empathically but firmly confront the impaired colleague and take appropriate action.

Ethics and research

The need for research in psychiatry, as for any other medical specialty, is obvious. The tremendous suffering and disability associated with severe psychiatric illness mandates ongoing efforts to broaden our understanding of mental illness and its causes, mechanisms, and treatments.

Research into mental illness carries with it particular risks. Patients undergoing some drug trials may be withdrawn from medications that are often beneficial and may relapse either before or during the trial of a new agent. This dilemma is hardly unique to psychiatry. However, for many psychiatric conditions, relapse may alter not only the subject's capacity to further participate in research but also his or her ability to consent to treatment once participation in the study is over. Human studies committees have an obligation to evaluate issues of informed consent and risks before approving such protocols.

Another issue of particular relevance to psychiatric research is the fact that highly sensitive, personal information—possibly involving behaviors that are illegal or otherwise socially condemned—may need to be gathered from research participants, with consequent concerns about confidentiality. However, patients with severe mental illnesses—the ones most in need of improved treatment—often lack the ability to truly understand the risks involved, whether breach of confidentiality or substantial worsening of illness, and are the least able to validly consent to research protocols.

Capacity to participate in research, as in other settings, has no clear threshold. It would seem that, at a minimum, in order to participate, potential research subjects should demonstrate a capacity to understand risks and benefits at least equivalent to that required for consent to treatment. But the dilemma noted above, that those most in need of improved treatments are often those least likely to demonstrate high levels of insight or grasp of the risks involved, suggests that the stringency of the capacity requirement might be altered depending on the nature, severity, and likelihood of the risks involved as well as on the potential value of the knowledge gained. Thus in some settings, after being informed of the nature of the project, it may suffice for the participant to exhibit the ability to evidence a choice. Next most stringent would be a requirement that the individual can demonstrate a factual understanding of the issues involved. An even stricter requirement would be that the individual not only has an adequate factual grasp but can rationally process the facts. Finally, the most restrictive standard would require that the individual can not only rationally process the relevant information but can relate it to his or her own situation. That is, the individual is aware of the personal implications of consenting or refusing, can rationally discuss the reasons for consenting and refusing, and can weigh the potential risk in relation to his or her own circumstances.

Conclusion

In this brief overview, a few ethical issues have been described that may arise in the practice of psychiatry, either in the office or in consultation with other professionals. Such an analysis may be of interest to primary care physicians faced with similar dilemmas. From the standpoint of psychiatry, an understanding of the varied manifestations of mental illness, as well as an appreciation of the limitations of psychiatric knowledge, can play a substantial role in how ethical questions are framed and decisions are made. While empirical study cannot take the place of rigorous analysis of the ethical issues and duties involved when troubling questions arise, we believe that properly conducted research can inform such decisions—and a frank acknowledgment of the absence of sound data can sometimes make ethical issues moot. Better decisions about allocation of scarce resources (such as in organ transplantation or which services a medical center should emphasize) may be made if good information is available about etiology, course, and treatment response of illness. In many cases, such empirical data are lacking. However, even in the absence of data, asking questions about the unexamined assumptions on which ethical decisions are founded may force the clinician to view the clinical problem in another light and thereby lead to more judicious choices.

Annotated bibliography

Bloch, S, Chodoff, P, and Green, SA (eds) (1999) *Psychiatric Ethics*, Third Edition, New York, Oxford University Press.
This multiauthored work provides a comprehensive overview of ethical issues affecting psychiatry.

Guze, SB (1992) *Why Psychiatry is a Branch of Medicine*, New York, Oxford University Press.
This is an excellent, concise, and clearly written explication of the medical model approach to psychiatry.

Bibliography

Chapter 1

Beck, AT and Freeman, AM (1990) *Cognitive Therapy of Personality Disorders*, New York, Guilford Press.

Brown, GW and Harris, T (1978) *Social Origins of Depression*, London, Tavistock Publications.

Damasio, AR (1994) *Descartes' Error: Emotion, Reason, and the Human Brain*, New York, G.P. Putnam.

Feighner, JP, et al. (1972) Diagnostic criteria for use in psychiatric research, *Arch Gen Psychiatry* 26:57–63.

Gabbard, GO (1990) *Psychodynamic Psychiatry in Clinical Practice*, Washington DC, American Psychiatric Press.

Gazzaniga, MS (ed.) (2000) *The Cognitive Neurosciences*, Cambridge, MA, MIT Press.

Gelenberg, AJ (1976) The catatonic syndrome, *Lancet* 2:1339–1341.

Goodwin, DW and Guze, SB (1989) *Psychiatric Diagnosis*, 4th Edition, New York, Oxford University Press.

Guze, SB (1979) Can the practice of medicine be fun for a lifetime?, *JAMA* 241:2021–2023.

Guze, SB (1970) The need for toughmindedness in psychiatric thinking, *South Med J* 63:662–671.

Headache Classification Committee of the International Headache Society (1988) Classification and diagnostic criteria for headache disorders, cranial neuralgias and facial pain, *Cephalalgia* 8 (Suppl 7):1–96.

Hudgens, RW (1993) The turning of American psychiatry, *Missouri Medicine* 90:283–291.

Meyer, A (1994) A short sketch of the problems of psychiatry [1897], *Am J Psychiatry* 151(suppl):43–47.

Murphy, GE (1975) The physician's responsibility for suicide: I. an error of commission, *Ann Int Med* 82:301–304.

Murphy, GE (1975) The physician's responsibility for suicide: II. errors of omission, *Ann Int Med* 82:305–309.

Murray, CJL and Lopez, AD (eds) (1996) *The global burden of disease and injury series, volume 1: a comprehensive assessment of mortality and disability from diseases, injuries, and risk factors in 1990 and projected to 2020*, Cambridge, MA, Harvard University Press, published by the Harvard School of Public Health on behalf of the World Health Organization and the World Bank.

Myerson, A (1994) Some trends of psychiatry [1944], *Am J Psychiatry* 151(suppl):55–63.

National Advisory Mental Health Council (1993) Health care reform for Americans with severe mental illnesses: report of the National Advisory Mental Health Council, *Am J Psychiatry* 150:1447–1465.

Szasz, TS (1961) *The Myth of Mental Illness*, New York, Hoeber-Harper.

U.S. Department of Health and Human Services. Mental Health: A Report of the Surgeon General, Rockville, MD, U.S. Department of Health and Human Services, Substance Abuse and Mental Health Services Administration, Center for Mental Health Services, National Institutes of Health, National Institute of Mental Health, 1999. Also available at http://www.surgeongeneral.gov/library/mentalhealth/home.html Accessed 3/12/04.

Weiner, WJ and Lang, AE (eds) (1995) *Advances in Neurology*, vol. 65, Behavioral neurology of movement disorders, New York, Raven Press.

Whitrow, M (1993) *Julius Wagner-Jauregg (1857–1940)*, London, Smith-Gordon.

Woodruff, RA Jr., Clayton, PJ, and Guze, SB (1971) Hysteria: studies of diagnosis, outcome, and prevalence, *JAMA* 215:425–428.

World Health Organization: The World Health Report 2001: Mental Health: New Understanding, New Hope, http://www.who.int/whr2001/, accessed 3/12/04.

Chapter 2

Akiskal, HS, The mental status examination, in Winokur, G and Clayton, PJ (eds) (1994) *The Medical Basis of Psychiatry*, Philadelphia, WB Saunders Co, pp 3–15.

American Psychiatric Association (2000) *Diagnostic and Statistical Manual of Mental Disorders, 4th Edition, text revision (DSM-IV-TR)*, Washington, D.C.

Barsky, AJ, Wyshak, G, and Klerman, GL (1992) Psychiatric comorbidity in DSM-III-R hypochondriasis, *Arch Gen Psychiatry* 49:101–108.

Bauer, MS and Dunner, DL (1993) Validity of seasonal pattern as a modifier for recurrent mood disorders for DSM-IV, *Compr Psychiatry* 34:159–170.

Brown, TA, Barlow, DH, and Liebowitz, MR (1994) The empirical basis of generalized anxiety disorder, *Am J Psychiatry* 151:1272–1280.

Corty, E, Lehman, AF, and Myers, CP (1993) Influence of psychoactive substance use on the reliability of psychiatric diagnosis, *J Consult Clin Psychol* 61:165–170.

Dunner, DL and Tay, LK (1993) Diagnostic reliability of the history of hypomania in bipolar II patients and patients with major depression, *Compr Psychiatry* 34:303–307.

Faraone, SV and Tsuang, MG (1994) Measuring diagnostic accuracy in the absence of a "gold standard," *Am J Psychiatry* 151:650–657.

Feighner, JP, et al. (1972) Diagnostic criteria for use in psychiatric research, *Arch Gen Psychiatry* 26:57–63.

Fennig, S, et al. (1994) Best-estimate versus structured interview-based diagnosis in first-admission psychosis, *Compr Psychiatry* 35:341–348.

Gauron, EF and Dickinson, JK (1966) Diagnostic decision making in psychiatry: I. information usage, *Arch Gen Psychiatry* 14:225–232.

Guze, SB (1992) Diagnosis, in *Why Psychiatry is a Branch of Medicine*, New York, Oxford, pp. 37–53.

Hatcher, S (1995) Decision analysis in psychiatry, *Br J Psychiatry* 166:184–190.

Headache Classification Committee of the International Headache Society (1988) Classification and diagnostic criteria for headache disorders, cranial neuralgias and facial pain, *Cephalalgia* 8 (Suppl 7):1–96.

Hyler, SE, Williams, JBW, and Spitzer, RL (1982) Reliability in the *DSM-III* field trials: interview *v* case summary, *Arch Gen Psychiatry* 39:1275–1278.

Jensen, P, et al. (1995) Test-retest reliability of the Diagnostic Interview Schedule for Children (DISC 2.1). Parent, child, and combined algorithms, *Arch Gen Psychiatry* 52:61–71.

North, CS, et al. (1993) *Multiple Personalities, Multiple Disorders: Psychiatric Classification and Media Influence*, New York, Oxford University Press.

Noyes, R Jr, et al. (1993) The validity of DSM-III-R hypochondriasis, *Arch Gen Psychiatry* 50:961–970.

Parker, G, et al. (1994) Defining melancholia: properties of a refined sign-based measure, *Br J Psychiatry* 164:316–326.

Reynolds, CF 3rd, et al. (1991) Subtyping DSM-III-R primary insomnia: a literature review by the DSM-IV Work Group on Sleep Disorders, *Am J Psychiatry* 148:432–438.

Rhea, SA, Nagoshi, CT, and Wilson, JR (1993) Reliability of sibling reports on parental drinking behaviours, *J Stud Alcohol* 54:80–84.

Robins, E and Guze, SB (1970) Establishment of diagnostic validity in psychiatric illness: its application to schizophrenia, *Am J Psychiatry* 126:983–987.

Rounsaville, BJ, et al. (1993) Cross system agreement for substance use disorders: DSM-III-R, DSM-IV and ICD-10, *Addiction* 88:337–348.

Spitzer, RL, Endicott, J, and Robins, E (1975) *Research Diagnostic Criteria (RDC) for a Selected Group of Functional Disorders*, New York, Biometrics Research, New York State Psychiatric Institute.

Spitzer, RL (1991) An outsider-insider's view about revising the DSMs, *J Abnormal Psychol* 100:294–296.

Wittchen, HU (1994) Reliability and validity studies of the WHO Composite International Diagnostic Interview (CIDI): a critical review, *J Psychiatr Res* 28:57–84.

Zanarini, MC, et al. (1991) The face validity of the DSM-III and DSM-III-R criteria sets for borderline personality disorder, *Am J Psychiatry* 148:870–874.

Chapter 3

Beckman, HB and Frankel, RM (1984) The effects of physician behavior on the collection of data, *Ann Intern Med* 101:692–696.

Cox, A, Hopkinson, K, and Rutter, M (1981) Psychiatric interviewing techniques II. Naturalistic study: Eliciting factual information, *Brit J Psychiatry* 138:283–291.

Cox, A, Holbrook, D, and Rutter, M (1981) Psychiatric interview techniques VI. Experimental study: Eliciting feelings, *Brit J Psychiatry* 139:144–152.

Cox, A, Rutter, M, and Holbrook, D (1988) Psychiatric interviewing techniques. A second experimental study: Eliciting Feelings, *Brit J Psychiatry* 152:64–72.

Saghir, MT (1971) A comparison of some aspects of structured and unstructured psychiatric interviews, *Am J Psychiatry* 128:72–76.

Chapter 4

American Psychiatric Association (2000) *Diagnostic and Statistical Manual of Mental Disorders*, 4th Edition, Text Revision (DSM-IV-TR), Washington, D.C.

Beitchman, JH and the Work Group on Quality Issues, AACAP (1998) Summary of the practice parameters for the assessment and treatment of children and adolescents with language and learning disorders, *Journal of the American Academy of Child and Adolescent Psychiatry*, 37(10), Suppl: 46S–62S, p. 47S.

Ben-Porath, YS, Butcher, JN, and Graham, JR (1991) Contribution of the MMPI-2 content scales to the differential diagnosis of schizophrenia and major depression, *Psychol Assessment* 3:634–640.

Boring, EG (1923) Intelligence as the tests test it, *New Republic* 35:35–37.

Carr, DB, Gray, S, Baty, J, and Morris, JC (2000) The value of informant versus individual's complaints of memory impairment in early dementia, *Neurology* 55:1724–1726.

Cohen, FW and Phelp, RE (1985) Incest markers in children's artwork, *Arts in Psychotherapy* 12:265–283.

Dahlstrom, WG, Welsh, GS, and Dahlstrom, LE (1972) *An MMPI Handbook: clinical interpretation*, vol 1, revised, Minneapolis, Minn., University of Minnesota Press.

Exner, JE Jr (1993) *The Rorschach: a comprehensive system*, 3rd Edition, New York, Wiley Interscience.

Eyde, LD, et al. (1993) *Responsible Test Use: case studies for assessing human behavior*, Washington, D.C., American Psychological Association.

Franzen, MD, Robbins, DE, and Sawicki, RF (1989) *Reliability and Validity in Neuropsychological Assessment*, New York, Plenum Press.

Greene, RL: Assessment of malingering and defensiveness by objective personality inventories in Rogers, R (ed.) (1988) *Clinical Assessment of Malingering and Deception*, New York, Guilford Press.

Grossman, HJ (ed.) (1983) *Classification in Mental Retardation*, revision, Washington, D.C., American Association on Mental Deficiency.

Hagood, MM (1992) Diagnosis or dilemma: drawings of sexually abused children, *Br J Projective Psychol* 37:22–33.

Holtzman, WH and Swartz, JD (1983) The Holtzman inkblot technique: a review of 25 years of research, *Zeitschrift für differentielle und diagnostische Psychologie* 4:241–259.

Keyes, DW, Edwards, WJ, and Derning, TJ (1998) Mitigating mental retardation and capital cases: finding the "invisible" defendant, *Mental and Physical Disability Law Reporter* 22:529–539.

Klein, RG: Questioning the clinical usefulness of projective psychological tests for children in Chess, S, Thomas, A, and Hertzig, M (eds) (1987) *Annual Progress in Child Psychiatry and Child Development*, New York, Brunner & Mazel.

Kline, P (1991) *Intelligence: the Psychometric View*, New York, Routledge.

Lyons, JA and Keane, TM (1992) Keane PTSD scale: MMPI and MMPI-2 update, *J Trauma Stress* 5:111–117.

Matarazzo, JD (1972) *Wechsler's Measurement and Appraisal of Adult Intelligence*, 5th Edition, Baltimore, Williams and Wilkins.

Mathes, PG and Denton, CA (2002) The prevention and identification of reading disability, *Seminars in Pediatric Neurology* 9:185–191.

Morris, JC, et al. (1991) Very mild Alzheimer's disease: informant-based clinical, psychometric, and pathologic distinction from normal aging, *Neurology* 41:469–478.

Morris, JC, et al. (2001) Mild cognitive impairment represents early-stage Alzheimer disease, *Arch Neurol* 58:397–405.

Nihara, K, et al. (1974) *AAMR Adaptive Behavior Scale*, Washington, D.C., American Association on Mental Deficiency.

North, CS, et al. (1993) *Multiple Personalities, Multiple Disorders: psychiatric classification and media influence*, New York, Oxford University Press.

Pulsifer, MB (1996) The neuropsychology of mental retardation, *Journal of the International Neuropsychological Society* 2:159–176.

Rapaport, D, Gill, MM, and Schafer R (1968) *Diagnostic Psychological Testing*, revised edition, Holt, RR (ed) Bern, International Universities Press.

Rorschach, H (1942) *Psychodiagnostik*, Bern, Hans Huber Verlag. Cited in Exner, JE Jr (1993) *The Rorschach: a comprehensive system*, 3rd Edition, New York, Wiley Interscience.

Rubin, EH, Veiel, LL, Kinscherf, DA, Morris, JC and Storandt, M (2001) Clinically significant depressive symptoms and very mild to mild dementia of the Alzheimer's type, *Int J Geriatr Psychiatry* 16(7):694–701.

Sparrow, SS, Balla, DA, and Cicchetti, DV (1984) *Vineland Adaptive Behavior Scales*, Circle Press, Minn., American Guidance Service.

Sparrow, SS and Carter, AS (1992) Mental retardation: current issues related to assessment in Rapin, I and Segalowitz, SJ (eds) *Handbook of Neuropsychology*, vol 6, Amsterdam, Elsevier Science Publishing Co.

Sparrow, SS and Cicchetti, DJ (1989) The Vineland adaptive behavior scales in Newmark, C (ed) *Major Psychological Assessment Instruments*, vol 2, Needham, Mass., Allyn & Bacon.

Welsh, GS and Dahlstrom, WG (eds) (1956) *Basic Readings on the MMPI in Psychology and Medicine*, Minneapolis, Minn., University of Minnesota Press.

Ziskin, J and Faust, D (1988) *Coping With Psychiatric and Psychological Testimony*, 4th Edition, Los Angeles, Law and Psychology Press.

Chapter 5

Brown, ES, Rush, AJ, Biggs, MM, Shores-Wilson, K, Carmody, TJ, and Suppes, T (2003) Clinical ratings vs. global ratings of symptom severity: a comparison of symptom measures in the bipolar disorder module, phase II, Texas Medication Algorithm Project, *Psychiatry Res* 117(2):167–175.

Drake, M, Butman, J, Fontan, L, Lorenzo, J, Harris P, Allegri, R, and Ollari, J (2003) Screening for mild cognitive impairment: usefulness of the 7-Minute Screen Test, *Actas Esp Psiquiatr* 31(5):252–255.

Haro, JM, Kamath, SA, Ochoa, S, Novick, D, Rele, K, Fargas, A, Rodriguez, MJ, Rele, R, Orta, J, Kharbeng, A, Araya, S, Gervin, M, Alonso, J, Mavreas, V, Lavrentzou, E, Liontos, N, Gregor, K, and Jones, PB, SOHO Study Group (2003) The Clinical Global Impression-Schizophrenia Scale: a simple instrument to measure the diversity of symptoms present in schizophrenia, *Acta Psychiatr Scand Suppl* (416):16–23.

Zimmerman, M (2003) What should the standard of care for psychiatric diagnostic evaluations be?, *J Nerv Ment Dis* 191(5):281–286.

Chapter 6

Abi-Dargham, A, Mawlawi, O, Lombardo, I, et al. (2002) Prefrontal dopamine D1 receptors and working memory in schizophrenia, *J Neurosci* 22:3708–3719.

Barch, DM, Carter, CS, Braver, TS, et al. (2001) Selective deficits in prefrontal cortex regions in medication naive schizophrenia patients, *Arch Gen Psychiatry* 50:280–288.

Baxter, LR, et al. (1989) Reduction of prefrontal cortex glucose metabolism common to three types of depression, *Arch Gen Psychiatry* 46:243–250.

Baxter, LR, et al. (1987) Local cerebral glucose metabolic rates in obsessive-compulsive disorder—A comparison with rates in unipolar depression and in normal controls, *Arch Gen Psychiatry* 44:211–218.

Bertolino, A, Esposito, G, Callicott, JH, et al. (2000) Specific relationship between prefrontal neuronal N-acetylaspartate and activation of the working memory cortical network in schizophrenia, *Am J Psychiatry* 157:26–33.

Biver, F, et al. (1994) Frontal and parietal metabolic disturbances in unipolar depression, *Biol Psychiatry* 36:381–388.

Botteron, KN, et al. (1995) Magnetic resonance imaging in childhood and adolescent bipolar affective disorder: A pilot investigation, *J Am Acad Child Adol Psychiatry* 34:742–749.

Botteron, KN, Raichle, ME, Drevets, WC, Heath, AC, and Todd, RD (2002) Volumetric reduction in left subgenual prefrontal cortex in early onset depression, *Biol Psychiatry* 51(4):342–344.

Brody AL, Saxena, S, Stoessel, P, Gillies, LA, Fairbanks, LA, Alborzian, S, Phelps, ME, Huang, SC, Wu, HM, Ho, ML, Ho, MK, Au, SC, Maidment, K, and Baxter, LR (2001) Regional brain metabolic changes in patients with major depression treated with either paroxetine or interpersonal therapy: preliminary findings, *Arch Gen Psychiatry* 58:631–640.

Callicott, JH, Bertolino, A, Mattay, VS, et al. (2000) Physiological dysfunction of the dorsolateral prefrontal cortex in schizophrenia revisited, *Cerebral Cortex* 10:1078–1092.

Callicott, JH, Egan, MF, Mattay, VS, et al. (2003) Abnormal fMRI response of the dorsolateral prefrontal cortex in cognitive intact siblings of patients with schizophrenia, *Am J Psychiatry* 160:709–719.

Carter, CS, MacDonald, AW III, Ross, LL, and Stenger, VA (2001) Anterior cingulate cortex activity and impaired self-monitoring of performance in patients with schizophrenia: an event-related fMRI study, *Am J Psychiatry* 158:1423–1428.

Castellanos, FX, et al. (1994) Quantitative morphology of the caudate nucleus in attention deficit hyperactivity disorder, *Am J Psychiatry* 151:1791–1796.

Cotter, D, Mackay, D, Beasley, C, Kerwin, R, and Everall, I (2000) Reduced glial density and neuronal volume in major depressive disorder and schizophrenia in the anterior cingulate cortex, *Schizophr Res* 41:106.

Cotter, D, Mackay, D, Chana, G, Beasley, C, Landau, S, and Everall, I (2002) Reduced neuronal size and glial cell density in Area 9 of the dorsolateral prefrontal cortex in subjects with major depressive disorder, *Cereb Cortex* 12:386–394.

Courchesne, E, et al. (1994) The brain in infantile autism, *Neurology* 44:214–223.

DeLisi, L, et al. (1985) Positron emission tomography in schizophrenic patients with and without neuroleptic medication, *J Cereb Blood Flow Metab* 5:201–206.

DiRocco, RJ, et al. (1989) The relationship between CNS metabolism and cytoarchitecture: a review of 14C-deoxyglucose studies with correlation to cytochrome oxidase histochemistry, *Comput Medical Imaging and Graphics* 13:81–92.

Drevets, WC, et al. (1992) A functional anatomical study of unipolar depression, *J Neurosci* 12:3628–3641.

Drevets, WC, Frank, E, Price, JC, Kupfer, DJ, Holt, D, Greer, PJ, Huang, H, Gautier, C, and Mathis, C (1999) PET imaging of serotonin 1A receptor binding in depression, *Biol Psychiatry* 46(10):1375–1387.

Drevets, WC, Bogers, W, and Raichle, ME (2002) Functional anatomical correlates of antidepressant drug treatment assessed using PET measures of regional glucose metabolism, *Eur Neuropsychopharmacol* 12:527–544.

Drevets, WC, Price, JL, Simpson, JR, Todd, RD, Reich, T, Vannier, M, and Raichle, ME (1997) Subgenual prefrontal cortex abnormalities in mood disorders, *Nature* 386:824–827.

Drevets, WC, Price, JL, Bardgett, ME, Reich, T, Todd, RD, and Raichle, ME (2002) Glucose metabolism in the amygdala in depression: relationship to diagnostic subtype and stressed plasma cortisol levels, *Pharmacol Biochem Behav* 71:431–447.

Drevets, WC and Raichle, ME (1998) Reciprocal suppression of regional cerebral blood flow during emotional versus higher cognitive processes: Implications for interactions between emotion and cognition, *Cognition and Emotion* 12(3):353–385.

Drevets, WC, et al. (1995) Regional blood flow changes in response to phobic anxiety and habituation, *J Cerebral Blood Flow and Metab* 15(1):S856.

Eastwood, SL and Harrison, PJ (2000) Hippocampal synaptic pathology in schizophrenia, bipolar disorder, and major depression: a study of complexin mRNAs, *Mol Psychiatry* 5:425–432.

Ebert, D, Feistel, H, and Barocka, A (1991) Effects of sleep deprivation on the limbic system and the frontal lobes in affective disorders: A study with Pc-99m-HMPAO SPECT, *Psychiatry Res: Neuroimaging* 40:247–251.

Elkis, H, Friedman, L, Wise, A, et al. (1995) Meta-analyses of studies of ventricular enlargement and cortical sulcal prominence in mood disorders—Comparisons with controls or patients with schizophrenia, *Arch Gen Psychiatry* 52:735–746.

Figiel, GS, et al. (1991) Subcortical hyperintensities on brain magnetic resonance imaging: A comparison of normal and bipolar subjects, *J Neuropsychiatry* 3:18–22.

Fox, PT, et al. (1988) Nonoxidative glucose consumption during focal physiologic neural activity, *Science* 241:462–464.

Heckers, S, Rauch, SL, Goff, D, et al. (1998) Impaired recruitment of the hippocampus during conscious recollection in schizophrenia, *Nat Neurosci* 1:318–323.

Heeger, DJ and Ress, D (2002) What does fMRI tell us about neuronal activity?, *Nat Rev Neurosci* 3:142–151.

Hirayasu, Y, Shenton, ME, Salisbury, DF, Kwon, JS, Wible, CG, Fischer, IA, Yurgelon-Todd, D, Zarate, C, Kikinis, R, Jolesz, FA, and McCarley, RW (1999) Subgenual cingulate cortex volume in first-episode psychosis, *Am J Psychiatry* 156(7):1091–1093.

Hynd, GW, et al. (1991) Corpus callosum morphology in attention deficit-hyperactivity disorder: morphometric analysis of MRI, *J Learning Dis* 24:141–146.

Kellner, C, et al. (1991) Brain MRI in obsessive-compulsive disorder, *Psychiatry Res* 36:45–49.

Ketter, TA, Kimbrell, TA, George, MS, Dunn, RT, Speer, AM, Benson, BE, Willis, MW, Danielson, A, Frye, MA, Herscovitch, P, and Post, RM (2001) Effects of mood and subtype on cerebral glucose metabolism in treatment-resistant bipolar disorder, *Biol Psychiatry* 49(2):97–109.

Krishnan, KRR, et al. (1992) Magnetic resonance imaging of the caudate nuclei in depression, *Arch Gen Psychiatry* 49:553–557.

Krishnan, KRR, McDonald, WM, Doraiswamy, PM, et al. (1993) Neuroanatomical substrates of depression in the elderly, *Eur Arch Psychiatry Neurosci* 243:41–46.

LaPlane, D, et al. (1989) Obsessive-compulsive and other behavioural changes with bilateral basal ganglia lesions, *Brain* 112:699–725.

Laruelle, M, Abi-Dargham, A, Gil, R, Kegeles, L, and Innis, R (1999) Increased dopamine transmission in schizophrenia: relationship to illness phases, *Biol Psychiatry* 46:56–72.

Liberzon, I, Taylor, SF, Amdur, R, Jung, TD, Chamberlain, KR, Minoshima, S, Koeppe, RA, and Fig, LM (1999) Brain activation in PTSD in response to trauma-related stimuli, *Biol Psychiatry* 45(7):817–826.

MacFall, JR, Payne, ME, Provenzale, JE, and Krishnan, KRR (2001) Medial orbital frontal lesions in late onset depression, *Biol Psychiatry* 49:803–806.

Magistretti, PJ and Pellerin, L (1999) Cellular mechanisms of brain imaging metabolism and their relevance to functional brain imaging, *Philosophical Transactions of the Royal Society of London—Series B: Biological Sciences* 354(1387):1155–1163.

Malizia, AL, Cunningham, VJ, Bell, CJ, Liddle, PF, Jones, T, and Nutt, DJ (1998) Decreased brain GABA(A)-benzodiazepine receptor binding in panic disorder: preliminary results from a quantitative PET study, *Arch Gen Psychiatry* 55(8):715–720.

Manji, H, Drevets, WC, and Charney, D (2001) The cellular neurobiology of depression, *Nat Med* 7(5):541–547.

Mayberg, HS, Brannan, SK, Mahurin, RK, Jerabek, PA, Brickman, JS, Tekell, JL, Silva, JA, McGinnis, S, Glass, TG, Martin, CC, and Fox, PT (1997) Cingulate function in depression: a potential predictor of treatment response, *NeuroReport* 8:1057–1061.

Mayberg, HS, Liotti, M, Brannan, SK, McGinnis, BS, Mahurin, RK, Jerabek, PA, et al. (1999) Reciprocal limbic-cortical function and negative mood: converging PET findings in depression and normal sadness, *Am J Psychiatry* 156:675–682.

Mayberg, HS, Starkstein, SE, Sadzot, B, Preziosi, T, Andrezejewski, PL, Dannals, RF, Wanger, HN Jr, and Robinson, RG (1990) Selective hypometabolism in the inferior frontal lobe in depressed patients with Parkinson's disease, *Ann Neurol* 28:57–64.

Mazziotta, JC, Phelps, ME, Plummer, D, and Kuhl, DE (1981) Quantitation in positron emission computed tomography. 5. Physical-anatomical effects, *J Comput Assist Tomogr* 5:734–743.

McDonald, WM, Krishnan, KRR, Doraiswamy, PM, et al. (1991) Occurrence of subcortical hyperintensities in elderly subjects with mania, *Psychiatry Res* 40:211–220.

McEwen, BS (1999) Stress and hippocampal plasticity, *Ann Rev Neurosci* 22:105–122.

Meyer, JH, Wilson, AA, Ginovart, N, Goulding, V, Hussey, D, Hood, K, and Houle, S (2001) Occupancy of serotonin transporters by paroxetine and citalopram during treatment of depression: A [(11)C] DASB PET imaging study, *Am J Psychiatry* 158(11):1843–1849.

Nemeroff, CB, Krishnan, KRR, Reed, D, et al. (1992) Adrenal gland enlargement in major depression: a computed tomographic study, *Arch Gen Psychiatry* 49:384–387.

Nobler, MS, Roose, S, Prohovnik, I, Moeller, JR, Louie, J, Van Heertum, RL, and Sackeim, HA (2000) Regional cerebral blood flow in mood disorders, V. Effects of antidepressant medication in late-life depression, *Am J Geriatr Psychiatry* 8:289–296.

Nobler, MS, Oquendo, MA, Kegeles, LS, Malone, KM, Campbell, C, Sackeim, HA, and Mann, JJ (2001) Decreased regional brain metabolism after ECT, *Am J Psychiatry* 158:305–308.

Öngür, D, Drevets, WC, and Price, JL (1998) Glial reduction in the subgenual prefrontal cortex in mood disorders, *Proc Nat Acad Sc* 95:13290–13295.

Pearlson, GD, et al. (1995) In vivo D2 dopamine receptor density in psychotic and nonpsychotic patients with bipolar disorder, *Arch Gen Psychiatry* 52:471–477.

Petersen SE, et al. (1989) Positron emission tomographic studies of the processing of single words, *J Cogn Neurosci* 1:153–170.

Peterson, B, et al. (1993) Reduced basal ganglia volumes in Tourette's syndrome using three-dimensional reconstruction techniques from magnetic resonance images, *Neurology* 43:941–949.

Phillips, ML, Drevets, WC, Rauch, SL, and Lane, RD (2003) Neurobiology of emotion perception I: the neural basis of normal emotion perception, *Biol Psychiatry* 54:504–514.

Phillips, ML, Drevets, WC, Rauch, SL, and Lane, RD (2003) Neurobiology of emotion perception II: implications for major psychiatric disorders, *Biol Psychiatry* 54:515–528.

Rajkowska, G, Miguel-Hidalgo, JJ, Wei, J, Dilley, G, Pittman, SD, Meltzer, HY, Overholser, JC, Roth, BL, and Stockmeier, CA (1999) Morphometric evidence for neuronal and glial prefrontal cell pathology in major depression, *Biol Psychiatry* 45(9):1085–1098.

Rauch, SL, Savage, CR, Alpert, NM, Fischman, AJ, and Jenike, MA (1997) The functional neuroanatomy of anxiety: A study of three disorders using positron emission tomography and symptom provocation, *Biol Psychiatry* 42:446–452.

Rauch, SL, Whalen, PJ, Shin, LM, McInerney, Macklin, ML, Lasko, NB, Orr, SP, and Pitman, RK (2000) Exaggerated amygdala response to masked facial stimuli in posttraumatic stress disorder: a functional MRI study, *Biol Psychiatry* 47:769–776.

Rauch, SL, Jenike, MA, Alpert, NM, Baer, L, Breiter, H, Savage, CR, and Fischman, AJ (1994) Regional cerebral blood flow measured during symptom provocation in obsessive-compulsive disorder using oxygen 15-labeled carbon dioxide and positron emission tomography, *Arch Gen Psychiatry* 51:62–70.

Reiman, EM, et al. (1989) Neuroanatomical correlates of a lactate-induced anxiety attack, *Arch Gen Psychiatry* 46:493–500.

Schwartz, JM, et al. (1987) The differential diagnosis of depression: relevance of positron emission tomography studies of cerebral glucose metabolism to the bipolar-unipolar dichotomy, *JAMA* 258:1368–1373.

Semrud-Clikeman, M, et al. (1994) Attention-deficit hyperactivity disorder: Magnetic resonance imaging morphometric analysis of the corpus callosum, *J Am Acad Child Adolesc Psychiatry* 33:875–881.

Sheline, YI, Sanghavi, M, Mintun, MA, and Gado, M (1999) Depression duration but not age predicts hippocampal volume loss in medically healthy women with recurrent major depression, *J Neurosci* 19:5034–5043.

Sheline, YI, Gado, MH, and Price, JL (1998) Amygdala core nuclei volumes are decreased in recurrent major depression, *Neuroreport* 9(9):2023–2028.

Shenton, ME, et al. (1992) Abnormalities of the left temporal lobe and thought disorder in schizophrenia, *New Eng J Med* 327:604–612.

Shenton, ME, Dickey, CC, Frumin, M, and McCarley, RW (2001) A review of MRI findings in schizophrenia, *Schizophrenia Research* 49:1–52.

Sheppard, G, et al. (1983) ^{15}O-Positron emission tomographic scanning in predominantly never-treated acute schizophrenic patients, *Lancet* 322:1448–1452.

Shergill, SS, Brammer, MJ, Fukuda, R, Williams, SC, Murray, RM, and McGuire, PK (2003) Engagement of brain areas implicated in processing inner speech in people with auditory hallucinations, *Br J Psychiatry* 182:525–531.

Shin, LM, McNally, RJ, Kosslyn, SM, Thompson, WL, Rauch, SL, Alpert, NM, Metzger, LJ, Lasko, NB, Orr, SP, and Pitman, RK (1999) Regional cerebral blood flow during script-driven imagery in childhood sexual abuse-related PTSD: A PET investigation, *Am J Psychiatry* 156(4):575–584.

Siegle, GJ, Steinhauer, SR, Thase, ME, Stenger, VA, and Carter, CC (2002) Can't shake that feeling: event-related fMRI assessment of sustained amygdala activity in response to emotional information in depressed individuals, *Biol Psychiatry* 51:693–707.

Singer, HS, et al. (1992) Volumetric MRI changes in basal ganglia of children with Tourette's syndrome, *Neurology* 43:950–956.

Soares, JC and Innis, RB (1999) Neurochemical brain imaging investigations of schizophrenia, *Biol Psychiatry* 46:600–615.

Starkstein, SE and Robinson, RG (1989) Affective disorders and cerebral vascular disease, *Br J Psychiatry* 154:170–182.

Suddath, R, et al. (1990) Anatomical abnormalities in the brains of monozygotic twins discordant for schizophrenia, *New Eng J Med* 322:789–794.

Suhara, T, Nakayama, K, Inoue, O, Fukuda, H, Shimizu, M, Mori, A, and Tateno, Y (1992) D1 dopamine receptor binding in mood disorders measured by PET, *Psychopharmacology* 106:14–18.

Swedo, SE, et al. (1989) Cerebral glucose metabolism in childhood-onset obsessive-compulsive disorder, *Arch Gen Psychiatry* 46:518–523.

Tamminga, CA, et al. (1992) Limbic system abnormalities identified in schizophrenia using positron emission tomography with fluorodeoxyglucose and neocortical alterations with deficit syndrome, *Arch Gen Psychiatry* 49:522–530.

Thomas, KM, Drevets, WC, Dahl, RE, Ryan, ND, Birmaher, B, Eccard, CH, Axelson, D, Whalen, PJ, and Casey, BJ (2001) Abnormal amygdala response to faces in anxious and depressed children, *Arch Gen Psychiatry* 58:1057–1063.

Volkow, ND, et al. (1990) Effects of chronic cocaine abuse on postsynaptic dopamine receptors, *Am J Psychiatry* 147:719–724.

Volkow, ND, Fowler, JS, Wolf, AP, Hitzemann, R, Dewey, S, Bendriem, B, Alpert, R, and Hoff, A (1991) Changes in brain glucose metabolism in cocaine dependence and withdrawal, *Am J Psychiatry* 148:621–626.

Vythilingam, M, Shen, J, Drevets, WC, and Innis, R: Nuclear magnetic resonance imaging: basic principles and exemplary findings in neuropsychiatric disorders, in *Kaplan and Sadock's Comprehensive Textbook of Psychiatry* (in press) 8th Edition, Baltimore, MD, Lippincott, Williams & Wilkins, Inc.

Weinberger, DR, et al. (1986) Physiologic dysfunction of dorsolateral prefrontal cortex in schizophrenia. I. Regional cerebral blood flow evidence, *Arch Gen Psychiatry* 43:114–124.

Wong, DF, et al. (1986) Positron emission tomography reveals elevated D2 dopamine receptors in drug-naive schizophrenics, *Science* 234:1558–1563.

Wu, JC, et al. (1992) Effect of sleep deprivation on brain metabolism of depressed patients, *Am J Psychiatry* 149:538–543.

Zakzanis, KK and Heinrichs, RW (1999) Schizophrenia and the frontal brain: a quantitative review, *J Int Neuropsychol Soc* 5:556–566.

Chapter 7

Benner, DG (2003) *Strategic Pastoral Counseling: A Short Term Structured Model*, 2nd Edition, Grand Rapids, Baker Academic.

Crum, RM, Cooper-Patrick, L, and Ford, DE (1994) Depressive symptoms among general medical patients: prevalence and one-year outcome, *Psychosom Med* 56:109–117.

Depression Guideline Panel (1993) *Clinical Practice Guideline No 5: depression in primary care*, vol 1: *Detection and diagnosis*, vol 2: *Treatment of major depression*, Agency for Health Care Policy and Research Publication 93–0551, Rockville, Md., U.S. Department of Health and Human Services, Public Health Service.

Faiver, C, Eisengart, S, and Colonna, R (2004) *The Counselor Intern's Handbook*, 3rd Edition, Belmont, CA, Brooks/Cole.

Fortinash, KM and Holoday-Worret, PA (2003) *Psychiatric Mental Health Nursing*, 3rd Edition, St. Louis, Mosby.

Hirschfeld, RMA and Russell, JM (1997) Assessment and treatment of suicidal patients, *New Engl J Med* 337:910–915.

Jacobs, DG (ed.) (1999) *The Harvard Medical School Guide to Suicide Assessment and Intervention*, San Francisco, Jossey-Bass.

Katon, W, et al. (1994) Methodological issues in randomized trials of liaison psychiatry in primary care, *Psychosom Med* 56:97–103.

Keller, MB, et al. (2000) A comparison of nefazodone, the cognitive behavioral-analysis system of psychotherapy, and their combination for the treatment of chronic depression, *New Engl J Med* 342:1462–1470.

Keyes, D (1998) *Beyond Identity*, Carlisle, UK, Paternoster Press.

Lefley, HP and Wasow, M (eds) (1994) *Helping Families Cope With Mental Illness*, Langhorne, Penn., Harwood Academic Publishers.

Mueser, KT and Gingerich, S (1994) *Coping With Schizophrenia*, Oakland, Calif., New Harbinger Publications.

Petrakis, IL, Gonzalez, G, Rosenheck, R, and Krystal, JH (2002) Comorbidity of Alcoholism and Psychiatric Disorders: An Overview, *Alcohol Research and Health*, vol. 26, no 2.

Regier, DA, Goldberg, ID, and Taube, CH (1988) The de facto U.S. mental health service system, *Arch Gen Psychiatry* 45:977–986.

Robins, LN and Regier, DA (eds) (1991) *Psychiatric Disorders in America*, New York, The Free Press.

Smith, MD, Hong, BA, and Robson, AM (1985) Diagnosis of depression in patients with end-stage renal disease, *Am J Med* 79:160–166.

Wise, MG and Rundell, JR (2002) *Textbook of Consultation-Liaison Psychiatry*, 2nd Edition, Washington, DC, American Psychiatric Publishing.

Whooley, MA and Simon, GE (2000) Managing depression in medical outpatients, *New Engl J Med* 343:1942–1950.

Chapter 8

American Psychiatric Association (2000) *Diagnostic and Statistical Manual of Mental Disorders, 4th Edition, Text Revision* (DSM-IV-TR). Washington, D.C., American Psychiatric Association.

Anderson, IM (2000) Selective serotonin reuptake inhibitors versus tricyclic antidepressants: a meta-analysis of efficacy and tolerability, *J Affect Disord* 58(1):19–36.

Babyak, M, Blumenthal, JA, Herman, S, Khatri, P, Doraiswamy, M, Moore, K, Craighead, WE, Baldewicz, TT, and Krishnan, KR (2000) Exercise treatment for major depression: maintenance of therapeutic benefit at 10 months, *Psychosomatic Medicine* 62(5):633–638.

Bauer, MS (2001) An evidence-based review of psychosocial treatments for bipolar disorder, *Psychopharmacol Bull* 35(3):109–134.

Bowden, CL, Brugger, AM, Swann, AC, Calabrese, JR, Janicak, PG, Petty, F, Dilsaver, SC, Davis, JM, Rush, AJ, Small, JG, et al. (1994) Efficacy of divalproex vs lithium and placebo in the treatment of mania, The Depakote Mania Study Group, *JAMA* 271:918–924.

Bradwejn, J, Shriqui, C, Koszycki, D, and Meterissian, G (1990) Double blind comparison of the effects of clonazepam and lorazepam in acute mania, *J Clin Psychopharmacol* 10:403–408.

Caspi, A, Sugden, K, Moffitt, TE, Taylor, A, Craig, IW, Harrington, H, McClay, J, Mill, J, Martin, J, Braithwaite, A, and Poulton, R (2003) Influence of life stress on depression: moderation by a polymorphism in the 5-HTT gene, *Science* 301(5631):291–293.

Charney, DS, Reynolds, CF 3rd, Lewis, L, Lebowitz, BD, Sunderland, T, Alexopoulos, GS, Blazer, DG, Katz, IR, Meyers, BS, Arean, PA, Borson, S, Brown, C, Bruce, ML, Callahan, CM, Charlson, ME, Conwell, Y, Cuthbert, BN, Devanand, DP, Gibson, MJ, Gottlieb, GL, Krishnan, KR, Laden, SK, Lyketsos, CG, Mulsant, BH, Niederehe, G, Olin, JT, Oslin, DW, Pearson, J, Persky, T, Pollock, BG, Raetzman, S, Reynolds, M, Salzman, C, Schulz, R, Schwenk, TL, Scolnick, E, Unutzer, J, Weissman, MM, and Young, RC (2003) Depression and Bipolar Support Alliance consensus statement on the unmet needs in diagnosis and treatment of mood disorders in late life, *Arch Gen Psychiatry* 60(7):664–672.

Cole, MG, Bellavance, F, and Mansour, A (1999) Prognosis of depression in elderly community and primary care populations: a systematic review and meta-analysis, *Am J Psychiatry* 156(8):1182–1189.

Coryell, W, Scheftner, W, Keller, M, Endicott, J, Maser, J, and Klerman, GL (1993) The enduring psychosocial consequences of mania and depression, *Am J Psychiatry* 150:720–727.

Drevets, WC, Videen, TO, Price, JL, Preskorn, SH, Carmichael, ST, and Raichle, ME (1992) A functional anatomical study of unipolar depression, *J Neuroscience* 12:3628–3641.

Drevets, WC, Price, JL, Simpson, JR, Todd, RD, Reich, T, Vannier, M, and Raichle, ME (1997) Subgenual prefrontal cortex abnormalities in mood disorders, *Nature* 386:824–827.

Drevets, WC, Frank, E, Price, JC, Kupfer, DJ, Holt, D, Greer, PJ, Huang, H, Gautier, C, and Mathis, C (1999) PET imaging of serotonin 1A receptor binding in depression, *Biol Psychiatry* 46(10):1375–1387.

Drevets, WC, Gadde, K, and Krishnan, R: Neuroimaging Studies of Depression, in Charney, DS, Nestler, EJ, and Bunney, BJ (eds) (in press) *The Neurobiological Foundation of Mental Illness*, 2nd Edition, New York, Oxford University Press.

Dubovsky, SL (2001) Rapid cycling bipolar disease: new concepts and treatments, *Curr Psychiatry Rep* 3(6):451–462.

Folstein, SE, Peyser, CE, Starkstein, SE, and Folstein, MF: Subcortical triad of Huntington's Disease: a model for a neuropathology of depression, dementia, and dyskinesia, in Carroll, BJ and Barrett, JE (eds) (1991) *Psychopathology and the Brain*, pp 65–75, New York, Raven Press, Ltd.

Frank, E and Thase, ME (1999) Natural history and preventative treatment of recurrent mood disorders, *Annu Rev Med* 50:453–468.

Gloaguen, V, Cottraux, J, Cucherat, M, and Blackburn, IM (1998) A meta-analysis of the effects of cognitive therapy in depressed patients, *J Affect Disord* 49(1):59–72.

Gold, PW, Drevets, WC, and Charney, DS (2002) New insights into the role of cortisol and the glucocorticoid receptor in severe depression, *Biol Psychiatry* 52(5):381–385.

Kathol, RG, Mutgi, A, Williams, J, Clamon, G, and Noyes, R (1990) Diagnosis of major depression in cancer patients according to four sets of criteria, *Am J Psychiatry* 147:1021–1024.

Keck, PE Jr, Mendlwicz, J, Calabrese, JR, Fawcett, J, Suppes, T, Vestergaard, PA, and Carbonell, C (2000) A review of randomized, controlled clinical trials in acute mania, *J Affect Disord* 59(Suppl 1):S31–S37.

Keller, MB, McCullough, JP, Klein, DN, Arnow, B, Dunner, DL, Gelenberg, AJ, Markowitz, JC, Nemeroff, CB, Russell, JM, Thase, ME, Trivedi, MH, and Zajecka, J (2000) A comparison of nefazodone, the cognitive behavioral-analysis system of psychotherapy, and their combination for the treatment of chronic depression, *N Engl J Med* 342(20):1462–1470.

Kupfer, DJ, Frank, E, Perel, JM, Cornes, C, Mallinger, AG, Thase, ME, McEachran, AB, and Grochocinski, VJ (1992) Five-year outcome for maintenance therapies in recurrent depression, *Arch Gen Psychiatry* 49(10):769–773.

Manji, HK and Zarate, CA (2002) Molecular and cellular mechanisms underlying mood stabilization in bipolar disorder: implications for the development of improved therapeutics, *Mol Psychiatry* 7(Suppl 1):S1–S7.

Manji, H, Drevets, WC, and Charney, D (2001) The cellular neurobiology of depression, *Nat Med* 7(5):541–547.

McHugh, PR (1989) The neuropsychiatry of basal ganglia disorders, *Neuropsych Neuropsychol Behav Neurol* 2:239–247.

Miller, NA and Gold, MS (1991) Abuse, addiction, tolerance and dependence to benzodiazepines in medical and nonmedical populations, *Am J Drug Alcohol Abuse* 17:27–37.

Mukherjee, S, Sackeim, HA, and Schnur, DB (1994) Electroconvulsive therapy of acute manic episodes: a review, *Am J Psychiatry* 151:169–176.

Müller-Oerlinghausen, B, Ahrens, B, Grof, E, Grof, P, Lenz, G, Schou, M, Simhandl, C, Thau, K, Volk, J, Wolf, R, et al. (1992) The effect of long-term lithium treatment on the mortality of patients with manic-depressive and schizoaffective illness, *Acta Psychiatr Scand* 86:218–222.

Müller-Oerlinghausen, B, Muser-Causemann, B, and Volk, J (1992) Suicides and parasuicides in a high risk patient group on and off lithium long-term medication, *J Affect Disord* 25:261–269.

Musselman, DL and Nemeroff, CB (1993) The role of corticotropin-releasing factor in the pathophysiology of psychiatric disorders, *Psychiatric Annals* 23:676–681.

Öngür, D, Drevets, WC, and Price, JL (1998) Glial reduction in the subgenual prefrontal cortex in mood disorders. *Proc Natl Acad Sci USA* 95:13290–13295.

Peet, M (1994) Induction of mania with selective serotonin reuptake inhibitors and tricyclic antidepresssants, *Br J Psychiatry* 164:549–550.

Post, RM (1992) Transduction of psychosocial stress into the neurobiology of recurrent affective disorder, *Am J Psychiatry* 149:999–1010.

Price, JL, Carmichael, ST, and Drevets, WC (1996) Networks related to the orbital and medial prefrontal cortex: a substrate for emotional behavior? *Prog Brain Res* 107:523–36.

Rice, J, Reich, T, Andreasen, N, Endicott, J, VanEerdewegh, M, Fishman, R, Herschfeld, R, and Klearman, G (1987) The familial transmission of bipolar illness, *Arch Gen Psychiatry* 44:441–447.

Robins, LN, Helzer, JE, Weissman, MM, Orvaschel, H, Gruenberg, E, Burke, JD Jr, and Regier, DA (1984) Lifetime prevalence of specific psychiatric disorders in three sites, *Arch Gen Psychiatry* 41:949–958.

Robinson, RG (2003) Poststroke depression: prevalence, diagnosis, treatment, and disease progression, *Biol Psychiatry* 54(3):376–387.

Roose, SP, Glassman, AH, Attia, E, and Woodring, S (1994) Comparative efficacy of selective serotonin reuptake inhibitors and tricyclics in the treatment of melancholia, *Am J Psychiatry* 151:1735–1739.

Sachs, GS, Thase, ME, Otto, MW, Bauer, M, Miklowitz, D, Wisniewski, SR, Lavori, P, Lebowitz, B, Rudorfer, M, Frank, E, Nierenberg, AA, Fava, M, Bowden, C, Ketter, T, Marangell, L, Calabrese, J, Kupfer, D, and Rosenbaum, JF (2003) Rationale, design, and methods of the systematic treatment enhancement program for bipolar disorder (STEP-BD), *Biol Psychiatry* 53(11):1028–1042.

Sackeim, HA, Prudic, J, Devanand, DP, Nobler, MS, Lisanby, SH, Peyser, S, Fitzsimons, L, Moody, BJ, and Clark, J (2000) A prospective, randomized, double-blind comparison of bilateral and right unilateral electroconvulsive therapy at different stimulus intensities, *Arch Gen Psychiatry* 57(5):425–434.

Schou, M (1988) Effects of long-term lithium treatment on kidney function: an overview, *J Psychiatry Res* 22:287–296.

Starkman, MN and Schteingart, DE (1981) Neuropsychiatric manifestations of patients with Cushing's Syndrome. Relationship to cortisol and adrenocorticotropic hormone levels, *Arch Intern Med* 141:215–219.

Starkstein, SE, Fedoroff, P, Berthier, ML, and Robinson, RG (1991) Manic-depressive and pure manic states after brain lesions, *Biol Psychiatry* 29:149–158.

Suppes, T, Baldessarini, RJ, Faedda, GL, and Tohen, M (1991) Risk of recurrence following discontinuation of lithium treatment in bipolar disorder, *Arch Gen Psychiatry* 48:1082–1088.

Taylor-Tavares, J, Drevets, WC, and Sahakian, BS (2003) Cognition in mania and depression, *Psychol Med* 33:959–967.

Thase, ME, Greenhouse, JB, Frank, E, Reynolds, CF 3rd, Pilkonis, PA, Hurley, K, Grochocinski, V, and Kupfer, DJ (1997) Treatment of major depression with psychotherapy or psychotherapy-pharmacotherapy combinations, *Arch Gen Psychiatry* 54(11):1009–1015.

Thase, ME, Simons, A, and Reynolds, C (1993) Psychobiological correlates of poor response to cognitive behavior therapy: potential indications for antidepressant pharmacotherapy, *Psychopharmacol Bull* 29:293–301.

Weissman, MM, Leaf, PJ, Tischler, GL, Blazer, DG, Karno, M, Bruce, ML, and Florio, LP (1988) Affective disorders in five United States communities, *Psychol Med* 18:141–153.

Winokur, G (1982) The development and validity of familial subtypes in primary unipolar depression, *Pharmacopsychiatr* 15:142–146.

Wisner, KL, Gelenberg, AJ, Leonard, H, Zarin, D, and Frank, E (1999) Pharmacologic treatment of depression during pregnancy, *JAMA* 282(13):1264–1269.

Chapter 9

Allgulander, C, et al. (2003) WCA recommendations for the long-term treatment of generalized anxiety disorder, *CNS Spectr* 8(8 Suppl 1):53–61.

American Psychiatric Association (1998) Practice Guideline for the treatment of patients with panic disorder, Work Group on Panic Disorder, *Am J Psychiatry* 155(5S):1–34.

Ballenger, JC, et al. (1998) Consensus statement on social anxiety disorder from the International Consensus Group on Depression and Anxiety, *J Clin Psychiatry* 59(17S):54–60.

Ballenger, JC, et al. (2001) Consensus statement on generalized anxiety disorder from the International Consensus Group on Depression and Anxiety, *J Clin Psychiatry* 62(11S):53–58.

Brown, TA, et al. (1994) The empirical basis of generalized anxiety disorder (Review), *Am J Psychiatry* 151(9):1272–1280.

Davidson, JR (2004) Use of benzodiazepines in social anxiety disorder, generalized anxiety disorder, and post-traumatic stress disorder, *J Clin Psychiatry* 65(5S):29–33.

Eaton, WW, et al. (1994) Panic and panic disorder in the United States, *Am J Psychiatry* 151(3):413–420.

Fyer, AJ, et al. (1993) A direct interview family study of social phobia, *Arch Gen Psychiatry* 50(4):286–293.

Gelernter, CS, et al. (1991) Cognitive-behavioral and pharmacological treatments of social phobia. A controlled study, *Arch Gen Psychiatry* 48(10):938–945.

Greenberg, PE, et al. (1999) The economic burden of anxiety disorders in the 1990s, *J Clin Psychiatry* 60(7):427–435.

Hettema, JM, et al. (2001) A review and meta-analysis of the genetic epidemiology of anxiety disorders, *Am J Psychiatry* 158(10):1568–1578.

Hettema, JM, et al. (2001) A population-based twin study of generalized anxiety disorder in men and women, *J Nerv Ment Dis* 189(7):413–420.

Kendler, KS, et al. (2003) The structure of genetic and environmental risk factors for common psychiatric and substance use disorders in men and women, *Arch Gen Psychiatry* 60(9):929–937.

Kessler, RC, et al. (1994) Lifetime and 12-month prevalence of DSM-III-R psychiatric disorders in the United States, *Arch Gen Psychiatry* 51:8–19.

Kessler, RC, et al. (1999) Lifetime co-morbidities between social phobia and mood disorders in the US National Comorbidity Survey, *Psychol Med* 29(3):555–567.

Magee, WJ, et al. (1996) Agoraphobia, simple phobia, and social phobia in the National Comorbity Survey, *Arch Gen Pyschiatry* 53(2):159–168.

Nagy, LM, et al. (1989) Clinical and medication outcome after short-term alprazolam and behavioral group treatment in panic disorder: 2.5 year naturalistic follow-up study, *Arch Gen Psychiatry* 46(11):993–999.

Nemeroff, CB (2003) The role of GABA in the pathophysiology and treatment of anxiety disorders, *Psychopharmacol Bull* 37(4):133–146.

Noyes, R Jr, et al. (1990) Outcome of panic disorder. Relationship to diagnostic subtypes and comorbidity, *Arch Gen Psychiatry* 47(9):809–818.

Pande, AC, et al. (2004) Efficacy of the novel anxiolytic pregabalin in social anxiety disorder: a placebo-controlled, multicenter study, *J Clin Psychopharmacol* 24(2):141–149.

Pollack, MH, et al. (2003) WCA recommendations for the long-term treatment of panic disorder, *CNS Spectr* 8(8 Suppl 1):17–30.

Regier, DA, et al. (1990) Comorbidity of mental disorders with alcohol and other drug abuse, *JAMA* 264(19):2511–2518.

Roy-Bryne, PP, et al. (2000) Lifetime panic-depression comorbidity in the National Comorbidity Survey. Association with symptoms, impairment, course and help-seeking, *Br J Psychiatry* 176:229–235.

Schneier, FR, et al. (1992) Social phobia. Comorbidity and morbidity in an epidemiologic sample, *Arch Gen Psychiatry* 49(4):282–288.

Weissman, MM, et al. (1989) Suicidal ideation and suicide attempts in panic disorder and attacks, *N Engl J Med* 321(18):1209–1214.

Wittchen, HU, et al. (1994) DSM-III-R generalized anxiety disorder in the National Comorbidity Survey, *Arch Gen Psychiatry* 51(5):355–364.

Chapter 10

Ackerman, DL and Greenland, S (2002) Multivariate meta-analysis of controlled drug studies for obsessive-compulsive disorder, *J Clin Psychopharmacol* 22:309–317.

American Psychiatric Association (2000) *Diagnostic and Statistical Manual of Mental Disorders*, 4th Edition, Text Revision. Washington, D.C., American Psychiatric Association Press.

Baer, L, Rauch, SL, Ballantine, H, et al. (1995) Cingulotomy for intractable obsessive-compulsive disorder: prospective long-term follow-up of 18 patients, *Arch Gen Psychiatry* 52:384–392.

Baxter, LR, et al. (1988) Cerebral glucose metabolic rates in non-depressed patients with obsessive-compulsive disorder, *Am J Psychiatry* 145:1560–1563.

Baxter, LR, et al. (1992) Caudate glucose metabolic rate changes with both drug and behavior therapy for obsessive-compulsive disorder, *Arch Gen Psychiatry* 49:681–689.

Bellodi, L, et al. (1992) Psychiatric disorders in the families of patients with obsessive-compulsive disorder, *Psychiatry Res* 42:111–120.

Berrios, GE (1989) Obsessive-compulsive disorder: Its conceptual history in France during the 19th century, *Compr Psychiatry* 30:283–295.

Black, DW, et al. (1992) A family study of obsessive-compulsive disorder, *Arch Gen Psychiatry* 49:362–368.

Bogetto, F, et al. (2000) Olanzapine augmentation of fluvoxamine-refractory obsessive-compulsive disorder (OCD): a 12-week open trial, *Psychiatry Res* 96:91–98.

Clomipramine Collaborative Study Group (1991) Clomipramine in the treatment of patients with obsessive-compulsive disorder, *Arch Gen Psychiatry* 48:730–738.

Cummings, JL and Cunningham, K (1992) Obsessive-compulsive disorder in Huntington's disease, *Biol Psychiatry* 31:263–270.

Denys, D, van Megen, H, and Westenberg, H (2002) Quetiapine addition to serotonin reuptake inhibitor treatment in patients with treatment-refractory obsessive-compulsive disorder: an open-label study, *J Clin Psychiatry* 63:700–703.

Dunner, DL (2001) Management of anxiety disorders: the added challenge of comorbidity, *Depress Anxiety* 13:57–71.

Foa, EB, et al. (1995) DSM-IV Field Trial: Obsessive-compulsive disorder, *Am J Psychiatry* 152:90–96.

Garvey, MA, Perlmutter, SJ, Allen, AJ, et al. (1999) A pilot study of penicillin prophylaxis for neuropsychiatric exacerbations triggered by streptococcal infections, *Biol Psychiatry* 45:1564–1571.

Giedd, JN, Rapoport, JL, Leonard, HL, et al. (1996) Case study: acute basal ganglia enlargement and obsessive-compulsive symptoms in an adolescent boy, *J Am Acad Child Adolesc Psychiatry* 35:913–915.

Giedd, JN, Rapoport, JL, Garvey, MA, et al. (2000) MRI assessment of children with obsessive-compulsive disorder or tics associated with streptococcal infection, *Am J Psychiatry* 157:281–283.

Gilbert, AR, Moore, GJ, Keshavan, MS, et al. (2000) Decrease in thalamic volumes of pediatric patients with obsessive-compulsive disorder who are taking paroxetine, *Arch Gen Psychiatry* 57:449–456.

Goodman, WK, et al. (1989) The Yale-Brown Obsessive Compulsive Scale, *Arch Gen Psychiatry* 46:1012–1016.

Goodman, WK, et al. (1996) Treatment of obsessive compulsive disorder with fluvoxamine: a multicentre, double-blind, placebo-controlled trial, *Int Clin Psychopharmacol* 11:21–29.

Goodwin, DW, Guze, SB, and Robins, E (1969) Follow-up studies in obsessional neurosis, *Arch Gen Psychiatry* 20:182–187.

Grabe, HJ, Meyer, C, Hapke, U, et al. (2001) Lifetime-comorbidity of obsessive-compulsive disorder and subclinical obsessive-compulsive disorder in northern Germany, *Eur Arch Pyschiatry Clin Neurosci* 251:130–135.

Greist JH, et al. (1995) Efficacy and tolerability of serotonin transport inhibitors in obsessive-compulsive disorder, *Arch Gen Psychiatry* 52:53–60.

Greist, J, Chouinard, G, DuBoff, E, et al. (1995) Double-blind parallel comparison of three dosages of sertraline and placebo in outpatients with obsessive-compulsive disorder, *Arch Gen Psychiatry* 52:289–295.

Hanna, GL, Veenstra-VanderWeele, J, Cox, NJ, et al. (2002) Genome-wide linkage analysis of families with obsessive-compulsive disorder ascertained through pediatric probands, *Am J Med Genet* 114:541–552.

Hembree, EA, Riggs, DS, Kozak, MJ, et al. (2003) Long-term efficacy of exposure and ritual prevention therapy and serotonergic medications for obsessive-compulsive disorder, *CNS Spectrums* 8:363–371, 381.

Himle, JA, Rassi, S, Haghighatgou, H, et al. (2001) Group behavioral therapy of obsessive-compulsive disorder: seven vs. twelve-week outcomes, *Depress Anxiety* 13:161–165.

Hohagen, F, Winkelmann, G, Rasche-Rauchle, H, et al. (1998) Combination of behaviour therapy with fluvoxamine in comparison with behaviour therapy and placebo: results of a multicentre study, *Br J Psychiatry* 173(35S):71–78.

Hollander, E, Bienstock, CA, Koran, LM, et al. (2002) Refractory obsessive-compulsive disorder: state-of-the-art treatment, *J Clin Psychiatry* 63(suppl 6):20–29.

Hudziak, JJ, van Beijsterveldt, CE, Althoff, RR, et al. (2004) Genetic and environmental contributions to the child behavior checklist obsessive-compulsive scale: a cross-cultural twin study, *Arch Gen Psychiatry* 61:608–16.

Jenike, MA, et al. (1991) Cingulotomy for refractory obsessive-compulsive disorder, *Arch Gen Psychiatry* 48:548–555.

Jonnal, AH, Gardner, CO, Prescott, CA, and Kendler, KS (2000) Obsessive and compulsive symptoms in a general population sample of female twins, *Am J Med Genet* 96:791–796.

Kampman, M, Keijsers, GPJ, Hoogduin, CAL, and Verbraak, MJPM (2002) Addition of cognitive-behaviour therapy for obsessive-compulsive disorder patients non-responding to fluoxetine, *Acta Psychiatr Scand* 106:314–319.

Koran, LM, McElroy, SL, Davidson, JRT, et al. (1996) Fluvoxamine versus clomipramine for obsessive-compulsive disorder: a double-blind comparison, *J Clin Psychopharmacol* 16:121–129.

Laplane, D, et al. (1989) Obsessive-compulsive and other behavioral changes with bilateral basal ganglia lesions: A neuropsychological, magnetic resonance imaging and positron tomography study, *Brain* 112:699–725.

Leonard, HL, et al. (1989) Treatment of obsessive-compulsive disorder with clomipramine and desipramine in children and adolescents: A double-blind crossover comparison, *Arch Gen Psychiatry* 46:1088–1092.

Lougee, L, Perlmutter, SJ, Nicolson, R, et al. (2000) Psychiatric disorders in first-degree relatives of children with pediatric autoimmune neuropsychiatric disorders associated with streptococcal infections (PANDAS), *J Am Acad Child Adolesc Psychiatry* 39:1120–1126.

Marks, IM, Baer, L, Greist, JH, et al. (1998) Home self-assessment of obsessive-compulsive disorder. Use of a manual and a computer-conducted telephone interview: two UK-US studies, *Br J Psychiatry* 172:406–412.

Mathew, SJ, Coplan, JD, Perko, KA, et al. (2001) Neuroendocrine predictors of response to intravenous clomipramine therapy for refractory obsessive-compulsive disorder, *Depress Anxiety* 14:199–208.

Mavissakalian, MR, Jones, B, and Olson, S (1990) Absence of placebo response in obsessive-compulsive disorder, *J Nerv Men Dis* 178:268–270.

McGuire, PK, et al. (1994) Functional anatomy of obsessive-compulsive phenomena, *Br J Psychiatry* 164:459–468.

McDougle, CJ, Epperson, CN, Pelton, GH, et al. (2000) A double-blind, placebo-controlled study of risperidone addition in serotonin reuptake inhibitor-refractory obsessive-compulsive disorder, *Arch Gen Psychiatry* 57:794–801.

Milos, G, Spindler, A, Ruggiero, G, et al. (2002) Comorbidity of obsessive-compulsive disorders and duration of eating disorders, *Int J Eat Disord* 31:284–289.

Mindus, P and Nyman, H (1991) Normalization of personality characteristics in patients with incapacitating anxiety disorders after capsulotomy, *Acta Psychiatr Scand* 83:283–291.

Montgomery, SA, Kasper, S, Stein, DJ, et al. (2001) Citalopram 20 mg, 40 mg and 60 mg are all effective and well tolerated compared with placebo in obsessive-compulsive disorder, *Int Clin Pharmaco* 16:75–86.

Murphy, ML and Pichichero, ME (2002) Prospective identification and treatment of children with pediatric autoimmune neuropsychiatric disorder associated with group A streptococcal infection (PANDAS), *Arch Pediatr Adolesc Med* 156:356–361.

Nestadt, G, Samuels, J, Riddle, M, et al. (2000) A family study of obsessive-compulsive disorder, *Arch Gen Psychiatry* 57:358–363.

Nestadt, G, Samuels, J, Riddle, MA, et al. (2001) The relationship between obsessive-compulsive disorder and anxiety and affective disorders: results from the Johns Hopkins OCD family study, *Psychol Med* 31:481–487.

Neziroglu, F, Yaryura-Tobias, JA, Walz, J, and McKay, D (2000) The effect of fluvoxamine and behavior therapy on children and adolescents with obsessive-compulsive disorder, *J Child Adolesc Psychopharmacol* 10:295–306.

Nuttin, BJ, Gabriels, LA, Cosyns, PR, et al. (2003) Long-term electrical capsular stimulation in patients with obsessive-compulsive disorder, *Neurosurgery* 52:1263–1272.

Pallanti, S, Quercioli, L, and Koran, LM (2002) Citalopram intravenous infusion in resistant obsessive-compulsive disorder: an open trial, *J Clin Psychiatry* 63:796–801.

Pato, MT, et al. (1988) Return of symptoms after discontinuation of clomipramine in patients with obsessive-compulsive disorder, *Am J Psychiatry* 145:1521–1525.

Pauls, DL, et al. (1986) Gilles de la Tourette's syndrome and obsessive-compulsive disorder: Evidence supporting a genetic relationship, *Arch Gen Psychiatry* 43:1180–1182.

Perlmutter, SJ, Leitman, SF, Garvey, MA, et al. (1999) Therapeutic plasma exchange and intravenous immunoglobulin for obsessive-compulsive disorder and tic disorders in childhood, *Lancet* 354:1153–1158.

Perugi, G, Toni, C, Frare, F, et al. (2002) Obsessive-compulsive-bipolar comorbidity: a systematic exploration of clinical features and treatment outcome, *J Clin Psychiatry* 63:1129–1134.

Rasmussen, SA and Tsuang, MT (1986) DSM-III obsessive compulsive disorder: Clinical characteristics and family history, *Am J Psychiatry* 143:317–322.

Rauch, SL, et al. (1995) A positron emission tomography study of simple phobic symptom provocation, *Arch Gen Psychiatry* 52:20–28.

Rauch, SL, Dougherty, DD, Cosgrove, GR, et al. (2001) Cerebral metabolic correlates as potential predictors of response to anterior cingulotomy for obsessive compulsive disorder, *Biol Psychiatry* 50:659–667.

Rauch, SL, Shin, LM, Dougherty, DD, et al. (2002) Predictors of fluvoxamine response in contamination-related obsessive compulsive disorder: a PET symptom provocation study, *Neuropsychopharmacology* 27:782–791.

Ricciardi, JN, et al. (1992) Changes in DSM-III-R Axis II diagnoses following treatment of obsessive-compulsive disorder, *Am J Psychiatry* 149:829–831.

Riddle, MA, et al. (1990) Obsessive compulsive disorder in children and adolescents: Phenomenology and family history, *J Am Acad Child Adolesc Psychiatry* 29(5):766–772.

Robins, LN, et al. (1984) Lifetime prevalence of specific psychiatric disorders in three sites, *Arch Gen Psychiatry* 41:949–958.

Rosqvist, J, Thomas, JC, and Egan, D (2002) Home-based cognitive-behavioral treatment of chronic, refractory obsessive-compulsive disorder can be effective. Single case analysis of four patients, *Behav Modif* 26:205–222.

Saxena, S, Brody, AL, Ho, ML, et al. (2002) Differential cerebral metabolic changes with paroxetine treatment of obsessive-compulsive disorder vs major depression, *Arch Gen Psychiatry* 59:250–261.

Saxena, S, Brody, AL, Ho, ML, et al. (2003) Differential brain metabolic predictors of response to paroxetine in obsessive-compulsive disorder versus major depression, *Am J Psychiatry* 160:522–532.

Shapiro, AK and Shapiro, E (1992) Evaluation of the reported association of obsessive-compulsive symptoms or disorder with Tourette's disorder, *Compr Psychiatry* 33:152–165.

Swedo, SE, et al. (1992) Cerebral glucose metabolism in childhood-onset obsessive-compulsive disorder: Revisualization during pharmacotherapy, *Arch Gen Psychiatry* 49:690–694.

Swedo, SE, et al. (1989) High prevalence of obsessive-compulsive symptoms in patients with Sydenham's chorea, *Am J Psychiatry* 146:246–249.

Swedo, SE (2002) Pediatric autoimmune neuropsychiatric disorders associated with streptococcal infections (PANDAS), *Molecular Psychiatry* 7(suppl 2):S24–S25.

Tollefson, GD, et al. (1994) A multicenter investigation of fixed-dose fluoxetine in the treatment of obsessive-compulsive disorder, *Arch Gen Psychiatry* 51:559–567.

Van Balkom, AJLM, De Haan, E, Van Oppen, P, et al. (1998) Cognitive and behavioral therapies alone versus in combination with fluvoxamine in the treatment of obsessive compulsive disorder, *J Nerv Ment Dis* 186:492–499.

Chapter 11

Aggleton, JP and Saunders, RC (1997) The relationship between temporal lobe and diencephalic structures implicated in anterograde amnesia, *Memory* 5:49.

Alluisi, EA, et al. (1973) Behavioral effects of tularemia and sandfly fever in man, *J Infect Dis* 128:710.

Ammoni, JM, Beer, S, and Kesselring, J (1992) Severe traumatic brain injury: epidemiology and outcome after 3 years, *Disabil Rehabil* 14:23.

Blansjaar, BA, Horjus, MC, and Nijhuis, HGJ (1987) Prevalence of the Korsakoff syndrome in The Hague, The Netherlands, *Acta Psychiatr Scand* 75:604.

Block, SD (2001) Psychological considerations, growth, and transcendence at the end of life: the art of the possible, *JAMA* 285:2898.

Breitbart, W, et al. (1996) A double-blind trial of haloperidol, chlorpromazine and lorazepam in the treatment of delirium in hospitalized AIDS patients, *Am J Psychiatry* 153:231.

Brown, TM and Boyle, MF (2002) ABC of psychological medicine: delirium, *BMJ* 325:644.

Burns, A, Gallagley, A, and Byrne, J (2004) Delirium, *J Neurol Neurosurg Psychiatry* 75:362.

Butters, N, Delis, DC, and Lucas, JA (1995) Clinical assessment of memory disorders in amnesia and dementia, *Annu Rev Psychol* 46:493.

Centeno, C, Sanz, A, and Bruera, E (2004) Delirium in advanced cancer patients, *Palliative Medicine* 18:184.

Cole, MG, et al. (1994) Systematic intervention for elderly inpatients with delirium: a randomized trial, *CMAJ* 151:965.

Cole, MG, et al. (2002) Systematic detection and multidisciplinary care of delirium in older medical inpatients: a randomized trial, *Can Med Assoc J* 167:753.

Cole, MG, et al. (2002) Symptoms of delirium among elderly medical inpatients with or without dementia, *J Neuropsychiatry Clin Neurosci* 14:167.

Crammer, JL (2002) Subjective experience of a confusional state, *Br J Psychiatry* 180:71.

Ernst, E (2003) Serious psychiatric and neurological adverse effects of herbal medicines—a systematic review, *Acta Psychiatr Scand* 108:83.

Eustache, F, et al. (2000) Functional neuroanatomy of amnesia: positron emission tomography studies, *Microsc Res Tech* 51:94.

Fama, R, Marsh, L, and Sullivan, EV (2004) Dissociation of remote and anterograde memory impairment and neural correlates in alcoholic Korsakoff syndrome, *J Int Neuropsychol Soc* 10(3):427–441.

Fann, JR, et al. (2002) Delirium in patients undergoing hematopoietic stem cell transplantation: incidence and pretransplantation risk factors, *Cancer* 95:1971.

Fields, SD (2003) Review: delirium predicts 12-month mortality independent of dementia status, *ACP Journal Club* 139:80.

Fontaine, DK (1994) Nonpharmacologic management of patient distress during mechanical ventilation, *Crit Care Clin* 10:695.

Francis, J and Kapoor, WN (1992) Prognosis after hospital discharge of older medical patients with delirium, *J Am Geriatr Soc* 40:601.

Francis, J, Martin, D, and Kapoor, WN (1990) A prospective study of delirium in hospitalized elderly, *JAMA* 263:1097.

Gallassi, R, et al. (1993) Transient global amnesia: neuropsychological findings after single and multiple attacks, *Eur Neurol* 33:297.

Geijerstam, J-L and Britton, M (2003) Mild head injury—mortality and complication rate: meta-analysis of findings in a systematic literature review, *Acta Neurochir* 145:843.

Goldstein, LH, et al. (1992) The effect of anticonvulsants on cognitive functioning following a probable encephalitic illness, *Br J Psychiatry* 160:546.

Good, MI (1989) Substance-induced dissociative disorders and psychiatric nosology, *J Clin Psychopharmacol* 9:88.

Goodwin, DW (1995) Alcohol amnesia, *Addiction* 90:315.

Hanrahan, JP and Gordon, MA (1984) Mushroom poisoning: case reports and a review of therapy, *JAMA* 251:1057.

Harper, C, et al. (1988) The Wernicke-Korsakoff syndrome in Sydney: a prospective necropsy study, *Med J Aust* 149:718.

Harper, CG and Kril, JJ (1990) Neuropathology of alcoholism, *Alcohol Alcohol* 35:207.

Hodges, JR (1994) Semantic memory and frontal executive function during transient global amnesia, *J Neurol Neurosurg Psychiatry* 57:605.

Hodges, JR and Warlow, CP (1990) Syndromes of transient amnesia: towards a classification, *J Neurol Neurosurg Psychiatry* 53:834.

Hopkins, RO, et al. (1999) Neuropsychological sequelae and impaired health status in survivors of severe acute respiratory distress syndrome, *Am J Respir Crit Care Med* 160:50.

Inouye, SKS, et al. (1993) A predictive model for delirium in hospitalized elderly medical patients based on admission characteristics, *Ann Intern Med* 119:474.

Johnson, R and Gleave, J (1987) Counting the people disabled by head injury, *Injury* 18:7.

Kapur, N (1991) Amnesia in relation to fugue states: distinguishing a neurological from a psychogenic basis, *Br J Psychiatry* 159:872.

Kopelman, MD (1987) Amnesia: organic and psychogenic, *Br J Psychiatry* 150:428.

Kopelman, MD, et al. (2001) Structural MRI volumetric analysis in patients with organic amnesia, 2: correlations with anterograde memory and executive tests in 40 patients, *J Neurol Neurosurg Psychiatry* 71:23.

Koski, KJ and Marttila, RJ (1990) Transient global amnesia: incidence in an urban population, *Acta Neurol Scand* 81:358.

Lerner, DM and Rosenstein, DL (2000) Neuroimaging in delirium and related conditions, *Semin Clin Neuropsychiatry* 5:98.

Levine, RL (1994) Pharmacology of intravenous sedatives and opioids in critically ill patients, *Crit Care Clin* 10:709.

Lewis, SL (1998) Aetiology of transient global amnesia, *Lancet* 352:397.

Lindesay, J, Rockwood, K, and Macdonald, A (eds) (2002) *Delirium in Old Age*, Oxford, Oxford University Press.

Manworren, RGB, Paulos, CL, and Pop, R (2004) Treating children for acute agitation in the PACU: differentiating pain and emergence delirium, *J Perianesth Nurs* 19:183.

Marcantonio, ER, et al. (1994) A clinical prediction rule for delirium after elective noncardiac surgery, *JAMA* 271:134.

Marcantonio, ER, et al. (1994) The relationship of postoperative delirium with psychoactive medications, *JAMA* 272:1518.

Mayo-Smith, MF, et al. (2004) Management of alcohol withdrawal delirium, *Arch Intern Med* 164:1405.

McCartney, JR and Boland, RJ (1994) Anxiety and delirium in the intensive care unit, *Crit Care Clin* 10:673.

McNicoll, L, et al. (2003) Delirium in the intensive care unit: occurrence and clinical course in older patients, *J Am Geriatr Soc* 51:591.

Meagher, DJ (2001) Delirium: optimizing management, *BMJ* 322:144.

Mulsant, BH, et al. (2003) Serum anticholinergic activity in a community-based sample of older adults, *Arch Gen Psychiatry* 60:198.

Nanji, AA (1983) Drug-induced electrolyte disorders, *Drug Intelligence Clin Pharm* 17:175.

Nettis, E, et al. (2003) Drug-induced aseptic meningitis, *Curr Drug Imm Endo Metab Disorders* 3:143.

Newton, NL and Janati, A (1986) Delirium, a study of 100 cases, *Stress Med* 2:267.

Oscar-Berman, M, et al. (2004) Comparisons of Korsakoff and non-Korsakoff alcoholics on neuropsychological tests of prefrontal brain functioning, *Alcohol Clin Exp Res* 28:667.

Packard, RC (2001) Delirium, *The Neurologist* 7:327.

Pantoni, L, Lamassa, M, and Unzitari, D (2000) Transient global amnesia: a review emphasizing pathogenic aspects, *Acta Neurol Scand* 102:275.

Pellman, EJ, et al. (2004) Concussion in professional football: epidemiological features of game injuries and review of the literature—part 3, *Neurosurgery* 54:81.

Preskorn, SH and Jerkovich, GS (1990) Central nervous system toxicity of tricyclic antidepressants: phenomenology, course, risk factors, and the role of therapeutic drug monitoring, *J Clin Psychopharmacol* 10:88.

Price, J, et al. (1987) The Wernicke-Korsakoff syndrome: a reappraisal in Queensland with special reference to prevention, *Med J Aust* 147:561.

Prieto, JM, et al. (2002) Psychiatric morbidity and impact on hospital length of stay among hematologic cancer patients receiving stem-cell transplantation, *J Clin Oncol* 20:1907.

Pritchard, PB, et al. (1985) Epileptic amnesic attacks: benefit from antiepileptic drugs, *Neurology* 35:1188.

Purdie, FR, Honigman, B, and Rosen, P (1981) Acute organic brain syndrome: a review of 100 cases, *Ann Emerg Med* 10:455.

Rees, PM (2003) Contemporary issues in mild traumatic brain injury, *Arch Phys Med Rehabil* 84:1885.

Schneir, AB, et al. (2003) Complications of diagnostic physostigmine administration to emergency department patients, *Ann Emerg Med* 42:14.

Schofield, I (1997) A small exploratory study of the reaction of older people to an episode of delirium, *J Adv Nurs* 25:942.

Singleton, CK and Martin, PB (2001) Molecular mechanisms of thiamine utilization, *Curr Mol Med* 1:197.

Sirois, F (1988) Delirium: 100 cases, *Can J Psychiatry* 33:375.

Smith, AJ, et al. (1988) The effects of experimentally induced respiratory virus infections on performance, *Psychol Med* 18:65.

Somprakit, P, et al. (2002) Mental state change after general and regional anesthesia in adults and elderly patients, a randomized clinical trial, *J Med Assoc Thai* 85:S875.

Squire, LR, Amaral, DG, and Press, GA (1990) Magnetic resonance imaging of the hippocampal formation and mammillary nuclei distinguish medial temporal lobe and diencephalic amnesia, *J Neurosci* 10:3106.

Stracciari, A, et al. (1994) Post-traumatic retrograde amnesia with selective impairment of autobiographical memory, *Cortex* 30:59.

Sullivan, EV and Marsh, L (2003) Hippocampal volume deficits in alcoholic Korsakoff's syndrome, *Neurology* 61:1716.

Thomson, AD, et al. (2002) The Royal College of Physicians report on alcohol: guidelines for managing Wernicke's encephalopathy in the Accident and Emergency Department, *Alcohol Alcoholism* 37:513.

Triebig, G and Lang, C (1993) Brain imaging techniques applied to chronically solvent-exposed workers: current results and clinical evaluation, *Environ Res* 61:239.

Verfaellie, M and Cermak, LS (1994) Acquisition of generic memory in amnesia, *Cortex* 30:293.

Verstappen, CCP, et al. (2003) Neurotoxic complications of chemotherapy in patients with cancer: clinical signs and optimal management, *Drugs* 63:1549.

Weber, JB, Coverdale, JH, and Kunik, ME (2004) Delirium: current trends in prevention and treatment, *Intern Med J* 34:115.

Williams, DH, Levin, HS, and Eisenberg, HM (1990) Mild head injury classification, *Neurosurgery* 27:422.

Zeleznik, J (2001) Delirium: still searching for risk factors and effective preventive measures, *J Am Geriatr Soc* 49:1729.

Zhang, Q and Sachdev, PS (2003) Psychotic disorder and traumatic brain injury, *Curr Psychiatry Rep* 5:197.

Chapter 12

Aisen, PS, et al. (2003) Effects of rofecoxib or naproxen vs. placebo on Alzheimer disease progression: a randomized controlled trial, *JAMA* 289:2819–2826.

American Psychiatric Association (2000) *Diagnostic and Statistical Manual of Mental Disorders,* 4th edition, text revision. Washington, D.C., American Psychiatric Association.

Barinaga, M (1995) Missing Alzheimer's gene found, *Science* 269:917–918.

Berg, L, et al. (1988) Mild senile dementia of the Alzheimer type: 2. Longitudinal assessment, *Annals of Neurology* 23:477–484.

Berg, L, et al. (1992) Mild senile dementia of the Alzheimer type: 4. Evaluation of intervention, *Annals of Neurology* 31:242–249.

Bonner, LT and Peskind, ER (2002) Pharmacologic treatments of dementia, *Med Clin N Am* 86:657–674.

Bullock, R (2002) New drugs for Alzheimer's disease and other dementias, *Br J Psychiatry* 180:135–139.

Chui, IH: Vascular dementia. In Morris JC, Galvin J, Holtzman D (eds) (in press) *Handbook of Dementing Illnesses,* 2nd Edition, New York, Marcel Dekker, Inc.

Clark, RF and Goate, AM (1993) Molecular genetics of Alzheimer's disease, *Archives of Neurology* 50:1164–1172.

Cummings, JL (2003) Use of cholinesterase inhibitors in clinical practice: evidence-based recommendations, *Am J Geriatr Psychiatry* 11:131–145.

Cummings, JL (ed.) (2003) *The Neuropsychiatry of Alzheimer's Disease and Related Dementias*, London, Martin Dunitz.

Cummings, JL and Cole, G (2002) Alzheimer disease, *JAMA* 287:2335–2338.

Doody, RS, et al. (2001) Practice parameter: management of dementia (an evidence-based review): report of the Quality Standards Subcommittee of the American Academy of Neurology, *Neurology* 56:1154–1166.

Drevets, WC and Rubin, EH (1989) Psychotic symptoms and the longitudinal course of senile dementia of the Alzheimer Type, *Biological Psychiatry* 25:39–48.

Folstein, ME, Folstein, SE, and McHugh, PR (1975) 'Mini-mental state.' A practical method for grading the cognitive state of patients for the clinician, *J Psychiatr Res* 12:189–198.

Galvin, JE: Dementia with Lewy bodies. In Morris JC, Galvin J, Holtzman D (eds) (in press) *Handbook of Dementing Illnesses*, 2nd Edition, New York, Marcel Dekker, Inc.

Games, D, et al. (1995) Alzheimer-type neuropathology in transgenic mice overexpressing V717F B-amyloid precursor protein, *Nature* 373:523–527.

Hebert, LE, et al. (1995) Age-specific incidence of Alzheimer's disease in a community population, *JAMA* 273:1354–59.

Jarvis, B and Figgitt, DP (2003) Memantine, *Drugs Aging* 20:465–476.

Katzman, R, et al. (1983) Validation of a short orientation-memory-concentration test of cognitive impairment, *Am J Psychiatry* 140:734–739.

Katzman, R and Kawas, C: The epidemiology of dementia and Alzheimer's disease. In Terry, RD, Katzman, R, Bick, KL (eds) (1994) *Alzheimer's Disease*, New York, Raven Press, Ltd.

Katzman, R: Apolipoprotein E4 as the major genetic susceptibility factor for Alzheimer disease. In Terry, RD, Katzman, R, Bick, KL (eds) (1994) *Alzheimer's Disease*, New York, Raven Press, Ltd.

Klunk, WE, et al. (2004) Imaging brain amyloid in Alzheimer's disease with Pittsburgh Compound-B, *Ann Neurol* 55:306–319.

Knopman, DS, et al. (2001) Practice parameter: diagnosis of dementia (an evidence-based review): report of the Quality Standards Subcommittee of the American Academy of Neurology, *Neurology* 56:1143–1153.

Kukull, WA: The epidemiology of dementia. In Morris JC, Galvin J, Holtzman D (eds) (in press) *Handbook of Dementing Illnesses*, 2nd Edition, New York, Marcel Dekker, Inc.

Levy-Lahad, E, et al. (1995) Candidate gene for the chromosome 1 familial Alzheimer's disease locus, *Science* 269:973–977.

Levy-Lahad, E, et al. (1995) A familial Alzheimer's disease locus on chromosome 1, *Science* 269:970–973.

Max, W (1993) The economic impact of Alzheimer's disease, *Neurology* 43(suppl 4):S6–S10.

McKeith, IG (2002) Dementia with Lewy bodies, *Br J Psychiatry* 180:144–147.

Miller, ER 3rd, Pastor-Barriuso, R, Dalal, D, Riemersma, RA, Appel, LJ, and Guallar, E (2005) Meta-analysis: high-dosage vitamin E supplementation may increase all-cause mortality, *Ann Intern Med* 142:37–46.

Miller, BL and Gustavson, A: Alzheimer's disease and frontotemporal dementia. In Coffey, CE and Cummings, JL (eds) (2000) *The American Psychiatric Press Textbook of Geriatric Neuropsychiatry*, 2nd Edition, Washington, D.C., American Psychiatric Press.

Miller, BL and Liu, W: Fronto-temporal dementia. In Morris JC,

Galvin J, Holtzman D (eds) (in press) *Handbook of Dementing Illnesses*, 2nd Edition, New York, Marcel Dekker, Inc.

Mirra, SS and Sheffield, LG: The neuropathology of dementia. In Morris, JC, Galvin, J, Holtzman, D (eds) (in press) *Handbook of Dementing Illnesses*, 2nd Edition, New York, Marcel Dekker, Inc.

Morris, JC (1993) The Clinical Dementia Rating (CDR): Current version and scoring rules, *Neurology* 43:2412–2414.

Morris, JC and Rubin, EH (1991) Clinical diagnosis and course of Alzheimer's disease, *Psychiatric Clinics of North America* 14(2):223–236.

Morris, JC: Alzheimer's disease. In Morris, JC, Galvin, J, Holtzman, D (eds) (in press) *Handbook of Dementing Illnesses*, 2nd Edition, New York, Marcel Dekker, Inc.

Morris, JC: Frontotemporal dementias. In Clark, CM, Trojanowski, JQ (eds) (2000) *Neurodegenerative Dementias: Clinical Features and Pathological Mechanisms*, New York, McGraw-Hill.

Mulnard, RA, et al. (2000) Estrogen replacement therapy for treatment of mild to moderate Alzheimer disease, *JAMA* 283:1007–1015.

Pearlson, GD: Late-life-onset psychoses. In Coffey, CE, Cummings, JL (eds) (2000) *The American Psychiatric Press Textbook of Geriatric Neuropsychiatry*, 2nd Edition, Washington, D.C., American Psychiatric Association.

Puglielli, L, Tanzi, RE, and Kovacs, DM (2003) Alzheimer's disease: the cholesterol connection, *Nat Neurosci* 6:345–351.

Rapp, SR, et al. (2003) Effect of estrogen plus progestin on global cognitive function in postmenopausal women: the Women's Health Initiative Memory Study: a randomized controlled trial, *JAMA* 289:2663–2672.

Reisberg, B, et al. (2003) Memantine in moderate-to-severe Alzheimer's disease, *N Engl J Med* 348:1333–1341.

Rubin, EH: Psychopathology of senile dementia of the Alzheimer Type. In Wurtman, RJ, Corkin, S, Growdon, JH (eds) (1990) *Advances in Neurology: Alzheimer's disease*, vol 51, New York, Raven Press, Ltd.

Rubin, EH: Depression and dementia. In Morris, JC, Galvin, J, Holtzman, D (eds) (in press) *Handbook of Dementing Illnesses*, 2nd Edition, New York, Marcel Dekker, Inc.

Schatzberg, AF and Nemeroff, CB (eds) (2004) *The American Psychiatric Press Textbook of Psychopharmacology*, 3rd Edition, Washington, D.C., American Psychiatric Press.

Schneider, EL and Guralnik, JM (1990) The aging of America, *JAMA* 263:2335–2340.

Shumaker, SA, et al. (2003) Estrogen plus progestin and the incidence of dementia and mild cognitive impairment in postmenopausal women: the Women's Health Initiative Memory Study: a randomized controlled trial, *JAMA* 289:2651–2662.

Snowden, JS, Neary, D, and Mann, DMA (2002) Frontotemporal dementia, *Br J Psychiatry* 180:140–143.

Stewart, R (2002) Vascular dementia: a diagnosis running out of time, *Br J Psychiatry* 180:152–156.

Wolfe, MS (2002) Therapeutic strategies for Alzheimer's disease, *Nat Rev Drug Discov* 1:859–866.

Chapter 13

Abi-Dargham, A, et al. (2000) Increased baseline occupation of D_2 receptors by dopamine in schizophrenia, *Proc Natl Acad Sci* 97(14):8104–8109.

Allebeck P and Wistedt, B. (1986) Mortality in schizophrenia: a ten-year follow-up on the Stockholm County inpatient register, *Arch Gen Psychiatry* 43:650–653.

Anand, A, et al. (2000) Attenuation of the neuropsychiatric effects of ketamine with lamotrigine: support for hyperglutamatergic effects of N-methyl-D-aspartate receptor antagonists, *Arch Gen Psychiatry* 57(3):270–276.

Andreasen, NC, et al. (1995) Symptoms of schizophrenia: methods, meanings, and mechanisms, *Arch Gen Psychiatry* 52:341–351.

Andreasen, NC, Arndt, S, and Swayze, V II, et al. (1994) Thalamic abnormalities in schizophrenia visualized through magnetic resonance image averaging, *Science* 266:294–298.

Andreasen, NC and Carpenter WT (1993) Diagnosis and classification of schizophrenia, *Schizophr Bull* 19:199–214.

Arnold, SE, et al. (1995) Smaller neuron size in schizophrenia in hippocampal subfields that mediate cortical-hippocampal interactions, *Am J Psychiatry* 152:738–748.

Baldessarini, RJ and Viguera, AC (1995) Neuroleptic withdrawal in schizophrenic patients, *Arch Gen Psychiatry* 52:189–192.

Benes, F, et al. (2003) DNA fragmentation decreased in schizophrenia but not bipolar disorder, *Arch Gen Psychiatry* 60:359–364.

Berman, KF, Zec, RF, and Weinberger, DR (1986) Physiological dysfunction of dorsolateral prefrontal cortex in schizophrenia: ii. role of neuroleptic treatment, attention, and mental effort, *Arch Gen Psychiatry* 43:126–135.

Bleuler, E (1950) *Dementia Praecox or the Group of Schizophrenias*, New York, International Universities Press.

Brake, W, Sullivan, R, and Gratton, A (2000) Perinatal stress leads to lateralized medial prefrontal cortical dopamine hypofunction in adult rats, *J Neuroscience* 20(14):5538–5543.

Caldwell, CB and Gottesman, II (1990) Schizophrenics kill themselves too: a review of risk factors for suicide, *Schizophr Bull* 16:571–589.

Cancro, R and Lehmann, HE: Schizophrenia: clinical features. In Sadock BJ, Sadock VA (eds) (2000) *Kaplan & Sadock's Comprehensive Textbook of Psychiatry/VII*, Philadelphia, Lippincott Williams & Wilkins.

Carr, D, et al. (2000) Dopamine terminals in the rat prefrontal cortex synapse on pyramidal cells that project to the nucleus accumbens, *J Neuroscience* 19(24):11049–11060.

Casey, DE, Haupt, DW, Newcomer, JW, Henderson, DC, Sernyak, MJ, Davidson, M, Lindenmayer, JP, Manoukian, SV, Banerji, MA, Lebovitz, HE, and Hennekens, CH (2004) Antipsychotic-induced weight gain and metabolic abnormalities: implications for increased mortality in patients with schizophrenia, *J Clin Psychiatry* 65(Suppl 7):4–18.

Chambers, R, Krystal, J, and Self, D (2001) A neurobiological basis for substance abuse comorbidity in schizophrenia, *Biol Psychiatry* 50(2):71–83.

Cloninger, CR, et al. (1985) Diagnosis and prognosis in schizophrenia, *Arch Gen Psychiatry* 42:15–25.

Cloninger, CR (2002) The discovery of susceptibility genes for mental disorders, *Proc Natl Acad Sci* 99(21):13365–13367.

Cohen, LJ, Test, MA, and Brocon, RL (1990) Suicide and schizophrenia: data from a prospective community treatment study, *Am J Psychiatry* 147:602–607, correction: 147:1110.

Cooper, JE, et al. (1969) Cross-national study of diagnosis of the mental disorders: some results from the first comparative investigation, *Am J Psychiatry* 125(suppl 10):21–29.

Csernansky, J, Mahmoud, R, and Brenner, R (2002) A comparison of risperidone and haloperidol for the prevention of relapse in patients with schizophrenia, *N Engl J Med* 346(1):16–22.

Deutsch, S, et al. (2003) Adjuvant topiramate administration: a pharmacologic strategy for addressing NMDA receptor hypofunction in schizophrenia, *Clinical Neuropharmacology* 26(4):199–206.

Dixon, L, et al. (1999) The association of medical comorbidity in schizophrenia with poor physical and mental health, *J Nerv Ment Dis* 187(8):496–502.

Docherty, JP, et al. (1978) Stages of onset of schizophrenic psychosis, *Am J Psychiatry* 135:420–426.

Drake, RE, et al. (1985) Suicide among schizophrenics: a review, *Compr Psychiatry* 26:90–100.

Dursun, S and Deakin, J (2001) Augmenting antipsychotic treatment with lamotrigine or topiramate in patients with treatment-resistant schizophrenia: a naturalistic case-series outcome study, *J Psychopharmacology* 15(4):297–301.

Egan, MF and Hyde, TM: Schizophrenia: neurobiology. In Sadock BJ, Sadock VA (eds) (2000) *Kaplan & Sadock's Comprehensive Textbook of Psychiatry/VII*, Philadelphia, Lippincott Williams & Wilkins.

Faraone, S, et al. (2002) Linkage of chromosome 13q32 to schizophrenia in a large Veterans Affairs Cooperative Study sample, *Am J Med Genetics* 114(6):598–604.

Flaum, M, et al. (1995) Effects of diagnosis, laterality, and gender on brain morphology in schizophrenia, *Am J Psychiatry* 152:704–714.

Friedman, J, et al. (2002) Correlates of change in functional status of institutionalized geriatric schizophrenic patients: focus on medical comorbidity, *Am J Psychiatry* 158(9):1388–1394.

Gilbert, PL, Harris, MJ, McAdams, LA, and Jeste, DV (1995) Neuroleptic withdrawal in schizophrenic patients: a review of the literature, *Arch Gen Psychiatry* 52:173–188.

Goff, D and Coyle, J (2001) The emerging role of glutamate in the pathophysiology and treatment of schizophrenia, *Am J Psychiatry* 158(9):1367–1377.

Gottesman, II (1991) *Schizophrenia Genesis: The Origins of Madness*, New York, W.H. Freeman & Company.

Gur, RE and Gur, RC: Schizophrenia: brain structure and function. In Sadock BJ, Sadock VA (eds) (2000) *Kaplan & Sadock's Comprehensive Textbook of Psychiatry/VII*, Philadelphia, Lippincott Williams & Wilkins.

Hafner, H, Gattaz, WF, and Janzarik, W (1987) *Search for the Causes of Schizophrenia*, Berlin, Springer-Verlag.

Hafner, H: Der Krankheitsbegriff in der Psychiatrie, in Degkwitz R, Siedow, H (eds) (1981) *Standorte der Psychiatrie*, Munich, Urban & Schwarzenberg, vol 2: Zum umstrittenen psychiatrischen Krankheitsbegriff.

Harris, MJ, Cullum, CM, and Jeste, DV (1988) Clinical presentation of late-onset schizophrenia, *J Clin Psychiatry* 49(9):356–360.

Hashimoto, T, et al. (2003) Gene expression deficits in a subclass of GABA neurons in the prefrontal cortex of subjects with schizophrenia, *J Neuroscience* 23(15):6315–6326.

Haywood, TW, et al. (1995) Predicting the 'revolving door' phenomenon among patients with schizophrenic, schizoaffective, and affective disorders, *Am J Psychiatry* 152:856–861.

Heckers, S, et al. (2002) Differential hippocampal expression of glutamic acid decarboxylase 65 and 67 messenger RNA in bipolar disorder and schizophrenia, *Arch Gen Psychiatry* 59:521–529.

Heinz, A, et al. (2003) Molecular brain imaging and the neurobiology and genetics of schizophrenia, *Pharmacopsychiatry* 36(Suppl.3): S152–S157.

Jeanblanc, J, Hoeltzel, A, and Louilot, A (2003) Differential involvement of dopamine in the anterior and posterior parts of the dorsal striatum in latent inhibition, *Neuroscience* 118(1):233–241.

Jeste, DV, et al. (1995) Clinical and neuropsychological characteristics of patients with late-onset schizophrenia, *Am J Psychiatry* 152:722–730.

Jones, H and Pilowsky, L (2002) Dopamine and antipsychotic drug action revisited, *Br J Psychiatry* 181:271–275.

Kapur, S (2003) Psychosis as a state of aberrant salience: a framework linking biology, phenomenology, and pharmacology in schizophrenia, *Am J Psychiatry* 160:13–23.

Kapur, S and Seeman, P (2002) Atypical antipsychotics, cortical D_2 receptors and sensitivity to endogenous dopamine, *Br J Psychiatry* 180:465–466.

Kapur, S and Seeman, P (2001) Does fast dissociation from the dopamine D2 receptor explain the action of atypical antipsychotics?: A new hypothesis, *Am J Psychiatry* 158(3):360–369.

Kapur, S and Seeman, P (2002) NMDA receptor antagonists ketamine and PCP have direct effects on the dopamine (D_2) and serotonin $5-HT_{(2)}$ receptors—implications for models of schizophrenia, *Molecular Psychiatry* 7(8):837–844.

Kay, SR (1991) *Positive and Negative Syndromes in Schizophrenia: Assessment and Research*, New York, Brunner/Mazel, Inc.

Kendler, KS: Schizophrenia: genetics. In Sadock BJ, Sadock VA (eds) (2000) *Kaplan & Sadock's Comprehensive Textbook of Psychiatry/VII*, Philadelphia, Lippincott Williams & Wilkins.

Kendler, K, McGuire, M, Gruenberg, A, and Walsh, D (1995) Examining the validity of DSM-III-R schizoaffective disorder and its putative subtypes in the Roscommon Family Study, *Am J Psychiatry* 152(5):755–764.

Kendler, KS, et al. (1993) The Roscommon Family Study: I. Methods, diagnosis of probands, and risks of schizophrenia in relatives, *Arch Gen Psychiatry* 50:527–540.

Kendler, KS, et al. (1993) The Roscommon Family Study: II. The risk of nonschizophrenic nonaffective psychoses in relatives, *Arch Gen Psychiatry* 50:645–652.

Kessler, RC, McGonagle, KA, Zhao, S, et al. (1994) Lifetime and 12–month prevalence of DSM-III-R psychiatric disorders in the United States, *Arch Gen Psychiatry* 51:8–19.

Ko, F, Seeman, P, Sun, W, and Kapur, S (2002) Dopamine D_2 receptors internalize in their low-affinity state, *NeuroReport* 13:1017–1020.

Koreen, AR, et al. (1993) Depression in first-episode schizophrenia, *Am J Psychiatry* 150(11):1643–1648.

Kraepelin, E (1971) *Dementia Praecox and Paraphrenia*, New York, Robert E. Krieger, GM Robertson (ed.).

Kramer, MS, et al. (1989) Antidepressants in 'depressed' schizophrenic inpatients: a controlled trial, *Arch Gen Psychiatry* 46:922–928.

Laurellio, J, et al. Schizoaffective disorder, schizoaffective disorder, and brief psychotic disorder. In Sadock BJ, Sadock VA (eds) (2000) *Kaplan & Sadock's Comprehensive Textbook of Psychiatry/VII*, Philadelphia, Lippincott Williams & Wilkins.

Leonard, S, et al. (2002) Association of promoter variants in the α7 nicotinic acetylcholine receptor subunit gene with an inhibitory deficit found in schizophrenia, *Arch Gen Psychiatry* 59:1085–1096.

Leucht, S, Pitschel-Walz, G, Abraham, D, and Kissling, W (1999) Efficacy and extrapyramidal side-effects of the new antipsychotics olanzapine, quetiapine, risperidone, and sertindole compared to conventional antipsychotics and placebo. A meta-analysis of randomized controlled trials, *Schiz Res* 35(1):61–68.

Levinson, DF, et al. (1995) Fluphenazine plasma levels, dosage, efficacy, and side effects, *Am J Psychiatry* 152:765–771.

Lewis, D (2002) In pursuit of the pathogenesis and pathophysiology of schizophrenia: where do we stand?, *Am J Psychiatry* 159(9):1467–1469.

Limosin, F, Rouillon, F, Payan, C, Cohen, JM, and Strub, N (2003) Prenatal exposure to influenza as a risk factor for adult schizophrenia, *Acta Psychiatr Scand* 107:331–335.

Lohr, J and Braff, D (2003) Value of referring to recently introduced antipsychotics as 'second generation,' *Am J Psychiatry* 160(8): 1371–1372.

Lyon, E (1999) A review of the effects of nicotine on schizophrenia and antipsychotic medications, *Psychiatric Services* 50(10):1346–1350.

Maj, M, et al. (2000) Reliability and validity of the DSM-IV diagnostic category of schizoaffective disorder: preliminary data, *J Affective Disorders* 57(1–3):95–98.

Manschreck, TC: Delusional disorder and shared psychotic disorder. In Sadock BJ, Sadock VA (eds) (2000) *Kaplan & Sadock's Comprehensive Textbook of Psychiatry/VII*, Philadelphia, Lippincott Williams & Wilkins.

Marder, SR: Schizophrenia: somatic treatment. In Sadock BJ, Sadock VA (eds) (2000) *Kaplan & Sadock's Comprehensive Textbook of Psychiatry/VII*, Philadelphia, Lippincott Williams & Wilkins.

Mellor, CS (1970) First rank symptoms of schizophrenia, *Br J Psychiatry* 117:15–23.

Meltzer, HY, et al. (1993) Cost effectiveness of clozapine in neuroleptic-resistant schizophrenia, *Am J Psychiatry* 150(11):1630–1638.

Miller, NE and Cohen, GD (1987) *Schizophrenia and Aging*, New York, The Guilford Press.

National Advisory Mental Health Council (1993) Health care reform for Americans with severe mental illnesses: report of the National Advisory Mental Health Council, *Am J Psychiatry* 150(10):1447–1465.

Newcomer, J, et al. (2002) Abnormalities in glucose regulation during antipsychotic treatment of schizophrenia, *Arch Gen Psychiatry* 59:337–345.

Newcomer, J, et al. (1999) Ketamine-induced NMDA receptor hypofunction as a model of memory impairment and psychosis, *Neuropsychopharmacology* 20(2):106–118.

Nicolson, R, et al. (2000) Lessons from childhood-onset schizophrenia, *Brain Research Reviews* 31:147–156.

Norquist, GS and Narrow WE: Schizophrenia: epidemiology. In Sadock BJ, Sadock VA (eds) (2000) *Kaplan & Sadock's Comprehensive Textbook of Psychiatry/VII*, Philadelphia, Lippincott Williams & Wilkins.

Olney, J and Farber N (1995) Glutamate receptor dysfunction and schizophrenia, *Arch Gen Psychiatry* 52(12):998–1007.

Olney, J, Newcomer, J, and Farber, N (1999) NMDA receptor hypofunction model of schizophrenia, *J Psychiatric Research* 33:523–533.

Pearlson, GD and Marsh, L (1993) Magnetic resonance imaging in psychiatry. In *American Psychiatric Press Review of Psychiatry*, vol 12, Washington D.C., American Psychiatric Press.

Petty, RG, et al. (1995) Reversal of asymmetry of the planum temporale in schizophrenia, *Am J Psychiatry* 152:715–721.

Pope, H, et al. (1980) 'Schizoaffective disorder': an invalid diagnosis? A comparison of schizoaffective disorder, schizophrenia, and affective disorder, *Am J Psychiatry* 137(8):921–927.

Pope, HG and Lipinski, JF (1978) Diagnosis in schizophrenia and manic-depressive illness: a reassessment of the specificity of "schizophrenic" symptoms in the light of current research, *Arch Gen Psychiatry* 35:811–828.

Regier, DA, et al. (1984) The NIMH Epidemiologic Catchment Area Program: historical context, major objectives, and study population characteristics, *Arch Gen Psychiatry* 41:934–941.

Robins, E and Guze, SB (1970) Establishment of diagnostic validity in psychiatric illness: its application to schizophrenia, *Am J Psychiatry* 126:983–987.

Robins, LN, et al. (1984) Lifetime prevalence of specific psychiatric disorders in three sites, *Arch Gen Psychiatry* 41:949–958.

Schneider, K (1939) *Psychischer Befund und Psychiatrische Diagnose; later editors renamed Klinische Psychopathologie*; Engl translation *Clinical Psychopathology*; New York, Grune & Stratton.

Seeman, P and Kapur, S (2000) Schizophrenia: more dopamine, more D_2 receptors, *Proc Natl Acad Sci* 97(14):7673–7675.

Siris, SF, et al. (1987) Adjunctive imipramine in the treatment of post-psychotic depression: a controlled study, *Arch Gen Psychiatry* 44:533–539.

Spitzer, RL, et al. (1994) *DSM-IV Casebook*, Washington, American Psychiatric Press, Inc.

Sydenham, T: Observations medicare (1676), in J Swan (ed.) (1742) *The Entire Works of Thomas Sydenham Newly Made English from the Originals*, London, Cave.

Thaker, G (2002) Sensory gating deficit in schizophrenia: is the nicotinic alpha–7 receptor implicated?, *J Nerv Ment Dis* 190:550–551.

Tsuang, D, et al. (2001) Examination of genetic linkage of chromosome 15 to schizophrenia in a large Veterans Affairs Cooperative Study sample, *Am J Med Genetics* 105(8):662–668.

Volk, D and Lewis, D (2002) Impaired prefrontal inhibition in schizophrenia: relevance for cognitive dysfunction, *Physiology & Behavior* 77(4–5):501–505.

Weinberger, DR, Berman, KF, and Torrey, EF (1992) Correlations between abnormal hippocampal morphology and prefrontal physiology in schizophrenia, *Clin Neuropharmacol* 15:393A–394A.

Weinberger, DR, Berman, KF, and Zec, RF (1986) Physiological dysfunction of dorsolateral prefrontal cortex in schizophrenia: I. regional cerebral blood flow (rCBF) evidence, *Arch Gen Psychiatry* 43:114–124.

Weinberger, DR, Wagner, R, and Wyatt, RJ (1983) Neuropathological studies of schizophrenia: a selective review, *Schizophr Bull* 9:193–212.

Weinberger, DR (1984) Brain disease and psychiatric illness: when should a psychiatrist order a CAT scan?, *Am J Psychiatry* 141:1521–1527.

Westermeyer, JF, Harrow, M, and Marengo, JT (1991) Risk for suicide in schizophrenia and other psychotic and non-psychotic disorders, *J Nerv Ment Dis* 179:259–266.

Wing, JK, Cooper, JE, and Sartorius, N (1974) *Measurement and Classification of Psychiatric Symptoms: An Instruction Manual for the Present State Examination and CATEGO Program*, Cambridge, Cambridge Press.

Wong, DF, et al. (1986) Positron emission tomography reveals elevated D_2 dopamine receptors in drug-naive schizophrenics, *Science* 234:1558–1563.

World Health Organization (1973) *Report on the International Pilot Study of Schizophrenia*, Geneva, World Health Organization.

Wyatt, RJ, et al. (1988) Schizophrenia, just the facts. What do we know, how well do we know it?, *Schizophr Res* 1:3–18.

Yesavage, JA (1984) Correlates of dangerous behavior by schizophrenics in hospital, *J Psychiatry Res* 18:225–231.

Zubin, J, Magaziner, J, and Steinhauer, SR (1983) The metamorphosis of schizophrenia: from chronicity to vulnerability, *Psychological Medicine* 13:551–571.

Chapter 14

Amass, L, Bicker, WK, Higgins, ST, et al. (1994) Alternate-day dosing during buprenorphine treatment opioid dependence, *Life Sci* 54:1215–1228.

American Psychiatric Association (1980) *Diagnostic and Statistical Manual of Mental Disorders*, 3rd Edition. Washington, D.C., American Psychiatric Association.

American Psychiatric Association (1987) *Diagnostic and Statistical Manual of Mental Disorders*, 3rd Edition, Revised. Washington, D.C., American Psychiatric Association.

American Psychiatric Association (2000) *Diagnostic and Statistical Manual of Mental Disorders*, 4th Edition, Text Revision. Washington, D.C., American Psychiatric Association.

Anglin, MD, Hser, Y, and Booth, MW (1994) Sex differences in addict careers, *Am J Drug and Alc Abuse* 13:253–280.

Babor, T (1988) *Alcohol: Customs and Rituals*, London, Burke Publishing.

Babor, TF, de la Fuente, JR, Saunders, J, and Grant, M (1992) *Audit — The Alcohol Use Disorders Identification Test: Guidelines for use in Primary Health Care*, Geneva, World Health Organization Programme on Substance Abuse.

Bohman, M, Sigvardsson, S, and Cloninger, CR (1981) Maternal inheritance of alcohol abuse: cross-fostering analysis of adopted women, *Arch Gen Psychiatry* 38:965–969.

Bohman, M (1978) Genetic aspects of alcoholism and criminality, *Arch Gen Psychiatry* 35:269–276.

Cadoret, RJ, Cain, CA, and Grove, WM (1979) Development of alcoholism in adoptees raised apart from alcoholic biologic relatives, *Arch Gen Psychiatry* 37:561–563.

Cadoret, RJ, Troughton, E, and O'Gorman, TW (1987) Genetic and environmental factors in alcohol abuse and antisocial personality, *J Stud Alcohol* 48:1–8.

Cloninger, CR, Bohman, M, and Sigvardsson, S (1981) Inheritance of alcohol abuse: cross-fostering analysis of adopted men, *Arch Gen Psychiatry* 38:861–868.

Compton, WM, Cottler, LB, Abdallah, AB, Cunningham-Williams, RM, and Spitznagel, EL (2000) The effects of psychiatric comorbidity on response to an HIV prevention intervention, *Drug Alcohol Depend* 58(3):247–257.

Compton, WM, Cottler, LB, Abdallah, AB, Phelps, DL, Spitznagel, EL, and Horton, JC (2000) Substance dependence and other psychiatric disorders among drug dependent subjects: Race and gender correlates, *Am J Addict* 9:113–125.

Compton, WM, Cottler, LB, Dinwiddie, SH, Spitznagel, EL, Mager, DE, and Asmus, GA (1994) Inhalant use: characteristics and predictors, *Am J Addict* 3:263–272.

Compton, WM, Grant, BF, Colliver, JD, Glantz, MD, and Stinson, FS (2004) Prevalence of marijuana use disorders in the United States: 1991–1992 and 2001–2002, *JAMA* 291:2114–2121.

Cotton, NS (1979) The familial incidence of alcoholism: a review, *J Stud Alcohol* 40:89–116.

D'Aunno, T and Pollack, HA (2002) Changes in methadone treatment practices: results from a national panel study, 1988–2000, *JAMA* 288(7):850–856.

Edwards, G, Gross, MM, Keller, M, Moser, J, and Room, R (1977) *Alcohol-related Disabilities*, Geneva, WHO.

Goodwin, D and Guze, SB (1989) *Psychiatric Diagnosis*, 4th Edition. New York, Oxford University Press.

Goodwin, DW, Crane, JB, and Guze, SB (1971) Felons who drink: an 8-year follow-up, *Q J Stud Alcohol* 32:136–147.

Goodwin, DW, Schulsinger, F, Hermansen, L, et al. (1973) Alcohol problems in adoptees raised apart from alcoholic biological parents, *Arch Gen Psychiatry* 28:238–243.

Goodwin, DW (1985) Alcoholism and genetics: the sins of the fathers, *Arch Gen Psychiatry* 42:171–174.

Grant, BF, et al. (2004) Prevalence and co-occurrence of substance use disorders and independent mood and anxiety disorders, *Arch Gen Psychiatry* 61:807–816.

Grotenhermen, F (2004) Pharmacology of cannabinoids, *Neuroendocrinology Letters* 25:14–23.

Guze, SB (1992) *Why Psychiatry is a Branch of Medicine*, New York, Oxford University Press.

Helzer, JE, Canino, GJ, Hwu, HG, et al. (1990) Alcoholism: North America and Asia, *Arch Gen Psychiatry* 47:313–319.

Helzer, JE, Robins, LN, Taylor, JR, et al. (1985) The extent of long-term moderate drinking among alcoholics discharged from medical and psychiatric treatment facilities, *N Engl J Med* 312:1678–1682.

Hrubec, Z and Omenn, GS (1981). Evidence of genetic predisposition to alcoholic cirrhosis and psychosis: twin concordances for alcoholism and its biological end points by zygosity among male veterans, *Alcoholism Clin Exp Res* 5:207–215.

http://www.drugabuse.gov/about/organization/genetics/Genetics6.html.

http://www.nida.nih.gov/

http://www.nida.nih.gov/DrugsofAbuse.html

http://www.samhsa.gov/

Hyman, MM (1976) Alcoholics 15 years later, *Ann NY Acad Sci* 273:613–623.

Ibrahim, MM, Deng, H, Zvonok, A, Cockayne, DA, Kwan, J, Mata, HP, Vanderah, TW, Porreca, F, Makriyannis, A, and Malan, TP (2003) Activation of CB2 cannabinoid receptors by AM1241 inhibits experimental neuropathic pain: pain inhibition by receptors not present in the CNS, *Proc Natl Acad Sci USA* 100(18):10529–10533.

Jellinek, EM (1952) Phases of alcohol addiction, *Q J Stud Alcohol* 13:673–684.

Jellinek, EM (1960) *The Disease Concept of Alcoholism*, New Haven, College and University Press.

Johnson, RE, Chutuape, MA, Strain, EC, et al. (2000) A comparison of levomethadyl acetate, buprenorphine, and methadone for opioid dependence, *N Engl J Med* 343:1290–1297.

Johnston, LD, O'Malley, PM, and Bachman, JG (2003) *Monitoring the Future: National Results on Adolescent Drug Use: Overview of Key Findings*, 2002. NIH Publication. Washington, DC: National Institute on Drug Abuse.

Kaij, L (1960) *Studies on the Etiology and Sequels of Abuse of Alcohol*, Lund, University of Lund.

Keller, M (1982) On defining alcoholism: with comment on some other relevant words. In: *Alcohol, Science and Society Revisited*, Ann Arbor, University of Michigan Press.

Kendler, KS, Prescott, CA, Myers, J, and Neale, MC (2003) The structure of genetic and environmental risk factors for common psychiatric and substance use disorders in men and women, *Arch Gen Psychiatry* 60(9):929–937.

Kessler, RC, McGonagle, KA, Zhao, S, Nelson, CB, Hughes, M, Eshleman, S, Wittchen, H-U, and Kendler, KS (1994) Lifetime and 12-month prevalence of DSM-III-R psychiatric disorders in the United States, *Arch Gen Psychiatry* 51:8–19.

Langbehn, DR, Cadoret, RJ, Caspers, K, Troughton, EP, and Yucuis, R (2003) Genetic and environmental risk factors for the onset of drug use and problems in adoptees, *Drug Alcohol Depend* 69(2):151–167.

Liebman, JM and Cooper, SJ (eds) (1989) *The Neuropharmacological Basis of Reward*, Oxford, Oxford University Press.

Ling, W, Charuvastra, C, Collins, JF, et al. (1998) Buprenorphine maintenance treatment of opioid dependence: a multicenter, randomized clinical trial, *Addiction* 93:475–486.

Lowinson, JH, Ruiz, P, Millman, RB, and Langrod, JG (eds) (2004) *Substance Abuse—A Comprehensive Textbook*, 4th Edition. Lippincott, Williams & Wilkins.

Mayo-Smith, MF, Beecher, LH, Fischer, TL, Gorelick, DA, Guillaume, JL, Hill, A, Jara, G, Kasser, C, and Melbourne, J (2004) Management of alcohol withdrawal delirium: an evidence-based guideline, *Arch Intern Med* 164:1405–1412.

National Survey on Drug Use and Health. http://www.samhsa.gov/centers/clearinghouse/clearinghouses.html

Newcomb, MD and Bentler, PM: Antecedents and consequences of cocaine use: a eight year study from early adolescence to young adulthood. In: Robins, LN and Rutter, M (eds) (1990) *Straight and Devious Pathways from Childhood to Adulthood*, Cambridge, UK, Cambridge University Press.

O'Malley, SS, Jaffe, AJ, Chang, G, Schottenfield, RS, Meyer, RE, and Rounsaville, B (1992) Naltrexone and coping skills therapy for alcohol dependence, *Arch Gen Psychiatry* 49:881–887.

Pemberton, DA (1967) A comparison of the outcome of treatment in female and male alcoholics, *Br J Psychiatry* 113: 367–373.

Quartilho, A, Mata, HP, Ibrahim, MM, Vanderah, TW, Porreca, F, Makriyannis, A, and Malan, TP (2003) Inhibition of inflammatory hyperalgesia by activation of peripheral CB2 cannabinoid receptors, *Anesthesiology* 99(4):955–960.

Regier, DA, Farmer, ME, Rae, DS, Locke, BZ, Keith, SJ, Judd, LL,

Goodwin, FK (1990) Comorbidity of mental disorders with alcohol and other drug abuse, *JAMA* 264:2511–2518.

Robins, LN and McEvoy, L (1990) Conduct problems as predictors of substance abuse. In: Robins LN, Rutter M (eds) *Straight and Devious Pathways from Childhood to Adulthood*, Cambridge, UK, Cambridge University Press.

Robins, LN and Regier, DA (eds) (1991) *Psychiatric Disorders in America*, New York, The Free Press.

Robins, LN (1993) Vietnam veterans' rapid recovery from heroin addiction: a fluke or normal expectation?, *Addiction* 88:1041–1054.

Rouche, B, (1960) *Alcohol*, New York, Grove Press.

Rush, B (1811) *An Inquiry into the Effects of Ardent Spirits upon the Human Body and Mind*, 6th Edition, New York.

Saitz, R, Mayo-Smith, MF, Roberts, MS, Redmond, HA, Bernard, DR, and Calkins, DR (1994) Individualized treatment for alcohol withdrawal. A randomized double-blind controlled trial, *JAMA* 272(7):519–523.

Shuckit, MA (1999) *Drug and Alcohol Abuse: A Clinical Guide to Diagnosis and Treatment,* 5th Edition. Kluwer Academic/Plenum Publishers.

Skinner, HA (1979) A multivariate evaluation of the MAST, *Journal of Studies on Alcohol* 40:831–844.

Skinner, HA (1982) The drug abuse screening test, *Addictive Behaviors* 7:363–371.

Spragg, SDS (1940) Morphine addiction in chimpanzees, *Comp Psychol Monogr* 15:1–132.

Substance Abuse and Mental Health Services Administration (2003) *Results from the 2002 National Survey on Drug Use and Health: National Findings* (Office of Applied Studies, NHSDA Series H–22, DHHS Publication No. SMA 03-3836). Rockville, MD.

Sullivan, JT, Sykora, K, Schneiderman, J, Naranjo, CA, and Sellers, EM (1989) Assessment of alcohol withdrawal: the revised Clinical Institute withdrawal assessment for alcohol scale (CIWA-AR), *Br J Addict* 84:1353–1357.

Tsuang, MT, Bar, JL, Harley, RM, and Lyons, MJ (2001) The Harvard Twin Study of Substance Abuse: what we have learned, *Harv Rev Psychiatry* 9(6):267–79.

Vaillant, GE (1973) A 20-year follow-up of New York narcotic addicts, *Arch Gen Psychiatry* 19:237–241.

Vaillant, GE (1983) *The Natural History of Alcoholism: Causes, Patterns, and Paths to Recovery*, Cambridge, Harvard University Press.

Volkow, ND and Swanson, JM (2003) Variables that affect the clinical use and abuse of methylphenidate in the treatment of ADHD, *Am J Psychiatry* 160:1909–1918.

Volpicelli, JR, Alterman, AI, Hayachida, M, and O'Brien, CP (1992) Naltrexone in the treatment of alcohol dependence, *Arch Gen Psychiatry* 49:876–880.

Warner, LA, Kessler, RC, Hughes, M, Anthony, JC, and Nelson, CB (1995) Prevalence and correlates of drug use and dependence in the United States: results from the National Comorbidity Survey, *Arch Gen Psychiatry* 52:219–229.

World Health Organization (1992) *The ICD-10 Classification of Mental and Behavioural Disorders*, Geneva, World Health Organization.

Zacny, J, Bigelow, G, Compton, P, Foley, K, Iguchi, M, and Sannerud, C (2003) College on Problems of Drug Dependence taskforce on prescription opioid non-medical use and abuse: position statement, *Drug Alcohol Depend* 69:215–232.

Chapter 15

American Dietetic Association (1994) Position on nutrition intervention in the treatment of anorexia nervosa, bulimia nervosa, and binge eating, *J Am Diet Assoc* 94:902–907.

American Psychiatric Association (2000) *Diagnostic and Statistical Manual of Mental Disorders*, 4th Edition, Text revision. Washington D.C., American Psychiatric Association.

American Psychiatric Association (1993) Practice guidelines for eating disorders, *Am J Psychiatry* 150:207–228.

Babarich, NC, et al. (2003) Neurotransmitter and imaging studies in anorexia nervosa: new targets for treatment, *Current Drug Targets: CNS & Neurological Disorders* 2(1):61–72.

Carter, JC, et al. (2003) Self-help for bulimia nervosa: a randomized controlled trial, *Am J Psychiatry* 160(5):973–978.

Deter, HC and Herzog, W (1994) Anorexia nervosa in a long term perspective: results of the Heidelberg-Mannheim Study, *Psychosom Med* 56:20–27.

Drewnowski, A, et al. (1994) Eating pathology and DSM-III-R bulimia nervosa: a continuum of behavior, *Am J Psychiatry* 151:1217–1219.

Ferguson, JM (1993) The use of electroconvulsive therapy in patients with intractable anorexia nervosa, *Int J Eat Disord* 13:195–201.

Field, AE, et al. (1999) Relation of peer and media influences to the development of purging behaviors among preadolescent and adolescent girls, *Arch Ped & Adolescent Med* 153(11):1184–1189.

Garner, DM, Garfinkel, PE (eds) (1997) *Handbook of Treatment for Eating Disorders*. New York, Guilford Press.

Giannini, AJ, Slaby, AE (eds) (1993) *The Eating Disorders*. New York, Springer-Verlag.

Goldstein, DJ (ed.) (1999) *Management of Eating Disorders and Obesity*. Totowa NJ, Humana Press.

Halmi, KA, et al. (2002) Relapse predictors of patients with bulimia nervosa who achieved abstinence with cognitive behavioral therapy, *Arch Gen Psychiatry* 59:1105–1109.

Holderness, CC, et al. (1994) Co-morbidity of eating disorders and substance abuse: review of the literature, *Int J Eat Disord* 16:1–34.

Johnson, JG, et al. (2002) Childhood adversities associated with risk for eating disorders or weight problems during adolescence or early adulthood, *Am J Psychiatry* 159:394–400.

Kaplan, AS, Garfinkel, PE (eds) (1993) *Medical Issues and the Eating Disorders: the Interface*, New York, Brunner/Mazel.

Katzman, DK, et al. (1997) A longitudinal magnetic resonance imaging study of brain changes in adolescents with anorexia nervosa, *Arch Ped & Adolescent Med* 151(8):793–797.

Keel, PK, et al. (2003) Predictors of mortality in eating disorders, *Arch Gen Psychiatry* 60(2):179–183.

Kendler, KS, et al. (1991) The genetic epidemiology of bulimia nervosa, *Am J Psychiatry* 148:1627–1637.

Kendler, KS (2001) Twin studies of psychiatric illness: an update, *Arch Gen Psychiatry* 58(11):1005–1014.

Lask, B and Bryant-Waugh, R (2000) *Anorexia Nervosa and Related*

Eating Disorders in Childhood and Adolescence, Hove, UK, Psychology Press.

Maj, M (ed.) (2003) *Eating Disorders,* Chichester UK, John Wiley & Sons.

McDowell BD, et al. (2003) Cognitive impairment in anorexia nervosa is not due to depressed mood, *Int J Eat Disord* 33(3):351–355.

(The) McKnight Investigators (2003) Risk factors for the onset of eating disorders in adolescent girls: results of the McKnight longitudinal risk factor study, *Am J Psychiatry* 160(2):248–254.

Mitchell, JE, et al. (2003) Drug therapy for patients with eating disorders, *Current Drug Targets—CNS & Neurological Disorders* 2(1):17–29.

Sharp, CW, et al. (1994) Clinical presentation of anorexia nervosa in males: 24 new cases, *Int J Eat Disord* 15:125–134.

Schocken, DD, et al. (1989) Weight loss and the heart: effects of anorexia nervosa and starvation, *Arch Int Med* 149(4):877–881.

Schork, EJ, et al. (1994) The relationship between psychopathology, eating disorder diagnosis, and clinical outcome at 10 year follow-up in anorexia nervosa, *Compr Psychiatry* 35:113–123.

Steinhausen, H-C (2002) The outcome of anorexia nervosa in the 20th century, *Am J Psychiatry* 159:1284–1293.

Szmulker, G, Dare, C, Treasure, J (eds) (1995) *Handbook of Eating Disorders: Theory, Treatment, and Research,* Chichester UK, John Wiley & Sons.

Theil, A, et al. (1995) Obsessive-compulsive disorder among patients with anorexia nervosa and bulimia nervosa, *Am J Psychiatry* 152:72–75.

Udovich, M (2002) A secret society of the starving, *The New York Times Magazine,* Sept. 8.

Woolsey, MM (2002) *Eating Disorders: a Clinical Guide to Counseling and Treatment,* Chicago, American Dietetic Association.

Zerbe, KJ (1993) *The Body Betrayed: Women, Eating Disorders and Treatment,* Washington D.C., American Psychiatric Press.

Chapter 16

Obesity

Allison, DB, Mentore, JL, Heo, M, et al. (1999) Antipsychotic-induced weight gain: A comprehensive research synthesis, *Am J Psychiatry* 156:1686–1696.

Andersen, RE, Wadden, TA, Bartlett, SJ, Zemel, B, Verde, TJ, and Franckowiak, SC (1999) Effects of lifestyle activity vs. structured aerobic exercise in obese women: A randomized trial, *JAMA* 28:335–340.

Aronne, LJ (2002) Classification of obesity and assessment of obesity-related health risks, *Obes Res* 10(Suppl 2):105S–115S.

Bocchieri, LE, Meana, M, and Fisher, BL (2002) A review of psychosocial outcomes of surgery for morbid obesity, *J Psychosom Res* 52:155–165.

Bravata, DM, Sanders, L, Huang, J, Krumholz, HM, Olkin, I, and Gardner, CD (2003) Efficacy and safety of low-carbohydrate diets: A systematic review, *JAMA* 289:1837–1850.

Bray, GA and Greenway, FL (1999) Current and potential drugs for treatment of obesity, *Endocr Rev* 20:805–875.

Bray, GA, Hollander, P, Klein, S, et al. (2003) A 6-month randomized, placebo-controlled, dose-ranging trial of topiramate for weight loss in obesity, *Obes Res* 11:722–733.

Brolin, RE (2002) Bariatric surgery and long-term control of morbid obesity, *JAMA* 288:2793–2796.

Brownell, KD (2000) *The LEARN Program for Weight Management 2000,* 10th Edition, Dallas, American Health Publishing Company.

Chagnon, YC, Rankinen, T, Snyder, EE, Weisnagel, SJ, Perusse, L, and Bouchard, C (2003) The human obesity gene map: The 2002 update, *Obes Res* 11:313–367.

Cooper, Z and Fairburn, CG (2001) A new cognitive behavioural approach to the treatment of obesity, *Behav Res Ther* 39:499–511.

Cummings, DE and Schwartz, MW (2003) Genetics and pathophysiology of human obesity, *Annu Rev Med* 54:453–471.

Davidson, MH, Hauptman, J, DiGirolamo, M, et al. (1999) Weight control and risk factor reduction in obese subjects treated for 2 years with orlistat: A randomized controlled trial, *JAMA* 281:235–242.

DiLillo, V, Siegfried, NJ, and West, DS (2003) Incorporating motivational interviewing into behavioral obesity treatment, *Cognitive and Behavioral Practice* 10:120–130.

Finer, N, James, WP, Kopelman, PG, Lean, ME, and Williams, G (2000) One-year treatment of obesity: A randomized, double-blind, placebo-controlled, multicentre study of orlistat, a gastrointestinal lipase inhibitor, *Int J Obes Relat Metab Disord* 24:306–313.

Flegal, KM, Carroll, MD, Ogdenm CL, and Johnson, CL (2002) Prevalence and trends in obesity among US adults, 1999–2000, *JAMA* 288:1723–1727.

Ford, ES, Giles, WH, and Dietz, WH (2002) Prevalence of the metabolic syndrome among US adults: Findings from the third National Health and Nutrition Examination Survey, *JAMA* 287:356–359.

Foster, GD, Wyatt, HR, Hill, JO, et al. (2003) A randomized trial of a low-carbohydrate diet for obesity, *N Engl J Med* 348:2082–2090.

Gadde, KM, Franciscy, DM, Wagner, HR, and Krishnan, KR (2003) Zonisamide for weight loss in obese adults: A randomized controlled trial, *JAMA* 289:1820–1825.

Galuska, DA, Will, JC, Serdula, MK, and Ford, ES (1999) Are health care professionals advising obese patients to lose weight?, *JAMA* 282:1576–1578.

Giacobino, JP (2002) Uncoupling proteins, leptin, and obesity: An updated review, *Ann N Y Acad Sci* 967:398–402.

Heshka, S, Anderson, JW, Atkinson, RL, et al. (2003) Weight loss with self-help compared with a structured commercial program: A randomized trial, *JAMA* 289:1792–1798.

Heymsfield, SB, Greenberg, AS, Fujioka, K, et al. (1999) Recombinant leptin for weight loss in obese and lean adults: A randomized, controlled, dose-escalation trial, *JAMA* 282:1568–1575.

Hill, JO and Wyatt, H (2002) Outpatient management of obesity: A primary care perspective, *Obes Res* 10(Suppl 2):124S–130S.

Hill, JO, Wyatt, HR, Reed, GW, and Peters, JC (2003) Obesity and the environment: Where do we go from here?, *Science* 299:853–855.

Hukshorn, CJ, Westerterp-Plantenga, MS, and Saris, WH (2003) Pegylated human recombinant leptin (PEG-OB) causes additional weight loss in severely energy-restricted, overweight men, *Am J Clin Nutr* 77:771–776.

James, WP, Astrup, A, Finer, N, et al. (2000) Effect of sibutramine on weight maintenance after weight loss: A randomised trial. STORM Study Group. Sibutramine Trial of Obesity Reduction and Maintenance, *Lancet* 356:2119–2125.

Koutsari, C, Karpe, F, Humphreys, SM, Frayn, KN, and Hardman, AE (2003) Plasma leptin is influenced by diet composition and exercise, *Int J Obes Relat Metab Disord* 27:901–906.

Krude, H, Biebermann, H, and Gruters, A (2003) Mutations in the human proopiomelanocortin gene, *Ann N Y Acad Sci* 994: 233–239.

Kushner, RF and Weinsier, RL (2000) Evaluation of the obese patient. Practical considerations, *Med Clin North Am* 84:387–399, vi.

Latner, JD, Stunkard, AJ, Wilson, GT, Jackson, ML, Zelitch, DS, and Labouvie, E (2000) Effective long-term treatment of obesity: A continuing care model, *Int J Obes Relat Metab Disord* 24:893–898.

Latner, JD, Wilson, GT, Stunkard, AJ, and Jackson, ML (2002) Self-help and long-term behavior therapy for obesity, *Behav Res Ther* 40:805–812.

Leung, WY, Neil Thomas, G, Chan, JC, and Tomlinson, B (2003) Weight management and current options in pharmacotherapy: Orlistat and sibutramine, *Clin Ther* 25:58–80.

Lowe, MR, Miller-Kovach, K, and Phelan, S (2001) Weight-loss maintenance in overweight individuals one to five years following successful completion of a commercial weight loss program, *Int J Obes Relat Metab Disord* 25:325–331.

Perusse, L and Bouchard, C (1999) Genotype-environment interaction in human obesity, *Nutr Rev* 57:S31–S38.

Phelan, S and Wadden, TA (2002) Combining behavioral and pharmacological treatments for obesity, *Obes Res* 10:560–574.

Podnos, YD, Jimenez, JC, Wilson, SE, Stevens, CM, and Nguyen, NT (2003) Complications after laparoscopic gastric bypass: A review of 3464 cases, *Arch Surg* 138:957–961.

Roberts, RE, Deleger, S, Strawbridge, WJ, and Kaplan, GA (2003) Prospective association between obesity and depression: Evidence from the Alameda County Study, *Int J Obes Relat Metab Disord* 27:514–521.

Rolls, BJ, Morris, EL, and Roe, LS (2002) Portion size of food affects energy intake in normal-weight and overweight men and women, *Am J Clin Nutr* 76:1207–1213.

Rossner, S, Sjostrom, L, Noack, R, Meinders, AE, and Noseda, G (2000) Weight loss, weight maintenance, and improved cardiovascular risk factors after 2 years treatment with orlistat for obesity. European Orlistat Obesity Study Group, *Obes Res* 8:49–61.

Rubenstein, RB (2002) Laparoscopic adjustable gastric banding at a U.S. center with up to 3-year follow-up, *Obes Surg* 12:380–384.

Schwartz, MB, Chambliss, HO, Brownell, KD, Blair, SN, and Billington, C (2003) Weight bias among health professionals specializing in obesity, *Obes Res* 11:1033–1039.

Serdula, MK, Khan, LK, and Dietz, WH (2003) Weight loss counseling revisited, *JAMA* 289:1747–1750.

Thompson, D and Wolf, AM (2001) The medical-care cost burden of obesity, *Obes Rev* 2:189–197.

Wadden, TA, Berkowitz, RI, Sarwer, DB, Prus-Wisniewski, R, and Steinberg, C (2001) Benefits of lifestyle modification in the pharmacologic treatment of obesity: A randomized trial, *Arch Intern Med* 161:218–227.

Wadden, TA and Phelan, S (2002) Assessment of quality of life in obese individuals, *Obes Res* 10(Suppl 1):50S–57S.

Wilding, J, Van Gaal, L, Rissanen, A, Vercruyesse, F, and Fitchet, M; OBES-002 Study Group (2004) A randomized double-blind placebo-controlled study of the long-term efficacy and safety of topiramate in the treatment of obese subjects, *Int J Obes Res* 28:1399–1410.

Woods, SC and Seeley, RJ (2002) Understanding the physiology of obesity: Review of recent developments in obesity research, *Int J Obes Relat Metab Disord* 26(Suppl 4):S8–S10.

Yanovski, SZ and Yanovski, JA (2002) Obesity, *N Engl J Med* 346:591–602.

Binge Eating Disorder

Agras, WS, Telch, CF, Arnow, B, Eldredge, K, and Marnell, M (1997) One-year follow-up of cognitive-behavioral therapy for obese individuals with binge eating disorder, *J Consult Clin Psychol* 65:343–347.

American Psychiatric Association Work Group on Eating Disorders (2000) Practice guideline for the treatment of patients with eating disorders (revision), *Am J Psychiatry* 157:1–39.

Appolinario, JC, Bacaltchuk, J, Sichieri, R, et al. (2003) A randomized, double-blind, placebo-controlled study of sibutramine in the treatment of binge-eating disorder, *Arch Gen Psychiatry* 60:1109–1116.

Arnold, LM, McElroy, SL, Hudson, JI, Welge, JA, Bennett, AJ, and Keck, PE (2002) A placebo-controlled, randomized trial of fluoxetine in the treatment of binge-eating disorder, *J Clin Psychiatry* 63:1028–1033.

Bulik, CM and Reichborn-Kjennerud, T (2003) Medical morbidity in binge eating disorder, *Int J Eat Disord* 34(Suppl):S39–S46.

Carter, JC and Fairburn, CG (1998) Cognitive-behavioral self-help for binge eating disorder: A controlled effectiveness study, *J Consult Clin Psychol* 66:616–623.

Carter, WP, Hudson, JI, Lalonde, JK, Pindyck, L, McElroy, SL, and Pope, HG, Jr (2003) Pharmacologic treatment of binge eating disorder, *Int J Eat Disord* 34(Suppl):S74–S88.

Craighead, LW and Allen, HN (1995) Appetite awareness training: A cognitive behavioral intervention for binge eating, *Cognitive and Behavioral Practice* 2:249–270.

Devlin, MJ, Goldfein, JA, and Dobrow, I (2003) What is this thing called BED? Current status of binge eating disorder nosology. *Int J Eat Disord* 34(Suppl):S2–S18.

de Zwaan, M (2001) Binge eating disorder and obesity, *Int J Obes Relat Metab Disord* 25(suppl 1):S51–S55.

Fairburn, CG (1995) *Overcoming Binge Eating*. New York, Guilford Press.

Fairburn, CG and Beglin, SJ (1994) Assessment of eating disorders: interview or self-report questionnaire?, *Int J Eat Disord* 16:363–370.

Fairburn, CG and Cooper, Z (1993) The eating disorder examination. In: Fairburn CG, Wilson GT, editors, *Binge Eating: Nature, Assessment, and Treatment*. London, The Guilford Press, pp. 317–360.

Fairburn, CG, Cooper, Z, Doll, HA, Norman, P, and O'Connor, M (2000) The natural course of bulimia nervosa and binge eating disorder in young women, *Arch Gen Psychiatry* 57:659–665.

Fairburn, CG, Doll, HA, Welch, SL, Hay, PJ, Davies, BA, and O'Connor, ME (1998) Risk factors for binge eating disorder: A community-based, case-control study, *Arch Gen Psychiatry* 55:425–432.

Grilo, CM and Masheb, RM (2000) Onset of dieting vs. binge eating in outpatients with binge eating disorder, *Int J Obes Relat Metab Disord* 24:404–409.

Hudson, JI, Carter, WP, and Pope, HG, Jr (1996) Antidepressant treatment of binge-eating disorder: Research findings and clinical guidelines, *J Clin Psychiatry* 57(Suppl 8):73–79.

Hudson, JI, McElroy, SL, Raymond, NC, et al. (1998) Fluvoxamine in the treatment of binge-eating disorder: A multicenter placebo-controlled, double-blind trial, *Am J Psychiatry* 155: 1756–1762.

Johnson, JG, Spitzer, RL, and Williams, JB (2001) Health problems, impairment and illnesses associated with bulimia nervosa and binge eating disorder among primary care and obstetric gynaecology patients, *Psychol Med* 31:1455–1466.

Nauta, H, Hospers, H, and Jansen, A (2001) One-year follow-up effects of two obesity treatments on psychological well-being and weight, *Br J Health Psychol* 6:271–284.

Peterson, CB, Crow, SJ, Nugent, S, Mitchell, JE, Engbloom, S, and Mussell, MP (2001) Predictors of treatment outcome for binge eating disorder, *Int J Eat Disord* 28:131–138.

Ricca, V, Mannucci, E, Mezzani, B, et al. (2001) Fluoxetine and fluvoxamine combined with individual cognitive-behaviour therapy in binge eating disorder: A one-year follow-up study, *Psychother Psychosom* 70:298–306.

Sherwood, NE, Jeffery, RW, and Wing, RR (1999) Binge status as a predictor of weight loss treatment outcome, *Int J Obes Relat Metab Disord* 23:485–493.

Spitzer, RL, Devlin, MJ, Walsh, BT, et al. (1992) Binge eating disorder: a multisite field trial of the diagnostic criteria, *Int J Eat Disord* 11:191–203.

Stice, E, Agras, WS, Telch, CF, Halmi, KA, Mitchell, JE, and Wilson, GT (2001) Subtyping binge eating-disordered women along dieting and negative affect dimensions, *Int J Eat Disord* 30:11–27.

Striegel-Moore, RH and Franko, DL (2003) Epidemiology of binge eating disorder, *Int J Eat Disord* 34(Suppl):S19–S29.

Stunkard, AJ and Allison, KC (2003) Two forms of disordered eating in obesity: Binge eating and night eating, *Int J Obes Relat Metab Disord* 27:1–12.

Stunkard, A, Berkowitz, R, Tanrikut, C, Reiss, E, and Young, L (1996) D-fenfluramine treatment of binge eating disorder, *Am J Psychiatry* 153:1455–1459.

Telch, CF, Agras, WS, and Linehan, MM (2001) Dialectical behavior therapy for binge eating disorder, *J Consult Clin Psychol* 69:1061–1065.

Wilfley, DE, Agras, WS, et al. (1993) Group cognitive-behavioral therapy and group interpersonal psychotherapy for the non-purging bulimic individual: A controlled comparison, *J Consult Clin Psychol* 61:296–305.

Wilfley, DE, Welch, RR, Stein, RI, et al. (2002) A randomized comparison of group cognitive-behavioral therapy and group interpersonal psychotherapy for the treatment of overweight individuals with binge eating disorder, *Arch Gen Psychiatry* 59:713–721.

Wonderlich, SA, de Zwaan, M, Mitchell, JE, Peterson, C, and Crow, S (2003) Psychological and dietary treatments of binge eating disorder: Conceptual implications, *Int J Eat Disord* 34(Suppl):S58–S73.

Yanovski, SZ (2003) Binge eating disorder and obesity in 2003: Could treating an eating disorder have a positive effect on the obesity epidemic?, *Int J Eat Disord* 34(Suppl):S117–S120.

Chapter 17

Abbey, SE and Garfinkel, PE (1991) Neurasthenia and chronic fatigue syndrome: the role of culture in the making of a diagnosis, *Am J Psychiatry* 148:1638–1646.

Bass, C and Benjamin, S (1993) The management of chronic somatisation, *Br J Psychiatry* 162:472–480.

Bibb, RC and Guze, SB (1972) Hysteria (Briquet's syndrome) in a psychiatric hospital: the significance of secondary depression, *Am J Psychiatry* 129:224–228.

Black, DW (1987) Somatization disorders, *Prim Care* 14:711–723.

Boffeli, TJ and Guze, SB (1992) The simulation of neurologic disease. *Psychiatr Clin North Am* 15:301–310.

Brown, FW, Golding, JM, and Smith, GR Jr (1990) Psychiatric comorbidity in primary care somatization disorder, *Psychosom Med* 52:445–451.

Brown, FW and Smith, GR Jr (1988) Somatization disorder in general medical settings, *Psychiatr Ann* 18:353–356.

Brown, FW and Smith, GR Jr (1991) Diagnostic concordance in primary care somatization disorder, *Psychosomatics* 32:191–195.

Cadoret, RJ (1978) Psychopathology in adopted-away offspring of biologic parents with antisocial behavior, *Arch Gen Psychiatry* 35:176–184.

Cadoret, RJ, et al. (1976) Studies of adoptees from psychiatrically disturbed biological parents. III. Medical symptoms and illnesses in childhood and adolescence, *Am J Psychiatry* 133:1316–1318.

Cloninger, CR and Guze, SB (1970) Psychiatric illness and female criminality: the role of sociopathy and hysteria in the antisocial woman, *Am J Psychiatry* 127:303–311.

Cloninger, CR, Reich, T, and Guze, SB (1975) The multifactorial model of disease transmission. II. Sex differences in the familial transmission of sociopathy (antisocial personality), *Br J Psychiatry* 127:11–22.

Cloninger, CR, et al. (1986) A prospective follow-up and family study of somatization in men and women, *Am J Psychiatry* 143:873–878.

Creed, F and Guthrie, E (1993) Techniques for interviewing the somatizing patient, *Br J Psychiatry* 162:467–471.

deGruy, F, et al. (1987) Somatization disorder in a family practice, *J Fam Pract* 25:579–584.

DeSouza, C, et al. (1988) Major depression and somatization disorder: the overlooked differential diagnosis, *Psychiatr Ann* 18:340–348.

Engel, GL (1970) Conversion symptoms. In MacBryde CM (ed.) *Sign and Symptoms: Applied Pathologic Physiology and Clinical Interpretation*, 5th Edition, Philadelphia, Lippincott.

Ford, CV and Folks, DG (1985) Conversion disorders: an overview, *Psychosomatics* 26:371–373.

Gatfield, PD and Guze, SB (1962) Prognosis and differential diagnosis of conversion reactions (a follow-up study), *Dis Nerv Sys* 23:1–8.

Guze, SB (1967) The diagnosis of hysteria: what are we trying to do?, *Am J Psychiatry* 124:77–84.

Guze, SB (1970) The role of follow-up studies: their contribution to diagnostic classification as applied to hysteria, *Semin Psychiatry* 2:392–402.

Guze, SB (1975) The validity and significance of the clinical diagnosis of hysteria (Briquet's syndrome), *Am J Psychiatry* 132:138–142.

Guze, SB (1993) Genetics of Briquet's syndrome and somatization disorder, *Ann Clin Psychiatry* 5:225–230.

Guze, SB and Perley, MJ (1963) Observations on the natural history of hysteria, *Am J Psychiatry* 119:960–965.

Guze, SB, Woodruff, RA, and Clayton, PJ (1971) Hysteria and antisocial behavior: further evidence of an association, *Am J Psychiatry* 127:133–136.

Guze, SB, Woodruff, RA, and Clayton, PJ (1971) A study of conversion symptoms in psychiatric outpatients, *Am J Psychiatry* 128:135–138.

Guze, SB, et al. (1986) A follow-up and family study of Briquet's syndrome, *Br J Psychiatry* 149:17–23.

Holt, RE and LeCann, AF (1984) Use of an integrative interview to manage somatization, *Psychosomatics* 25:663–665; 668–669.

Lazare, A (1978) Hysteria. In Hackett, TP, Cassem, NH (eds) *Massachusetts General Hospital Handbook Of General Hospital Psychiatry*, St. Louis, Mosby.

Lazare, A (1981) Conversion symptoms, *N Engl J Med* 305:745–748.

Lipowski, ZJ (1988) Somatization: the concept and its clinical application, *Am J Psychiatry* 145:1358–1368.

Liskow, B, et al. (1986) Is Briquet's syndrome heterogeneous disorder?, *Am J Psychiatry* 143:626–629.

Ljungberg, L (1957) Hysteria: a clinical, prognostic, and genetic study, *Acta Psychiatr Neurol Scand Suppl* 112:1–62.

Mai, FM and Merskey, H (1980) Briquet's treatise on hysteria, *Arch Gen Psychiatry* 37:1401–1405.

Martin, RL (1988) Problems in the diagnosis of somatization disorder: effects on research and clinical practice, *Psychiatr Ann* 18:357–362.

Martin, RL, et al. (1953) Excessive surgery in hysteria, *JAMA* 151:977–986.

Monson, RA and Smith, GR Jr (1983) Somatization disorder in primary care, *N Eng J Med* 308:1464–1465.

Morrison, JR (1978) Management of Briquet syndrome (hysteria), *West J Med* 128:482–487.

Morrison, JR (1989) Managing depression in a woman with somatization disorder, *Ann Clin Psychiatry* 1:255–257.

Murphy, GE (1982) The clinical management of hysteria, *JAMA* 247:2559–2564.

North, CS, et al. (1993) *Multiple Personalities, Multiple Disorders: Psychiatric Classification and Media Influence*, New York, Oxford University Press.

Othmer, E (1988) Somatization disorder, *Psychiatr Ann* 18:330–331.

Pendergrast, M (1995) *Victims of Memory: Incest Accusations and Shattered Lives*, Hinesburg, Vt., Upper Access Books.

Pennebaker, JW and Watson, D: The psychology of somatic symptoms. In Kirmayer, LJ, Robbins, JM (eds) (1991) *Current Concepts of Somatization: Research and Clinical Perspectives*, Washington, D.C., American Psychiatric Press.

Perley, MJ and Guze, SB (1962): Hysteria the stability and usefulness of clinical criteria, *N Engl J Med* 266:421–426.

Purtell, JJ, Robins, E, and Cohen, ME (1951) Observations on clinical aspects of hysteria, *JAMA* 146:902–909.

Quill, TE (1985) Somatization disorder: one of medicine's blind spots, *JAMA* 252:3075–3079.

Rust, KM, et al. (1992) The comorbidity of *DSM-III-R* personality disorders in somatization disorder, *Gen Hosp Psychiatry* 14:322–326.

Simon, GE and VonKorff, M (1991) Somatization and psychiatric disorder in the NIMH epidemiologic catchment area study, *Am J Psychiatry* 148:1494–1500.

Smith, GR Jr (1992) The epidemiology and treatment of depression when it coexists with somatoform disorders, somatization or pain, *Gen Hosp Psychiatry* 14:265–272.

Smith, GR Jr (1994) The course of somatization and its effects on utilization of health care resources, *Psychosomatics* 35:263–267.

Smith, GR Jr, Miller, LM, and Monson, RA (1986) Consultation-liaison intervention in somatization disorder, *Hosp Comm Psychiatry* 37:1207–1210.

Smith, GR Jr, Monson, RA, and Livingston, RL (1985) Somatization disorder in men, *Gen Hosp Psychiatry* 7:4–8.

Smith, GR Jr, Monson, RA, and Ray, DC (1986) Psychiatric consultation in somatization disorder, *N Engl J Med* 314:1407–1413.

Stewart, DE (1990) The changing faces of somatization, *Psychosomatics* 31:153–158.

Swartz, M, et al. (1991) Somatization disorder. In Robins, LN, Regier, DA (eds): *Psychiatric Disorders in America: the Epidemiologic Catchment Area Study*, New York, The Free Press.

Tomasson, K, Kent, D, and Coryell, W (1991) Somatization and conversion disorders: comorbidity and demographics at presentation, *Acta Psychiatr Scand* 84:288–293.

Torgerson, S (1986) Genetics of somatoform disorders, *Arch Gen Psychiatry* 43:502–505.

Wetzel, RD, et al. (1994) Briquet's syndrome (hysteria) is both a somatoform and a 'psychoform' illness: a Minnesota Multiphasic Personality Inventory study, *Psychosom Med* 56:564–569.

Woerner, PI and Guze, SB (1968) A family and marital study of hysteria, *Br J Psychiatry* 114:161–168.

Woodruff, RA, Clayton, PJ, and Guze, SB (1971) I Hysteria: studies of diagnosis outcome, and prevalence, *JAMA* 215:425–428.

Young, SJ, et al. (1976) Psychiatric illness and the irritable bowel syndrome, *Gastroenterology* 70:162–166.

Zoccolillo, M and Cloninger, CR (1986) Somatization disorder: psychologic symptoms, social disability and diagnosis, *Compr Psychiatry* 27:65–73.

Chapter 18

Aduan, RP, et al. (1979) Factitious fever and self-induced infection: a report of 32 cases and review of the literature, *Ann Intern Med* 90:230–242.

Asher, R (1951) Munchausen's syndrome, *Lancet* 1:339–341.

Barker, JC (1962) The syndrome of hospital addiction (Munchausen syndrome): a report on the investigation of seven cases, *J Ment Sci* 108:167–182.

Bliss, EL (1980) Multiple personalities: a report of 14 cases with implications for schizophrenia and hysteria, *Arch Gen Psychiatry* 37:1388–1397.

Bliss, EL (1986) *Multiple Personality, Allied Disorders, and Hypnosis,* New York, Oxford University Press.

Bowers, MK, Brecher-Marer, S, and Newton, BW (1971) Therapy of multiple personality, *Int J Clin Exp Hypn* 19:57–65.

Braun, BG (1984) Hypnosis creates multiple personality: myth or reality? *Int J Clin Exp Hypn* 32:191–197.

Braun, BG (1984) Towards a theory of multiple personality and other dissociative phenomena, *Psychiatr Clin North Am* 7:171–193.

Bursten, B (1965) On Munchausen's syndrome, *Arch Gen Psychiatry* 13:261–268.

Carney, MWP (1980) Artefactual illness to attract medical attention, *Br J Psychiatry* 136:542–547.

Chapman, JS (1957) Peregrination problem patients—Munchausen's syndrome, *JAMA* 165:927–933.

Clarke, E and Melnick, SC (1958) The Munchausen syndrome or the problem of hospital hoboes, *Am J Med* 25:6–12.

Coons, PM (1980) Multiple personality: diagnostic considerations, *J Clin Psychiatry* 41:330–336.

Coons, PM (1984) The differential diagnosis of multiple personality: a comprehensive review, *Psychiatr Clin North Am* 7:51–67.

Coons, PM (1986) The prevalence of multiple personality disorder, *Newsletter International Society of Study of Multiple Personality Dissociation* 4:6–7.

Coons, PM, Bowman, ES, and Milstein, V (1988) Multiple personality disorder: a clinical investigation of 50 cases, *J Nerv Ment Dis* 175:519–527.

Coryell, W (1983) Single case study: multiple personality and primary affective disorder, *J Nerv Ment Dis* 171:388–390.

Cutler, B and Reed, J (1975) Multiple personality: a single case study with a 15 year follow-up, *Psychol Med* 5:18–26.

Decker, HS: The lure of nonmaterialism in materialist Europe: Investigations of dissociative phenomena, 1880–1915. In Quen, JM (ed.) (1986) *Split Minds/Split Brains: Historical and Current Perspectives,* New York, New York University Press.

Dinwiddie, SH, North, CS, and Yutzy, SH (1993) Multiple personality disorder: scientific and medicolegal issues, *Bull Am Acad Psychiatry Law* 21:69–79.

Eisendrath, SJ: *Factitious Disorder with Physical Symptoms.* In American Psychiatric Association (1989) *Treatments of Psychiatric Disorders: a Task Force Report of the American Psychiatric Association,* Washington, D.C., American Psychiatric Press.

Enoch, MD and Trethowan, WH (1979) *Uncommon Psychiatric Syndromes,* 2nd Edition, Bristol, England, John Wright & Sons.

Fahy, TA, Abas, M, and Brown, JC (1989) Multiple personality: a symptom of psychiatric disorder, *Br J Psychiatry* 154:99–101.

Feighner, JP, et al. (1972) Diagnostic criteria for use in psychiatric research, *Arch Gen Psychiatry* 26:57–62.

Ford, CV (1973) The Munchausen syndrome: a report of four new cases and a review of psychodynamic considerations, *Int J Psychiatry Med* 4:31–45.

Fras, I and Coughlin, BE (1971) The treatment of factitial disease, *Psychosomatics* 12:117–122.

Ganaway, GK (1989) Historical versus narrative truth: clarifying the role of exogenous trauma in the etiology of MPD and its variants, *Dissociation* 2:205–220.

Gorman, CA, Wahner, HW, and Tauxe, WN (1970) Metabolic malingerers: patients who deliberately induce or perpetrate a hypermetabolic or hypometabolic state, *Am J Med* 48:708–714.

Greaves, GB (1980) Multiple personality: 165 years after Mary Reynolds, *J Nerv Ment Dis* 168:577–596.

Gruenewald, D (1977) Multiple personality and splitting phenomena: a reconceptualization, *J Nerv Ment Dis* 164:385–393.

Hacking, I (1991) Two souls in one body, *Crit Inquir,* 17:838–867.

Hawkings, JR, et al. (1956) Deliberate disability, *Br Med J* 1:361–367.

Hollender, MH and Hersh, SP (1970) Impossible consultation made possible, *Arch Gen Psychiatry* 23:343–345.

Horevitz, RP and Braun, BG (1984) Are multiple personalities borderline? An analysis of 33 cases, *Psychiatr Clin North Am* 7:69–87.

Ireland, P, Sapira, JD, and Templeton, B (1967) Munchausen's syndrome: review and report of an additional case, *Am J Med* 43:579–592.

Jonas, JM and Pope, HG (1985) The dissimulating disorders: a single diagnostic entity?, *Compr Psychiatry* 26:58–62.

Kasl, SV, Chisholm, RE, and Eskenazi, B (1981) The impact of the accident at Three Mile Island on the behavior and well-being of nuclear workers, *Am J Pub Health* 71:472–495.

Kluft, RP (1982) Varieties of hypnotic interventions in the treatment of multiple personality, *Am J Clin Hypn* 24:230–240.

Kluft, RP (1984) An introduction to multiple personality disorder, *Psychiatr Ann* 14:19–24.

Kluft, RP (1984) Treatment of multiple personality disorder: a study of 33 cases, *Psychiatr Clin North Am* 7:9–29.

Kluft, RP (1985) Making the diagnosis of multiple personality disorder (MPD), *Dir Psychiatry,* 5:1–12.

Kluft, RP (1988) The postunification treatment of multiple personality disorder: first findings, *Am J Psychother* 42:212–228.

Kluft, RP (1991) Clinical presentations of multiple personality disorder, *Psychiatr Clin North Am* 14:605–629.

Kohlenberg, RJ (1973) Behavioristic approach to multiple personality: a case study, *Behav Ther* 4:137–140.

Meadow, R (1977) Munchausen's syndrome by proxy: the hinterland of child abuse, *Lancet* 2:343–345.

Nadelson, T (1979) The Munchausen spectrum: borderline character features, *Gen Hosp Psychiatry* 1:11–17.

Nijenhuis, ER, et al. (2003) Evidence for associations among somatoform dissociation, psychological dissociation and reported trauma in patients with chronic pelvic pain. *J Psychosom Obstet Gynaecol* 24:87–98.

North, CS, et al. (1993) *Multiple Personalities, Multiple Disorders: Psychiatric Classification and Media Influence,* New York, Oxford University Press.

Pankratz, L (1981) A review of the Munchausen syndrome, *Clin Psychol Rev* 1:65–78.

Patterson, R (1988) The Munchausen syndrome: Baron von Munchausen has taken a bum rap, *Can Med Assoc J* 139:566–569.

Piper, A (1994) Multiple personality disorder, *Br J Psychiatry* 164:600–612.

Piper, A Jr (1994) Treatment for multiple personality disorder: at what cost?, *Am J Psychother* 48:392–400.

Putnam, FW: The scientific investigation of multiple personality disorder. In Quen, JM (ed.) (1986) *Split Minds/Split Brains: Historical and Current Perspectives,* New York, New York University Press.

Putnam, FW (1989) *Diagnosis and Treatment of Multiple Personality Disorder,* New York, Guilford Press.

Putnam, FW (1991) Recent research on multiple personality disorder, *Psychiatr Clin North Am* 14:489–502.

Putnam, FW, et al. (1986) The clinical phenomenology of multiple personality disorder: review of 100 recent cases, *J Clin Psychiatry* 47:285–293.

Raspe, RE, et al. (1948) *Singular Travels, Campaigns, and Adventures of Baron Munchausen*, London, Cresset Press.

Reich, P and Gottfried, LA (1983) Factitious disorders in a teaching hospital, *Ann Intern Med* 99:240–247.

Robins, E and Guze, SB (1970) Establishment of diagnostic validity in psychiatric illness: its application to schizophrenia, *Am J Psychiatry* 126:983–987.

Rogers, R (ed.) (1997) *Clinical Assessment of Malingering and Deception*, 2nd Edition, New York, Guilford Press.

Rosenberg, DA (1987) Web of deceit: a literature review of Munchausen syndrome by proxy, *Child Abuse Negl* 11:547–563.

Ross, CA (1989) *Multiple Personality Disorder. Diagnosis, Clinical Features, and Treatment*, New York, Wiley.

Ross, CA (1991) Epidemiology of multiple personality disorder and dissociation, *Psychiatr Clin North Am* 14:503–517.

Ross, CA, Miller, SD, and Reagor, P (1990) Structured interview data on 102 cases of multiple personality from four centers, *Am J Psychiatry* 147:596–601.

Roth, M (1962) The desire to be ill, *Univ Durham Med Gaz* 57:1–18.

Saltman, V and Solomon, RS (1982) Incest and the multiple personality, *Psychol Rep* 50:1127–1141.

Serban, G (1992) Multiple personality: an issue for forensic psychiatry, *Am J Psychother* 46:269–280.

Sergi, JS, Murray, M, and Cotanch, PH (1989) An understudied population: the homeless, *Oncol Nurs Forum* 16:113–114.

Simpson, MA (1988) Multiple personality disorder (letter), *J Nerv Ment Dis* 176:535.

Sneed, RC and Bell, RF (1976) The dauphin of Munchausen: factitious passage of renal stones in a child, *Pediatrics* 58:127–130.

Spanos, NP, Weekes, JR, and Bertrand, LD (1985) Multiple personality: a social psychological perspective, *J Abnorm Psychol* 94:362–376.

Spiegel, D (1984) Multiple personality as a post-traumatic stress disorder, *Psychiatr Clin North Am* 7:101–110.

Spiro, HR (1968) Chronic factitious illness: Munchausen's syndrome, *Arch Gen Psychiatry* 18:569–579.

Stafne, WA and Moe, AE (1951) Hypoprothrombinemia due to Dicumarol in a malingerer: a case report, *Ann Intern Med* 35:910–911.

Stone, MH (1977) Factitious illness: psychological findings and treatment recommendations, *Bull Menninger Clin* 41:239–254.

Taylor, WS and Martin, MF (1944) Multiple personality, *J Abnorm Soc Psychol* 39:281–300.

Thigpen, CH and Cleckley, HM (1984) On the incidence of multiple personality disorder: a brief communication, *Int J Clin Exp Hypn* 32:63–66.

Wallach, J (1994) Laboratory diagnosis of factitious disorders, *Arch Intern Med* 154:1690–1696.

Chapter 19

American Psychiatric Association (2000) *Diagnostic and Statistical Manual*, 4th Edition, Text Revision. (DSM-IV-TR), Washington, DC, American Psychiatric Association Press.

Bayon, C, Hill, K, et al. (1996) Dimensional assessment of personality in an outpatient sample: Relations of the systems of Millon and Cloninger, *Journal of Psychiatric Research* 30:341–352.

Cloninger, CR (1986) A unified biosocial theory of personality and its role in the development of anxiety states, *Psychiatric Developments* 3:167–226.

Cloninger, CR (1987) A systematic method for clinical description and classification of personality variants: a proposal, *Archives of General Psychiatry* 44:573–587.

Cloninger, CR (1994) Temperament and personality, *Current Opinion in Neurobiology* 4:266–273.

Cloninger, CR (1998) The genetics and psychobiology of the seven factor model of personality. In *The Biology of Personality Disorders*. KR Silk (ed.) Washington, D.C., American Psychiatric Press: 63–84.

Cloninger, CR (1999) A new conceptual paradigm from genetics and psychobiology for the science of mental health, *Australian and New Zealand Journal of Psychiatry* 33:174–186.

Cloninger, CR (ed.) (1999) *Personality and Psychopathology*. Washington, D.C., American Psychiatric Press.

Cloninger, CR (2000) Biology of personality dimensions, *Current Opinions in Psychiatry* 13:611–616.

Cloninger, CR (2002) Functional neuroanatomy and brain imaging of personality and its disorders. In *Biological Psychiatry*. H D'haenen, JA den Boer and P. Willner. Chichester, England, John Wiley & Sons, Ltd. 2:1377–1385.

Cloninger, CR (2003) Completing the psychobiological architecture of human personality development: Temperament, Character, & Coherence. In *Understanding Human Development: Dialogues with lifespan psychology*. UM Staudinger and UER Lindenberger. Boston, Kluwer Academic Publishers: 159–182.

Cloninger, CR, Bayon, C, et al. (1998) Measurement of temperament and character in mood disorders: A model of fundamental states as personality types, *Journal of Affective Disorders* 51:21–32.

Cloninger, CR, Sigvardsson, S, et al. (1988) Childhood personality predicts alcohol abuse in young adults, *Alcoholism: Clinical & Experimental Research* 12:494–505.

Cloninger, CR and Svrakic, DM (1997) Integrative psychobiological approach to psychiatric assessment and treatment, *Psychiatry* 60:120–141.

Cloninger, CR, Svrakic, DM, et al. (1993) A psychobiological model of temperament and character, *Archives of General Psychiatry* 50:975–990.

Cloninger, CR, Svrakic, DM, et al. (1997) Role of personality self-organization in development of mental disorder and disorder, *Development and Psychopathology* 9:881–906.

Cloninger, CR, Sigvardsson, S, Bohman, M, and von Knorring, AL (1982) Predisposition to petty criminality in Swedish adoptees II. Cross-fostering analysis of gene-environment interaction, *Arch Gen Psychiatry* 39:1242–1247.

Cloninger, CR: Antisocial Behavior. In: Smith-Grahame, DG, Hippius, H, Winokur, G (eds) *Psychopharmacology*, vol 1, Excerpta Medica, Amsterdam, 353, 1983.

Cloninger, CR, Svrakic, DM, and Przybeck, TR (1993) A psychobiological model of temperament and character, *Arch Gen Psychiatry* 50:975–990.

Constantino, JN, Cloninger, CR, et al. (2002) Application of the seven-factor model of personality to early childhood, *Psychiatry Research* 109(3):229–243.

Cowdry, RW (1987) Psychopharmacology of borderline personality disorder: A review, *J Clin Psyc* 48:8 (Suppl)15–22.

Cowdry, RW and Gardner, DL (1988) Pharmacotherapy of borderline personality disorder. *Arch Gen Psychiatry* 45:11–119.

Deltito, J and Stam, M (1989) Psychopharmacological treatment of avoidant personality disorder, *Compr Psych* 30(6):498–504.

Derksen, J (1995) *Personality Disorders: Clinical and Social Perspectives*, New York, John Wiley & Sons.

Ekselius, L (1994) *Personality Disorders in the DSM-III-R*. Acta of the University of Uppsala, Dissertation 484.

Faltus, FJ (1984) The positive effects of alprazolam in the treatment of three patients with borderline personality disorder, *Am J Psychiatry* 141:802–803.

Gardner, DL and Cowdry, RW (1989) Pharmacotherapy of borderline personality disorder: An overview, *Psychopharmacology Bull* 25(4):515–523.

Gillespie, NA, Cloninger, CR, et al. (2003) The genetic and environmental relationship between Cloninger's dimensions of temperament and character, *Personality & Individual Differences* 35:1931–1946.

Gusnard, DA, Ollinger, JM, et al. (2003) Persistence and brain circuitry, *Proceedings of the National Academy of Sciences USA* 100(6):3479–3484.

Gusnard, DA, Ollinger, JM, et al. (2001) Personality differences in functional brain imaging, *Society of Neuroscience Abstracts* 27(80):11.

Heath, AC, Cloninger, CR, et al. (1994) Testing a model for the genetic structure of personality: A comparison of the personality systems of Cloninger and Eysenck, *Journal of Personal and Social Psychology* 66:762–775.

Heatherton, TF and Weinberger, JL (eds) (1994) *Can Personality Change?*, Washington, DC, American Psychological Association.

Hedberg, DL, Houck, JH, and Glueck, BC (1971) Tranylcypromine-trifluoperazine combination in the treatment of schizophrenia, *Am J Psychiatr* 127:1141–1146

Joyce, PR, Mulder, RT, et al. (1994) Temperament predicts clomipramine and desipramine response in major depression, *Journal of Affective Disorders* 30:35–46.

Joyce, PR, Mulder, RT, and Cloninger, CR (1994) Temperament and hypercortisolemia in depression, *Am J Psychiatry* 151:195.

Klar, H and Siever, L (1984) The psychopharmacologic treatment of personality disorders, *Psych Clin North Amer* 7(4):791–801.

Klein, D (1968) Psychiatric diagnosis and a typology of clinical drug effects, *Psychopharmacologia* 13:359–386.

Klein, D, Gittelman, R, Quitkin, F, et al. (1980) Clinical management of affective disorders. In: Klein D, Davis J (eds) *Diagnosis and Drug Treatment of Psychiatric Disorders*, Williams & Wilkins, Baltimore.

Liebowitz, MR (1987) Discussions arising from: Cloninger, CR: A unified biosocial model of personality and its role in the development of anxiety states, *Psych Develop* 4:385–387.

Liebowitz, M, Fyer, AJ, Gorman, JM, et al. (1986) Phenelzine in social phobias, *J Clin Psychopharmac* 6:93–98.

Liebowitz, M, Gorman, JM, Fyer, AJ, et al. (1988) Pharmacotherapy of social pphobia: An interim report of a placebo-controlled comparison of phenelzine and atenolol, *J Clin Psychiatry* 49:252–257.

Liebowitz, M and Klein, D (1979) Hysteroid dysphoria. *Psych Clin North Amer* 2(3):555–575.

Links, P, Steiner, M, Bolago, I, et al. (1990) Lithium therapy for borderline patients: Preliminary findings, *J Pers Dis* 4(3):173–181.

Menza, MA, Globe, LI, Cody, RA, and Forman, NE (1993) Dopamine-related personality traits in Parkinson's disease, *Neurology* 43:505–508.

Mulder, RT, Joyce, PR, et al. (1996) Towards an understanding of defense style in terms of temperament and character, *Acta Psychiatrica Scandinavica* 99:99–104.

Myers, JK and Weissman, MM (1980) Use of a self-report symptom scale to detect depression in a community sample, *Am J Psychiatry* 137:1081–1084.

Norden, MJ (1989) Fluoxetine in borderline personality disorder, *Prog Neuropsychopharmacol Biol Psychiatry* 13:885–893.

Parsons, B, Quitkin, F, McGrath, P, et al. (1989) Phenelzine, imipramine, and placebo in borderline patients meeting criteria for atypical depression, *Psychopharmacology Bull* 25(4):524–534.

Radloff, LS (1977) The CES-D scale: A self-report depression scale for research in the general population, *Applied Psychological Measurement* 1:385.

Reich, J and Yates, W (1988) A pilot study of treatment of social phobia with alprazolam. *Am J Psychiatry* 145:590–594.

Reyntjens, AM (1972) A series of multicentric pilot trials with pimozide in psychiatric practice. I Pimozide in treatment of personality disorders, *Acta Psych Belgica* 72:653–661.

Rifkin, A, Quitkin, F, Carrilo, C, et al. (1972) Lithium carbonate in emotionally unstable character disorders, *Arch Gen Psychiatry* 27:519–523.

Robins, L (1966) *Deviant Children Grown Up: A Sociological and Psychiatric Study of Sociopathic Personality*, Baltimore, Williams & Wilkins.

Selzer, ML, Vinokur, A, and van Rooijen, L (1975) A self-administered short michigan alcoholism screening Test (SMAST), *J Studies Alcohol* 36:117–126.

Sheard, MH (1976) Lithium in the treatment of aggression, *J Nerv Ment Dis* 160:108–112.

Sheard, MH, Marini, JL, Bridges, CI, et al. (1976) The effect of lithium on impulsive aggressive behavior in man, *Am J Psychiatry* 133:1409–1412.

Sheehan, DV, Ballenger, J, and Jacobson, G (1980) Treatment of endogenous anxiety with phobic hysterical and hypochondriacal symptoms, *Arch Gen Psychiatry* 37:51–59.

Siassi, I (1982) Lithium treatment of impulsive behavior in children, *J Clin Psych* 43:482–484.

Sigvardsson, S, Bohman, M, et al. (1987) Structure and stability of childhood personality: prediction of later social adjustment, *Journal of Child Psychology and Psychiatry* 28:929–946.

Soloff, P (1990) What's new in personality disorders? An update on pharmacologic treatment, *J Pers Dis* 4(3):233–243.

Soloff, P: Psychopharmacologic therapies in borderline personality disorder. In Tasman, A, Hales, E, Frances, A (eds) (1989) *American Psychiatric Press Review of Psychiatry*, vol. 8, pp. 65–83.

Soloff, P, George, A, Nathan, RS, et al. (1989) Amitriptyline versus Haloperidol in borderlines: final outcomes and predictors of response, *J Clin Psychopharmacol* 9:238–246.

Soloff, PH, George, A, Nathan, RS, et al. (1986) Paradoxical effects of amitriptyline in borderline patients, *Am J Psychiatry* 143:1603–1605.

Stallings, MC, Hewitt, JK, et al. (1996) Genetic and environmental structure of the Tridimensional Personality Questionnaire: three or four temperament dimensions?, *Journal of Personal and Social Psychology* 70:127–140.

Stewart, AL, Hays, RD, and Ware, JE Jr (1988) The Medical Outcome Study (MOS) short-form General Health Survey: Reliability and validity in a patient population, *Med Care* 26:724–735.

Stringer, AY and Josef, NC (1983) Methylphenidate in the treatment of aggression in two patients with antisocial personality disorder, *Am J Psychiatry* 140:1365–1366.

Svrakic, DM, Whitehead, C, et al. (1993) Differential diagnosis of personality disorders by the seven factor model of temperament and character, *Arch Gen Psychiatry* 50:991–999.

Svrakic, NM, Svrakic, DM, et al. (1996) A general quantitative theory of personality development: Fundamentals of a self-organizing psychobiological complex, *Development and Psychopathology* 8:247–272.

Thapar, A and McGuffin, P (1993) Is personality disorder inherited? An overview of the evidence, *J Psychopathology Behav Assessment* 15:325.

Tome, MB, Cloninger, CR, et al. (1997) Serotonergic autoreceptor blockade in the reduction of antidepressant latency: personality and response to paroxetine and pindolol, *Journal of Affective Disorders* 44:101–109.

Vedeniapin, AB, Anokhin, AA, et al. (2001) Visual P300 and the self-directedness scale of the temperament-character inventory, *Psychiatry Research* 101:145–156.

Zuckerman, M and Cloninger, CR (1996) Relationships between Cloninger's, Zuckerman's, and Eysenck's dimensions of personality, *Personality & Individual Differences* 21:283–285.

Chapter 20

Abenhaim, L (1992) Study of civilian victims of terrorist attacks (France 1982–1987), *J Epidemiol* 45:103–109.

Archibald, HC and Tuddenham, RD (1965) Persistent stress reaction after combat, *Arch Gen Psychiatry* 12:475–481.

Bass, E and Davis, L (1992) *The Courage to Heal: A Guide for Women Survivors of Child Sexual Abuse*, New York, Harper Perennial.

Bremner, JD, et al. (1992) Dissociation and post-traumatic stress disorder in Vietnam combat veterans, *Am J Psychiatry* 149:328–332.

Breslau, N and Davis, GC (1992) Posttraumatic stress disorder in an urban population of young adults: risk factors for chronicity, *Am J Psychiatry* 149:671–675.

Breslau, N, et al. (1991) Traumatic events and posttraumatic stress disorder in an urban population of young adults, *Arch Gen Psychiatry* 48:216–222.

Briere, A, et al. (1987) Controllable and uncontrollable stress in humans: alterations in mood and neuroendocrine and psychophysiological function, *Am J Psychiatry* 144:1419–1425.

Buydens-Branchey, L, Noumair, D, and Branchey, M (1990) Duration and intensity of combat exposure and posttraumatic stress disorder in Vietnam veterans, *J Nerv Ment Dis* 178:582–587.

Centers for Disease Control (1988) Health status of Vietnam veterans. I. Psychosocial characteristics, *JAMA* 259:2701–2708.

Chambers, RA, et al. (1999) Glutamate and posttraumatic stress disorder: toward a psychobiology of dissociation, *Sem Clin Neuropsychiatry* 4:274–281.

Cottler, LB, et al. (1992) Posttraumatic stress disorder among substance users from the general population, *Am J Psychiatry* 149:664–670.

Davidson, J, et al. (1985) A diagnostic and family study of posttraumatic stress disorder, *Am J Psychiatry* 142:90–93.

Dobbs, D and Wilson, WP (1960) Observations on persistence of war neurosis, *Dis Nerv Sys* 21:686–691.

Dodge, KA, Bates, JE, and Pettit, GS (1990) Mechanisms in the cycle of violence, *Science* 250:1678–1683.

Engdahl, BE, et al. (1991) Comorbidity of psychiatric disorders and personality profiles of American World War II prisoners of war, *J Nerv Ment Dis* 179:181–187.

Epstein, RS (1989) Posttraumatic stress disorder: a review of diagnostic and treatment issues, *Psychiatr Ann* 19:556–563.

Friedman, MJ (1988) Toward rational pharmacotherapy for posttraumatic stress disorder: an interim report, *Am J Psychiatry* 145:281–285.

Green, BL (1990) Defining traumas: terminology and generic stressor dimensions, *J Appl Soc Psychology* 20:1632–1641.

Green, BL, et al. (1990) Buffalo Creek survivors in the second decade: stability of stress symptoms, *Am J Orthopsychiatry* 60:43–54.

Helzer, JE, Robins, LN, and McEvoy, L (1987) Posttraumatic stress disorder in the general population, *New Engl J Med* 317:1630–1634.

Horowitz, MJ (1985) Disasters and psychological responses to stress, *Psychiatr Ann* 15:161–167.

Institute of Medicine (2003) *Preparing for the Psychological Consequences of Terrorism: A Public Health Strategy*. Washington, DC: National Academy of Science.

Javitt, DC, and Zukin, SR (1991) Recent advances in the phencyclidine model of schizophrenia. *Am J Psychiatry* 148:1301–1308.

Kolb, LC (1987) A neuropsychological hypothesis explaining posttraumatic stress disorders, *Am J Psychiatry* 144:989–995.

Kolb, LC (1993) The psychobiology of PTSD: perspectives and reflections on the past, present, and future, *J Traum Stress* 6, 293–304.

Kramer, M and Kinney, L (1985) Is sleep a marker of vulnerability to delayed posttraumatic stress disorder?, *Sleep Res* 14:181.

Kramer, M, Kinney, L, and Scharf, M (1982) Sleep in delayed stress victims, *Sleep Res* 11:113.

Krause, N (1987) Exploring the impact of a natural disaster on the health and psychological well-being of older adults, *J Hum Stress* 2:61–69.

Lavie, P, et al. (1979) Long-term effects of traumatic war-related events on sleep, *Am J Psychiatry* 136:175–178.

Madakasira, S and O'Brien, KF (1987) Acute posttraumatic stress disorder in victims of a natural disaster, *J Nerv Ment Dis* 175:286–290.

Mason, JW, et al. (1988) Elevation of urinary norepinephrine-cortisol ratio in posttraumatic stress disorder, *J Nerv Ment Dis* 176:498–502.

McCaffrey, RJ, Hickling, EJ, and Marrazo, MJ (1989) Civilian-related posttraumatic stress disorder: assessment-related issues, *J Clin Psychology* 45:72–76.

McCarroll, JE, et al. (1993) Handling bodies after violent death: strategies for coping, *Am J Orthopsychiatry* 63:209–214.

Mitchell, JT (1988) Stress: development and functions of a critical incident stress debriefing team, *J Emerg Med Serv* 13:42–46.

Mullen, PE, et al. (1993) Childhood sexual abuse and mental health in adult life, *Br J Psychiatry* 163:721–732.

Norris, FH (1992) Epidemology of trauma: frequency and impact of different potentially traumatic events on different demographic groups, *J Cons Clin Psychology* 60:409–418.

North, CS (1995) Human response to violent trauma, *Balliere's Clin Psychiatry* 1:225–245.

North, CS, et al. (1999) Psychiatric disorders among survivors of the Oklahoma City bombing, *JAMA* 282:755–762.

North, CS, Smith, EM, and Spitznagel, EL (1994) Posttraumatic stress disorder in survivors of a mass shooting, *Am J Psychiatry* 151:82–88.

North, CS, Tivis, L, McMillen, JC, Pfefferbaum, B, Spitznagel, EL, Cox, J, Nixon, S, Bunch, KP, and Smith, EM (2002) Psychiatric disorders in rescue workers after the Oklahoma City bombing, *Am J Psychiatry*, 159:857–859.

North, CS and Pfefferbaum, B (2002) Research on the mental health effects of terrorism, *JAMA*, 288:633–636.

Pitman, RK, et al. (1990) Naloxone-reversible analgesic response to combat-related stimuli in posttraumatic stress disorder. A pilot study, *Arch Gen Psychiatry* 47:541–544.

Ramsay, R (1990) Posttraumatic stress disorder: a new clinical entity?, *J Psychosom Res* 34:355–365.

Robert, JA, et al. (1985) MCMI characteristics of DSM-III posttraumatic stress disorder in Vietnam veterans, *J Pers Assess* 49:226–230.

Robins, LN (1990) Steps toward evaluating posttraumatic stress reaction as a psychiatric disorder, *J Appl Soc Psychology* 20:1674–1677.

Rubonis, AV and Bickman, L (1991) Psychological impairment in the wake of disaster: the disaster-psychopathology relationship, *Psychol Bull* 109:384–399.

Schlossberg, A and Benjamin, M (1978) Sleep patterns in three acute combat fatigue cases, *J Clin Psychiatry* 39:546–549.

Shalev, A (2000) Auditory startle response in trauma survivors with posttraumatic stress disorder: a prospective study, *Am J Psychiatry* 157:255–261.

Shore, JH, Tatum, EL, and Vollmer, WM: The Mount St. Helens stress response syndrome. In Shore, JH (ed.) (1986) *Disaster Stress Studies: New Methods and Findings* (pp. 77–97), Washington, D.C., American Psychiatric Press.

Sierles, FS, et al. (1986) Concurrent psychiatric illness in non-Hispanic outpatients diagnosed as having posttraumatic stress disorder, *J Nerv Ment Dis* 174:171–173.

Smith, EM and North, CS: Posttraumatic stress disorder in natural disasters and technological accidents. In Wilson, JP, Raphael, B (eds) (1993) *International Handbook of Traumatic Stress Syndromes*, New York, Plenum Press.

Smith, EM, et al. Psychosocial consequences of a disaster. In Shore, JH (ed.) (1986) *Disaster Stress Studies: New Methods and Findings*, Washington, D.C., American Psychiatric Press.

Solomon, SD and Canino, GJ (1990) Appropriateness of DSM-III-R criteria for posttraumatic stress disorder, *Compr Psychiatry* 31:227–237.

Solomon, SD, et al. (1987) Social involvement as a mediator of disaster-induced stress, *J Appl Soc Psychology* 17:1092–1112.

Southwick, SM, et al. (1999) Neurotransmitter alterations in PTSD: catecholamines and serotonin, *Sem Clin Neuropsychiatry* 4:242–248.

Southwick, SM, Yehuda, R, and Giller, EL (1993) Personality disorders in treatment-seeking combat veterans with posttraumatic stress disorder, *Am J Psychiatry* 150:1020–1023.

Southwick, SM, et al. (1993) Trauma-related symptoms in veterans of Operation Desert Storm: a preliminary report, *Am J Psychiatry* 150:1524–1528.

Spiegel, D (1984) Multiple personality as a posttraumatic stress disorder, *Psychiatr Clin North Am* 7:101–110.

Steinberg, D (2001) Understanding stress disorder takes on urgency, *Scientist* 15:1.

Sutker, PB, Allain, AN, and Winstead, DK (1993) Psychopathology and psychiatric diagnoses of World War II Pacific theater prisoner of war survivors and combat veterans, *Am J Psychiatry* 150:240–245.

Watson, IPB, Hoffman, L, and Wilson, GV (1988) The neuropsychiatry of posttraumatic stress disorder, *Br J Psychiatry* 152:164–173.

Yehuda, R, et al. (1991) Lymphocyte glucocorticoid receptor number in posttraumatic stress disorder, *Am J Psychiatry* 148:499–504.

Chapter 21

American Heritage Dictionary of English Language (1996) 3rd Edition, Boston, Houghton Mifflin.

Barlow, DH (2001) *Clinical Handbook of Psychological Disorders: a step-by-step treatment manual*, 3rd Edition, New York, Guilford Press.

Bloom, BL (1997) *Planned Short-term Psychotherapy: A clinical handbook*, 2nd Edition, Boston, Pearson Allyn & Bacon.

Dewald, PA (1973) *Psychotherapy: a dynamic approach*, New York, Basic Books Inc., Publishers.

Dorland's Illustrated Medical Dictionary, 28th Edition, Philadelphia, 1994, W.B. Saunders.

Egan, G (2002) *The Skilled Helper—a problem-management and opportunity-development approach to helping*, 7th Edition, Monterey, CA, Brooks/Cole Publishing Company.

Guze, SB (1992) *Why Psychiatry is a Branch of Medicine*, New York, Oxford University Press.

Insel, TR and Charnet, DS (2003) Research on major depression: strategies and priorities, *JAMA* 289:3167–3168.

Lipkin, M, Putnam, SM, and Lazare, A (1995) *The Medical Interview: Clinical care, education, and research*, New York, Springer-Verlag.

Lustman, PJ and Clouse, RE (2002) Treatment of depression in diabetes: impact on mood and medical outcome, *J Psychosom Res* 52:917–924.

Nathan, PE and Gorman, JM (2002) *A Guide to Treatments That Work*, 2nd Edition, New York, Oxford University Press.

Oxford English Dictionary, 2nd Edition, Oxford, 1989, Oxford University Press.

Rosenzweig, S (1951) Idiodynamics in personality theory with special reference to projective methods, *Psychological Review* 58:213–223.

Spiegler, MD and Guevremont, DC (2003) *Contemporary Behavior Therapy*, 4th Edition, Pacific Grove, CA, Brooks/Cole Publishing Company.

Chapter 22

Allison, DB, Mentore, JL, Heo, M, Chandler, LP, Cappelleri, JC, Infante, MC, and Weiden, PJ (1999) Antipsychotic-induced weight gain: A comprehensive research synthesis, *Am J Psychiatry* 156:1686–1696.

Arana, GW and Rosenbaum, JF (2000) *Handbook of Psychiatric Drug Therapy*, 4th Edition, Philadelphia, Lippincott, Williams & Wilkins. (Note: the 5th edition of this text is scheduled to be released May 2005.)

Bruce, SE, Vasile, RG, Goisman, RM, Salzman, C, Spencer, M, Machan, JT, and Keller, MB (2003) Are benzodiazepines still the medication of choice for patients with panic disorder with or without agoraphobia?, *Am J Psychiatry* 160:1432–1438.

Csernansky, JG, Brenner, R, Mahmoud, R, and the RIS-79 Study Group (2002) Reducing relapse rates in schizophrenia: A long-term double-blind comparison of risperidone and haloperidol, *New Eng J Med*, 346:16–22.

Davis, JM, Chen, N, and Glick, ID (2003) A meta-analysis of the efficacy of second-generation antipsychotics, *Arch Gen Psychiatry* 60:553–564.

Keck, PE, Nelson, EB, and McElroy, SL (2003) Advances in the treatment of bipolar depression, *Biol Psychiatry* 53:671–679.

Schatzberg, AF and Nemeroff, CB (2004) *The American Psychiatric Publishing Textbook of Psychopharmacology*, 3rd Edition, Washington DC, American Psychiatric Publishing.

Tohen, M, Vieta, E, Calabrese, J, Ketter, TA, Sachs, G, Bowden, C, Mitchell, PB, Centorrino, F, Risser, R, Baker, RW, Evans, AR, Beymer, K, Dube, S, Tollefson, GD, and Breier, A (2003) Efficacy of olanzapine and olanzapine-fluoxetine combination in the treatment of bipolar I depression, *Arch Gen Psychiatry* 60:1079–1088.

Chapter 23

Abrams, R (2000) *Electroconvulsive Therapy*, 4th Edition, New York, 2002, Oxford University Press.

American Psychiatric Association (2002) Practice guideline for the treatment of patients with major depressive disorder, 2nd Edition, *Am J Psychiatry* 157:(4 suppl):1–45.

American Psychiatric Association (2002) Practice guideline for the treatment of patients with bipolar disorder, 2nd Edition, *Am J Psychiatry* 159 (4 suppl):1–50.

American Psychiatric Association, Committee on Electroconvulsive Therapy (2001) *The Practice of Electroconvulsive Therapy: recommendations for treatment, training and privileging*, 2nd Edition, Washington D.C., American Psychiatric Association.

Devanand, DP, Dwork, AJ, Hutchinson, ER, Bolwig, TG, and Sackeim, HA (1994) Does ECT alter brain structure? *Am J Psychiatry* 151:957–970.

George, MS, Nahas, Z, Kozel, FA, Li, X, Denslow, S, Yamanaka, K, Mishory, A, Foust, MJ, and Bohning, DE (2002) Mechanisms and state of the art of transcranial magnetic stimulation, *J ECT* 18:170–181.

Gershon, AA, Dannon, PN, and Grunhaus, L (2003) Transcranial magnetic stimulation in the treatment of depression, *Am J Psychiatry* 160:835–845.

Hoffman, RE, Hawkins, KA, Gueorguieva, R, Boutros, NN, Rachid, F, Carroll, K, and Krystal, JH (2003) Transcranial magnetic stimulation of left temporoparietal cortex and medication-resistant auditory hallucinations, *Arch Gen Psychiatry* 60:49–56.

Lafferty, JE, North, CS, Spitznagel, E, and Isenberg, K (2001) Laboratory screening prior to ECT, *J ECT* 17:158–165.

Lisanby, SH, Maddox, JH, Prudic, J, Devanand, DP, and Sackeim, HA (2000) The effects of electroconvulsive therapy on memory of autobiographical and public events, *Arch Gen Psychiatry* 57:581–590.

McCall, WV, Reboussin, DM, Weiner, RD, and Sackeim, HA (2000) Titrated moderately suprathreshold vs. fixed high-dose right unilateral electroconvulsive therapy: acute antidepressant and cognitive effects, *Arch Gen Psychiatry* 57:438–444.

Mukherjee, S, Sackeim, HA, and Schnur, DB (1994) Electroconvulsive therapy of acute manic episodes: a review of 50 years' experience, *Am J Psychiatry* 151:169–176.

Sackeim, HA, Haskett, RF, Mulsant, BH, Thase, ME, Mann, JJ, Pettinati, HM, Greenberg, RM, Crowe, RR, Cooper, TB, and Prudic, J (2001) Continuation pharmacotherapy in the prevention of relapse following electroconvulsive therapy: a randomized controlled trial, *JAMA* 285:1299–1307.

Sackeim, HA, Long, J, Luber, B, Moeller, JR, Prohovnik, I, Devanand, DP, and Nobler, MS (1994) Physical properties and quantification of the ECT stimulus: I. Basic principles, *Convulsive Ther* 10:93–123.

Sackeim, HA, Prudic, H, Devanand, DP, Kiersky, JE, Fitzsimons, L, Moody, BJ, McElhiney, MC, Coleman, EA, and Settembrino, JM (1993) Effects of stimulus intensity and electrode placement on the efficacy and cognitive effects of electroconvulsive therapy, *N Engl J Med* 328:839–846.

Sackeim, HA, Prudic, H, Devanand, DP, Nobler, MS, Lisanby, SH, Peyser, S, Fitzsimons, L, Moody, BJ, and Clark, J (2000) A prospective, randomized, double-blind comparison of bilateral and right unilateral electroconvulsive therapy at different stimulus intensities, *Arch Gen Psychiatry* 57:425–434.

Schwarz, T, Loewenstein, J, and Isenberg, KE (1995) Maintenance ECT: indications and outcome, *Convulsive Ther* 11:14–23.

UK ECT Review Group (2003) Efficacy and safety of electroconvulsive therapy in depressive disorders: a systematic review and meta-analysis, *Lancet* 361:799–808.

Chapter 24

Anonymous (1995) Statement on use of apolipoprotein E testing for Alzheimer's disease. American College of Medical Genetics/American Society of Human Genetics Working Group on ApoE and Alzheimer's disease, *JAMA*, 274:1627–1629.

Ansell, SM, Ackerman, MJ, Black, JL, et al. (2003) Primer on medical genomics. Part VI: Genomics and molecular genetics in clinical practice, *Mayo Clinic Proceedings* 78:307–317.

Badano, JL and Katsanis, N (2002) Beyond Mendel: an evolving view of human genetic disease transmission, *Nature Reviews Genetics* 3:779–789.

Biesecker, BB (2001) Goals of genetic counseling, *Clinical Genetics*, 60:323–330.

Biesecker, BB and Peters, KF (2001) Process studies in genetic counseling: peering into the black box, *American Journal of Medical Genetics* 106:191–198.

Boomsma, D, Busjahn, A, and Peltonen, L (2002) Classical twin studies and beyond, *Nature Reviews Genetics* 3:872–882.

Burke, W and Emery, J (2002) Genetics education for primary-care providers, *Nature Reviews Genetics* 3:561–566.

Ciarleglio, LJ, Bennett, RL, Williamson, J, et al. (2003) Genetic counseling throughout the life cycle, *Journal of Clinical Investigation* 112:1280–1286.

Collins, FS, Green, ED, Guttmacher, AE, et al. (2003) A vision for the future of genomics research, *Nature* 422:835–847.

Collins, FS, Guttmacher, AE (2001) Genetics moves into the medical mainstream, *JAMA* 286:2322–2324.

Cooper, B (2001) Nature, nurture and mental disorder: old concepts in the new millennium, *British Journal of Psychiatry* 178 (Suppl 40):S91–S101.

Craddock, N and Jones, I (1999) Genetics of bipolar disorder, *Journal of Medical Genetics* 36:585–594.

Desmond, DW, Moroney, JT, Lynch, T, et al. (1999) The natural history of CADASIL: a pooled analysis of previously published cases [see comment], *Stroke* 30:1230–1233.

Ensenauer, RE, Reinke, SS, Ackerman, MJ, et al. (2003) Primer on medical genomics. Part VIII: Essentials of medical genetics for the practicing physician, *Mayo Clinic Proceedings* 78:846–857.

Guttmacher, AE and Collins, FS (2002) Genomic medicine—a primer [see comment], *New England Journal of Medicine* 347:1512–1520.

Insel, TR and Collins, FS (2003) Psychiatry in the genomics era, *American Journal of Psychiatry* 160:616–620.

Joutel, A, Corpechot, C, Ducros, A, et al. (1996) Notch3 mutations in CADASIL, a hereditary adult-onset condition causing stroke and dementia [see comment] *Nature* 383:707–710.

Joyce, CA, Dennis, NR, Cooper, S, et al. (2001) Subtelomeric rearrangements: results from a study of selected and unselected probands with idiopathic mental retardation and control individuals by using high-resolution G-banding and FISH, *Human Genetics* 109:440–451.

Liddell, MB, Lovestone, S, and Owen, MJ (2001) Genetic risk of Alzheimer's disease: advising relatives [see comment], *British Journal of Psychiatry* 178:7–11.

Lindsay, EA (2001) Chromosomal microdeletions: dissecting del22q11 syndrome, *Nature Reviews Genetics* 2:858–868.

Pardanani, A, Wieben, ED, Spelsberg, TC, et al. (2002) Primer on medical genomics. Part IV: Expression proteomics, *Mayo Clinic Proceedings* 77:1185–1196.

Post, SG, Whitehouse, PJ, Binstock, RH, et al. (1997) The clinical introduction of genetic testing for Alzheimer's disease. An ethical perspective [see comment], *JAMA* 277:832–836.

Roses, AD (1997) Genetic testing for Alzheimer's disease. Practical and ethical issues, *Archives of Neurology* 54:1226–1229.

Scheuner, MT, Wang, SJ, Raffel, LJ, et al. (1997) Family history: a comprehensive genetic risk assessment method for the chronic conditions of adulthood, *American Journal of Medical Genetics* 71:315–324.

Tabor, HK, Risch, NJ, and Myers, RM (2002) Opinion: Candidate-gene approaches for studying complex genetic traits: practical considerations, *Nature Reviews Genetics* 3:391–397.

Yoon, PW, Olney, RS, Khoury, MJ, et al. (1997) Contribution of birth defects and genetic diseases to pediatric hospitalizations. A population-based study [see comment], *Archives of Pediatrics & Adolescent Medicine* 151:1096–1103.

Yoon, PW, Scheuner, MT, and Khoury, MJ (2003) Research priorities for evaluating family history in the prevention of common chronic diseases, *American Journal of Preventive Medicine* 24:128–135.

Yoon, PW, Scheuner, MT, Peterson-Oehlke, KL, et al. (2002) Can family history be used as a tool for public health and preventive medicine? *Genetics in Medicine* 4:304–310.

Chapter 25

Barkley, RA, et al. (1990) The adolescent outcome of hyperactive children diagnosed by research criteria. I. An 8-year prospective follow-up study, *J Am Acad Child Adolesc Psychiatry* 26:317–325.

Brent, DA, et al. (1993) Psychiatric risk factors for adolescent suicide: a case control study, *J Am Acad Child Adolesc Psychiatry* 32:521–529.

Cicchetti, D and Toth, SL (1995) A developmental psychopathology perspective on child abuse and neglect, *J Am Acad Child Adolesc Psychiatry* 34:541–565.

Costello, EJ, et al. (1988) Psychopathology in pediatric primary care: the new hidden morbidity, *Pediatrics* 82:415–424.

Costello, EJ, et al. (1993) How can epidemiology improve mental health services for children and adolescents? *J Am Acad Child Adolesc Psychiatry* 32:1106–1113.

Emslie, GJ, et al. (2002) Fluoxetine for acute treatment of depression in children and adolescents: a placebo-controlled, randomized clinical trial, *J Am Acad Child Adolesc Psychiatry* 41(10):1205–1215.

Glowinski, AL, et al. (2003) Genetic epidemiology of self-reported lifetime DSM-IV major depressive disorder in a population-based twin sample of female adolescents, *J Child Psychol Psychiatry* 44(7):988–986.

Hacker, DJ (1994) An existential view of adolescence, *J Early Adolesc* 14(3):300–327.

Henggeler, SW, et al. (2003) One-year follow-up of multisystemic therapy as an alternative to the hospitalization of youths in psychiatric crisis, *J Am Acad Child Adolesc Psychiatry* 42(5):543–551.

Jones, MB and Offord, DR (1989) Reduction in antisocial behavior in poor children by non-school skill-development, *J Child Psychol Psychiatry* 30:737–750.

Kazdin, AE (ed.) (1987) *Conduct disorders in childhood and adolescence*, Newbury Park, Calif., Sage.

Kazdin, AE (1993) Adolescent mental health: prevention and treatment programs, *Am Psychol* 48:127–141.

Kazdin, AE (2000) Treatments for aggressive and antisocial children, *Child Adolesc Psychiatr Clin N Am* 9(4):841–58.

Kovacs, M, Ho, V, and Pollock, MH (1995) Criterion and predictive validity of the diagnosis of adjustment disorder: a prospective study of youths with new-onset insulin-dependent diabetes mellitus, *Am J Psychiatry* 152:523–528.

Kovacs, M, et al. (1984) Depressive disorders in childhood, *Arch Gen Psychiatry* 41:229–237.

Kramer, TL, et al. (2003) Detection and outcomes of substance use disorders in adolescents seeking mental health treatment, *J Am Acad Child Adolesc Psychiatry* 42(11):1318–1326.

Leonard, HL, (ed.) (1993) Anxiety disorders, *Child Adolesc Psychiatr Clin North Am* 2:563–838.

Lewis, DO (1992) From abuse to violence: psychophysiological consequences of maltreatment, *J Am Acad Child Adolesc Psychiatry* 31:383–391.

Mannuzza, S, et al. (1993) Adult outcome of hyperactive boys: educational achievement, occupational rank, and psychiatric status, *Arch Gen Psychiatry* 50:565–576.

Martin, A, Scahill, L, Charney, DS, Leckman, JT (eds) (2003) *Pediatric Psychopharmacology: Principles and Practice*, New York, Oxford.

Mattison, RE and Spitznagel, EL (1999) Long-term stability of Child Behavior Checklist profile types in a child psychiatric clinic population, *J Am Acad Child Adolesc Psychiatry* 38:700–707.

McConaughy, SH (1993) Evaluating behavioral and emotional disorders with the CBCL, TRF, and YSR cross-informant scales, *J Emotion Behav Disord* 1:40–52.

Offer, D and Schonert-Reich, KA (1992) Debunking the myths of adolescence: findings from recent research, *J Am Acad Child Adolesc Psychiatry* 31:1003–1014.

Reiff, MI, et al. (2003) Attention-deficit/hyperactivity disorder evaluation and diagnosis: a practical approach in office practice, *Pediatr Clin North Am* 50(5):1019–1048.

Rotheram-Borus, MJ, et al. (1994) Brief cognitive-behavioral treatment for adolescent suicide attempters and their families, *J Am Acad Child Adolesc Psychiatry* 33:508–517.

Shaffer, D, et al. (1988) Preventing teenager suicide: a critical review, *J Am Acad Child Adolesc Psychiatry* 27:675–687.

Wilson, MD and Joffe, A (1995) Adolescent medicine, *JAMA* 273:1657–1659.

Chapter 26

Barraclough, BM (1971) Suicide in the elderly, *Br J Psychiatry* (Special supplement 6, Recent Developments in Psychogeriatrics):87–97.

Blank, K and Duffy, JD (2000) Medical therapies. In Coffey, CE, Cummings, JL (eds) *The American Psychiatric Press Textbook of Geriatric Neuropsychiatry*, 2nd Edition, Washington, D.C., American Psychiatric Press.

Blazer, DG, Bachar, JR, and Manton, KG (1986) Suicide in late life. Review and commentary, *J Am Geriatr Soc* 34:519–525.

Blumenthal, SJ and Kupfer, DJ (eds) (1990) *Suicide Over the Life Cycle: Risk factors, assessment, and treatment of suicidal patients*, Washington, D.C., American Psychiatric Press, Inc.

Conwell, Y (1997) Management of suicidal behavior in the elderly, *Psychiatr Clin North Am* 20:667–683.

Copeland, AR (1987) Suicide among the elderly—The Metro-Dade County experience, 1981–83, *Med Sci Law* 27:32–36.

Cummings, JL and Cole, G (2002) Alzheimer disease, *JAMA* 287:2335–2338.

Drevets, WC and Rubin, EH (1989) Psychotic symptoms and the longitudinal course of senile dementia of the Alzheimer type, *Biol Psychiatry* 25:39–48.

Drevets, WC, et al. (1992) A functional anatomical study of unipolar depression, *J Neurosci* 12:3628–3641.

Federal Interagency Forum on Aging-Related Statistics (2000) Older Americans 2000: key indicators of well-being. Federal Interagency Forum on Aging-Related Statistics, Washington, DC, Government Printing Office, August. http://www.agingstats.gov/chartbook2000/default.htm, accessed 12/11/03.

Folstein, MF, Folstein, SE, and McHugh, PR (1975) 'Mini-mental state.' A practical method for grading the cognitive state of patients for the clinician, *J Psychiatr Res* 12:189–198.

Foster, JR (1988) Normal aging—biological aspects. In Lazarus, LW (ed.) *Essentials of Geriatric Psychiatry. A guide for health professionals*, New York, Springer Publishing Company.

Frasure-Smith, N, Lesperance, F, and Talajic, M (1993) Depression following myocardial infarction, *JAMA* 270:1819–1825.

Gazini, L, Nelson, HD, Schmidt, TA, Kraemer, DF, Delorit, MA, and Lee, MA (2000) Physicians' experiences with the Oregon Death with Dignity Act, *N Engl J Med* 342:557–563.

Greenblatt, D (1993) Basic pharmacokinetic principles and their application to psychotropic drugs, *J Clin Psychiatry* 54:9(suppl)8–13.

Hirano, A and Llena, J: Structure of neurons in the aging nervous system. In Calne, D (ed.) (1994) *Neurodegenerative Diseases*, Philadelphia, W. B. Saunders Company.

Katz, IR (1998) Diagnosis and treatment of depression in patients with Alzheimer's disease and other dementias, *J Clin Psychiatry* 59(suppl 9):38–44.

Katzman, R, et al. (1983) Validation of a short orientation-memory-concentration test of cognitive impairment, *Am J Psychiatry* 140:734–739:1542.

Kay, DWK, Cooper, AF, Garside, RF, and Roth, M (1976) The differentiation of paranoid from affective psychoses by patients' premorbid characteristics, *Br J Psychiatry* 129:207–215.

Kelly, BD and McLoughlin, DM (2002) Euthanasia, assisted suicide and psychiatry: a Pandora's box, *Br J Psychiatry* 181:278–279.

Levanthal, EA: Biology of Aging. In Sadavoy, J, Lazarus, LW, Jarvik, LF, Grossberg, GT (eds) (1996) *Comprehensive Review of Geriatric Psychiatry—II*, 2nd Edition, Washington, D.C., American Psychiatric Press.

Lieberman, A (1998) Managing the neuropsychiatric symptoms of Parkinson's disease, *Neurology* 50(suppl 6):S33–S38.

Lustman, PJ, et al. (1992) Depression in adults with diabetes, *Diabetes Care* 15:1631–1639.

Lyness, JM, King, DA, Cox, C, Yoediono, Z, and Caine, ED (1999) The importance of subsyndromal depression in older primary care patients: prevalence and associated functional disability, *J Am Geriatr Soc* 47:647–652.

Malmgren, R (2000) Epidemiology of aging. In Coffey, CE, Cummings, JL (eds) *The American Psychiatric Press Textbook of Geriatric Neuropsychiatry*, 2nd Edition, Washington, D.C., American Psychiatric Press.

McIntosh, JL (1992) Epidemiology of suicide in the elderly. In *Suicide and life-threatening behavior*, vol 22(1), Spring, The American Association of Suicidology.

McKeith, IG (2002) Dementia with Lewy bodies, *Br J Psychiatry* 180:144–147.

Miller, M (1979) *Suicide After Sixty. The final alternative*, New York, Springer Publishing Company.

Morris, JC (2000) The nosology of dementia, *Neurol Clin* 18:773–788.

Pearlson, GD: Late-life-onset psychoses. In Coffey, CE, Cummings, JL (eds) (2000) *The American Psychiatric Press Text-*

book of Geriatric Neuropsychiatry, 2nd Edition, Washington, D.C., American Psychiatric Press.

Powers, RE: Neurobiology of aging. In Coffey, CE, Cummings, JL (ed) (2000) *The American Psychiatric Textbook of Geriatric Neuropsychiatry*, 2nd Edition, Washington, D.C., American Psychiatric Press.

Preskorn, S (1993) Pharmacokinetics of antidepressants: why and how they are relevant to treatment, *J Clin Psychiatry* 54:9(suppl)14–33.

Robins, E (1981) *The Final Months*. New York, Oxford University Press.

Rubin, EH, et al. (1991) The influence of major depression on clinical and psychometric assessment of senile dementia of the Alzheimer type, *Am J Psychiatry* 148:1164–1171.

Rubin, EH: Depression and dementia. In Morris, JC, Galvin, J, Holtzman, D (eds) (in press) *Handbook of Dementing Illnesses*, 2nd Edition, New York, Marcel Dekker, Inc.

Rubin, EH and Kinscherf, DA (1989) Psychopathology of very mild dementia of the Alzheimer type, *Am J Psychiatry* 146:1017–1021.

Rubin, EH, Veiel, LL, Kinscherf, DA, Morris, JC, and Storandt, M (2001) Clinically significant depressive symptoms and very mild to mild dementia of the Alzheimer type, *Int J Geriatr Psychiatry* 16:694–701.

Rubin, EH, Zorumski, CF, and Burke, WJ (1988) Overlapping symptoms of geriatric depression and Alzheimer type dementia, *Hospital Community Psychiatry* 39:1074–1079.

Sadavoy, J, Lazarus, LW, Jarvik, LF, and Grossberg, GT (1996) *Comprehensive Review of Geriatric Psychiatry-II*, Washington, D.C., American Psychiatric Press.

Schneider, EL and Guralnik, JM (1990) The aging of America, *JAMA* 263:2335–2340.

Shulman, K (1978) Suicide and parasuicide in old age: a review, *Age Ageing* 7:201–209.

von Moltke, LL, Abernethy, DR, and Greenblatt, DJ: Kinetics and dynamics of psychotropic drugs in the elderly. In Salzman, C (ed.) (1998) *Clinical Geriatric Psychopharmacology*, 3rd Edition, Baltimore, Williams & Wilkins.

Troster, AI, Fields, JA, and Koller, WC: Parkinson's disease and Parkinsonism. In Coffey, CE, Cummings, JL (eds) (2000) *The American Psychiatric Press Textbook of Geriatric Neuropsychiatry*, 2nd Edition, Washington, D.C., American Psychiatric Press.

Zaubler, TS and Sullivan, MD (1996) Psychiatry and physician-assisted suicide, *Psychiatr Clin North Am* 19:413–427.

Chapter 27

Atkinson, JH and Grant, I (1994) Natural history of neuropsychiatric manifestations of HIV disease, *Psychiatric Clinics of North America* 17(1):17–33.

Black, KJ (1995) Diagnosing depression after stroke, *South Med J* 88(7):699–708.

Bright, DA (1994) Postpartum mental disorders, *American Family Physician* 50(3):595–598.

Brockington, IF and Meakin, CJ (1994) Clinical clues to the aetiology of puerperal psychosis, *Prog Neuro-Psychopharmacol Biol Psychiatry* 18:417–429.

Carney, RM, et al. (1993) Ventricular tachycardia and psychiatric depression in patients with coronary artery disease, *Am J Med* 95:23–28.

Clouse, RE (1988) Anxiety and gastrointestinal illness, *Psychiatric Clinics of North America* 11(2):399–417.

Clouse, RE and Lustman, PJ (1989) Gastrointestinal symptoms in diabetic patients: lack of association with neuropathy, *Am J Gastroenterol* 84(8):868–872.

Cozza, KL, Armstrong, SC, and Oesterheld, JR (2003) *Drug Interaction Principles for Medical Practice: Cytochrome P450s, UGTs, P-Glycoproteins*, 2nd Edition. Washington D.C., American Psychiatric Publishing, Inc.

Craven, JL, et al. (1987) The diagnosis of depression in renal dialysis patients, *Psychosom Med* 49:482–492.

Craven, JL, Rodin, GM, and Littlefield, C (1988) The Beck Depression Inventory as a screening device for major depression in renal dialysis patients, *Int J Psychiatry Med* 18(4):365–374.

Csernansky, JG, Black, KJ, and Faustman, WO: The interface between standard psychiatric and neuropsychological diagnoses. In: Maruish, ME, Moses, JA Jr (eds) (1997) *Theoretical Foundations of Clinical Neuropsychology for Clinical Practitioners*. Mahwah, NJ: Lawrence Erlbaum Associates, pp. 311–346.

Cunningham, LA (1994) Depression in the medically ill: Choosing an antidepressant, *J Clin Psychiatry*, 55(9, Suppl A):90–97.

DeVane, CL (1994) Pharmacogenetics and drug metabolism of newer antidepressant agents, *J Clin Psychiatry* 55(12 suppl): 38–47.

Dobie, SA and Walker, EA (1992) Depression after childbirth, *J Am Board Fam Pract* 5:303–311.

Freedland, KE, et al. (1992) Underdiagnosis of depression in patients with coronary artery disease: The role of nonspecific symptoms, *Int J Psychiatry Med* 22(3):221–229.

Freidman, JH and Factor, SA (2000) Atypical antipsychotics in the treatment of drug-induced psychosis in Parkinson's disease, *Mov Disord* 15:201–211.

Gavard, JA, Lustman, PJ, and Clouse, RE (1993) Prevalence of depression in adults with diabetes, *Diabetes Care* 16(8):1167–1178.

Goldberg, RJ (1995) Diagnostic dilemmas presented by patients with anxiety and depression, *Am J Med* 98:278–284.

Goodnick, PJ (2001) Use of antidepressants in treatment of comorbid diabetes mellitus and depression as well as in diabetic neuropathy, *Ann Clin Psychiatry* 13:31–41.

Guengerich, FP (1994) Catalytic selectivity of human cytochrome P450 enzymes: relevance to drug metabolism and toxicity, *Toxicology Letters* 70:133–138.

Heilman, KM, Leon, SA, and Rosenbek, JC (2004) Affective aprosodia from a medial frontal stroke, *Brain Lang* 89:411–416.

Henrickson, GA, et al. (1989) Depression in hemodialysis patients, *Psychosomatics* 30:284–285.

Jorge, RE, et al. (1993) Depression and anxiety following traumatic brain injury, *J Neuropsychiatry Clin Neurosci* 5:369–374.

Kendler, KS, et al. (1995) Stressful life events, genetic liability, and onset of an episode of major depression in women, *Am J Psychiatry* 152:833–842.

Kennedy, SH, Craven, JL, and Roin, GM (1989) Major depression in renal dialysis patients: an open trial of antidepressant therapy, *J Clin Psychiatry* 50:60–63.

Lane, EA (1991) Renal function and the disposition of antidepressants and their metabolites, *Psychopharmacology Bulletin* 27(4): 533–540.

Leigh, H and Kramer, SI (1984) The psychiatric manifestations of endocrine disease, *Adv Intern Med* 29:413–445.

Lishman, WA (1987) *Organic Psychiatry: The Psychological Consequences of Cerebral Disorder*, 2nd Edition, Boston, Blackwell Scientific Publications.

Lloyd, GG and Cawley, RH (1983) Distress or illness? A study of psychological symptoms after myocardial infarction, *Br J Psychiatry* 142:120–125.

Lustman, PJ (1988) Anxiety disorders in adults with diabetes mellitus, *Psychiatric Clinics of North America* 11(2):419–432.

Lustman, PJ, et al. (1992) Depression in adults with diabetes, *Diabetes Care* 15(11):1631–1639.

Lustman, PJ, et al. (2000) Fluoxetine for depression in diabetes: A randomized double-blind placebo-controlled trial, *Diabetes Care* 23(5):618–623.

McDaniel, JS, et al. (1995) Depression in patients with cancer, *Arch Gen Psychiatry* 52:89–99.

McDonald, WM, Richard, IH, and DeLong, MR (2003) Prevalence, etiology, and treatment of depression in Parkinson's disease, *Biol Psychiatry* 54:363–375.

Migliorelli, R, et al. (1995) Prevalence and correlates of dysthymia and major depression among patients with Alzheimer's disease, *Am J Psychiatry* 152:37–44.

Minden, SL and Schiffer, RB (1990) Affective disorders in multiple sclerosis: review and recommendations for clinical research, *Arch Neurol* 47:98–104.

Newport, DJ, Fisher, A, Graybeal, S, and Stowe, ZN: Psychopharmacology during pregnancy and lactation. In: Schatzberg, AF, Nemeroff, CB (2004) *The American Psychiatric Textbook of Psychopharmacology*, 3rd Edition, American Psychiatric Publishing, pp. 1109–1146.

Platz, C and Kendell, RE (1988) A matched-control follow-up and family study of "Puerperal Psychoses," *Br J Psychiatry* 153:90–94.

Pons, G, Rey, E, and Matheson, I (1994) Excretion of psychoactive drugs into breast milk, *Clin Pharmacokinet* 27(4):270–289.

Potash, M and Breitbart, W (2002) Affective disorders in advanced cancer, *Hematology/Oncology Clinics of North America* 16:671–700.

Price, JS (1978) Chronic depressive illness, *Br Med J* 1:1200–1201.

Richard, IH, Schiffer, RB, and Kurlan, R (1996) Anxiety and Parkinson's disease. *J Neuropsychiatry Clin Neurosci* 8:383–392.

Rifkin, A (1992) Depression in physically ill patients, *Postgraduate Medicine* 92(3):147–154.

Schleifer, SJ, et al. (1989) The nature and course of depression following myocardial infarction, *Arch Intern Med* 149:1785–1789.

Smith, MD, Hong, BA, and Robson, AM (1985) Diagnosis of depression in patients with end-stage renal disease, *American Journal of Medicine* 79:160–166.

Starkstein, SE and Robinson, RG (eds) (1993) *Depression in Neurologic Disease*. Baltimore, Johns Hopkins University Press.

Trzepacz, PT, et al. (1993) Psychopharmacologic issues in organ transplantation. Part I: Pharmacokinetics in organ failure and psychiatric aspects of immunosuppressants and anti-infectious agents. *Psychosomatics* 34(3):199–207.

Turkington, RW (1980) Depression masquerading as diabetic neuropathy, *JAMA* 243(11):1147–1150.

Videbech, P and Gouliaev, G (1995) First admission with puerperal psychosis: 7–14 years of follow-up, *Acta Psychiatr Scand* 91:167–173.

Weiner, WJ and Lang, AE (eds) (1995) Behavioral Neurology of Movement Disorders. *Adv Neurol* vol. 65.

Wise, MG and Rundell, JR (2002) *The American Psychiatric Publishing Textbook of Consultation-Liaison Psychiatry*, 2nd Edition, Washington, D.C., APPI.

Chapter 28

Aben, I, et al. (2003) A comparative study into the one year cumulative incidence of depression after stroke and myocardial infarction, *J Neurol Neurosurg Psychiatry* 74:581–585.

Abramson, J, et al. (2001) Depression and risk of heart failure among older persons with isolated systolic hypertension, *Arch Intern Med* 161:1725–1730.

Anderson, RJ, et al. (2001) The prevalence of comorbid depression in adults with diabetes: a meta-analysis, *Diabetes Care* 24:1069–1078.

Barefoot, JC, et al. (2000) Depressive symptoms and survival of patients with coronary artery disease, *Psychosom Med* 62:790–795.

Beekman, AT, et al. (1998) Depression in survivors of stroke: a community-based study of prevalence, risk factors and consequences, *Soc Psychiatry Psychiatr Epidemiol* 33:463–470.

Berkman, LF, et al. (2003) Effects of treating depression and low perceived social support on clinical events after myocardial infarction: the Enhancing Recovery in Coronary Heart Disease Patients (ENRICHD) Randomized Trial. *JAMA* 289:3106–3116.

Brummett, BH, et al. (2003) Effect of smoking and sedentary behavior on the association between depressive symptoms and mortality from coronary heart disease, *Am J Cardiol* 92:529–532.

Carnethon, MR, et al. (2003) Symptoms of depression as a risk factor for incident diabetes: findings from the National Health and Nutrition Examination Epidemiologic Follow-up Study, 1971–1992, *Am J Epidemiol* 158:416–423.

Carney, RM, et al. (1988) Major depressive disorder predicts cardiac events in patients with coronary artery disease, *Psychosom Med* 50:627–633.

Carney, RM, et al. (2000) Change in heart rate and heart rate variability during treatment for depression in patients with coronary heart disease, *Psychosom Med* 62:639–647.

Carney, RM, et al. (2001) Depression as a risk factor for coronary heart disease mortality, *Arch Gen Psychiatry* 58:229–230.

Carney, RM, et al. (2001) Depression, heart rate variability, and acute myocardial infarction, *Circulation* 104:2024–2028.

Carney, RM, et al. (2002) Depression as a risk factor for cardiac mortality and morbidity: a review of potential mechanisms, *J Psychosom Res* 53:897–902.

Carney, RM and Freedland, KE (2002) Psychological distress as a risk factor for stroke-related mortality, *Stroke* 33:5–6.

Carney, RM and Freedland, KE (2003) Depression, mortality, and medical morbidity in patients with coronary heart disease, *Biol Psychiatry* 54:241–247.

Carson, AJ, et al. (2000) Depression after stroke and lesion location: a systematic review, *Lancet* 356:122–126.

Chemerinski, E, et al. (2001) The effect of remission of poststroke depression on activities of daily living in a double-blind randomized treatment study, *J Nerv Ment Dis* 189:421–425.

Ciechanowski, PS, et al. (2000) Depression and diabetes: impact of depressive symptoms on adherence, function, and costs, *Arch Intern Med* 160:3278–3285.

Classen, C, et al. (2001) Supportive-expressive group therapy and distress in patients with metastatic breast cancer: a randomized clinical intervention trial, *Arch Gen Psychiatry* 58:494–501.

Clouse, RE, et al. (2003) Depression and coronary heart disease in women with diabetes, *Psychosom Med* 65:376–383.

de Groot, M, et al. (2001) Association of depression and diabetes complications: a meta-analysis, *Psychosom Med* 63:619–630.

Desai, MM, et al. (2002) Mental disorders and quality of diabetes care in the Veterans Health Administration, *Am J Psychiatry* 159:1584–1590.

Diabetes Control and Complications Trial Research Group (1993) The effect of intensive treatment of diabetes on the development and progression of long-term complications in insulin-dependent diabetes mellitus, *N Engl J Med* 329:977–986.

Eaton, WW (2002) Epidemiologic evidence on the comorbidity of depression and diabetes, *J Psychosom Res* 53:903–906.

Everson, SA, et al. (1996) Hopelessness and risk of mortality and incidence of myocardial infarction and cancer, *Psychosom Med* 58:113–121.

Faris, R, et al. (2002) Clinical depression is common and significantly associated with reduced survival in patients with non-ischaemic heart failure, *Eur J Heart Fail* 4:541–551.

Ferketich, AK, et al. (2000) Depression as an antecedent to heart disease among women and men in the NHANES I study. National Health and Nutrition Examination Survey, *Arch Intern Med* 160:1261–1268.

Fisch, MJ, et al. (2003) Fluoxetine versus placebo in advanced cancer outpatients: a double-blinded trial of the Hoosier Oncology Group, *J Clin Oncol* 21:1937–1943.

Frasure-Smith, N, et al. (1993) Depression following myocardial infarction. Impact on 6-month survival, *JAMA* 270:1819–1825.

Frasure-Smith, N, et al. (1995) Depression and 18-month prognosis after myocardial infarction, *Circulation* 91:999–1005.

Frasure-Smith, N and Lesperance, F (2003) Depression and other psychological risks following myocardial infarction, *Arch Gen Psychiatry* 60:627–636.

Freedland, KE, et al. (1991) Depression in elderly patients with congestive heart failure, *J Geriatr Psychiatry* 24:59–71.

Freedland, KE, et al. (2003) Prevalence of depression in hospitalized patients with congestive heart failure, *Psychosom Med* 65:119–128.

Gillen, R, et al. (2001) Depressive symptoms and history of depression predict rehabilitation efficiency in stroke patients, *Arch Phys Med Rehabil* 82:1645–1649.

Glassman, AH, et al. (2002) Sertraline treatment of major depression in patients with acute MI or unstable angina, *JAMA* 288:701–709.

Grigsby, AB, et al. (2002) Prevalence of anxiety in adults with diabetes: a systematic review, *J Psychosom Res* 53:1053–1060.

Hays, RD, et al. (1995) Functioning and well-being outcomes of patients with depression compared with chronic general medical illnesses, *Arch Gen Psychiatry* 52:11–19.

Holland, JC, et al. (1998) A controlled trial of fluoxetine and desipramine in depressed women with advanced cancer, *Psycho-Oncology* 7:291–300.

Jiang, W, et al. (2001) Relationship of depression to increased risk of mortality and rehospitalization in patients with congestive heart failure, *Arch Intern Med* 161:1849–1856.

Jonas, BS and Mussolino, ME (2000) Symptoms of depression as a prospective risk factor for stroke, *Psychosom Med* 62:463–471.

Kessler, RC, et al. (2003) The epidemiology of major depressive disorder: results from the National Comorbidity Survey Replication (NCS-R), *JAMA* 289:3095–3105.

Kishi, Y, et al. (2001) Suicidal ideation among patients with acute life-threatening physical illness, *Psychosomatics* 42:382–390.

Knowler, WC, et al. (2002) Reduction in the incidence of type 2 diabetes with lifestyle intervention or metformin, *New Engl J Med* 346:393–403.

Koenig, HG (1998) Depression in hospitalized older patients with congestive heart failure, *Gen Hosp Psychiatry* 20:29–43.

Kotila, M, et al. (1999) Post-stroke depression and functional recovery in a population-based stroke register: The Finnstroke study, *Eur J Neuro* 6:309–312.

Krishnan, KR (2000) Depression as a contributing factor in cerebrovascular disease, *Am Heart J* 140:Supp1–6.

Larson, SL, et al. (2001) Depressive disorder, dysthymia, and risk of stroke: thirteen-year follow-up from the Baltimore Epidemiologic Catchment Area Study, *Stroke* 32:1979–1983.

Lustman, PJ, et al. (1997) Effects of nortriptyline on depression and glycemic control in diabetes: results of a double-blind, placebo-controlled trial, *Psychosom Med* 59:241–250.

Lustman, PJ, et al. (1998) Cognitive behavior therapy for depression in type 2 diabetes mellitus. A randomized, controlled trial, *Ann Intern Med* 129:613–621.

Lustman, PJ, et al. (2000) Fluoxetine for depression in diabetes: a randomized double-blind placebo-controlled trial, *Diabetes Care* 23:618–623.

Lustman, PJ, et al. (2000) Depression and poor glycemic control: a meta-analytic review of the literature, *Diabetes Care* 23:934–942.

Lustman, PJ and Clouse, RE (2002) Treatment of depression in diabetes: impact on mood and medical outcome, *J Psychosom Res* 53:917–924.

Miller, GE, et al. (2002) Clinical depression and inflammatory risk markers for coronary heart disease, *Am J Cardiol* 90:1279–1283.

Narushima, K, et al. (2003) Does cognitive recovery after treatment of poststroke depression last? A 2-year follow-up of cognitive function associated with poststroke depression, *Am J Psychiatry* 160:1157–1162.

Ostir, GV, et al. (2001) The association between emotional well-being and the incidence of stroke in older adults, *Psychosom Med* 63:210–215.

Penninx, BW, et al. (1998) Chronically depressed mood and cancer risk in older persons, *J Natl Cancer Inst* 90:1888–1893.

Penninx, BW, et al. (1998) Depressive symptoms and physical decline in community-dwelling older persons, *JAMA* 279:1720–1726.

Penninx, BW, et al. (2001) Depression and cardiac mortality: results from a community-based longitudinal study, *Arch Gen Psychiatry* 58:221–227.

Pratt, LA, et al. (1996) Depression, psychotropic medication, and risk of myocardial infarction. Prospective data from the Baltimore ECA follow-up, *Circulation* 94:3123–3129.

Robinson, RG, et al. (2000) Nortriptyline versus fluoxetine in the treatment of depression and in short-term recovery after stroke: a placebo-controlled, double-blind study, *Am J Psychiatry* 157:351–359.

Robinson, RG (2003) Poststroke depression: prevalence, diagnosis, treatment, and disease progression, *Biol Psychiatry* 54:376–387.

Roose, SP, et al. (2001) Relationship between depression and other medical illnesses, *JAMA* 286:1687–1690.

Rumsfeld, JS, et al. (2003) History of depression, angina, and quality of life after acute coronary syndromes, *Am Heart J* 145:493–499.

Ruo, B, et al. (2003) Depressive symptoms and health-related quality of life: the Heart and Soul Study, *JAMA* 290:215–221.

Rutledge, T, et al. (2001) Psychosocial variables are associated with atherosclerosis risk factors among women with chest pain: the WISE study, *Psychosom Med* 63:282–288.

Serebruany, VL, et al. (2003) Platelet/endothelial biomarkers in depressed patients treated with the selective serotonin reuptake inhibitor sertraline after acute coronary events: the Sertraline AntiDepressant Heart Attack Randomized Trial (SADHART) Platelet Substudy, *Circulation* 108:939–944.

Spertus, JA, et al. (2000) Association between depression and worse disease-specific functional status in outpatients with coronary artery disease, *Am Heart J* 140:105–110.

Spiegel D, et al. (1981) Group support for patients with metastatic cancer. A randomized outcome study, *Arch Gen Psychiatry* 38:527–533.

Spiegel, D (2001) Mind matters—group therapy and survival in breast cancer, *New Engl J Med* 345:1767–1768.

Sullivan, M, et al. (2002) Depression-related costs in heart failure care, *Arch Intern Med* 162:1860–1866.

Watkins, LL, et al. (2003) Cognitive and somatic symptoms of depression are associated with medical comorbidity in patients after acute myocardial infarction, *Am Heart J* 146:48–54.

Wells, KB, et al. (1989) The functioning and well-being of depressed patients. Results from the Medical Outcomes Study, *JAMA* 262:914–919.

Williams, SA, et al. (2002) Depression and risk of heart failure among the elderly: a prospective community-based study, *Psychosom Med* 64:6–12.

Wing, RR, et al. (2002) The role of adherence in mediating the relationship between depression and health outcomes, *J Psychosom Res* 53:877–881.

Ziegelstein, RC, et al. (2000) Patients with depression are less likely to follow recommendations to reduce cardiac risk during recovery from a myocardial infarction, *Arch Intern Med* 160:1818–1823.

Chapter 29

Allgulander, C (1994) Suicide and mortality patterns in anxiety neurosis and depressive neurosis, *Arch Gen Psychiatry* 51:708–712.

Allgulander, C, Allebeck, P, Przybeck, TR, and Rice, JP (1992) Risk of suicide by psychiatric diagnosis in Stockholm County. A longitudinal study of 80,970 psychiatric inpatients, *European Arch Psychiatry and Clinical Neuroscience* 241:323–326.

Allgulander, C and Lavori, PW (1991) Excess mortality among 3302 patients with 'pure' anxiety neurosis, *Arch Gen Psychiatry* 48:599–602.

Appleby, L, Cooper, J, Amos, T, and Faragher, B (1999) Psychological autopsy study of suicides by people aged under 35, *Br J Psychiatry* 175:168–174.

Arató, M, Demeter, E, Rihmer, Z, and Somogyi, E (1988) Retrospective psychiatric assessment of 200 suicides in Budapest, *Acta Psychiatr Scand* 77:454–456.

Asgård, U (1990) A psychiatric study of suicide among urban Swedish women, *Acta Psychiatr Scand* 82:115–124.

Barraclough, B, Bunch, J, Nelson, B, and Sainsbury, P (1974) A hundred cases of suicide: clinical aspects, *Br J Psychiatry* 125:355–373.

Beskow, J (1979) Suicide and mental disorder in Swedish men, *Acta Psychiatr Scand* 277(suppl):1–138.

Blackburn, IM, Bishop, S, Glen, AI, Whalley, LJ, and Christie, JE (1981) The efficacy of cognitive therapy in depression: a treatment trial using cognitive therapy and pharmacotherapy, each alone and in combination, *Br J Psychiatry* 139:181–189.

Blair-West, GW, Mellsop, GW, and Eyeson-Annan, ML (1997) Down-rating lifetime suicide risk in major depression, *Acta Psychiatr Scand* 95:259–263.

Brent, DA, Johnson, BA, Perper, J, Connolly, J, Bridge, J, Bartle, S, and Rather, C (1994) Personality disorder, personality traits, impulsive violence, and completed suicide in adolescents, *J Am Acad Child Adolesc Psychiatry* 33:1080–1086.

Brent, DA, Perper, JA, Goldstein, CE, Kolko, DJ, Allan, MJ, Allman, CJ, and Zelenak, JP (1988) Risk factors for adolescent suicide: a comparison of adolescent suicide victims with suicidal inpatients, *Arch Gen Psychiatry* 45:581–588.

Brent, DA, Perper, JA, Moritz, G, Allman, C, Friend, A, Roth, C, Schweers, J, Balach, L, and Baugher, M (1993) Psychiatric risk factors for adolescent suicide: a case control study, *J Am Acad Child Adolesc Psychiatry* 32:521–529.

Caldwell, CB and Gottesman, II (1990) Schizophrenics kill themselves too: a review of risk factors for suicide, *Schizophrenia Bull* 16:571–589.

Carlson, GA, Rich, CL, Grayson, P, and Fowler, RC (1991) Secular trends in psychiatric diagnoses of suicide victims, *J Affect Disord* 21(2):127–132.

Cavanagh, JTO, Owens, DGC, and Johnstone, EC (1999) Suicide and undetermined death in south east Scotland. A case-control study using the psychological autopsy method, *Psychological Medicine* 29:1141–1149.

Cheng, ATA (1995) Mental illness and suicide: a case-control study in Taiwan, *Arch Gen Psychiatry* 52:594–603.

Cheng, ATA, Mann, AH, and Chan, KA (1997) Personality disorder and suicide. A case-control study, *Br J Psychiatry* 170:441–446.

Chynoweth, R, Tonge, JI, and Armstrong, J (1980) Suicide in Brisbane: a retrospective psychosocial study, *Austr N Z J Psychiatry* 14:37–45.

Clendenin, WW and Murphy, GE (1971) Wrist cutting: new epidemiological findings, *Arch Gen Psychiatry* 25:465–469.

Conwell, Y, Duberstein, PR, Cox, C, Herrmann, JH, Forbes, NT, and Caine, ED (1996) Relationships of age and Axis I diagnoses in victims of completed suicide: a psychological autopsy study, *Am J Psychiatry* 153:1001–1008.

Dannenberg, AL, McNeil, JG, Brundage, JF, and Brookmeyer, R (1996) Suicide and HIV infection. Mortality follow-up of 4147 HIV-seropositive military service applicants, *JAMA* 276(21): 1743–1746.

Delong, WB and Robins, E (1961) The communication of suicidal intent prior to psychiatric hospitalization: a study of 87 patients, *Am J Psychiatry* 117:695–705.

Di Maio, L, Squitieri, F, Napolitano, G, Campanella, G, Trofatter, JA, and Conneally, PM (1993) Suicide risk in Huntington's disease, *J Med Genetics* 30:293–295.

Dorpat, TL and Ripley, HS (1960) A study of suicide in the Seattle area, *Compr Psychiatry* 1:349–359.

Fawcett, J (1972) Suicidal depression and physical illness, *JAMA* 219:1303–1306.

Foster, T, Gillespie, K, and McClelland, R (1997) Mental disorders and suicide in Northern Ireland, *Br J Psychiatry* 170:447–452.

Fowler, RC, Rich, CL, and Young, D (1986) San Diego Suicide Study. II. Substance abuse in young cases, *Arch Gen Psychiatry* 43:962–965.

Friedman, RC and Downey, JI (1994) Homosexuality, *New Engl J Med* 331(14):923–930.

Guze, SB and Robins, E (1970) Suicide and primary affective disorders, *Br J Psychiatry* 117:437–438.

Haberlandt, WF (1967) Aportacion a La Genetica del Studio (Datos ei gemelos y hallazgoes familiares), *Folio Clinica Internacional* 17:319–322.

Hagnell, O and Rorsman, B (1979) Suicide in the Lundby study: a comparative investigation of clinical aspects, *Neuropsychobiology* 5:61–73.

Harris, EC and Barraclough, B (1998) Excess mortality of mental disorder, *Br J Psychiatry* 173:11–53.

Heilä, H, Isometsä, ET, Henriksson, MM, Heikkinen, ME, Marttunen, MJ, and Lönnqvist, JK (1997) Suicide and schizophrenia: A nationwide psychological autopsy study on age and sex-specific clinical characteristics of 92 suicide victims with schizophrenia, *Am J Psychiatry* 154:1235–1242.

Henriksson, MM, Aro, HM, Marttunen, MJ, Heikkinen, ME, Isometsä, ET, Kuoppasalmi, KI, and Lönnqvist, JK (1993) Mental disorders and comorbidity in suicide, *Am J Psychiatry* 150: 935–994.

Henriksson, MM, Marttunen, MJ, Isometsä, ET, Heikkinen, ME, Aro, IIM, Kuoppasalmi, KI, and Lönnqvist, JK (1995) Mental disorders in elderly suicides, *International Psychogeriatrics* 7:275–286.

Henriksson, MM, Isometsä, ET, Kuoppasalmi, KI, Heikkinen, ME, Marttunen, MJ, and Lönnqvist, JK (1996) Panic disorder in completed suicide, *J Clin Psychiatry* 57:275–281.

Inskip, HM, Harris, EC, and Barraclough, B (1998) Lifetime risk of suicide for affective disorder, alcoholism and schizophrenia, *Br J Psychiatry* 172:35–37.

Isacsson, G, Boëthius, G, and Bergman, U (1992) Low level of antidepressant prescription for people who later commit suicide: 15 years of experience from a population-based drug database in Sweden, *Acta Psychiatr Scand* 85:444–448.

Isacsson, G, Bergman, U, and Rich, CL (1994) Antidepressants, depression and suicide: an analysis of the San Diego study, *J Affect Disord* 32:277–286.

Isometsä, ET, Aro, HM, Henriksson, MM, Heikkinen, ME, and Lönnqvist, JK (1994) Suicide in major depression in different treatment settings, *J Clin Psychiatry* 55:523–527.

Isometsä, ET, Heikkinen, ME, Marttunen, MJ, Henriksson, MM, Aro, HM, and Lönnqvist, JK (1995) The last appointment before suicide: Is suicide intent communicated? *Am J Psychiatry* 152:919–922.

Isometsä, ET, Henriksson, MM, Heikkinen, ME, and Lönnqvist, JK (1996) Completed suicide and recent electroconvulsive therapy in Finland, *Convulsive Therapy* 12:152–155.

Kapamadzija, B, Biro, M, and Sovljanski, M (1982) Sociopsihijatrijska i patomorfoloska analiza, 100 izvrsenih samoubistava, *Soc Psihijat* 10:35–56.

Kelly, TM and Mann, JJ (1996) Validity of DSM-III-R diagnosis by psychological autopsy: a comparison with clinician antemortem diagnosis, *Acta Psychiatr Scand* 94:337–343.

Lesage, AD, Boyer, R, Grunberg, F, Vanier, C, Morisette, R, Ménard-Buteau, C, and Loyer, M (1994) Suicide and mental disorders: a case-control study of young men, *Am J Psychiatry* 151:1063–1068.

Litman, RE, Curphey, T, Shneidman, ES, Farberow, NL, and Tabachnick, N (1963) Investigations of equivocal suicides, *JAMA* 184(12):924–929.

Mann, JJ and Kapur, S (1991) The emergence of suicidal ideation and behavior during antidepressant pharmacotherapy, *Arch Gen Psychiatry* 48:1027–1033.

Marttunen, MJ, Aro, HM, Henriksson, MM, and Lönnqvist, JK (1991) Mental disorders in adolescent suicide. *DSM-III-R* Axes I and II diagnoses in suicides among 13- to 19-year-olds in Finland, *Arch Gen Psychiatry* 48:834–839.

Marttunen, MJ, Aro, HM, Henriksson, MM, and Lönnqvist, JK (1994) Antisocial behaviour in adolescent suicide, *Acta Psych Scand* 89:167–173.

Marttunen, MJ, Aro, HM, Henriksson, MM, and Lönnqvist, JK (1994) Psychosocial stressors more common in adolescent suicides with alcohol abuse compared with depressive adolescent suicides, *J Am Acad Child Adolesc Psychiatry* 33:490–497.

Marzuk, PM, Tierney, H, Tardiff, K, Gross, EM, Morgan, EB Hsu, MA, and Mann, JJ (1988) Increased risk of suicide in persons with AIDS, *JAMA* 259:1333–1337.

McGuffin, P, Maruši, A, and Farmer, A (2001) What can psychiatric genetics offer suicidology? *Crisis* 22:61–65.

Mitterauer, B (1981) Mehrdimensionale Diagnostik von 121 Suiziden im Bundesland Salzburg im Jahre 1978, *Wien Med Wochenschr* 9:229–234.

Muehrer, P (1995) Suicide and sexual orientation: a critical summary of recent research and directions for future research, *Suicide Life Threat Behav* 25 (suppl):72–81.

Murphy, GE and Robins, E (1967) Social factors in suicide, *JAMA* 199:303–308.

Murphy, GE (1975) The physician's responsibility for suicide. II. Errors of omission, *Ann Intern Med* 82:305–309.

Murphy, GE, Armstrong, JW, Hermele, SL, Fischer, JR, and Clendenin, WW (1979) Suicide and alcoholism. Interpersonal loss confirmed as a predictor, *Arch Gen Psychiatry* 36:65–69.

Murphy, GE, Wetzel, RD, Robins, E, McEvoy, L (1992) Multiple risk factors predict suicide in alcoholism, *Arch Gen Psychiatry* 49:459–463.

Murphy, GE and Wetzel, RD (1990) The lifetime risk of suicide in alcoholism, *Arch Gen Psychiatry* 47:383–392.

Noyes, RN (1991) Suicide and panic disorder: a review, *J Affect Disord* 22:1–11.

Phillips, MR, Yang, G, Zhang, Y, Wang, L, Ji, H, and Zhou, M (2002)

Risk factors for suicide in China: a national case-control psychological autopsy study, *Lancet* 360:1728–1736.

Regier, DA, Farmer, ME, Rae, DS, Locke, BZ, Keith, SJ, Judd, LL, and Goodwin, FK (1990) Comorbidity of mental disorders with alcohol and other drug abuse, *JAMA* 264:2511–2518.

Renaud, J, Brent, DA, Birmaher, B, Chiappetta, L, and Bridge, J (1999) Suicide in adolescents with disruptive disorders, *J Am Acad Child Adolesc Psychiatry* 38:846–851.

Rich, CL, Fowler, RC, Fogarty, LA, and Young, D (1988) San Diego Suicide Study. III. Relationships between diagnoses and stressors, *Arch Gen Psychiatry* 45:589–592.

Rich, CL and Runeson, BS (1992) Similarities in diagnostic comorbidity between suicide among young people in Sweden and the United States, *Acta Psychiatr Scand* 86:335–339.

Rich, CL, Sherman, M, and Fowler, RC (1990) San Diego Suicide Study: The adolescents, *Adolescence* 25:855–865.

Rich, CL, Young, D, and Fowler, RC (1986) San Diego Suicide Study. I: Young vs old subjects, *Arch Gen Psychiatry* 43:577–582.

Robins, E, Gassner, S, Kayes, J, Wilkinson, RH, and Murphy, GE (1959) The communication of suicidal intent: a study of 134 consecutive cases of successful (completed) suicide, *Am J Psychiatry* 115:724–733.

Robins, E, Murphy, GE, Wilkinson, RH, Gassner, S, and Kayes, J (1959) Some clinical considerations in the prevention of suicide based on a study of 134 successful suicides, *Am J Public Health* 49:888–899.

Robins, LN, Locke, BZ, and Regier, DA (1991) *Psychiatric Disorders in America*, New York, The Free Press.

Roy, A (1993) Genetic and biologic risk factors for suicide in depressive disorders, *Psychiatr Q* 64:345–358.

Roy, A, Rylander, G, and Sarchiapone, M (1997) Genetics of suicide. Family studies and molecular genetics, *Ann NY Acad Sci* 836:135–157.

Runeson, B (1989) Mental disorder in youth suicide: DSM-III-R axes I and II, *Acta Psychiatr Scand* 79:490–497.

Shaffer, D, Fisher, P, Hicks, RH, Parides, M, and Gould, M (1995) Sexual orientation in adolescents who commit suicide, *Suicide Life Threat Behav* 25(Suppl):64–71.

Shaffer, D, Gould, MS, Fisher, P, Trautman, P, Moreau, D, Kleinman, M, and Flory, M (1996) Psychiatric diagnosis in child and adolescent suicide, *Arch Gen Psychiatry* 53:339–348.

Shafii, M, Carrigan, S, Whittinghill, JR, and Derrick, A (1985) Psychological autopsy of completed suicide in children and adolescents, *Am J of Psychiatry* 142:1061–1064.

Starace, F (1993) Suicidal behaviour in people infected with human immunodeficiency virus: A literature review, *Int J Soc Psychiatry* 39(1):64–70, Spr.

Stengel, E, Cook, NG, with the assistance of Kreeger, IS (1958) *Attempted Suicide: its social significance and effects*. London, Chapman & Hall.

Tanney, BL: Mental disorders, psychiatric patients and suicide. In Maris, RW, Berman, AL, Maltsberger, JT, Yufit, RI (eds) (1992) *Assessment and Prediction of Suicide*. New York: Guilford Press, pp 277–320.

Teicher, MH, Glod, C, and Cole, Jo (1990) Emergence of intense suicidal preoccupation during fluoxetine treatment, *Am J Psychiatry* 147:207–210.

Tsuang, MT (1977) Genetic factors in suicide, *Diseases of the Nervous System* 38:498–501.

van Haastrecht, HJ, Mientjes, GH, van den Hoek, AJ, and

Coutinho, RA (1994) Death from suicide and overdose among drug injectors after disclosure of first HIV test result, *AIDS* 8(12):1721–1725.

Vijayakumar, L and Rajkumar, S (1999) Are risk factors for suicide universal? A case-control study in India, *Acta Psychiatra Scand* 99:407–411.

Wender, PH, Kety, SS, Rosenthal, D, Schulsinger, F, Ortmann, J, and Lunde, I (1986) Psychiatric disorders in the biological and adoptive families of adopted individuals with affective disorders, *Arch Gen Psychiatry* 43(10):923–929.

Zhang, J, Conwell, Y, Wieczorek, WF, Jiang, C, Jia, S, and Zhou, L (2003) Studying Chinese suicide with proxy-based data: reliability and validity of the methodology and instruments in China, *J Nerv Ment Dis* 191:450–457.

Zhang, J, Wieczorek, WF, Jiang, C, Zhou, L, Jia, S, Sun, Y, Jin, S, and Conwell, Y (2002) Studying suicide with psychological autopsy: social and cultural feasibilities of the methodology in China, *Suicide Life Threat Behav* 32:370–379.

Chapter 30

American Academy of Psychiatry and the Law Ethical Guidelines for the Practice of Forensic Psychiatry (1995). Available at www.aapl.org/ethics.htm, accessed June 22, 2004.

American Medical Association (1997) *Code of Medical Ethics, Current Opinions with Annotations*. Available at www.ama-assn.org/ama/pub/category/2503.html, accessed June 22, 2004.

American Psychiatric Association (2001) *The Principles of Medical Ethics with Annotations Especially Applicable to Psychiatry*. Available at www.psych.org/psych_pract/ethics/ppaethics.pdf, accessed June 22, 2004.

Gutheil, TG and Appelbaum, PS (2000) *Clinical Handbook of Psychiatry and the Law*, 3rd Edition, Philadelphia, Lippincott, Williams & Wilkins.

Health Insurance Portability and Accountability Act of 1996. Public Law 104–191, August 21, 1996.

Kaplan, HI and Sadock, BJ (2000) *Comprehensive Textbook of Psychiatry*, 7th Edition, Philadelphia, Lippincott, Williams & Wilkins.

Missouri Revised Statutes, 2003.

Rosner, R (2003) *Principles and Practice of Forensic Psychiatry*, 2nd Edition, New York, Oxford University Press Inc.

Simon, RI (2001) *Concise Guide to Psychiatry and Law for Clinicians*, 3rd Edition, Washington D.C., American Psychiatric Press.

Chapter 31

Appelbaum, PS and Roth, LS (1982) Competency to consent to research, *Arch Gen Psychiatry* 39:951–958.

Brody, BA (1993) Assessing empirical research in bioethics, *Theor Med* 14:211–219.

Burstajn, HJ, et al. (1991) Beyond cognition: the role of disorder affective states in impairing competence to treatment, *Bull Am Acad Psychiatry Law* 19:383–388.

Carithers, RL Jr (2000) Liver transplantation. American Association for the Study of Liver Diseases, *Liver Transpl* 6(1): 122–135.

DiMartini, A, Weinrieb, R, and Fireman, M (2002) Liver transplantation in patients with alcohol and other substance use disorders, *Psychiatric Clin NA* 25(1):195–209.

Dinwiddie, SH (1992) Physician-assisted suicide: epistemological problems, *Int J Med Law* 11:345–352.

Dinwiddie, SH (1999–2000) Potential psychodynamic factors in physician-assisted suicide, *Omega* 40(1):101–108.

Dinwiddie, SH and Briska, W (2004) Prosecution of violent psychiatric inpatients: theoretical and practical issues, *International Journal of Law and Psychiatry* 27:17–29.

Dinwiddie, SH, Staples, N, and Meyers, D: Using information to manage cultural change: establishing the medical model for inpatient care. In Reid, WH, Silver, SB (eds) (2003) *Handbook of Mental Health Administration and Management*, New York, Brunner-Routledge, pp. 397–408.

Emanuel, EJ and Emanuel, LL (1992) Four models of the physician-patient relationship, *JAMA* 267:2221–2226.

Goldman, MJ and Gutheil, TG (1994) The misperceived duty to report patients' past crimes, *Bull Am Acad Psychiatry Law* 22:407–410.

Gutheil, TG and Gabbard, GO (1993) The concept of boundaries in clinical practice: theoretical and risk management dimensions, *Am J Psychiatry* 150:188–196.

Guze, SB (1970) The need for toughmindedness in psychiatric thinking, *South Med J* 63:662–671.

Guze, SB (1992) *Why Psychiatry is a Branch of Medicine*, New York, Oxford University Press.

Martens, W (2001) Do alcoholic liver transplantation candidates merit lower medical priority than non-alcoholic candidates? *Transp Int* 14(3):170–175.

Mushkin, PR (1998) The request to die: role for a psychodynamic perspective on physician-assisted suicide, *JAMA* 279(4):323–328.

Pellegrino, ED and Thomasma, DC (1988) *For the Patient's Good*, Oxford, England, Oxford University Press.

Strasburger, LH, Gutheil, TG, and Brodsky, A (1997) On wearing two hats: role conflict in serving as both psychotherapist and expert witness, *Am J Psychiatry* 154(4):448–456.

Index

Note: page numbers in **bold** refer to tables, boxes and case studies; those in *italics* refer to figures.

cognitive impairment
  amnestic disorder 180
  delirium 167
  depression 37
  elderly patients 379–80
  neuropsychological dysfunction screening
    38
  schizophrenia 201–2
  tricyclic antidepressants 123
cognitive psychology 6
cognitive–behavioral theories 92
cognitive–behavioral therapy 6
  adolescents 368, 369
  binge eating disorder 255, 257
  depression 321
  major depressive disorder 118–20
  outcome 120
  panic disorder 133
  personality disorder 301
colon cancer, gene mutation 349
communication
  disturbances 25
  physician-to-physician 77
  psychotherapy 319
  suicide 416–17
community
  mental health professionals 77
  mental health services 80
  response to catastrophe 314–15
  support in substance abuse 232–3
  support workers 82
Comparative Genomic Hybridization 353
competency of patient 38, 422–3, 434
complaints
  chief 26
  presenting 24–5
compliance 83–4
  difficult patients 434
Composite International Diagnostic
    Interview (CIDI) 20
compulsions 27
  diagnostic criteria **143**
  obsessive–compulsive disorder differential
    diagnosis 145
  primary **144**
  primary care 77
computed tomography (CT) 45, 46
  amnestic disorder 178
  delirium 167
  dementia 186
concentration
  disturbances 25
  impaired 37
conduct disorder in adolescents 369–70
confidentiality 424, **425**, 432–3
  breaches 422, 432, 433
  research 436
confusion
  ECT-induced 342
  elderly patients 121
congestive heart failure, depression
    comorbidity 406
Conners rating scale of ADHD 367
consanguinity 355

consent to treatment 422–3, 430
conservatorship 423–4
constipation, major depressive disorder 97
consultation
  psychiatric 427–8
  psychological 30, 32
conversion disorder 266–8
  differential diagnosis 267–8
  epidemiology 268
  family history 268
  genetics 268
  history 261–2
  natural history 266–7
  prognosis 267
conversion symptoms 103, 262
  dissociative disorder differential diagnosis
    279
  pseudoneurological 266
cooperativeness 292, 293, 297, 299
coronary heart disease
  depression comorbidity 402, 405–6
  diabetes mellitus comorbidity 403
  major depressive disorder 395
  obesity 248
corpus callosum, mood disorders 63
cortex
  β-adrenoceptors in suicide victims 117
  atrophy in Korsakoff's syndrome 179
  cocaine dependence 74
  functional neuroimaging 54
  temporopolar 73
  see also cingulate cortex; insular cortex;
    orbital cortex; prefrontal cortex
cortical-striatal-pallidal-thalamic circuitry
    70
corticosteroids
  delirium-causing 168
  substance-induced mood disorder 105
corticotrophin-releasing hormone
  depression 116
  mood disorders 67
cortisol, depression 67, 116
counselors
  genetic 360–1
  pastoral 79
  professional 80
counter-transference 301
  negative/positive 300
crack cocaine abuse 224
criminal behavior, personality disorder 297
criminal matters
  competency 422
  confidentiality 433
criminal responsibility 425–7
critical incident stress management 314–15
cultural models 7
Cushing's syndrome
  clinical features 116
  depressive syndrome 104, 392
custody disputes 433
cyclothymic disorder 105
  age of onset 109
  course 109
  diagnostic criteria 92, 107

emotional manifestations 108
  impairments 110
  mood-stablizing drugs 330–1
cytochrome P450 (CYP) system 387
  SSRIs 395
cytogenetic analysis 357

day care centers 84
day programs 84
  outpatients 86
death
  bipolar disorder 110
  preoccupation with in major depressive
    disorder 97
  see also suicide
dehydration, major depressive disorder 102
deletions, genetic 358
delirium 154–72
  agitation 193
  amnestic disorder differential diagnosis
    176–7
  cancer 171
  case study **157**
  causes 159–65, 169
  cerebral insufficiency 167
  cholinergic hypothesis 167–8
  classification 158
  clinical features 155–6, 158–65
  cognitive impairment 167
  death 165
  dementia association 165–6
  diagnosis 154–5
  diagnostic categories 159
  diagnostic criteria 158
  differential diagnosis 166
  drug intoxication 159–63
  epidemiology 166–7
  family history 166
  genetics 166
  head trauma 175–6
  hyperthyroidism 399
  imaging 167
  management 170, 180
  multifactorial 165
  natural history 165–6
  neurohumoral hypotheses 168
  patient evaluation 171
  prevention 168–9
  psychometric evaluation 158–9
  suicide 413–14
  terminal illness 171
  treatment 169–71
  tricyclic antidepressants 123
delirium tremens 158
  alcohol withdrawal 230
  drug withdrawal 162–3
delusional disorder 197, 268
  diagnostic criteria **219**
delusions 27
  antipsychotics 328
  bipolar disorder 105, 108
  delirium 158
  elderly patients 381, 382

Index **487**

case study **148, 151**
comorbidity 144
conversion syndrome differential diagnosis 268
cortical-striatal-pallidal-thalamic circuitry 70
definitions 142–3
diagnostic criteria **143**
differential diagnosis 144–5
ECT 337
epidemiology 144
family practice setting 151–2
family studies 145–6
Freud 146
gender ratio 144
major depressive disorder differential diagnosis 102–3
molecular genetic studies 145–6
neuroimaging 70, 150–1
neurologic illness association 150
PANDAS 145, 146, 147, 150
panic attacks 144–5
pathophysiology 150–1
PET 70
pharmacotherapy 146–7
prefrontal cortex 69
psychosurgery 149–50
PTSD differential diagnosis 310–11
rating scales 42
referral 152
ruminations 144
shared features with depression 70
SSRIs in adolescents 369
substance abuse 144
treatment 146–50
twin studies 145–6
olanzapine
bipolar disorder 127
bulimia nervosa 240
delirium treatment 170
obsessive–compulsive disorder 147
Parkinson's disease 393
schizophrenia 213
weight gain 217, 249
oligogenic disorders 352
opioid abuse 223
detoxification 232
methadone substitution 233
overdose 230
treatment 233
withdrawal 232
opioids, delirium-causing 161–2
oral contraceptives 105
oral intake in major depressive disorder 102
orbital cortex
depression 66
obsessive–compulsive disorder association 151
phobias 71, 72
post-traumatic stress disorder 73
orbital undercutting 149
organ transplantation 435
organic solvents, delirium 165
orlistat 252

outpatients, day program 86
oxazepam
alcohol withdrawal 230, 232
delirium treatment 171
oxcarbamazepine 77
personality disorder 303
oxycodone abuse 223
oxygen metabolism, PET measures 51

pain
chronic syndromes 273
control 86
major depressive disorder 97
management 86
pancreatic cancer, major depressive disorder 394
PANDAS (pediatric autoimmune neuropsychiatric disorders) 145, 146
obsessive–compulsive disorder association 150
treatment 147
panic attacks 130–4, **139**
comorbid personality disorder **298**
management 77
obsessive–compulsive disorder 144–5
recurrent 131
somatoform disorders 272
panic disorder 130–4
antidepressants 103
brain metabolism imaging 70–1
clinical features 130–2
depression association 131
diagnosis **131**
differential diagnosis 132
epidemiology 132–3
family history 132
major depressive disorder 131
differential diagnosis 103
medical disorders 396–7
neuroimaging 70–1
obsessive–compulsive disorder comorbidity 144
prefrontal cortex 71
serotonin type 1A receptor binding 46
substance abuse 131
suicidal thoughts 131–2
suicide 413
treatment 133
parahippocampal gyrus in schizophrenia 55
paranoia, bipolar disorder 105
parens patriae 420, 421
parents of adolescents 364, 365
parkinsonism
antipsychotic medication side-effects 211
dementia 185, 187
Parkinson's disease
antidepressants 393
antipsychotics 393
with dementia 186–7
depressive syndrome 104–5, 115, 116, 379, 390, 392–4
disinhibition 394
ECT 337–8, 393
major depressive disorder 104

psychosis 393
social phobia 394
paroxetine 122
adolescents 368
Alzheimer's disease 192
breast-feeding 397
obsessive–compulsive disorder 147
panic disorder 328
Parkinson's disease 393
PTSD 314
somatization disorder 273
pastoral counselors 79
paternalism 429–31
patient education
Alzheimer's disease 190
binge eating disorder 258
obesity 258
patient–physician relationship
confidentiality 424
ethics 430
psychotherapy 319
somatoform disorders 269–71
patient-rated scales 40
patients
attorney 426
difficult 433–4
exploitation 431–3, 435
financial advantage taking 432
information about 25–6
medical model of psychiatry 8
physician relationship 17, 28
sexual exploitation 432
unified general approach 10
payees 83
penetrance 353–4
perception disturbances 25
delirium 156, 158
peregrination 286
peripheral neuropathy, alcohol detoxification 232
persistence 293
personal growth 301
personalities, fusion 281
Personality Assessment Inventory 35
personality dimensions 292–5
heritability 298
personality disorder 290–304, **305**
age 296, 297
clinical features 290–8
cognitive-behavioral therapy 301
comorbidity 279, 297–8
criminal behavior 297
diagnosis
qualitative 290–2
quantitative 292–5
differential diagnosis 297
dynamic therapies 301
epidemiology 295–6
family history 298
genetics 298
maladaptive behavior 291
natural history 296–7
noncompliance 434
obsessive–compulsive disorder 144